Abdominal Imaging

Bernd Hamm • Pablo R. Ros
Editors

Abdominal Imaging

Volume 4

With 2233 Figures and 119 Tables

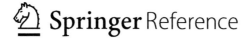 Springer Reference

Editors
Bernd Hamm
Department of Radiology
Charité - Universitätsmedizin Berlin
Berlin, Germany

Pablo R. Ros
Department of Radiology
Case Western Reserve University
University Hospitals Case Medical Center
Cleveland, OH, USA

ISBN 978-3-642-13326-8   ISBN 978-3-642-13327-5 (eBook)
ISBN 978-3-642-15139-2 (print and electronic bundle)
DOI 10.1007/978-3-642-13327-5
Springer Heidelberg New York Dordrecht London

Library of Congress Control Number: 2013931108

Printed on acid-free paper

Springer is part of Springer Science+Business Media (www.springer.com)

To all the medical students, residents, fellows, and radiologists we had the privilege to teach throughout our careers. You are the biggest source of enjoyment in our professional lives.

Preface

We are proud of this Abdominal Imaging handbook, which responds to the need to have in a single publication a comprehensive review on the entire field of Abdominal Radiology, including both Gastrointestinal and Genitourinary Systems. Although several excellent handbooks are available in both Gastrointestinal and Genitourinary Radiology, a comprehensive reference was desirable for abdominal images. Traditionally Gastrointestinal and Genitourinary Radiology developed independently based upon fundamentally different plain radiography procedures, such as barium studies for the gastrointestinal tract and excretory urography for the urinary system. With the development of cross-sectional imaging studies, however, the two subspecialties are coming closer and have already merged in the USA.

Today, in both academic and private practice, abdominal radiologists use all diagnostic imaging modalities ranging from plain radiography classic procedures, to ultrasonography, computed tomography, nuclear medicine/hybrid imaging and magnetic resonance imaging (MRI). They also perform image guided interventional procedures and therapies using the different imaging modalities. This unifying movement between Gastrointestinal and Genitourinary Radiology has been implemented in our organizations and in our daily practice.

Thus, this handbook on Abdominal Imaging aims to fill the gap and provide a source of reference not only for trainees and practitioners in Radiology, but also to others interested in Abdominal Imaging such as gastroenterologists, urologists, oncologic surgeons, digestive and general surgeons, gynecologists, oncologists, hepatologists, endocrinologists, family practitioners, internists, etc. Of course, this handbook also aims to be a reference to medical students and other professionals training in healthcare.

Another remarkable feature of this handbook is its global focus since its inception. This recognizes the global approach in radiology, medicine and so many other walks of life, which is so much part of the 21st century. With today's means of communication, electronic databases, and overall globalization, knowledge in a particular medical field is universal. Likewise, challenges, opportunities and solutions are apparent on a global basis and not the province anymore of a limited number of elite centers or even countries. Therefore, spurred by the challenging brief provided to us by our publishers at Springer, we decided from the beginning to enlist section editors and authors throughout the world.

The book is organized by organs, enabling the reader to approach one topic at a time or to look up specific diseases by organ and organ system. The book is logically divided into two main parts: Gastrointestinal and Genitourinary. Each of these organ systems is further divided into sections. A key element in the development process of this Abdominal Imaging handbook was to select section editors who are experts in their particular areas and are able to organize their sections into appropriate chapters and recruit the best authors on a global scale.

The gastrointestinal part includes sections for both hollow and solid viscera. As tradition dictates, it starts with pharynx and esophagus and follows with stomach and duodenum, small bowel, and colon. Liver, gallbladder and biliary tree, pancreas, spleen, mesentery, peritoneum and abdominal wall complete this part. The genitourinary organ system starts with the retroperitoneum, followed by kidney and renal pelvis, and then prostate, scrotum and penis, ureter and urethra, ovary and anexa, uterus, vagina and vulva. It ends with a section on imaging in pregnancy.

The organization of each section varies somewhat to fit the particular organ to be discussed. In general, each section has chapters devoted to technique, congenital anomalies and normal variance, inflammatory and infectious diseases, benign neoplasms, malignant neoplasms, and miscellaneous abnormalities covering metabolic, systemic disorders and other topics. The tailoring of each section to the area covered is important. In major organs, for instance the liver, there are chapters dedicated to different modalities such as Ultrasound, CT, MRI, molecular and hybrid imaging and interventional imaging.

We have provided this handbook a practical focus, including differential diagnosis and emphasis on the key features that allow the imaging characterization of disorders. Where it makes sense, we have offered the appropriate sequence of imaging studies and/ or invasive image guided techniques to guide the readership towards the meaningful utilization of imaging resources. The overall result is a handbook with over 150 chapters, several hundred authors, and more than 2,000 high quality images of the gastrointestinal tract, abdominal viscera, and genitourinary organs.

We believe this book reflects real life, taking actual cases from the extensive teaching collections of all of the authors and section editors. It reflects the work going on in hundreds of departments of radiology throughout the world and presents the interactions between faculty and trainees on hundreds of thousands of cases. At the end, this should serve as a tool to further learn abdominal imaging and build into the future of our subspecialty.

We had great pleasure in selecting section editors, approving the sectional table of contents, accepting authors, reviewing chapters, and of course, going over hundreds of emails to put all of this work together, so we could offer it to all its readers.

Finally, we are delighted that our Abdominal Imaging handbook will be accessible to a wider audience through SpringerReference (www.springerreference.com), the new publishing platform for Springer's major reference works which seek to address the needs of students, researchers and academics in all scientific disciplines in the 21st century.

In summary, we hope the readers enjoy accessing all different aspects of Abdominal Imaging in a single handbook. The global origins of the authors help to provide a universal approach to the dissemination of knowledge in this important area of Radiology. The entire authorship and publishing teams are delighted to put this work in your hands. We look forward to receiving comments regarding this comprehensive handbook and the potential ways to improve it in the future.

Bernd Hamm
Pablo R. Ros

Acknowledgments

This Abdominal Imaging handbook would have never seen the light without the efforts of many key people we would like to acknowledge. First of all is Ute Heilmann, PhD, Editorial Director for Clinical Medicine, Springer and actually the major reason this book is now a reality. Ute convinced us of the need for a comprehensive reference on Abdominal Imaging, it seems ages ago. Ute was able to provide a solution for each one of our arguments, stressing the resources and organization skills available to us as editors for such a comprehensive work with hundreds of chapters and authors.

Our heartfelt thanks go for sure to our Section Editors; we are indebted to each and every one of them. Drs. Carucci, Ekberg, Malone, Yee, Vilgrain, Soto, Mortele, Hahn, Shirkhoda, Herrmann, Heinz-Peer, Hallscheidt, Schlemmer, Derchi, Mueller-Lisse, Forstner, Sala, Rockall, and Avni are the backbone of this work. All of them are internationally recognized experts in their field, come from extremely prestigious institutions in their respective countries, and are major contributors to published knowledge in their areas of expertise. Of course our thanks also go to the chapter authors. Many of them have written their own textbooks in GI, GU, or modalities such as MR or CT. Despite this, they generously contributed to this Abdominal Imaging handbook.

Our acknowledgement also goes to the many residents, fellows, and faculty of the institutions where these chapters and sections originated. They truly represent the reason why the authors were able to contribute their chapters. All of them directly or indirectly have contributed to this book either by donating cases or helping out to formulate differential diagnosis to the overall content of the book.

We would also like to extend our gratitude to the many clinical colleagues and the radiological technologists around the world who provided the clinical material that resulted in the knowledge that ultimately is distilled in this work. Without their help, this book would have not been possible either.

On a more personal level we would like to thank our executive assistants that have helped us in our offices to keep the deadlines, communicate with the publisher, section editors and authors, filed the chapters, reminded us of the many to-dos and in general kept us afloat. At Case Western Reserve University and University Hospitals Case Medical Center we have to recognize Carla DiNunzio, Molly McGinnis and especially Marianne Chaloupek. At Charité – Universitätsmedizin Berlin, our thanks are due to Gabriele Förster and Bettina Herwig.

There are also many people on the Springer team who have throughout provided invaluable help, among them we have to highlight Wilma McHugh, Sylvana Freyberg, Andrew Spencer, Mauricio Quinones, Abhijit Baroi, and we are sure many others.

We are likely leaving out many other people deserving our acknowledgment, but as expressed before, we truly would like to thank the many that through their efforts have made this handbook possible and brought it to light. We take great pleasure in handing over this work to its contributors and readers.

Bernd Hamm
Pablo R. Ros

About the Editors

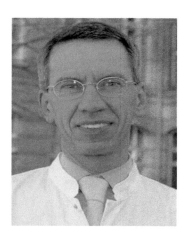

Bernd Hamm studied medicine at the Free University of Berlin and received his MD in 1982. Following his studies, he stayed in Berlin, becoming first a resident, then a senior staff member, and finally an Associate Professor of Radiology at Benjamin Franklin University Hospital.

After the fall of the Berlin Wall and German reunification, Dr. Hamm was offered, in 1992, the unique chance of becoming Chair of the Department of Radiology of the renowned Charité Medical School in East Berlin. In this position, he was involved in completely restructuring the provision of radiology services, teaching, and research. This challenging task has kept Dr. Hamm in Berlin ever since, although he was offered attractive positions as Professor and Chairman at the universities in Essen and Frankfurt. In the process of reorganization of university medicine in Berlin, both university hospitals of the Free University of Berlin merged with Charité Medical School, which is affiliated with Humboldt University. With this merger, Dr. Hamm became Chair of all three radiological departments, which together now constitute Germany's largest Department of Radiology. In addition, he is head of five outpatient healthcare centers of the Charité Medical School in the field of radiology and nuclear medicine and of two imaging centers in Berlin.

In Germany, Dr. Hamm served as President of the Berlin Society of Radiology and the German Society of Radiology. Since 2002, he has been a member of the board of the professional association of German radiologists. He was President of the 2011 annual meeting of the German Radiology Society. At the European level, Dr. Hamm served as President of the European Society of Urogenital Radiology, and he is currently Vice President of the European Congress of Radiology. He is a member of the Executive Council of the European Society of Radiology. He is an honorary member of the Austrian, Swiss, and Japanese radiological societies.

Since 2005, Dr. Hamm has been Editor of Germany's most prestigious radiological journal—*Fortschritte auf dem Gebiet der Röntgenstrahlen und der modernen bildgebenden Verfahren*. He is a reviewer for the German Research Foundation, the country's largest research funding organization.

Dr. Hamm's publications include over 450 peer-reviewed original articles, over 80 review articles and editorials, and 10 textbooks. His main clinical and research interests are imaging of liver tumors, cross-sectional imaging of the female pelvis and MR imaging of the prostate, molecular imaging including the development of iron oxide nanoparticles, and the development of drug-eluting balloons for interventional radiology.

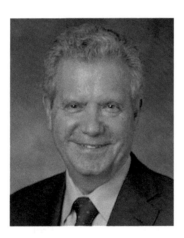

Pablo R. Ros received his MD and PhD, from the Autonomous University of Barcelona, in his native city. He completed his Residency and Fellowship at Mount Sinai Medical Center/University of Miami, Florida. He later obtained a Master of Public Heath (Health Care Policy and Management) at the Harvard School of Public Health. After finishing his training, Dr. Ros became Chief of Gastrointestinal Radiologic Pathology at the Armed Forces Institute of Pathology (AFIP), continuing his association with the AFIP for over 20 years. He became the Founding Director of the Division of Abdominal Imaging at the University of Florida (UF) and Director of Magnetic Resonance Imaging. At UF, Dr. Ros was promoted to Professor of Radiology and appointed Associate Chairman.

In 1998, Dr. Ros was named Professor of Radiology at Harvard Medical School and Executive Vice-Chair and Associate Radiologist-in-Chief at the Brigham and Women's Hospital. In Boston, he also served as Director and Chief Operating Officer of Partners Radiology and Chief of Radiology at the Dana Farber Cancer Institute.

In 2009, Dr. Ros was appointed Theodore J. Castele University Professor and Chairman of the Department of Radiology at University Hospitals Case Medical Center and Case Western Reserve University and Radiologist-in-Chief of the University Hospitals Health System.

Dr. Ros has served or serves as President, Committee Chair or in the Board of Directors of several radiological societies, such as The Radiological Society of North America (RSNA), Association of University Radiologists, Inter-American College of

Radiology, Society of Gastrointestinal Radiologists, American College of Radiology (ACR), New England Roentgen Ray Society and the Academy of Radiology Research. He is a Fellow of the ACR, Society of Abdominal Radiology (SAR) and Honorary Fellow of the European Society of Gastrointestinal and Abdominal Radiology (ESGAR).

Dr. Ros has published more than 300 papers and 18 textbooks primarily in Abdominal and Oncologic Imaging, focusing on liver, pancreatic, mesenteric, and gastrointestinal cross-sectional imaging with pathologic correlation. Dr. Ros is the Editor of textbooks such as *CT and MRI of the Abdomen and Pelvis*, *Radiologic-Pathologic Correlations from Head to Toe*, *Learning Diagnostic Imaging*, *Learning Abdominal Imaging*, *Learning GU and Pelvic Imaging* and the of the series *Imaging for Clinicians*. Other research areas include Magnetic Resonance Imaging, the development of liver-specific and oral contrast agents for MRI, CT and PET-CT imaging, and Radiology Services Research. He holds eleven editorial positions including past Associate Editor of *Radiology* and Consultant to the Editor of the same journal.

Section Editors

Fred E. Avni, Department of Medical Imaging, Erasme Hospital, Brussels, Belgium

Fred Avni is with the Department of Medical Imaging at the Erasme Hospital in Brussels, Belgium.

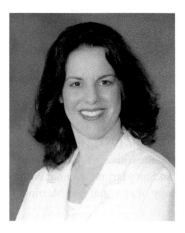

Laura R. Carucci, Department of Radiology, Virginia Commonwealth University Medical Center, Richmond, VA, USA

Laura R. Carucci is an Associate Professor and Director of Computed Tomography and Magnetic Resonance Imaging in the Department of Radiology at the Virginia Commonwealth University School of Medicine in Richmond, Virginia, USA. She graduated from Cornell University with a degree in microbiology and earned her medical doctorate at the State University of New York, Upstate Medical Center in Syracuse, New York. She is a fellowship-trained gastrointestinal radiologist specializing in fluoroscopy, computed tomography, and magnetic resonance imaging of the abdomen and pelvis and specifically the GI tract.

Dr. Carucci's main area of clinical and research interest is the luminal GI tract. Following completion of her diagnostic radiology residency at the University of Pennsylvania, Dr. Carucci completed a GI radiology fellowship at the same institution. She has been on faculty at the Virginia Commonwealth University for the past 10 years. She is an active member of the Society of Abdominal Radiology, Radiologic Society of North America, American Roentgen Ray Society, and the American College of Radiology. She is currently on the Editorial Board of the journal *Radiographics* and a member of the ACR Appropriateness Committee for GI.

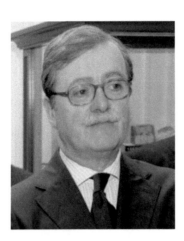

Lorenzo E. Derchi, Department of Radiology, University of Genoa, Genoa, Italy

Lorenzo E. Derchi graduated in Medicine in 1975 at the University of Genoa, Italy, and was Board certified in Radiology in 1979. He served as Staff Radiologist at Hospital San Martino, Genoa, in 1981. He was appointed Professor in Radiology at the Faculty of Medicine at the University of Genoa in 1994, and Chair of one of the Radiology units of Hospital San Martino, Genoa, in the same year. He was Chair of the Department of Radiology of Hospital San Martino, Genoa from January 2004 to September 2011.

Dr. Derchi started working in diagnostic ultrasound in 1975 and in Doppler techniques in 1984. He was Member of the Board of Directors of the Italian Society of Ultrasound in Medicine and Biology (SIUMB) during 1987 to 1989, and was President of the same society in the 1995-1997 period. He was Member of the Board of Directors of the Italian Society of Radiology (SIRM) from 1996 to 2000. At present, he is President of the Ultrasound Section of the same society. He has been Member of the Board of the European Society of Urogenital Radiology (ESUR) from 2000, and was its President from 2004 to 2006.

Dr. Derchi has been Chair of the Working Group on Ultrasound of the European Society of Radiology (ESR) since March 2009 and of the Communication and External Affairs Committee of ESR since March 2011. He was Co-Chair of the Categorical Course on Ultrasound held at the European Congress of Radiology (ECR) in Vienna in 2001-2002, of the "Hands-on" Workshops on Musculoskeletal US held at ECR in the following four years, and of the Categorical Course in Urogenital Radiology held at ECR 2012 and 2013. He was Chair of the combined meeting of ESUR and SUR (Society of Uroradiology) in Genoa in 2002.

Dr. Derchi has published 192 papers and a number of chapters in Italian and international textbooks. Most papers deal with diagnostic imaging using ultrasound and Doppler techniques and with topics on the genitourinary system, with special attention to renal and testicular diseases.

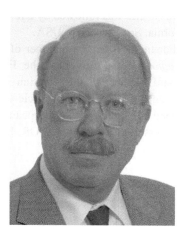

Olle Ekberg, Department of Diagnostic Radiology, Lund University, Malmö, Sweden

Olle Ekberg received his professional education at the Medical Faculty of Lund University in Sweden. He graduated in 1972 and received his Ph.D. in 1981. Dr. Ekberg has held several faculty appointments including Resident, Instructor, Assistant Professor, and Associate Professor of Radiology in Malmö, Sweden. He was Visiting Professor, Department of Radiology, Hospital of the University of Pennsylvania in Philadelphia, Pennsylvania, USA, between 1988 and 1990.

Since 1997, Dr. Ekberg has been Professor of Diagnostic Radiology in the Department of Diagnostic Radiology of Lund University in Malmö, Sweden. He was Chair of the Department of Radiology and Physiology of Lund University between 1997 and 2005. Dr. Ekberg has been Chair of the Department of Medical Radiology, IKVM, of Lund University since 2006. His has 315 publications, including peer-reviewed articles, reviews, and one textbook. Of these, 155 are related to swallowing.

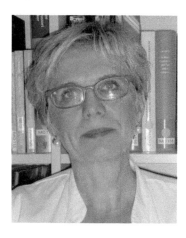

Rosemarie Forstner, Department of Radiology, Landeskrankenhaus Salzburg, Paracelsus Medical University, Salzburg, Austria

Rosemarie Forstner is Associate Professor at the Department of Radiology at the Landeskrankenhaus Salzburg, Paracelsus Medical University, Austria. She specializes in gynecologic and oncologic imaging with emphasis on CT and MRI.

Dr. Forstner's residency in Austria was followed by a fellowship in Abdominal MRI at the University of California, San Francisco, USA.

For many years, Dr. Forstner has been a member of the Editorial Board of the *Journal of European Radiology* and Editor of the Female Imaging section in *EuroRad*. She is also Board Member of the Austrian Roentgen Ray Society and the female imaging subgroup of the European Society of Urogenital Radiology. Dr. Forstner has been invited to lecture for the European Congress of Radiology for many years, for Erasmus courses, as well as for ESOR, ESUR, and AAF courses.

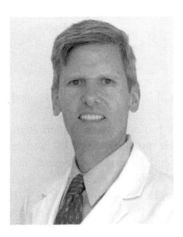

Peter F. Hahn, Massachusetts General Hospital, Boston, MA, USA

Peter F. Hahn is Radiologist at Massachusetts General Hospital (MGH) in Boston and Associate Professor of Radiology at Harvard Medical School in Boston, USA. He graduated from Harvard Medical School and has been a member of the Division of Abdominal Imaging and Interventional Radiology at MGH since 1987. Dr. Hahn's interests include MR contrast agents, cross-sectional imaging of the abdomen, and radiology utilization. Prior to entering medicine, he earned his Ph.D. in mathematics from Harvard and was a member of the faculty at the University of California, Berkeley. Dr. Hahn has 8 publications in mathematics and more than 250 related to radiology.

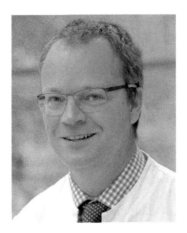

Peter Hallscheidt, Radiologie Darmstadt, Alice Hospital, Darmsadt, Germany

Peter Hallscheidt is with Radiologie Darmstadt at Alice Hospital in Darmstadt, Germany. Dr. Hallscheidt did his internship in radiology and residency in urology at the University of Heidelberg Medical School. Between 1996 and 1998, he was with the Department of Diagnostic Radiology in the same institution. In 2000, he received Fellowship at the German Cancer Research Center (DKFZ). In 2001, Dr. Hallscheidt cleared the Board examination in Diagnostic Radiology and became a senior physician in the Department of Diagnostic Radiology at the University of Heidelberg Medical School. In 2005, he was appointed Associate Professor of Radiology and in 2007 became Professor of Radiology at the University of Heidelberg. In 2011, Dr. Hallscheidt became Partner at Radiologie Darmstadt.

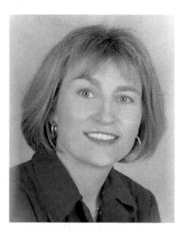

Gertraud Heinz-Peer, Institute of Diagnostic and Interventional Radiology, Medical University Hospital, Saint Poelten, Austria

Gertraud Heinz-Peer is Head of the Institute of Diagnostic and Interventional Radiology of the Medical University Hospital in Saint Poelten, Austria. She did her graduation at the Medical University of Vienna and her residency training at the Department of Radiology of the same institution. She received her Board Certification in radiology in 1996. Dr. Heinz-Pee was Staff Member at the Department of Radiology, Section Head of Genitourinary Radiology, and Interceding Section Head of Breast Imaging and Intervention at the General and Pediatric Department of Radiology of the Medical University of Vienna. She has been Associate Professor of Radiology since 1999. Dr. Heinz-Peer underwent postgraduate training for Leadership in Medical Profession at the University of Salzburg and in Health Care Management at the Medical University of Vienna (2009-2011), graduating with the MBA degree. She also has teaching appointments at the Medical School of Radiology (ESOR) and the ESUR Global Educational Program on the Safe Use of Contrast Media. Dr. Heinz-Peer holds Guest Professorships at the University of Sheffield, UK, and at the National Research Center of Mother and Child Health in Astana, Kazakhstan.

Dr. Heinz-Peer's areas of scientific interest and emphasis include urogenital imaging and interventions, breast imaging and interventions, oncologic imaging and interventions, and contrast media. She is a Board Member of ESUR and was its President between 2010 and 2012. Dr. Heinz-Peer is a member of several radiology societies (ESR, RSNA, ESUR, CMSC, and EAU). She has won several national and international awards (Austrian Roentgen Ray Society, SUR/SAR). Dr. Heinz-Peer is a reviewer for several international scientific journals. She is Member of the Advisory Board of *European Radiology* and Co-Editor of *Insight into Imaging*. Dr. Heinz-Peer has authored more than 90 papers in peer-reviewed scientific journals, written 18 book chapters, provided 11 book reviews, and given 220 lectures. She has been an organizer of several scientific meetings.

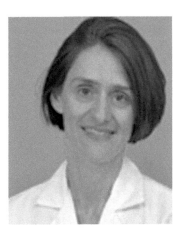

Karin A. Herrmann, Department of Radiology, University Hospitals, Cleveland, OH, USA

Karin A. Herrmann is Visiting Associate Professor of Radiology at University Hospitals (UH) of Cleveland, and Diagnostic Radiologist at UH Case Medical Center, Cleveland, Ohio, USA.

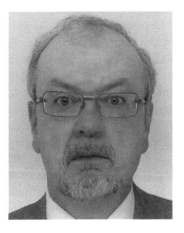

Dermot E. Malone, University College Dublin School of Medicine, Dublin, Ireland

Dermot E. Malone trained in medicine and radiology in Ireland and then trained in abdominal radiology in Canada. He is a Fellow of the Faculty of Radiologists,

RCSI (1986); Royal College of Radiologists (1987); and Royal College of Physicians of Canada (1988). Dr. Malone was a Staff Radiologist and Associate Professor of Radiology in McMaster University (1990-95), where he did an MD thesis on US monitoring of hepatic laser ablation. He returned to Ireland in 1996 as a Consultant Radiologist in St. Vincent's University Hospital (SVUH).

Dr. Malone's clinical interests are abdominal imaging and intervention, and academic interests are the application of Evidence-Based Medicine methods to radiology, liver imaging, imaging in Crohn's disease, and imaging the acute abdomen. He has more than 75 peer-reviewed publications and 12 book chapters, as well as many non-peer-reviewed publications. Dr. Malone is an Associate Clinical Professor in the University College Dublin School of Medicine, and a Board Member and Honorary Secretary of the Faculty of Radiologists, RCSI. Internationally, he has worked on committees of the European Society of Radiology, the European Society of Gastrointestinal and Abdominal Radiologists, and the Radiology Alliance for Health Services Research.

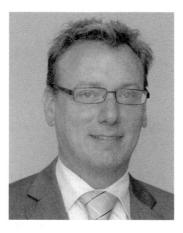

Koenraad J. Mortele, Division of Clinical MRI, Beth Israel Deaconess Medical Center, Harvard Medical School, Boston, MA, USA

Koenraad J. Mortele is Staff Radiologist, Abdominal Imaging and Body MRI, at Beth Israel Deaconess Medical Center (BIDMC) in Boston, USA. He is Director of the Division of Clinical MRI and Associate Professor of Radiology at Harvard Medical School.

Dr. Mortele received his MD degree from and completed his radiology training at Ghent University in Ghent, Belgium. In 2000, he completed a fellowship in Radiology Management at Brigham and Women's Hospital (BWH) in Boston, after which he joined the Faculty in the Division of Abdominal Imaging and Intervention. At BWH, Dr. Mortele served as Associate Director of the Division of Abdominal Imaging and Intervention, as Director of Abdominal and Pelvic MRI, as Director of Continuing Medical Education in the Department of Radiology, as Director of the BWH Contrast Agent Safety Committee, and as Assistant Fellowship Director in the Division of Abdominal Imaging and Intervention.

A prolific lecturer and author of over 150 scientific papers, Dr. Mortele has a particular interest in imaging of the pancreas, the hepatobiliary system, and the GI tract. Dr. Mortele has received numerous awards, including the Society of Gastrointestinal Radiology Visiting Professorship Award in 2009 and two BWH Radiology George Marina Teaching Awards. Dr. Mortele has edited a textbook on CT and MRI of the abdomen and pelvis, authored 15 book chapters, and is frequently invited to lecture and present workshops nationally and internationally.

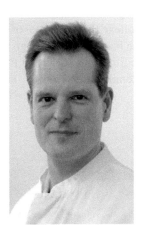

Ullrich G. Mueller-Lisse, Department of Clinical Radiology, University of Munich Hospitals, Munich, Germany

Ullrich G. Mueller-Lisse is Professor of Radiology and Attending Radiologist at the Department of Clinical Radiology of University of Munich Hospitals in Munich, Germany. He studied biology at Ripon College, Ripon, Wisconsin, USA; medicine at the universities of Bonn in Germany; Bristol in England, UK; and California in San Francisco, USA; outcomes research and clinical epidemiology at the University of California in San Francisco, USA; and health care management at the University of Applied Sciences, Deggendorf, Germany. Dr. Mueller-Lisse pursued residency training in urology, radiology, and neuroradiology at the University of Munich Hospitals, Germany, and worked as a clinical instructor and research fellow in radiology at the University of California in San Francisco, USA.

Besides his medical degree, full medical license, and board license in radiology, Dr. Mueller-Lisse holds a B.A. in biology and an MBA in health care management. He has been Attending Radiologist since 2002, Attending PET-CT Radiologist since 2012, and Professor of Radiology since 2012 at the University of Munich Hospitals, Germany. Dr. Mueller-Lisse has served as a reviewer for different national and international medical journals and is an active member of different national and international medical societies. His research interests include MRI, CT, and PET-CT of the urogenital system, the chest and lung, and the head and neck.

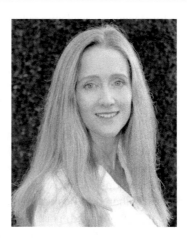

Andrea G. Rockall, Imperial College Healthcare NHS Trust, London, UK

Andrea G. Rockall graduated from King's College Hospital, London, UK, in 1990. She trained in internal medicine at Charing Cross Hospital and obtained her MRCP in 1993. She then started training in radiology at St. Mary's Hospital and University College Hospital, London, and was awarded the Gold Medal of the Royal College of Radiologists for the FRCR examination in 1997. Dr. Rockall was appointed Senior Lecturer in Diagnostic Imaging at Queen Mary University of London and Honorary Consultant Radiologist at Barts and the London NHS Trust in 2000. She became Professor of Cancer Imaging in 2009.

Dr. Rockall has a special interest in gynecologic, urologic, and endocrine imaging as well as functional imaging in genitourinary cancer. She is currently the Chair of the Female Pelvic Imaging Group of the European Society of Uroradiology. Dr. Rockall has recently taken up the position of Consultant Radiologist and Professor of Radiology at Imperial College Healthcare NHS Trust.

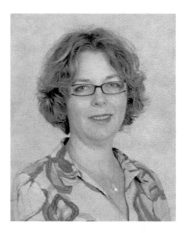

Evis Sala, Memorial Sloan-Kettering Cancer Center, New York, NY, USA

Evis Sala is an internationally recognized academic radiologist with a special interest in Cancer Imaging. She is currently the Director of Gynecologic Imaging at the Memorial Sloan-Kettering Cancer Center in New York, USA. Before joining the Center in July 2012, Dr. Sala was a University Lecturer in Radiology and Specialty Teaching Director (Radiology) at the University of Cambridge, UK, as well as an Honorary Consultant Radiologist and the Lead for Gynaecology Imaging at Addenbrooke's Hospital, Cambridge, UK.

Dr. Sala obtained her Ph.D. from the University of Cambridge, UK, in 2000 and completed her training in Clinical Radiology at Cambridge, UK, in 2005. She is an established researcher with more than 100 peer-reviewed papers and more than 80 invited lectures, and has been a principal investigator on multiple research grants. Dr. Sala has edited 3 books and authored 14 book chapters. She is an Editorial Board member and Head of Oncology Section of European Society of Radiology. Dr. Sala's research focuses on the development and validation of functional, multi-parametric, and quantitative MR imaging techniques in the evaluation of early treatment response in genitourinary malignancies, aimed at transferring these techniques from the laboratory to clinical use.

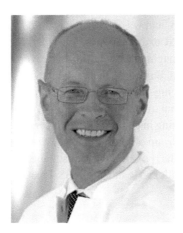

Heinz-Peter Schlemmer, Medical Faculty, Heidelberg, University, Heidelberg, Germany

Heinz-Peter Schlemmer is physicist, physician, and Full Professor of Radiodiagnostic Oncology at the University of Heidelberg, Germany. At the German Cancer Research Center (DFKZ), he is Director of the Department of Radiology and Coordinator of the research program "Imaging and Radiooncology." As a radiologist, Dr. Schlemmer has been actively involved for many years in the development and clinical application of novel imaging technologies in oncology. He started his career as a Physicist, and was engaged in basic research in nuclear magnetic resonance in physics/biophysics at the Max Planck Institute for Medical Research in Heidelberg.

During his academic studies in medicine and his residency in radiology, Dr. Schlemmer worked in several national and international university hospitals and continuously focused his research on clinical scientific applications of novel MR methods in oncology. His particular research is in advanced cross-sectional imaging methods, including morphological and functional MR at conventional 1.5 T up to ultra-high 7.0 T magnetic field strengths, dual-energy CT, hybrid imaging with PET/CT and PET/MRI, as well as US. Dr. Schlemmer's special scientific interest is currently focused on particular tumor entities: prostate cancer, lung cancer, multiple myeloma, and malignant melanoma. His clinical activities are performed in close cooperation within the departments of the research program as well as the Departments of Radiology, Neuroradiology, Nuclear Medicine, and Radiooncology of the Heidelberg University Hospital. His clinical activities include the operation of tumor boards at the National Center for Tumor Diseases (NCT) in Heidelberg. Dr. Schlemmer is President-Elect of the International Cancer Imaging Society and is currently developing an Oncologic Radiology Program of the German Roentgen Ray Society.

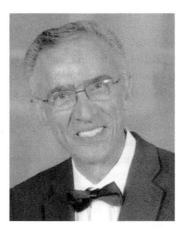

Ali Shirkhoda, Department of Radiology, University of California, Irvine, CA, USA

Ali Shirkhoda was trained as a Radiologist at George Washington University Hospital in Washington, DC, USA, and completed a Body Imaging Fellowship at the University of North Carolina in Chapel Hill. Currently he is a Clinical Professor of Radiology at the University of California in Irvine and works as an attending Radiologist at VA Health Care System in Long Beach, California.

Dr. Shirkhoda has just completed 25 years of service as Director of Diagnostic Imaging and Program Director of Fellowships at William Beaumont Hospital in Royal Oak, Michigan. He was formerly Professor of Radiology at the University of Texas MD Anderson Cancer Center. Dr. Shirkhoda's main field of interest continues to be gastrointestinal and genitourinary oncological imaging and intervention. He is the author or coauthor of over 150 scientific papers, has given over 200 lectures worldwide, and is the author of three textbooks, one of which—*Variants and Pitfalls in Body Imaging*—has been published in three languages.

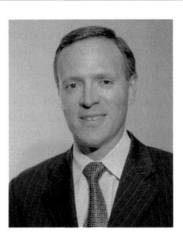

Jorge A. Soto, Department of Radiology, Boston University Medical Center, Boston, MA, USA

Jorge A. Soto completed medical and radiology residency training at the Instituto de Ciencias de la Salud in Medellin, Colombia, and a Fellowship in Body Imaging at Boston University Medical Center, Boston, USA. He is Professor of Radiology in Boston University School of Medicine and Vice-Chair of the Department of Radiology in Boston Medical Center.

Dr. Soto's main academic interests are in the fields of pancreatico-biliary imaging and traumatic and non-traumatic abdominal emergencies. He has published 120 peer-reviewed articles, numerous reviews, and book chapters, and edited five books. Dr. Soto serves as Committee Member and Officer in the Radiological Society of North America, American Roentgen Ray Society, Society of Abdominal Radiology, and American Society of Emergency Radiology. He is a member of the Editorial Board of the journal *Radiology*.

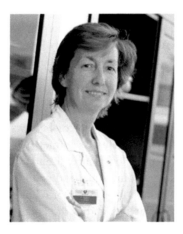

Valerie Vilgrain, Department of Radiology, Beaujon University Hospital, Université Paris Diderot, Sorbonne Paris Cité, France

Valerie Vilgrain is Chair of the Department of Radiology at the Beaujon University Hospital, and Professor of Radiology at the Université Paris Diderot, Sorbonne Paris Cité, France. Dr. Vilgrain received her MD from the Medical School of Paris Descartes University in 1985. She was Resident in Radiology at Paris University and completed a Fellowship in Radiology at the Beaujon University Hospital, Clichy, France, from 1987 to 1988. Her major research interests are diagnostic and interventional imaging of the liver, pancreas, and bile ducts with special interest in multidetector CT and MR imaging.

Dr. Vilgrain is member of several national and international societies such as Radiological Society of North America (RSNA), European Society of Radiology (ESR), European Society of Gastro and Abdominal Radiology (ESGAR), European Association for the Study of Liver (EASL), and French Radiological Society (SFR). She was Chair of the Education Program Committee of the French annual meeting from 2000 to 2008 and is Vice-Chair of the French Radiological Society since 2010. Dr. Vilgrain is member of the European Congress of Radiology (ECR) Congress Committee. She has published numerous peer-reviewed papers. Dr. Vilgrain is Associate Editor of the journal *Radiology*, and a reviewer for many national and international journals, including *European Radiology*, *Liver Transplantation*, *Hepatology*, *Journal of Hepatology*, *European Journal of Radiology*, *JCAT*, and *European Journal of Cancer*.

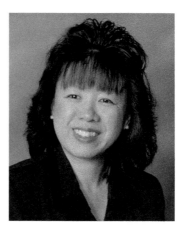

Judy Yee, Department of Radiology and Biomedical Imaging, University of California, San Francisco, USA

Judy Yee is Professor and Vice-Chair of the Department of Radiology and Biomedical Imaging at the University of California, San Francisco, USA. She is also Chief of Radiology at San Francisco VA Medical Center. Dr. Yee is an accomplished abdominal and gastrointestinal radiologist with a focus on CT colonography, as well as liver and pancreatic imaging using CT and MR. She has published multiple landmark studies in the field of CT colonography and continues to carry out research in the area.

Dr. Yee holds numerous leadership positions in major radiology organizations and serves on the Editorial Boards of respected journals. She is Chair of the

American College of Radiology Colon Cancer Committee, Chair of the RSNA Public Information Committee, and is on the Board of Directors of the Society of Abdominal Radiology. Dr. Yee provides numerous invited lectures nationally and internationally. She is a well-respected educator, having instructed and mentored multiple trainees in abdominal imaging. She is the recipient of many awards, including the Excellence in Teaching Award from the Academy of Medical Educators and the Visiting Professorship Award from the Society of Gastrointestinal Radiologists.

Contents

Volume 2

Volume 4

List of Contributors

S. Aasen Department of Radiology, Oslo University Hospital, Oslo, Norway

Helen Clare Addley Department of Radiology, McGill University Health Center, Montreal General Hospital, Montreal, Quebec, Canada

Fatih Akisik Department of Radiology, Indiana University School of Medicine, Indianapolis, IN, USA

Lauren F. Alexander University of Alabama at Birmingham, Birmingham, AL, USA

Jarrah Ali Al-Tubaikh Department of Clinical Radiology, Sabah Hospital, Kuwait City, Kuwait

Marco Amendola Department of Radiology, University of Miami, Miami, FL, USA

Stephan W. Anderson Department of Radiology, Boston University Medical Center, Boston, MA, USA

Laghi Andrea Dipartimento di Scienze Radiologiche, Oncologiche, Anatomo-Patologiche, Sapienza University of Rome – Polo Pontino, Latina, Italy

Marina-Portia Anthony Department of Diagnostic Radiology, The University of Hong Kong, Queen Mary Hospital, Hong Kong

Halil Arslan Department of Radiology, Yildirim Beyazit University School of Medicine, Ankara, Turkey

Fred E. Avni Department of Medical Imaging, Erasme Hospital, Brussels, Belgium

Nami Azar University Hospitals Case Medical Center, Cleveland, OH, USA

I. Baglio Department of Radiology, Azienda Ospedaliera Universitaria Integrata, Verona, Italy

Mark E. Baker Section, Abdominal Imaging, Imaging Institute and Digestive Disease Institute, Cleveland Clinic, Cleveland, OH, USA

Susanne Baroud Department of Radiology, Medical University of Vienna, Vienna, Austria

Libero Barozzi Emergency, Surgery and Transplants, Department – Radiology Unit – S. Orsola-Malpighi, University Hospital, Bologna, Italy

Tristan Barrett Department of Radiology, School of Clinical Medicine, Addenbrooke's Hospital and University of Cambridge, Cambridge, UK

Carlo Bartolozzi Department of Diagnostic and Interventional Radiology, University of Pisa, Pisa, PI, Italy

Clive I. Bartram Department of Radiology, The Princess Grace Hospital, London, UK

Ahmed Ba-Ssalamah Department of Radiology, Medical University of Vienna, Vienna, Austria

Valentina Battaglia Department of Diagnostic and Interventional Radiology, University of Pisa, Pisa, PI, Italy

Bernard Beber Department of Radiology, University of Miami, Miami, FL, USA

Marie-France Bellin University Paris Sud, AP-HP, Hôpital de Bicêtre, Le Kremlin-Bicêtre, France

Jonathan W. Berlin Department of Radiology, North Shore University Health System, University of Chicago, Evanston Hospital, Evanston, IL, USA

Antonio Bernardes Department of Anatomy, University of Coimbra, Coimbra, Portugal

Michele Bertolotto Department of Radiology, University of Trieste, Trieste, Italy

Nishat Bharwani Imaging, Bart's Cancer Centre, King George V Wing St Bartholomew's Hospital, West Smithfield, London, UK

Department of Radiology, St Mary's Hospital, Imperial College Healthcare NHS Trust, London, UK

Christian Bieg Institute of Radiology, Baden, Switzerland

Ennio Biscaldi Department of Radiology, Galliera Hospital, Genoa, Italy

Ola Björgell Diagnostic Centre of Imaging and Functional Medicine, Skåne University Hospital, Malmö, Sweden

Michael A. Blake Department of Abdominal Imaging and Intervention, Massachusetts General Hospital, Boston, MA, USA

Roberto Blasbalg Department of Radiology, University of Sao Paulo, School of Medicine, Sao Paulo, SP, Brazil

Thomas Bollen St. Antonius Hospital Nieuwegein, Nieuwegein, Netherlands

David Bonekamp The Russell H. Morgan Department of Radiology and Radiologic Science, The Johns Hopkins University, Baltimore, MD, USA

Peyman Borghei Department of Radiology, University of Alabama at Birmingham, Birmingham, AL, USA

Doumit S. BouHaidar Department of Radiology, Virginia Commonwealth University Medical Center, Richmond, VA, USA

Elena Bozzi Department of Diagnostic and Interventional Radiology, University of Pisa, Pisa, PI, Italy

Olga R. Brook Department of Radiology, Beth Israel Deaconess Medical Center, Harvard Medical School, Boston, MA, USA

A. Bucci Department of Radiology, Azienda Ospedaliera Universitaria Integrata, Verona, Italy

Helen Bungay National Health Service, Oxford, UK

Irene A. Burger Divison of Nuclear Medicine, Department of Medical Radiology, University Hospital Zurich, Zurich, Switzerland

Angela Caiado Department of Radiology, University of Sao Paulo, School of Medicine, Sao Paulo, SP, Brazil

Rafael O. P. de Campos Department of Radiology, University of North Carolina Hospitals, Chapel Hill, NC, USA

Cheri L. Canon Witten-Stanley Endowed Chair of Radiology, University of Alabama at Birmingham, Birmingham, AL, USA

Vito Cantisani Dirigente Medico Radiologo I livello, Dipartimento di Scienze Radiologiche, Oncologiche, Anatomo-Patologiche, Policlinico Umberto I, Sapienza University of Rome, Rome, Italy

Giovanni Carbognin Department of Radiology, Sacro Cuore Hospital, Verona, Negrar, Italy

Pablo Caro Children's University Hospital, Dublin 1, Ireland

Anne G. Carroll Department of Radiology, St. Vincent's University Hospital and University College Dublin, Dublin, Ireland

Laura R. Carucci Department of Radiology, Virginia Commonwealth University Medical Center, Richmond, VA, USA

Filipe Caseiro-Alves Department of Radiology, University of Coimbra, Coimbra, Portugal

Victor Javier Casillas Department of Radiology, University of Miami, Miami, FL, USA

Innovative Cancer Institue, South Miami, FL, USA

Marie Cassart Department of Medical Imaging (FEA, AM and MC) and Fetal Medicine (RL), University Clinics of Brussels, Erasme Hospital, Brussels, Belgium

German Castrillon Department of Radiology and Gastrohepatology, Universidad de Antioquia, Medellin, Colombia

Onofrio A. Catalano SDN, Institute for Nuclear and Diagnostic Imaging, Naples, Italy

Marco Cavallaro Department of Radiology, University of Trieste, Trieste, Italy

Victoria O. Chan Department of Radiology, St. Vincent's University Hospital, Dublin, Ireland

Jeanette Y. Chun University of Massachusetts, Worcester, MA, USA

Rachel Connor South Glasgow University Hospitals, The Victoria Infirmary, Glasgow, UK

João Filipe Costa Department of Radiology, University of Coimbra, Coimbra, Portugal

Diego A. Covarrubias Department of Abdominal Imaging and Intervention, Massachusetts General Hospital, Boston, MA, USA

Carmel Cronin Department of Radiology, Mater Misericordiae Hospital, Dublin, Ireland

David W. Crook Department of Medical Radiology, University Hospital Zürich, Zürich, Switzerland

Davide Bellini Department of Medical-Surgical Sciences and Biotechnologies, Sapienza University of Rome, Polo Pontino, Latina, Italy

Riccardo De Robertis Lombardi Istituto di Radiologia, Policlinico GB Rossi, Azienda Ospedaliera Universitaria Integrata Verona, Verona, Italy

Farrokh Dehdashti Division of Nuclear Medicine, Edward Mallinckrodt Institute of Radiology, Washington University School of Medicine, St. Louis, MO, USA

Lorenzo E. Derchi Department of Radiology, University of Genoa, Genoa, Italy

N. M. DeSouza Cancer Research UK and EPSRC Cancer Imaging Centre, Institute of Cancer Research and Royal Marsden NHS Foundation Trust, Sutton, UK

MRI Unit, Royal Marsden Hospital, Sutton, Surrey, UK

Nuno Dias Vascular Center, Skåne University Hospital Malmö, Malmö, Sweden

Alexander Ding Department of Radiology, Harvard Medical School/Massachusetts General Hospital, Boston, MA, USA

David J. DiSantis Department of Radiology, University of Kentucky College of Medicine Chandler Hospital, Lexington, KY, USA

Vikram S. Dogra Department of Imaging Sciences, School of Medicine and Dentistry, University of Rochester, Rochester, NY, USA

K. Downey Cancer Research UK and EPSRC Cancer Imaging Centre, Institute of Cancer Research and Royal Marsden NHS Foundation Trust, Sutton, UK

Ryan T. Downey Department of Radiology, University of California – San Francisco, San Francisco, CA, USA

David M. Einstein Section, Abdominal Imaging, Imaging Institute and Digestive Disease Institute, Cleveland Clinic, Cleveland, OH, USA

David Eiss University Paris V, AP-HP, Hôpital Necker, Paris, France

Sukru Mehmet Erturk Department of Radiology, Sisli Etfal Training and Research Hospital, Istanbul, Turkey

Negar Fakhrai Department of Radiology, Medical University of Vienna, Vienna, Austria

Peter F. Faulhaber University Hospitals of Cleveland, Cleveland, OH, USA

Claes-Henrik Florén Department of Internal Medicine, Division of Clinical Sciences, Skåne University Hospital, Lund University, Lund, Sweden

Rosemarie Forstner Department of Radiology, Landeskrankenhaus Salzburg, Paracelsus Medical University, Salzburg, Austria

Eric Frampas Central Department of Radiology and Medical Imaging, Hôtel-Dieu, Teaching Hospital Nantes, Nantes, Cedex 1, France

Alan H. Freeman Department of Radiology, Addenbrooke's Hospital, Cambridge, UK

Susan J. Freeman University Department of Radiology, Addenbrooke's Hospital, Cambridge, UK

Jürgen J. Fütterer Radboud University Medical Centre Nijmegen, Nijmegen, Netherlands

Toshifumi Gabata Department of Radiology, Kanazawa University Graduate School of Medical Science, Kanazawa University Hospital, Kanazawa, Japan

Suvranu Ganguli Massachusetts General Hospital/Harvard Medical School, Boston, MA, USA

Sangeet Ghai Department of Medical Imaging, University of Toronto, Toronto General Hospital, Toronto, ON, Canada

Richard M. Gore Department of Radiology, North Shore University Health System, University of Chicago, Evanston Hospital, Evanston, IL, USA

Sofia Gourtsoyianni N. Papanikolaou & Associates, Science and Technology Park of Crete, Heraklion, Crete, Greece

Department of Computed Tomography, Konstantopouleion General Hospital, Athens, Greece

Laurent Guibaud Center of Fetal Medicine, Hospital Femme Mère Enfant, Univeristé Claude Bernard, Lyon 1, France

Department of Pediatric and Fetal Imaging, Hospital Femme Mère Enfant, Univeristé Claude Bernard, Lyon 1, France

Boris Guiu Department of Radiology, University Hospital of Dijon, Dijon, France

B. Hadaschik Department of Urology, University Hospital Heidelberg, Heidelberg, Germany

Peter Hallscheidt Radiologie Darmstadt, Alice Hospital, Darmstadt, Germany

Robert A. Halvorsen, Jr. Department of Radiology, Virginia Commonwealth University Medical Center, Richmond, VA, USA

Anthony Hanbidge Department of Medical Imaging, University of Toronto, Toronto, ON, Canada

Randy A. Hawkins Department of Radiology, The University of California San Francisco, San Francisco, CA, USA

Gertraud Heinz-Peer Institute of Diagnostic and Interventional Radiology, Medical University Hospital, Saint Poelten, Austria

Karin A. Herrmann Department of Radiology, University Hospitals, Cleveland, OH, USA

Chandra P. Hewavitharana Department of Diagnostic & Interventional Radiology, Royal Perth Hospital, Perth, Western Australia, Australia

Olivier Hélénon University Paris V, AP-HP, Hôpital Necker, Paris, France

Richard Ho Department of Diagnostic and Interventional Radiology, Royal Perth Hospital, Perth, Western Australia, Australia

Peter Humphrey Lahey Clinic, Burlington, MA, USA

M. De Iorio Tecnomed (private practice), Verona, Italy

Tracy Jaffe Department of Radiology, Duke University Medical Center, Durham, NC, USA

Hyun-Jung Jang Department of Medical Imaging, Toronto General Hospital, University of Toronto, Toronto, ON, Canada

Taylor R. Jordan Department of Radiology & Biomedical Imaging, University of California, San Francisco, CA, USA

Eric Jordan Albert Einstein College of Medicine, NY, USA

Adam Jung Department of Radiology and Biomedical Imaging, University of California, San Francisco, CA, USA

Toufic Kachaamy Department of Radiology, Virginia Commonwealth University Medical Center, Richmond, VA, USA

Avinash R. Kambadakone Department of Abdominal Imaging and Intervention, Massachusetts General Hospital, Boston, MA, USA

Robert A. Kane Department of Radiology, Beth Israel Deaconess Medical Center, Harvard Medical School, Boston, MA, USA

Korosh Khalili Department of Medical Imaging, Toronto General Hospital, University of Toronto, Toronto, ON, Canada

Pek-Lan Khong Department of Diagnostic Radiology, The University of Hong Kong, Queen Mary Hospital, Hong Kong

Aoife Kilcoyne Department of Radiology, St. Vincent's University Hospital, Dublin, Ireland

Hee Jin Kim Department of Radiology, University of North Carolina Hospitals, Chapel Hill, NC, USA

Mi Jeong Kim Department of Radiology, University of North Carolina Hospitals, Chapel Hill, NC, USA

Seong Hyun Kim Department of Radiology, University of North Carolina Hospitals, Chapel Hill, NC, USA

Jung Hoon Kim Department of Radiology and Institute of Radiation Medicine, Seoul National University College of Medicine, Seoul, Chongno-gu, South Korea

Bohyun Kim Department of Radiology, Mayo Clinic College of Medicine, Rochester, MN, USA

Seung Hyup Kim Department of Radiology, Seoul National University Hospital, Seoul National University, College of Medicine, Chongno-gu, Seoul, South Korea

Chan Kyo Kim Department of Radiology and Center for Imaging Science, Samsung Medical Center, Sungkyunkwan University School of Medicine, Seoul, South Korea

Young H. Kim University of Massachusetts, Worcester, MA, USA

Tae Kyoung Kim Department of Medical Imaging, Toronto General Hospital, University of Toronto, Toronto, ON, Canada

Satoshi Kobayashi Department of Radiology, Kanazawa University Graduate School of Medical Science, Kanazawa University Hospital, Kanazawa, Japan

Wataru Koda Department of Radiology, Kanazawa University Graduate School of Medical Science, Kanazawa University Hospital, Kanazawa, Japan

Koenraad J. Mortele Division of Clinical MRI, Beth Israel Deaconess Medical Center, Harvard Medical School, Boston, MA, USA

Kazuto Kozaka Department of Radiology, Kanazawa University Graduate School of Medical Science, Kanazawa University Hospital, Kanazawa, Japan

Bernd J. Krause Klinik und Poliklinik für Nuklearmedizin, Zentrum für Radiologie, Universitätsklinikum Rostock, Rostock, Germany

Jonathan B. Kruskal Department of Radiology, Beth Israel Deaconess Medical Center, Harvard Medical School, Boston, MA, USA

Rahel A. Kubik-Huch Institute of Radiology, Baden, Switzerland

Naveen M. Kulkarni Department of Radiology, Harvard Medical School/ Massachusetts General Hospital, Boston, MA, USA

T. H. Kuru Department of Urology, University Hospital Heidelberg, Heidelberg, Germany

David Kurzencwyg McGill University, Jewish General Hospital, Montreal, QC, Canada

David Leiva Department of Radiology, Bellvitge University Hospital, Barcelona, Spain

Rosine Lejeune Department of Medical Imaging (FEA, AM and MC) and Fetal Medicine (RL), University Clinics of Brussels, Erasme Hospital, Brussels, Belgium

Marc S. Levine Department of Radiology, Hospital of the University of Pennsylvania, University of Pennsylvania School of Medicine, University of Pennsylvania Medical Center, Philadelphia, PA, USA

Angela D. Levy Department of Radiology, Georgetown University Hospital, Washington, DC, USA

Pr. Maïté Lewin Department of Radiology, Paul Brousse Hospital, Villejuif, France

Sara Lewis Department of Radiology, Mount Sinai School of Medicine, New York, NY, USA

Shilpa Liyanage Imaging, Bart's Cancer Centre, King George V Wing St Bartholomew's Hospital, West Smithfield, London, UK

Vincent H. S. Low Department of Medicine, University of Western Australia, Crawley, WA, Australia

K. E. A. Lundin Department of Gastroenterology, Centre for Immune Regulation, Oslo University Hospital, Oslo, Norway

Katarzyna J. Macura The Russell H. Morgan Department of Radiology, The Johns Hopkins University, Baltimore, MD, USA

Michael Maher University College Cork, Cork, Ireland

Martin Malina Vascular Center, Skåne University Hospital Malmö, Malmö, Sweden

Anil T. Maliyekkel University Case Medical Center, Cleveland, OH, USA

Dermot E. Malone University College Dublin School of Medicine, Dublin, Ireland

Bahar Mansoori University Hospitals Case Medical Center, Cleveland, OH, USA

Carina Mari Aparici Department of Radiology, The University of California San Francisco, San Francisco, CA, USA

Ciolina Maria Dipartimento di Scienze Radiologiche, Oncologiche, Anatomo-Patologiche, Sapienza University of Rome – Policlinico Umberto I, Rome, Italy

Daniele Marin Duke University Medical Center, Durham, NC, USA

Laura Martínez Department of Radiology, Bellvitge University Hospital, Barcelona, Spain

Jérôme Massardier Center of Fetal Medicine, Hospital Femme Mère Enfant, Univeristé Claude Bernard, Lyon 1, France

Anne Massez Department of Medical Imaging (FEA, AM and MC) and Fetal Medicine (RL), University Clinics of Brussels, Erasme Hospital, Brussels, Belgium

Mona Massoud Center of Fetal Medicine, Hospital Femme Mère Enfant, Univeristé Claude Bernard, Lyon 1, France

Osamu Matsui Department of Radiology, Kanazawa University Graduate School of Medical Science, Kanazawa University Hospital, Kanazawa, Japan

Colin J. McCarthy Department of Radiology, St Vincent's University Hospital, Dublin 4, Ireland

Jonathan E. McConathy Division of Nuclear Medicine, Edward Mallinckrodt Institute of Radiology, Washington University School of Medicine, St. Louis, MO, USA

Shaunagh McDermott Department of Abdominal Imaging and Intervention, Massachusetts General Hospital, Boston, MA, USA

Patrick McLaughlin University College Cork, Cork, Ireland

Uday K. Mehta Department of Radiology, North Shore University Health System, University of Chicago, Evanston Hospital, Evanston, IL, USA

Matthias Meissnitzer Department of Radiology, Landeskrankenhaus Salzburg, Paracelsus Medical University, Salzburg, Austria

Richard M. Mendelson Department of Diagnostic & Interventional Radiology, Royal Perth Hospital, University of Western Australia, Perth, Western Australia, Australia

Ur Metser Department of Medical Imaging, University of Toronto, UHN Princess Margaret Hospital, Toronto, ON, Canada

Tetsuya Minami Department of Radiology, Kanazawa University Graduate School of Medical Science, Kanazawa University Hospital, Kanazawa, Japan

Min Hoan Moon Department of Radiology, Seoul Metropolitan Boramae Medical Center, Seoul National University, College of Medicine, Dongjak-Gu, Seoul, South Korea

Desiree Morgan University of Alabama at Birmingham, Birmingham, AL, USA

Martina M. Morrin Beaumont Hospital, Dublin 9, Ireland

Penelope Moyle Department of Radiology, Hinchingbrooke Hospitals NHS Trust, Huntingdon, Cambridgeshire, UK

Ulrike L. Mueller-Lisse Department of Urology, University of Munich Hospitals, Muenchen, Germany

Ullrich G. Mueller-Lisse Department of Clinical Radiology, University of Munich Hospitals, Munich, Germany

Joe Murphy Department of Radiology, University College Hospital Galway, National University of Ireland, Galway, Galway, Ireland

Sergio Murrone Radiology Unit, Hospital of Brindisi, Brindisi, Italy

Dean A. Nakamoto University Hospitals, Cleveland, OH, USA

P. Narayanan Department of Diagnostic Imaging, Royal Marsden Hospital, London, UK

Rendon Nelson Duke University Medical Center, Durham, NC, USA

Geraldine M. Newmark Department of Radiology, North Shore University Health System, University of Chicago, Evanston Hospital, Evanston, IL, USA

Patricia Noël Department of Radiology, Universite Laval, Quebec, Canada

Owen J. O'Connor Department of Abdominal Imaging and Intervention, Massachusetts General Hospital, Boston, MA, USA

University College Cork, Cork, Ireland

E. J. O'Donovan Department of Diagnostic Imaging, Royal Marsden Hospital, London, UK

Renata Ogawa Department of Radiology, University of Sao Paulo, School of Medicine, Sao Paulo, SP, Brazil

Martin O'Malley Department of Medical Imaging, Toronto General Hospital, University of Toronto, Toronto, ON, Canada

Siobhan B. O'Neill University College Cork, Cork, Ireland

Mehmet Ruhi Onur University of Rochester, Rochester, NY, USA

Sascha Pahernik Urologische Klinik und Poliklinik, Universität Heidelberg, Heidelberg, Germany

Ricci Paolo Dipartimento di Scienze Radiologiche, Oncologiche, Anatomo-Patologiche, Sapienza University of Rome – Policlinico Umberto I, Rome, Italy

Nickolas Papanikolaou N. Papanikolaou & Associates, Science and Technology Park of Crete, Heraklion, Crete, Greece

Raj Mohan Paspulati University Hospitals Case Medical Center, Cleveland, OH, USA

Indravadan Patel University Hospitals Case Medical Center, Cleveland, OH, USA

Pietro Pavlica Department of Radiology, Villalba Hospital, Bologna, Italy

Pedro Sebastian Paz Autonoma University of Guadalajara, Miami, FL, USA

Vincent Pelsser McGill University, Jewish General Hospital, Montreal, QC, Canada

A. Persson Department of Radiology of Medical and Health Sciences (IMH), Center for Medical Image Science and Visualization (CMIV) University of Linkoping, Linköping, Sweden

Andrea Phillips Royal United Hospital Bath, Bath, UK

Ali Pirasteh Case Western Reserve University School of Medicine, Cleveland, OH, USA

Roberto Pozzi Mucelli Istituto di Radiologia, Policlinico GB Rossi, Azienda Ospedaliera Universitaria Integrata Verona, Verona, Italy

Srinivasa R. Prasad University of Texas M.D. Anderson Cancer Center, Houston, TX, USA

J. David Prologo University Hospitals Case Medical Center, Cleveland, OH, USA

Parvati Ramchandani Hospital of the University of Pennsylvania, University of Pennsylvania School of Medicine, Philadelphia, PA, USA

Caroline Reinhold Department of Radiology, McGill University Health Center, Montreal General Hospital, Montreal, Quebec, Canada

Jonathan Richenberg Brighton and Sussex University Hospitals, Brighton, UK

Clare Roche Department of Radiology, University College Hospital Galway, National University of Ireland, Galway, Galway, Ireland

Andrea G. Rockall Imperial College Healthcare NHS Trust, London, UK

M. Roethke Department of Radiology, German Cancer Research Center, Heidelberg, Germany

Gian Andrea Rollandi Department of Radiology, Galliera Hospital, Genoa, Italy

Maxime Ronot Department of Radiology, Assistance Publique des Hopitaux de Paris APHP, Hôpital Beaujon, University Paris 7, Clichy, France

Luis Ros Mendoza Hospital General Royo Villanova, Zaragoza, Spain

Cristina Rossi Radiology Unit, University Hospital of Parma, Parma, Italy

Stephen E. Rubesin Department of Radiology, MRI Center, University of Pennsylvania School of Medicine, Hospital of the University of Pennsylvania, Philadelphia, PA, USA

Sandra Ruiz Department of Radiology, Bellvitge University Hospital, Barcelona, Spain

Stephanie Ryan Children's University Hospital, Dublin 1, Ireland

E. Ronan Ryan Department of Radiology, St Vincent's University Hospital, Dublin 4, Ireland

Yasuji Ryu Department of Radiology, Kanazawa University Graduate School of Medical Science, Kanazawa University Hospital, Kanazawa, Japan

Mariangela Sabato Emergency Radiology Unit, University Hospital of Parma, Parma, Italy

Dushyant V. Sahani Massachusetts General Hospital, Boston, MA, USA

Anju Sahdev Department of Radiology, St Bartholomew's Hospital, Barts and The London NHS Trust and Queen Mary's School of Medicine and Dentistry, London, UK

Department of Diagnostic Imaging, King George V wing, St Bartholomew's Hospital, London, UK

Nisha I. Sainani Department of Abdominal Imaging and Intervention, Brigham and Women's Hospital and Harvard Medical School, Boston, MA, USA

Sanjay Saini Department of Radiology, Harvard Medical School/Massachusetts General Hospital, Boston, MA, USA

Anthony Sajewicz Redwood Regional Medical Group, Santa Rosa, CA, USA

Evis Sala Memorial Sloan-Kettering Cancer Center, New York, NY, USA

Giuseppe Salerno Pa.ma.fi.r. Medical Center, Palermo, Italy

Marco Salvatore Univeristy of Naples "Federico ll", Naples, Italy

R. Salvia Department of Pancreatic Surgery, Azienda Ospedaliera Universitaria Integrata, Verona, Italy

Jun-ichirou Sanada Department of Radiology, Kanazawa University Graduate School of Medical Science, Kanazawa University Hospital, Kanazawa, Japan

Isabel Schifferdecker Department of Diagnostic and Interventional Radiology, University Hospital Heidelberg, Heidelberg, Germany

Heinz-Peter Schlemmer Medical Faculty, Heidelberg University, Heidelberg, Germany

Florian Schneider Radiologische Klinik, Abteilung Diagnostische und Interventionelle Radiologie, Heidelberg, Germany

Sarah Schwarzenböck Klinik und Poliklinik für Nuklearmedizin, Zentrum für Radiologie, Universitätsklinikum Rostock, Rostock, Germany

Miguel Seco Department of Radiology, University of Coimbra, Coimbra, Portugal

Mattia Di Segni Dipartimento di Scienze Radiologiche, Oncologiche, Anatomo-Patologiche, Sapienza University of Rome – Policlinico Umberto I, Rome, Italy

Richard C. Semelka Department of Radiology, University of North Carolina Hospitals, Chapel Hill, NC, USA

Julia G. Seol Department of Abdominal Imaging and Intervention, Brigham and Women's Hospital and Harvard Medical School, Boston, MA, USA

Giovanni Serafini Department of Radiology, S. Corona Hospital, Pietra Ligure, Italy

Fergus Shanahan University College Cork, Cork, Ireland

Alampady K. Shanbhogue University of Texas Health Science Center at San Antonio, San Antonio, TX, USA

Ashley S. Shaw Department of Radiology, Addenbrooke's Hospital, Cambridge, UK

Steven Shay Department of Gastroenterology and Hepatology, Digestive Disease Institute, Cleveland Clinic, Cleveland, OH, USA

Ali Shirkhoda Department of Radiology, University of California, Irvine, CA, USA

Paul B. Shyn Department of Abdominal Imaging and Intervention, Brigham and Women's Hospital and Harvard Medical School, Boston, MA, USA

Paul S. Sidhu Department of Radiology, King's College London, King's College Hospital, London, UK

Henrik Simán Department of Internal Medicine, Växjö Central Hospital, Växjö, Sweden

A. Slater Oxford University Hospital Trust, Oxford, UK

S. A. Sohaib Department of Diagnostic Imaging, Royal Marsden Hospital, London, UK

Farnoosh Sokhandon Department of Radiology, William Beaumont Hospital, Royal Oak, MI, USA

Sat Somers Department of Radiology, McMaster University Medical Centre, Dundas, ON, Canada

M. J. Soo Imaging, Bart's Cancer Centre, King George V Wing, St Bartholomew's Hospital, London, UK

Andrea Soricelli University of Naples "Parthenope", Naples, Italy

Jorge A. Soto Department of Radiology, Boston University Medical Center, Boston, MA, USA

Michael Souvatzoglou Klinik und Poliklinik für Nuklearmedizin, Technische Universität München, München, Germany

Sathi Anandan Sukumar University Hospital of South Manchester, Manchester, UK

Maryellen Sun Department of Radiology, Beth Israel Deaconess Medical Center, Harvard Medical School, Boston, MA, USA

Naoki Takahashi Mayo Clinic, Rochester, MN, USA

Bachir Taouli Department of Radiology, Mount Sinai School of Medicine, New York, NY, USA

Tirkes Temel Indiana Radiology Partners Department of Radiology, Indiana University School of Medicine, Indianapolis, IN, USA

Kiran H. Thakrar Department of Radiology, North Shore University Health System, University of Chicago, Evanston Hospital, Evanston, IL, USA

Ruedi F. Thoeni Department of Radiology and Biomedical Imaging, The University of California, San Francisco, CA, USA

Henrik Thorlacius Department of Clinical Sciences, Section of Surgery, Skåne University Hospital, Lund University, Malmö, Sweden

Eavan Thornton Beaumont Hospital, Dublin 9, Ireland

Temel Tirkes Department of Radiology, Indiana University School of Medicine, Indianapolis, IN, USA

Drew Torigian University of Pennsylvania Medical Center and Perelman School of Medicine at the University of Pennsylvania, Philadelphia, PA, USA

William Toscano Department of Radiology, University of Trieste, Trieste, Italy

Ahmet Tuncay Turgut Department of Radiology, Ankara Training and Research Hospital, Ankara, Turkey

Paola Vagli Department of Diagnostic and Interventional Radiology, University of Pisa, Pisa, PI, Italy

Massimo Valentino Emergency Radiology Unit, University Hospital of Parma, Parma, Italy

Carlos Valls Department of Radiology, Bellvitge University Hospital, Barcelona, Spain

Hebert A. Vargas Radiology Department, Memorial Sloan-Kettering Cancer Center, New York, NY, USA

Valerie Vilgrain Department of Radiology, University Beaujon Hospital, Université Paris Diderot, Sorbonne, Paris Cité, France

Peter Vilmann Department of Surgical Gastroenterology, Hellerup, Denmark

Gustav K. von Schulthess Department of Medical Radiology and Director Nuclear Medicine, University Hospital Zürich, Zürich, Switzerland

Emily M. Webb Department of Radiology & Biomedical Imaging, University of California, San Francisco, CA, USA

Stefanie Weinstein Department of Radiology, The University of California, San Francisco, CA, USA

Daniel R. Wenzke Department of Radiology, North Shore University Health System, University of Chicago, Evanston Hospital, Evanston, IL, USA

C. Jason Wilkins Department of Radiology, King's College London, King's College Hospital, London, UK

Martin Willemink University Medical Center Utrecht, Utrecht, Netherlands

Ozge Yapici Department of Radiology, Sisli Etfal Training and Research Hospital, Istanbul, Turkey

Hooman Yarmohammadi University Hospitals, Case Medical Center, Cleveland, USA

Judy Yee Department of Radiology and Biomedical Imaging, University of California, San Francisco, CA, USA

Benjamin M. Yeh Department of Radiology, University of California – San Francisco, San Francisco, CA, USA

Giulia Zamboni Istituto di Radiologia, Policlinico GB Rossi, Azienda Ospedaliera Universitaria Integrata Verona, Verona, Italy

Patrik Zamecnik Department of Radiology, German Cancer Research Center, Heidelberg, Germany

Imaging Techniques and Normal Anatomy: Scrotum

Michele Bertolotto, Massimo Valentino, and Lorenzo E. Derchi

Scrotal Anatomy

The scrotum is a fibromuscular sac divided into two compartments by a median raphe. Its wall is composed (from superficial to deep) by skin, superficial fascia, dartos muscle, external spermatic fascia, cremasteric fascia, and internal spermatic fascia. The raphe is continuous with the dartos muscle. Beneath the internal spermatic fascia, there is the tunica vaginalis, a mesothelial layer which outlines a sac containing a testis, epididymis, and spermatic cord, usually together with a small amount of fluid. The layer of the tunica vaginalis lining the scrotal wall is defined as the parietal layer; the one extending over the testis and epididymis is called the visceral one. The two layers join at the posterolateral aspect of the testis, where the tunica attaches to the scrotal wall. Beneath the visceral layer of the tunica vaginalis is the tunica albuginea, an inelastic structure which covers the testis and, at its posterior surface, projects into the inner part to form an incomplete septum, the mediastinum; from there, multiple thin fibrous septa extend into the testicular parenchyma, dividing it into 200–400 lobules. Each lobule contains one to three seminiferous tubules which, at the mediastinum, open via the tubuli recti into dilated spaces called the rete testis and then drain into the epididymis through 10–15 efferent ductules. The epididymis, a tubular structure consisting of a head, body, and tail, is located superior to and contiguous with the posterior aspect of the testis. After entering the epididymal head, the ductules from the rete testis form a single duct, the ductus epididymis, which has very tortuous course from the head to the tail (up to 6 m). The ductus finally becomes the vas deferens and continues in the spermatic cord (Dogra et al. 2003; Garriga et al. 2009; Sidhu et al. 2011; Liguori et al. 2012).

Five testicular appendages, remnants of the degenerating mesonephric and paramesonephric ducts, are formed during development of the male genitourinary tract. The testicular and epididymal ones, found at the upper pole of the testis and at the head of the epididymis, respectively, are the most common and are usually visible macroscopically (Sahni et al. 1996; Sellars and Sidhu 2003).

Vascular supply to the scrotum arises from three arteries: the testicular, cremasteric, and ductus deferens ones. The testicular artery goes to the testis, piercing the tunica albuginea in a layer termed the tunica vasculosa and giving rise to branches which enter the testis running along the septa to converge on the mediastinum; there they give rise to recurrent branches to the parenchyma (Martinoli et al. 1992; Dogra et al. 2003; Sidhu et al. 2011). A transmediastinal arterial branch of the testicular artery is present in about 50% of normal testes; it runs through the mediastinum to supply the capsular arteries and is usually accompanied by a large vein (Martinoli et al. 1992; Middleton and Bell 1993). Veins exit the testes at the mediastinum, join the veins draining the epididymis, and form the

M. Bertolotto (✉)
Department of Radiology, University of Trieste, Trieste, Italy

M. Valentino
Emergency Radiology Unit, University Hospital of Parma, Parma, Italy

L.E. Derchi
Department of Radiology, University of Genova, Genoa, Italy

B. Hamm, P. R. Ros (eds.), *Abdominal Imaging*, DOI 10.1007/978-3-642-13327-5_204,
© Springer-Verlag Berlin Heidelberg 2013

pampiniform plexus at the superior aspect of the testes. The cremasteric plexus (which drains from extratesticular scrotal structures) lies posterior to the pampiniform one. The right testicular vein goes directly into the inferior vena cava, below the right renal vein; the left testicular vein drains into the left renal vein. These vessels are loosely held together by connective tissue along with nerves, lymphatics, and the vas deferens in the spermatic cord. The spermatic cord runs from the deep inguinal ring into the scrotum. Although it is not possible to identify specifically each artery within the spermatic cord, Doppler techniques allow to recognize three separate arteries and to identify the testicular one by showing significantly lower resistive index (RI) in it. Within the testis, intraparenchymal arteries present low-resistance flow (Paltiel et al. 1994; Dogra et al. 2003).

Testicular size varies with age and stage of sexual development. At birth, the testes measure approximately 1.5 cm in length and 1 cm in width. They grow slowly until puberty and, on clinical grounds, a male individual is considered to have reached puberty once the testis achieves a volume of 4 cm^3. The postpubertal testes are symmetric ovoid structures and measure approximately $5 \times 3 \times 2$ cm (Dogra et al. 2003; Garriga et al. 2009; Sidhu et al. 2011; Liguori et al. 2012).

Penile Anatomy

The penis has two corpora cavernosa, which function as the main erectile bodies, and the midline ventral corpus spongiosum, which contains the urethra (Bella et al. 2008). The cavernous tissue consists of interconnected sinusoids separated by smooth muscle trabeculae surrounded by collagen and elastic fibers. The crura of the corpora cavernosa flare laterally to attach to the ischiopubic rami. Skin is continuous with that of the lower abdominal wall; it folds back on itself and attaches at the coronal sulcus forming the prepuce. The corpora cavernosa and the corpus spongiosum are surrounded by the tunica albuginea which consists of two layers, the outer of which is oriented longitudinally, and the inner consisting of circular fibers. The inner layer of the albuginea contains struts, the intracavernous pillars, that course the cavernosal space and serve to augment the support provided by the intracavernosal septum. The corpus spongiosum lacks both the outer albugineal layer as well as the struts. The Buck's fascia covers the corpora cavernosa and the corpus spongiosum.

Blood supply to the penis is usually through the internal pudendal artery, a branch of the internal iliac artery. In many instances, however, accessory arteries arise from the external iliac, obturator, vesical, and/or femoral arteries, and may occasionally become the dominant or only arterial supply to the corpus cavernosum (Bella et al. 2008). The internal pudendal artery becomes the common penile artery after giving off a branch to the perineum. The three branches of the penile artery are the dorsal, bulbourethral, and cavernous arteries. The cavernous artery is responsible for tumescence of the corpus cavernosum and the dorsal artery for engorgement of the glans penis during erection. The bulbourethral artery supplies the bulb and corpus spongiosum. The cavernous artery enters the corpus cavernosum where the two crura merge. Along its course, it gives off many helicine arterioles, which supply the trabecular erectile tissue and the sinusoids.

The venous drainage of the penis originates in venules leading from the peripheral sinusoids immediately beneath the tunica albuginea that form the subtunical venular plexus before exiting as the emissary veins. Outside the tunica albuginea drainage is toward superficial and deep systems, which usually communicate via small anastomoses.

Penile and Scrotal Ultrasound

Ultrasound is the imaging modality of choice in patients referred for penile and scrotal problems. The examination is performed with high-frequency/high-resolution transducers with color and spectral Doppler capabilities. The transducer must have enough penetration capability to cover the entire region of interest. To avoid contraction of the cremasteric muscle, warm coupling gel has to be applied. The scrotum is usually elevated by a towel placed behind the sac, and the penis is held against the abdominal wall by the patient. Both axial and sagittal views have to be obtained; of special importance is to obtain a view of both testes in the axial plane to allow comparison of testicular parenchymal echostructure

Fig. 118.1 Gray-scale ultrasound appearance of the testis. (**a**) Homogeneous echogenic appearance in a 33-year-old male. The mediastinum testis (*curved arrow*) appears as a triangular-shaped echogenic area. (**b**) Age-related testicular fibrosis in an 86-year-old male resulting in a striated pattern

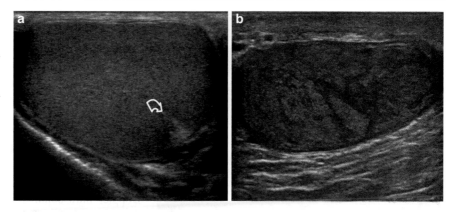

(the so-called spectacle view) (Dogra et al. 2003; Sidhu et al. 2011). Examination of the scrotal content has to be performed with simultaneous palpation to correlate clinical findings to images. If the study fails to identify a reported lesion, the patient should be asked to find it, guide the examiner, and be reevaluated (Sidhu et al. 2011). Ultrasound images have a field of view which is limited by the probe width. In patients with large lesions or with testes larger than the probe, the problem may be overcome by special techniques which allow reproduction in their full extent of targets larger than the rectangular field of view of the transducer (Bertolotto et al. 2012).

Penile ultrasound should be carried out while the penis is flaccid and after intracavernosal injection of vasoactive drugs (Doubilet et al. 1991; Bertolotto et al. 2008). Prostaglandin E1 injection at the dosage of 10 micrograms is usually adequate to obtain a suitable erectile response in potent patients (Bertolotto and Neumaier 1999). Color Doppler interrogation and spectral analysis is performed with slow flows settings which are tuned during the examination on minimal PRF values that do not determine aliasing. Spectral interrogation of the cavernosal arteries is obtained at the base of the penis under the guidance of color Doppler signal, and the angle correction cursor is adjusted to match the correct axis of flow. Steering is used to obtain a good angular correction.

Ultrasound Scrotal Anatomy

The testes appear at US as oval-shaped organs with a homogeneous structure made of fine, medium level echoes (Dogra et al. 2003; Sidhu et al. 2011). Prepuberal testes have lower echogenicity (McAlister and Sisler 1990). In old patients, the testicular parenchyma may have a "striated" pattern which is thought as due to atrophy of glandular elements accompanied by an increase in interstitial fibrosis (Fig. 118.1) (Loberant et al. 2010). The mediastinum testis is easily visible as an echogenic line of variable thickness and length parallel to the testicular main axis in sagittal images and as a triangular-shaped hyperechogenic area at the periphery of the testis in axial images (Dogra et al. 2003; Sidhu et al. 2011). The tunica albuginea can be seen as a thin echogenic line around the testis. When the testis is surrounded by a small amount of fluid, a double echogenic line corresponding to the two layers, the tunica albuginea and the tunica vaginalis can be detected (Fig. 118.2) (Migaleddu et al. 2012). In patients with transmediastinal testicular arteries, a hypoechoic triangular area below the vessel can be seen; this pattern has been described as the "two-tone testis" and has been related to a refraction artifact from the edges of the transmediastinal artery (Fig. 118.3) (Nicolaou and Cooperberg 1995; Bushby et al. 2007). The epididymis is best evaluated on longitudinal views. The head can be seen as a pyramidal structure of about 10 mm lying atop the superior pole of the testis. It is usually isoechoic or slightly hyperechoic to the testis, and its echotexture may be coarser. The body of the epididymis (2–4 mm in diameter) is usually slightly hypoechoic to the testis and can be difficult to distinguish from the surrounding peritesticular tissue; the tail is about 2–5 mm in diameter and can be seen as a curved hypoechoic

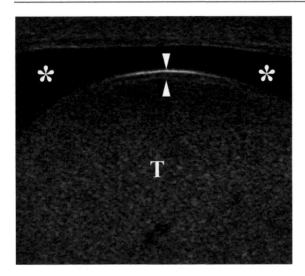

Fig. 118.2 Gray-scale ultrasound appearance of the scrotal content in a patient with hydrocele (*). The testis (*T*) presents with homogeneous echoes, surrounded by the tunica albuginea and by the visceral layer of the tunica vaginalis (*arrowheads*), which are stuck together and appear as parallel echogenic lines

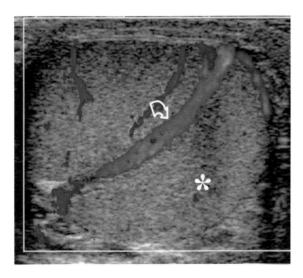

Fig. 118.3 Two-tone testis. Color Doppler image showing a low reflective area (*) produced below a transtesticular artery (*curved arrow*) with oblique course

structure at the inferior pole of the testis, where it becomes the proximal portion of the ductus deferens (Fig. 118.4) (Dogra et al. 2003; Sidhu et al. 2011). Variants in the position of the epididymis, with the body positioned posteriorly to the testis on longitudinal views or with the head located below the lower

pole of the testis, can be encountered and recognized (Puttemans et al. 2006).

The normal appendix testis and the appendix epididymis are seen when surrounded by fluid. The appendix testis appears as an ovoid structure in the groove between the testis and the epididymis. It is isoechoic to the testis and may appear as a small cystic nodule. The appendix epididymis is more often pedunculated (Fig. 118.5) (Sellars and Sidhu 2003; Kantarci et al. 2005).

Testicular vessels are easily identified with color Doppler ultrasound. Capsular arteries are visible at the outer margins of the testis. Intratesticular arteries have a relatively straight course and are best seen along some "vascular" planes (generally oblique to the standard axial and sagittal examination planes). In many cases, both centripetal arteries and their recurrent rami can be identified (Fig. 118.6). They have low-resistance flow pattern, with a mean RI of 0.61 (range 0.48–0.75). Prepuberal children have higher resistive indices which lower approaching to puberty (Martinoli et al. 1992; Middleton and Bell 1993; Paltiel et al. 1994; Dogra et al. 2003; Sidhu et al. 2011; Migaleddu et al. 2012). Transtesticular arteries are visible in about 50% of men, often paired with a transtesticular vein (Middleton and Bell 1993). Intratesticular veins are difficult to see in normal testes, and only small portions of them can be identified.

The spermatic cord can be recognized in the inguinal region as a ribbon-like structure containing echogenic fat, the vas deferens, and the spermatic arteries and veins. It is surrounded by a thin hyperechoic line representing its three fascial layers. The blood vessels can be differentiated at color Doppler by presence of flow and veins recognized by their compressibility; the vas deferens can be recognized by its cord-like structure within which its luminal walls can be often appreciated, and by its noncompressibility. It is about 2 mm thick (Kim et al. 2009; Middleton et al. 2009; Migaleddu et al. 2012).

Ultrasound Penile Anatomy

In the flaccid state, the corpora present as cylindrical structures with intermediate echogenicity and homogeneous echotexture. The echogenicity of the corpora cavernosa progressively decreases during tumescence

Fig. 118.4 Longitudinal gray-scale views showing normal epididymal anatomy. (**a**) The head (*curved arrow*) and the body (*arrowheads*) of the epididymis are respectively isoechoic and hypoechoic to the testis (*T*). (**b**) The tail of the epididymis (***) is seen at the inferior pole of the testis (*T*) anterior to the vas deferens (*small arrows*)

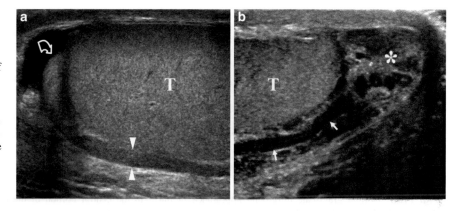

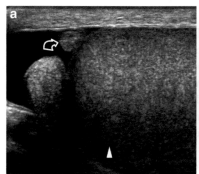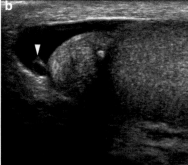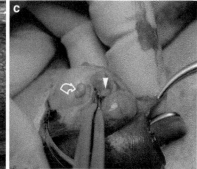

Fig. 118.5 Sonographic appearance of appendages. Patient presenting with a small palpable nodule in the left hemiscrotum. Longitudinal gray-scale views show appendix testis (**a**, *curved arrow*), which was palpable, and a cystic appendix epididymis (**b**, *arrowhead*) surrounded by a small amount of hydrocele. (**c**) Surgical view of the same testis showing the appendix testis (*curved arrow*) and epididymis (*arrowhead*)

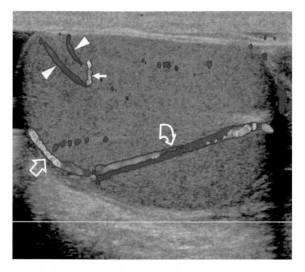

Fig. 118.6 Normal appearance of testicular vessels at color Doppler interrogation. Transmediastinal artery and vein (*curved arrow*); capsular vessels (*large arrow*); centripetal branches (*arrowheads*); recurrent artery (*small arrow*)

starting from the region surrounding the cavernosal arteries because of sinusoids dilatation (Fig. 118.7).

The tunica albuginea and the Buck's fascia are stuck together and appear as a thin echogenic line surrounding the corpora which became thinner during erection. The penile septum appears as an echogenic structure with back attenuation. The intracavernous pillars are recognizable on transverse scans as straight echogenic lines which run from one side to the other of the tunica albuginea. Several penile vessels can be identified at gray-scale ultrasound as well. In particular, the cavernosal arteries appear as a pair of dots located slightly medially in each corpus cavernosum. On longitudinal scans, they present as a narrow tubular structures with echogenic wall (Quam et al. 1989). The diameter of the normal cavernosal arteries ranges from 0.3 to 0.5 mm in the flaccid state and increases to 0.6–1.0 mm after an intracavernosal injection of a vasoactive agents.

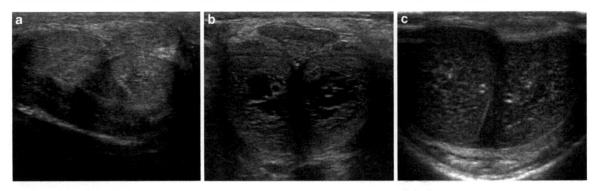

Fig. 118.7 Normal gray-scale ultrasound appearance of the penis. (**a**) In the flaccid state, the penile bodies are echogenic with homogeneous echotexture. (**b**) Distension of the sinusoids in the central portion of the corpora during the onset of the erection. (**c**) When complete erection is achieved, a fine echogenic network is appreciable

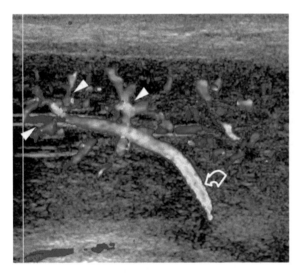

Fig. 118.8 Longitudinal color Doppler view of the penis during the onset of erection showing the helicine arterioles (*arrowheads*) branching from the cavernosal artery (*curved arrow*)

A full evaluation of penile arteries is obtained during the onset of erection (Fig. 118.8). In this phase, it is possible to study the pathway of the cavernosal, dorsal, and urethral arteries and to identify presence of anatomical variations. A variety of arterial communications are appreciable among the different arteries of the penis. Communications between the cavernosal arteries and cavernosal-spongiosal communications are identified in virtually all patients. Helicine arterioles cannot be identified during flaccidity due to insufficient blood flow. They become evident during the onset of erection and become progressively less visible while the penis is fully erect.

Depiction of penile veins at color Doppler ultrasound is inconstant in normal subjects due to low flow regimen both while flaccid and during erection (Kim et al. 2001). Veins are best identified during turgescence and especially during detumescence.

Cavernosal arteries present during the onset of erection with characteristic progression of Doppler waveform reflecting blood pressure changes within the cavernosal bodies (Fig. 118.9) (Fitzgerald et al. 1991; Schwartz et al. 1991; Kim 2002). In general, velocity values are highest at proximal sites and decrease progressively at distal sites of measurement (Chiou et al. 1999). As a consequence, standardization of the sampling location is needed to reduce variability of duplex Doppler interrogation, which is performed at the origin, where they angle posteriorly toward the crus, and a favorable Doppler angle is obtained (Kim 2002). In the flaccid state (phase 0), monophasic waveforms are recognized in the cavernosal arteries with low-velocity, high-resistance flow, typically of 15–25 cm/s. With the onset of erection (phase 1), there is an increase in systolic and diastolic flows. Peak systolic velocity >35 cm/s and diastolic velocity >8 cm/s are usually recorded in normal subjects in this phase. When the blood pressure within the corpora cavernosa begins to rise, a dicrotic notch appears at end systole and a progressive decrease of the diastolic flow is observed (phase 2). When the cavernosal pressure equals the diastolic pressure, diastolic flow declines to zero. Holodiastolic flow reversal (phase 4) reflects cavernosal pressure above the diastolic pressure and full erection. During rigid erection, the systolic envelope is narrowed and diastolic flow disappears (phase 5). The systolic peak reduces or even disappears, reflecting cavernosal

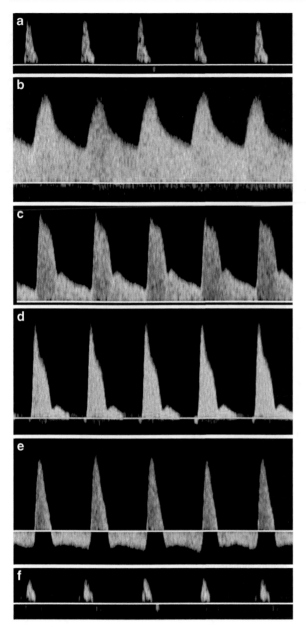

Fig. 118.9 Normal waveform changes in the cavernosal arteries during the onset of erection. (**a**) Phase 0. Monophasic flow with minimal or no diastolic flow occurring in the flaccid state. (**b**) Phase 1. Increased systolic and diastolic flow. (**c**) Phase 2. Dicrotic notch appearance at the end of the systole and progressive decrease of the diastolic flow. (**d**) Phase 3. End diastolic flow disappearance. (**e**) Phase 4. Diastolic flow reversal during full erection. (**f**) Phase 5. Reduction of the systolic peak during rigid erection

pressure approaching or exceeding blood systolic pressure. Cavernosal phase 5 requires contraction of the bulbocavernous muscles and is not commonly observed after pharmacologically induced erection.

MR Imaging of the Scrotum and Penis

A MR study of the penis and of the scrotal content is indicated when ultrasound findings are inconclusive, when there are discrepancies between the results of clinical and ultrasound examinations or when there is suspicion of pathologies producing diffuse tissue involvement. In clinical practice, the role of this technique is growing.

The best results can be obtained by the use of a surface coil or of a multichannel phased-array coil for parallel imaging, such as cardiac coils, which provide high definition images with excellent signal-to-noise ratio; however, the image quality provided by conventional body coils can be high enough for the diagnosis in many cases.

Appropriate patient positioning facilitates MR imaging of the scrotum and penis. The penis is dorsiflexed against the abdominal wall in the midline and taped in position to reduce organ motion during the examination, and the scrotum is lifted up and fixed on the tights. Both T1- and T2-weighted sequences are used; contrast-enhanced imaging is commonly used to image the scrotum, since it can provide useful informations about testicular perfusion, and is especially important when plain T1- and T2-weighted images are equivocal (Watanabe 2012a). For penile MR studies, contrast administration is necessary in selected cases only. In most of instances, it is desirable to image the penis during tumescence. Pharmacologically induced erection is contraindicated when imaging penile trauma and priapism.

MR Scrotal Anatomy

The testis appears with a homogeneous intermediate signal intensity on T1-weighted images and with high signal intensity in T2-weighted images (Fig. 118.10). The tunica albuginea is a thin hypointense line covering the testis. The mediastinum testis is hypointense, with a linear shape on longitudinal images and a triangular appearance on axial planes. The epididymis can be easily recognized, with a signal intensity similar to that of the testis in T1-weighted images, and hypointense to the testis in T2-weighted sequences. A small quantity of fluid in the tunica vaginalis is

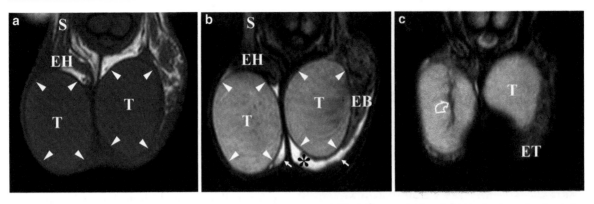

Fig. 118.10 Normal MR appearance of the scrotal content in a 29-year-old healthy volunteer. (**a**) T1-weighted coronal image. (**b**) Fat-suppressed (FS) T2-weighted coronal image. (**c**) FS-T2-weighted coronal image at the posterior level to the image-b. *T* testis, *EH* epididymal head, *EB* epididymal body, *ET* epididymal tail, *S* spermatic cord, *arrowheads* tunica albuginea and visceral layer of tunica vaginalis, *small arrow* parietal layer of the tunica vaginalis, *curved arrow* mediastinum testis, *Asterisk* fluid in the tunica vaginalis cavity

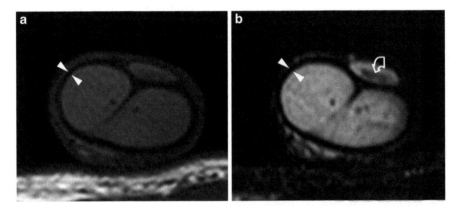

Fig. 118.11 Normal MR anatomy of the penis in a 30-year-old patient. T1-weighted (**a**) and fat-suppressed T2-weighted (**b**) axial images of the penile shaft obtained after intracavernosal prostaglandin injection. The erectile bodies display intermediate signal intensity on the T1-weighted image and high signal intensity on the T2-weighted image. Cavernosal arteries are depicted as paired hypointense dots within the cavernosal bodies. The tunica albuginea and the Buck's fascia (*arrowheads*) are hypointense to corpora. The urethra (*curved arrow*) is displayed on the T2-weighted image as a hypointense band within the corpus spongiosum

normally seen, and it appears of very high signal intensity in T2-weighted images (Baker et al. 1987; Watanabe 2012a, b).

MR Penile Anatomy

In normal individuals, the three erectile bodies exhibit intermediate signal intensity on T1-weighted MR images and high signal intensity on T2-weighted images (Fig. 118.11) (Choi et al. 2000; Pretorius et al. 2001; Vossough et al. 2002; Singh et al. 2005). Variable layering effects are a normal finding in the tumescent corpora cavernosa. Occasionally, T2 signal intensity of the corpora cavernosa is different from that of the corpus spongiosum, likely reflecting blood flow differences (Vossough et al. 2002).

The tunica albuginea and Buck's fascia are imaged as a rim of low signal intensity surrounding the corpora on T1- and T2-weighted images. The Buck's fascia usually cannot be distinguished from the adjacent albuginea. On axial T2-weighted images, the cavernosal arteries are depicted as small, round areas of hypointensity (due to faster flow) within the cavernosal bodies. The dorsal arteries and deep dorsal vein are seen as low signal intensity dots between Buck's fascia (Kirkham et al. 2008). If not dilated or distended, the anterior urethra is difficult to see at MR imaging. The muscular walls can be visualized on T2-weighted images as a band of relative hypointensity compared with the bright corpus spongiosum (Pretorius et al. 2001).

After gadolinium contrast media administration, the enhancement of the corpus spongiosum occurs almost immediately. Enhancement of the corpora cavernosa proceeds from the region surrounding the cavernosal arteries to the periphery, and from the proximal to the distal part (Kaneko et al. 1994; Pretorius et al. 2001; Vossough et al. 2002; Singh et al. 2005).

References

Baker LL, Hajek PC, et al. MR imaging of the scrotum: normal anatomy. Radiology. 1987;163:89–92.

Bella AJ, Brant WO, et al. Penile Anatomy. Springer-Verlag: Color Doppler US of the Penis. M. Bertolotto. Berlin Heidelberg; 2008. p. 11–14.

Bertolotto M, Lissiani A, et al. US anatomy of the penis: common findings and anatomical variations. In: Bertolotto M, editor. Color doppler US of the penis. Berlin Heidelberg: Springer-Verlag; 2008. p. 25–37.

Bertolotto M, Martinoli C, et al. Instrumentation, technical requirements: US. In: Bertolotto M, Trombetta C, editors. Scrotal pathology. Berlin Heidelberg: Springer-Verlag; 2012. p. 1–15.

Bertolotto M, Neumaier CE. Penile sonography. Eur Radiol. 1999;9(Suppl 3):S407–12.

Bushby LH, Sellars ME, et al. The "two-tone" testis: spectrum of ultrasound appearances. Clin Radiol. 2007;62:1119–23.

Chiou RK, Alberts GL, et al. Study of cavernosal arterial anatomy using color and power Doppler sonography: impact on hemodynamic parameter measurement. J Urol. 1999;162:358–60.

Choi MH, Kim B, et al. MR imaging of acute penile fracture. Radiographics. 2000;20:1397–405.

Dogra VS, Gottlieb RH, et al. Sonography of the scrotum. Radiology. 2003;227:18–36.

Doubilet PM, Benson CB, et al. The penis. Semin ultrasound CT MR. 1991;12:157–75.

Fitzgerald SW, Erickson SJ, et al. Color Doppler sonography in the evaluation of erectile dysfunction: patterns of temporal response to papaverine. AJR. 1991;157:331–6.

Garriga V, Serrano A, et al. US of the tunica vaginalis testis: anatomic relationships and pathologic conditions. Radiographics. 2009;29:2017–32.

Kaneko K, De Mouy EH, et al. Sequential contrast-enhanced MR imaging of the penis. Radiology. 1994;191:75–7.

Kantarci F, Ozer H, et al. Cystic appendix epididymis: a sonomorphologic study. Surg Radiol Anat. 2005;27:557–61.

Kim B, Kawashima A, et al. Imaging of the seminal vesicle and vas deferens. Radiographics. 2009;29:1105–21.

Kim JM, Joh YD, et al. Doppler sonography of the penile cavernosal artery: comparison of intraurethral instillation

and intracorporeal injection of prostaglandin E1. J Clin Ultrasound. 2001;29:273–8.

Kim SH. Doppler US evaluation of erectile dysfunction. Abdom Imaging. 2002;27:578–87.

Kirkham AP, Illing RO, et al. MR imaging of nonmalignant penile lesions. Radiographics. 2008;28:837–53.

Liguori G, Ollandini G, et al. Anatomy of the scrotum. In: Bertolotto M, Trombetta C, editors. Scrotal pathology. Berlin Heidelberg: Springer-Verlag; 2012. p. 27–34.

Loberant N, Bhatt S, et al. Striated appearance of the testes. Ultrasound Q. 2010;26:37–44.

Martinoli C, Pastorino C, et al. Color-Doppler echography of the testis. Study technique and vascular anatomy. Radiol Med. 1992;84:785–91.

McAlister WH, Sisler CL. Scrotal sonography in infants and children. Curr Probl Diagn Radiol. 1990;19:201–42.

Middleton WD, Bell MW. Analysis of intratesticular arterial anatomy with emphasis on transmediastinal arteries. Radiology. 1993;189:157–60.

Middleton WD, Dahiya N, et al. High-resolution sonography of the normal extrapelvic vas deferens. J Ultrasound Med. 2009;28:839–46.

Migaleddu V, Virgilio G, et al. Sonographic scrotal anatomy. In: Bertolotto M, Trombetta C, editors. Scrotal pathology. Berlin Heidelberg: Springer-Verlag; 2012. p. 41–54.

Nicolaou S, Cooperberg PL. The two-tone testis due to refractive shadowing of the intratesticular artery. J Ultrasound Med. 1995;14:963–5.

Paltiel HJ, Rupich RC, et al. Maturational changes in arterial impedance of the normal testis in boys: Doppler sonographic study. AJR. 1994;163:1189–93.

Pretorius ES, Siegelman ES, et al. MR imaging of the penis. Radiographics. 2001;21:S283–S298. Spec No: S283-298; discussion S298-289.

Puttemans T, Delvigne A, et al. Normal and variant appearances of the adult epididymis and vas deferens on high-resolution sonography. J Clin Ultrasound. 2006;34:385–92.

Quam JP, King BF, et al. Duplex and color Doppler sonographic evaluation of vasculogenic impotence. AJR. 1989;153:1141–47.

Sahni D, Jit I, et al. Incidence and structure of the appendices of the testis and epididymis. J Anat. 1996;189:341–8.

Schwartz AN, Lowe M, et al. Assessment of normal and abnormal erectile function: color Doppler flow sonography versus conventional techniques. Radiology. 1991;180:105–9.

Sellars ME, Sidhu PS. Ultrasound appearances of the testicular appendages: pictorial review. Eur Radiol. 2003;13:127–35.

Sidhu PS, Brkljacic B, et al. Ultrasound of the scrotum. In: Dietrich CF, editor. EFSUMB European Course Book. London, UK: EFSUMB; 2011.

Singh AK, Saokar A, et al. Imaging of penile neoplasms. Radiographics. 2005;25:1629–38.

Vossough A, Pretorius ES, et al. Magnetic resonance imaging of the penis. Abdom Imaging. 2002;27:640–59.

Watanabe Y. Instrumentation, technical requirements: MRI. In: Bertolotto M, Trombetta C, editors. Scrotal pathology. Berlin Heidelberg: Springer-Verlag; 2012a. p. 17–26.

Watanabe Y. Scrotal anatomy at MRI. In: Bertolotto M, Trombetta C, editors. Scrotal pathology. Berlin Heidelberg: Springer-Verlag; 2012b. p. 55–66.

Acute Scrotum

119

Ahmet Tuncay Turgut, Halil Arslan, and Vikram S. Dogra

Introduction

Acute scrotum is the most common urological emergency. Majority of patients of acute scrotal pain are usually young adults but any age group may be affected. Acute scrotal pain accounts for 0.5% of the total emergency department visits (Blaivas et al. 2001). Patients with acute scrotal pain often present a diagnostic dilemma even to the experienced clinicians because of the diverse etiologies and extreme local tenderness, which makes clinical examination extremely difficult (Cavusoglu et al. 2005). In one study conducted on patients presenting with acute scrotal pain, testicular torsion, torsion of a testicular appendage, and epididymitis were found to represent 94% of all final diagnoses (Knight and Vassy 1984). A significant challenge for an appropriate diagnosis is that the aforementioned etiologies can overlap in both signs and symptoms. Clinically, decreased or absent cremasteric reflex has been noted to be the best clinical predictor of testicular torsion (Yang et al. 2011; Kadish and Bolte 1998). However, a normal cremasteric reflex may infrequently be insufficient to exclude testicular

torsion and absent cremasteric reflex may be noticed in patients without torsion (Yang et al. 2011). Therefore, traditional reliance on medical history and physical examination alone may not be enough to differentiate between several of these etiologies. The main goal in these patients is to make distinction between surgical emergencies and nonsurgical problems, which is very critical, as testicular torsion necessitates surgical intervention, while several other etiologies like epididymitis are treated with medical management. Importantly, up to 70–90% of patients with acute scrotum do not require surgery (Kass et al. 1993; Yang et al. 2011). On the other hand, missed cases of testicular torsion are still a major concern for the emergency physicians, though testicular torsion is seen in less than 25% of these patients presenting with acute acrotum (Cass et al. 1980; Anderson et al. 1989). Misdiagnosis can result in testicle infarction, testicular atrophy, infertility, and significant morbidity. Some studies still recommend surgical exploration in all cases of acute scrotum (Murphy et al. 2006).

Etiology

Torsion

Testicular Torsion
Intravaginal Torsion
Testicular torsion is defined as "rotation of the testis in the longitudinal axis of the spermatic cord" (Micallef et al. 2000). It is the leading cause of acute scrotal pain. Extravaginal torsion is rare and occurs in newborns when the tunica vaginalis has abnormal attachment. Intravaginal torsion accounts for 65–80%

A.T. Turgut (✉)
Department of Radiology, Ankara Training and Research Hospital, Ankara, Turkey

H. Arslan
Department of Radiology, Yildirim Beyazit University School of Medicine, Ankara, Turkey

V.S. Dogra
Department of Imaging Sciences, School of Medicine and Dentistry, University of Rochester, Rochester, NY, USA

B. Hamm, P. R. Ros (eds.), *Abdominal Imaging*, DOI 10.1007/978-3-642-13327-5_206,
© Springer-Verlag Berlin Heidelberg 2013

of the cases (Favorito et al. 2004). Affecting 1 in 125 males, it is most common in adolescent boys (Williamson 1976). Interestingly, familial occurrence of testicular torsion has also been reported (Shteynshlyuger and Freyle 2011). Anatomically, a long mesorchium, implying a long intrascrotal portion of the spermatic cord, as is the case with cryptorchidism, predisposes to testicular torsion. Furthermore, bell-clapper deformity implying resemblance to a clapper inside a bell refers to tunica vaginalis completely encircling the epididymis, distal spermatic cord, and testis rather than attaching to the posterolateral aspect of the testis, which is often the underlying abnormality in patients with intravaginal testicular torsion (Dogra 2003). This deformity with 12% prevalence may be bilateral as well and is accepted as another predisposing condition for the twisting of the spermatic cord and testis (Parenti et al. 2009). From diagnostic point of view, US has a great accuracy for revealing the bell-clapper deformity particularly in the presence of moderate degree of hydrocele surrounding the distal portion of the spermatic cord and testis. Surgically, anchoring both testes with an orchiopexy is recommended as a precaution against a future twisting in patients with bell-clapper deformity.

Clinical Considerations

Torsion of the testis and the spermatic cord is accepted as the most critical cause of scrotal pain because a delay in intervention may cause irreversible testicular damage. Clinically, sudden onset of severe scrotal pain coming on at rest, during activity, or after trauma and worsening at night, followed by nausea, vomiting, and a low grade fever is the typical presentation (Dogra et al. 2006). The physical examination reveals a swollen and tender hemiscrotum, near-horizontal lie of the testis in the standing position, and a high-riding testicle. High-riding testicle is defined as the elevation of the testis toward the inguinal canal due to the shortening of the torsed spermatic cord (Angell 1963; Dogra et al. 2006). Elevation of scrotum above the level of symphysis pubis relieves pain in patients with epididymo-orchitis (A positive Prehn's sign) but does not relieve pain in patients with testicular torsion (Negative Prehn's sign) (Cassar et al. 2008). The absence of the cremasteric reflex is the most sensitive physical examination finding in patients with testicular torsion (Kadish and Bolte 1998; Kass and Lundak 1997). Owing to the fact that testicular salvage rate strongly

depends on the duration of ischemia, prompt diagnosis of testicular torsion is critical to avoid any delay in surgical intervention. In this regard, testicular salvage rate is quite high if surgical detorsion is performed as early as 4–6 h after the onset of the symptoms, whereas salvagable rate decreases beyond 6 h and it is virtually irreversible after 24 h of delay (Oyen 2002). It is noteworthy that unilateral testicular injury, causing testicular necrosis, may have an insult on the uninvolved testis through an autoimmune response (Dogra et al. 2006; Donohue and Utley 1978).

Ultrasound

Broadband high-frequency gray-scale US, combined with color and pulsed Doppler modes, is the method of choice in the management of patients with acute scrotal pain. As the US findings strongly depend on the duration of torsion and the degree of twisting of the spermatic cord, the patients may present with either the typical or atypical US features. In general, gray-scale US findings of testicular torsion are nonspecific. It reveals no abnormality immediately after the onset of the torsion, though a progressive hypoechogenicity associated with edema develops over time. The lobar architecture of the affected testis becomes more prominent because of the progressive interstitial and septal edema (Prando 2009). In general, a normal testicular echogenicity implies the viability of the testicular tissue, though it necessitates further evaluation with color and spectral Doppler US (Middleton et al. 1997). After 4–6 h, the predominant finding is an enlarged testis with decreased echogenicity. Nevertheless, a focal or partially hypoechoic pattern secondary to a partial infarct can be detected as well. Late or missed torsion refers to a phase of torsion characterized by diffuse, focal, or multifocal heterogeneous testicular echotexture secondary to hemorrhage and infarction developing after 24 h. Epididymis may be affected in upto 80% of patients with testicular torsion. On transverse gray-scale US, the appearence of an enlarged, heterogeneous epididymis with abnormally positioned mediastinum testis in close distal proximity to the inguinal canal occurring due to conversion of the long axis of the testis to an oblique or even horizontal position can be detected (Prando 2002, 2009). In a similar fashion, a well-identified and thickened mediastinum, which is less echogenic than the uninvolved testis, can also be detected (Prando 2002). Interestingly, "whirlpool sign" referring to the real-time,

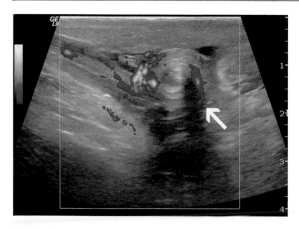

Fig. 119.1 Testicular torsion. Longitudinal color Doppler US scan demonstrates a whirlpool sign (*arrow*) resembling a snail shell, referring to concentric layers of coiled cord vessels formed by the twisting of the spermatic cord, which is highly specific for torsion

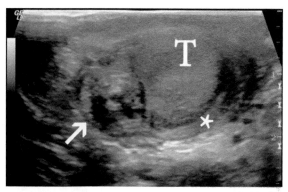

Fig. 119.2 Chronic testicular torsion. Longitudinal gray-scale US image shows an atrophic and torsed testis (*T*) with heterogeneous echotexture and a paratesticular, irregular mass (*arrow*) implying the twisting of the spermatic cord and the vascular structures. Note the increased thickness of peritesticular soft tissues (*asterisk*)

sonographic detection of a mass consisting of concentric layers of coiled cord vessels formed by the twisting of the spermatic cord has been found to be highly accurate in identifying the exact site of torsion (Vijayaraghavan 2006) (Fig. 119.1). The entity is also described as a "snail shell" or a "doughnut shape." Furthermore, increased thickness of paratesticular soft tissues and scrotal skin and a reactive hydrocele can be detected on US (Prando 2002, 2009). The sonographic appearance of an atrophic and diffusely hypoechoic testis with an extratesticular hyperechoic mass formed by twisted extratesticular structures may be consistent with chronic torsion (Prando 2002, 2009) (Fig. 119.2).

During the assessment of testicular perfusion, color Doppler US can typically demonstrate the presence of blood flow and early perfusion changes in the testis reliably, though power Doppler US enables better assessment of the diminished testicular blood (Dogra et al. 2006). Accordingly, the lack of blood flow in the involved testis, which is usually consistent with a twisting degree of the spermatic cord exceeding 450°, in contrast with the normal flow in the contralateral testis strongly suggests ischemia and is highly presumptive for testicular torsion (Fig. 119.3). However, arterial flow may not necessarily be absent for torsion to be present (Dogra et al. 2006) (Fig. 119.4). In this regard, a diminished arterial velocity and an increased RI consistent with a high-resistance blood flow and a decrease or reversal of diastolic flow on spectral Doppler evaluation can also be seen in the torsed testis with a small amount of residual arterial flow and represents early or incomplete torsion (Dogra and Bhatt 2004; Dogra et al. 2004). Nevertheless, the aforementioned flow pattern can also be a sequela of severe epididymo-orchitis, though it is characterized by increased overall blood flow to the involved side in contrast with torsion (Dogra et al. 2004). Less frequently, only a small arterial signal can be detected in the testis and this should not preclude the diagnosis of torsion, particularly in the appropriate clinical setting (Dogra et al. 2006). Notably, an accompanying hypervascularity in the extratesticular soft tissues can also be associated with testicular infarction (Dogra et al. 2006).

Magnetic Resonance Imaging

In acute torsion, the signal intensity of the testis is normal on MRI. However, the testis appears enlarged with areas of high signal intensity on T1-weighted images representing hemorrhagic areas with mixed signal intensity changes on T2-weighted images. In chronic torsion, the testis usually appears small with a decreased signal on T2-weighted images (Andipa et al. 2004). In the beginning, nonenhancement of the spermatic cord was accepted as the most sensitive and specific finding for torsion, which can help to differentiate torsion from epididymitis (Trambert et al. 1990). On the other hand, dynamic contrast-enhanced MRI can play an important role in the diagnosis of testicular torsion, thanks to its efficacy for the assessment the testicular perfusion (Watanabe et al. 2000, 2007; Watanabe 2002; Choyke 2000). Based on testicular

Fig. 119.3 Testicular torsion. Transverse color Doppler US image shows complete absence of blood flow within the symptomatic, torsed, left testis compared to the asymptomatic right testis. Note the enlarged and edematous appearance of the involved testis

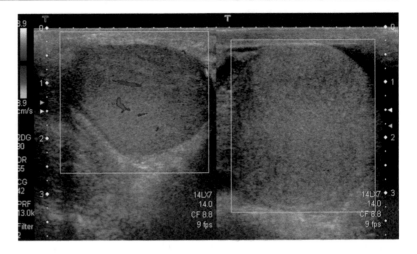

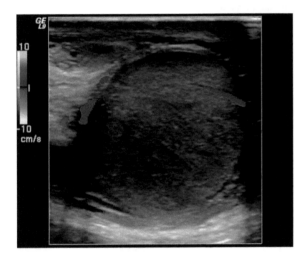

Fig. 119.4 Testicular torsion. Transverse color Doppler US image demonstrates heterogeneous echotexture of the testicular parenchyma with decreased vascularization

contrast-enhancement patterns, the technique can enable the differentiation of testicular torsion from other scrotal disorders (Watanabe et al. 2000). Furthermore, contrast-enhanced subtraction MRI has been found highly accurate in the diagnosis of testicular torsion (Terai et al. 2006). More importantly, low and very low signal intensities with spotty or streaky patterns on preoperative and follow-up T2-weighted MRI images can be helpful for demonstrating testicular hemorrhagic necrosis (Watanabe et al. 2007).

Partial or Incomplete Testicular Torsion

Basically, the torsion of the spermatic cord is not necessarily an all-or-nothing phenomenon (Prando 2009).

Partial testicular torsion, which is also called as incomplete torsion, is associated with a degree of twisting of the vascular pedicle less than 360°, whereas complete torsion refers to a rotation of more than 360° (Hörmann et al. 2004). Gray-scale US usually reveals no abnormal finding in patients with partial torsion (Cassar et al. 2008). Besides, the arterial blood flow is not necessarily absent on color Doppler US. Accordingly, asymmetry of the color flow Doppler findings in the involved testis consistent with decreased intratesticular flow compared to the contralateral testis as well as the persistence of intratesticular flow can be detected (Hörmann et al. 2004). Nevertheless, spectral Doppler evaluation revealing the variability of the amplitude of the spectral Doppler waveform relative to the uninvolved testis or within the same testis is particularly useful in detecting subtle flow asymmetry in the presence of typical clinical findings (Sanelli et al. 1999). In order to determine this variability, particular attention should be paid for including the upper, mid, and lower poles of each testis to the spectral Doppler evaluation. The other findings on spectral Doppler analysis that may help in establishing a proper diagnosis are increased resistance to arterial flow due to the decrease in the diastolic flow velocities and reversal of diastolic flow (Cassar et al. 2008). When a transient torsion manifests with a mild increase in testicular and extratesticular blood flow, the sonographic differentiation of the entity from epididymoorchitis becomes impossible. In such a case, the acute onset of symptoms and the abrupt resolution should suggest transient torsion (Herbener 1996).

Intermittent Torsion (Torsion-Detorsion Syndrome)

As the name implies, intermittent torsion refers to the recurrent self-limited episodes of acute and sharp unilateral testicular pain and scrotal swelling, with long lasting symptom-free intervals. On physical examination, a very mobile or horizontally positioned testis, an anteriorly located epididymis, and bulky spermatic cord can be detected. Among the US findings encountered are a normal or enlarged testis, horizontal testicular position, and focal or segmental hypoechoic testicular infarcts, which may or may not be present depending on the timing of the examination (Dogra et al. 2006, 2004). In the asymptomatic period, or immediately after the regression of the symptoms, paradoxically, increased blood flow with a decreased arterial resistance can be detected on color Doppler US (Dogra et al. 2004). Surgical exploration and orchiopexy is the preferred mode of treatment for intermittent torsion.

Torsion of Epididymis

Isolated torsion of the epididymis is very rare (Dibilio et al. 2006; Elert et al. 2002) Anomalies of the testicular-epididymal junction or the presence of a long and tortuous epididymis with a long mesorchium may cause a predisposition for the entity (Dogra 2003). Cryptorchidism is accepted as a predisposing condition for epididymal torsion. Sonographically, a normal testis with normal blood flow, an enlarged, heterogeneous epididymis with only a few or no vascular signals, and a highly vascularized epididymal head with twisting vessels may suggest the diagnosis (Dibilio et al. 2006; Lee et al. 2008).

Torsion of Appendages

More than 90% of twisted appendices involve the appendix testis (Dogra et al. 2006). The entity is more common in childhood. The clinical presentation for the torsion of appendix testis and appendix epididymis may be similar to that of testicular torsion, despite being less common. On physical examination "blue dot" sign representing a small, firm, and bluish palpable nodule on the superior aspect of the testis can be detected (Skoglund et al. 1970). The main role of US in the management of patients with the torsion of testicular appendix is to exclude testicular torsion or epididymo-orchitis. Sonographically, a circular and enlarged (>5.6 mm) hyperechoic or hypoechoic mass

of appendix testis without any internal blood flow and increased periappendiceal vascular signals strongly suggests torsion of appendix testis (Dogra et al. 2006; Oyen 2002; Yang et al. 2005). An enlarged epididymal head, increased testicular blood flow secondary to the inflammatory response, scrotal skin thickening, and reactive hydrocele are additional US findings (Karmazyn et al. 2006). A conservative approach with pain management is the preferred mode of treatment in cases with torsion of appendages.

Epididymitis and Epididymo-orchitis

Epididymitis is the most common cause of painful scrotal swelling over 18 years of age (Oyen 2002). It usually presents with a sudden onset of pain simulating testicular torsion, though the patients may be asymptomatic or have milder symptoms. It usually develops secondary to an ascending infection from the urinary tract, though the primary infection can less commonly be of hematogenous or traumatic origin (Gorman and Caroll 2005). Symptoms of lower urinary tract infection with fever and leukocytosis may be helpful for the differentiation of the entity from testicular torsion (Liguori et al. 2011). The involvement of the epididymal tail is followed by the spread of the inflammatory process to the body and the head of the epididymis, whereas testicular involvement occurs in 20–40% of the patients by direct extension of the infection. Focal involvement can infrequently be detected in both the testis and epididymis, though they are mostly diffusely affected (Dogra 2003; Micallef et al. 2000). In adolescents and men younger than 35 years, sexually transmitted *Chlamydia trachomatis* and *Neisseria gonorrhoeae* are the main causative agents and *Escherichia coli* and *Proteus mirabilis* are usually encountered in prepubertal boys and men over 35 years of age (Dogra 2003). Less frequently, the inflammatory process develops secondary to granulomatous diseases as sarcoidosis, brucellosis, and tuberculosis (Cook and Dewbury 2000). Among the complications of acute epididymo-orchitis are abscess, infarct, gangrene, infertility, atrophy, and pyocele (Dogra 2003; Micallef et al. 2000).

The gray-scale US findings for isolated epididymitis are nonspecific and include enlarged epididymis with hypoechoic or hyperechoic appearance, reactive hydrocele or pyocele, and scrotal wall thickening (Fig. 119.5).

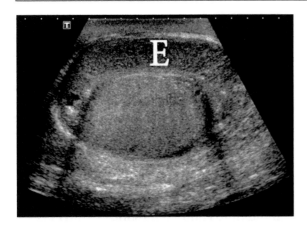

Fig. 119.5 Isolated epididymitis. Longitudinal gray-scale US image shows an enlarged epididymis (*E*) with hypoechoic appearance consistent with isolated epididymitis. Color Doppler US scan demonstrated epididymal hypervascularity (not shown)

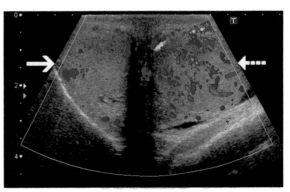

Fig. 119.6 Transverse color Doppler US image reveals increased blood flow within the left testis (*dashed arrow*) as a component of epididymo-orchitis contrary to the right testis with normal blood flow (*arrow*)

The testicular component of epididymo-orchitis developing secondary to contiguous spread of the infection manifests sonographically as edematous testicular enlargement, inhomogeneously hypoechoic or heterogeneous appearance for diffuse involvement, and as multiple hypoechoic lesions for focal involvement (Dogra 2003; Herbener 1996; See et al. 1988). It is noteworthy that the focal testicular involvement is mostly located adjacent to an inflamed epididymis (Liguori et al. 2011). Focal heterogeneous intratesticular lesions accompanying epididymo-orchitis should undergo sonographic follow-up to their complete resolution to exclude underlying tumor (Dogra 2003). Color flow Doppler evaluation in patients with acute epididymitis reveals marked increase in the blood flow as compared to the normal epididymis.

Color or power Doppler US typically reveals increased blood flow in the affected testis in acute epididymo-orchitis resulting in a high-flow, low-resistance flow pattern on spectral Doppler analysis, and comparison with the contralateral testis would also enhance the diagnostic accuracy (Fig. 119.6). The accompanying epididymal involvement may enable to exclude a neoplastic lesion in the presence of a focal hypoechoic, hypervascular lesion presumed to be focal orchitis (Micallef et al. 2000). However, infiltrative neoplasms like lymphoma and leukemia, which present with diffusely increased vascularization, as is the case for epididymo-orchitis, may be a challenge for establishing a correct diagnosis. Spectral Doppler

analysis reveals at least 1.7–2 fold increase in peak systolic velocity in intratesticular arteries (Oyen 2002). In accordance with decreased vascular resistance associated with the inflammation, a decrease in RI values can be detected in testicular and epididymal arteries that can rarely be less than 0.5–0.7, respectively (Oyen 2002; Jee et al. 1997). Furthermore, sonographic detection of increased venous flow, which may even be undetectable in healthy individuals, is also suggestive of orchitis (Horstman 1997).

In inconclusive cases, MRI can potentially be helpful to make a distinction between epididymo-orchitis and neoplasm (Woodward et al 2002). On MRI, isolated epididymitis is characterized by enlargement and intermediate signal intensity on T2-weighted images (Andipa et al. 2004; Kim et al. 2007) (Fig. 119.7). Nevertheless, increased signal intensity on both T1- and T2-weighted images has also been reported (Sica and Teeger 1996). Testicular involvement is depicted on T2-weighted images as ill-defined areas of low signal intensity, though high signal intensity has rarely been reported in cases with advanced disease (Andipa et al. 2004; Kim et al. 2007). On contrast-enhanced T1-weighted images, intense enhancement of the epididymis and the spermatic cord can be detected, whereas testicular involvement is characterized by inhomogeneous enhancement interspersed with hypointense bands (Kim et al. 2007) (Fig. 119.7b). Additional MRI findings supporting the diagnosis are ill-defined testicular borders, normal or thickened testicular septations, reactive hydrocele, and scrotal skin thickening (Baker et al. 1987).

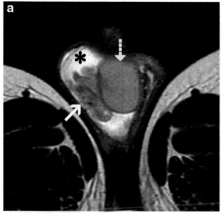
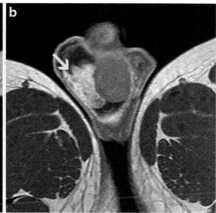

Fig. 119.7 Isolated epididymitis in a 13-year-old boy with a previous history of left orchiectomy presenting with acute painful scrotum. (**a**) Axial T2-weighted MRI scan demonstrates enlarged and irregular epididymis with intermediate signal intensity consistent with isolated epididymitis (*arrow*). Note the normal high signal intensity of the adjacent testis and higher signal intensity of the reactive hydrocele. (**b**) Contrast-enhanced T1-weighted MRI reveals intense enhancement of the epididymis (*arrow*)

Intratesticular Abscess

Intratesticular abscess is a significant complication of epididymo-orchitis. The clinical evaluation is usually unreliable during the early infection for making a differentiation between the two entities. Later, the diagnosis of testicular abscess should be considered for patients with persistent clinical findings consistent with epididymo-orchitis, which do not resolve despite having appropriate antibiotic treatment. Classically, the detection of a lesion with irregular walls, low level internal echoes, and rarely hypervascular margins on US suggests the diagnosis, though the whole testicular parenchyma can infrequently be replaced by the abscess tissue (Dogra et al. 2001) (Fig. 119.8). Recently, contrast-enhanced US has been proposed as a complemantary imaging tool in such patients for the investigation of the complications of epididymo-orchitis like abscess formation and/or testicular torsion. This may apparently suggest the need for surgical exploration or permit the urologists to avoid surgery, which is especially critical in older patients with other significant life-limiting medical conditions (Moschouris et al. 2009; Berman et al. 1996; Feld and Middleton 1992). Presence of strong rim enhancement with or without enhancing septa with a necrotic center on ultrasound contrast enhanced study is highly suggestive of an abscess (Muttarak and Lojanapiwat 2005).

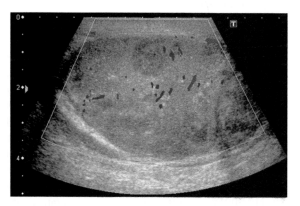

Fig. 119.8 Longitudinal color Doppler US image of a 58-year-old male patient after having an antibiotic treatment for epididymo-orchitis. The findings reveal diffuse involvement of the testis with abscess having a heterogeneous appearance

Tumor

Testicular or paratesticular tumors usually present with a painless lump on a testicle, though they infrequently may cause scrotal pain or discomfort, which is usually associated with intratumoral hemorrhage or epididymo-orchitis (Dogra and Bhatt 2004). The patients may suffer from a sharp and intermittent pain, though chronic pain associated with tumor growth is not rare.

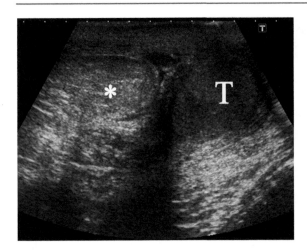

Fig. 119.9 Inguinal hernia. Transverse gray-scale US image demonstrates an echogenic paratesticular mass representing omental herniation (*asterisk*) into the scrotum. The diagnosis was supported by the displacement of the hernia content during Valsalva maneuver (T = testis)

Inguinal Hernia

The diagnosis of inguinal hernia is based on clinical evaluation and the role of US is limited to equivocal cases. The patients with incarcerated bowel usually present with a painful and erythematous groin swelling (Dogra 2003). Typical US appearance of a hernial sac containing bowel is a fluid- or air-filled bowel loop with valvulae or haustra in the scrotum with real-time visualization of peristaltic activity (Dogra 2003; Oyen 2002), though the lack of peristaltic activity can be detected implying bowel strangulation (Varsamidis et al. 2001). A diffusely echogenic paratesticular mass, on the other hand, represents omental content within the hernia (Ragheb and Higgins 2002; Cokkinos et al. 2011) (Fig. 119.9).

Iatrogenic or Postoperative Injuries

Injury to the testis and scrotal sac is a rare complication of inguinal herniorrhaphy. The underlying mechanisms are intraoperative transection of the spermatic cord or cord compression caused by intraoperative handling of the vas, excessively tight placement of the mesh arms around the spermatic cord, or mesh-induced delayed fibrosis resulting in ischemia (Dogra 2003). US has been reported to be much more sensitive (86%) than clinical examination (36%) for detecting

postoperative complications such as ischemia, infarction, hematoma, hydrocele, hematocele, and infection (Dattola et al. 2002). Rarely, iatrogenic testicular atrophy can be detected after open hernia repair (Howlett et al. 2000). Besides, inguinal hernia may cause minor degree of impairment in testicular volume and blood flow attributable to the intermittent mechanical compression effect on the funiculus spermaticus in the inguinal canal (Turgut et al. 2007).

Acute Idiopathic Scrotal Edema

Idiopathic scrotal edema, being quite rare in adults, is the leading cause of acute scrotum in children under 10 years of age (Shah et al. 2004; Najmaldin and Burge 1987). The presentation is sudden and can mimic other causes of acute scrotum. From imaging point of view, US may play a role mainly for its differentiation from various entities with a similar presentation including testicular torsion, torsion of the appendages, epididymo-orchitis, trauma, Fournier's gangrene, cellulitis, and testicular tumor (Rabinowitz and Hulbert 1995). Sonographically, marked echogenic thickening of scrotal skin and subcutaneous tissues and increased vascularization of the scrotal wall can be detected (Grainger et al. 1998). On US, the scrotal wall appears as several concentric rings with thin bands of high reflectivity separated by bands of low reflectivity (Shah et al. 2004). MRI, revealing hypointensity on T1-weighted and hyperintensity on T2-weighted images for the aforementioned morphological changes, may also be helpful by excluding pelvic causes of scrotal edema in doubtful cases and confirming the diagnosis especially when the clinical history and US findings are not entirely typical (Venkatanarasimha et al. 2009). This is a self-limiting disease.

Segmental Testicular Infarct

Segmental testicular infarct, mostly occurring in young men 20–40 years old, is an uncommon complication of epididymo-orchitis, scrotal trauma, transient torsion with subsequent detorsion, inguinal hernia repair, or an embolic phenomenon (Cassidy et al. 2010; Lentini et al. 1989; Liguori et al. 2011). Hematological diseases like vasculitis, sickle-cell disease, and polycythemia are accepted as predisposing factors

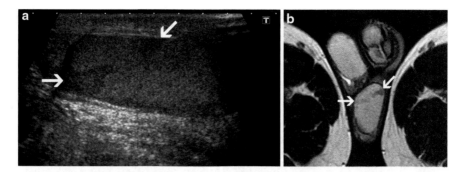

Fig. 119.10 Segmental infarct. (**a**) Longitudinal gray-scale US image of a 41-year-old male patient with acute onset of scrotal pain shows wedge-shaped areas of low echogenicity with their vertices directed toward the mediastinum testis (*arrows*) and complete absence of flow within the lesions on color Doppler images (not shown here). (**b**) On T2-weighted MRI, the infarct appears as segmental areas of low signal intensity (*arrows*)

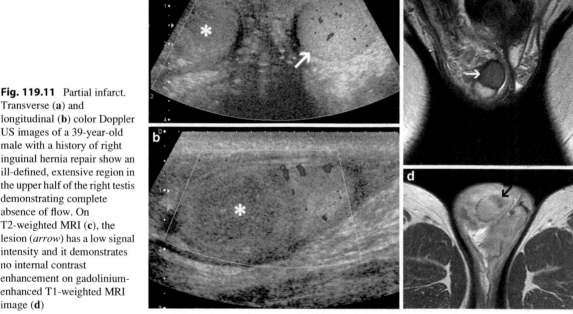

Fig. 119.11 Partial infarct. Transverse (**a**) and longitudinal (**b**) color Doppler US images of a 39-year-old male with a history of right inguinal hernia repair show an ill-defined, extensive region in the upper half of the right testis demonstrating complete absence of flow. On T2-weighted MRI (**c**), the lesion (*arrow*) has a low signal intensity and it demonstrates no internal contrast enhancement on gadolinium-enhanced T1-weighted MRI image (**d**)

(Chin et al. 1998; Sriprasad et al. 2001). It usually manifests with scrotal pain (Cassidy et al. 2010). Classically, a wedge-shaped or geographic area of low echogenicity on US with its vertex directed toward the mediastinum testis and complete absence of flow within the lesion on color Doppler images in the appropriate clinical context implies segmental testicular infarct (Kim et al. 2007; Cassidy et al. 2010) (Fig. 119.10a). Recently, contrast-enhanced US has been reported by Bertolotto et al. to improve conspicuity of segmental testicular infarct and depict anatomic characteristics (Bertolotto et al. 2011). Accordingly, detection of lobular morphologic characteristics and perilesional rim enhancement has been noted to improve the confidence in diagnosis (Bertolotto et al. 2011). The authors also added that changes in lesion features during follow-up, such as size and vascularization, may enable differentiation from other testicular lesions preventing unnecessary orchiectomy (Bertolotto et al. 2011).

MRI may also be helpful to rule out malignancy in doubtful cases (Madaan et al. 2008) (Fig. 119.10b).

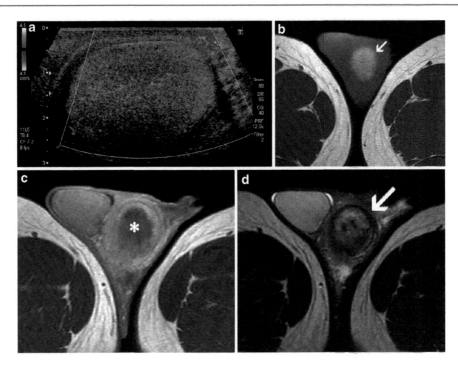

Fig. 119.12 Postinfectious hemorrhagic infarct. A 17-year-old asymptomatic male with a recent history of epididymo-orchitis was referred for US examination after having antibiotic treatment. (**a**) Transverse color Doppler US image shows diffusely heterogeneous parenchymal echotexture and complete absence of blood flow. On T1-weighted MRI (**b**), the lesion shows increased signal intensity, which is prominent peripherally. The central aspect of the lesion demonstrates no enhancement on gadolinium-enhanced T1-weighted MR image (**c**), suggesting postinfectious hemorrhagic infarct. Note that the lesion has a heterogeneous signal intensity on T2-weighted MRI (**d**) with a low signal intensity secondary to hemosiderin deposition within macrophages suggesting the chronic nature of the hemorrhage

A testicular infarct may atypically appear as a mass, which may be misinterpreted as a testicular neoplasm especially if it is small in size (Flanagan and Fowler 1995; Doebler and Norburt 1999). On MRI, infarcts may appear isointense to testicular parenchyma, whereas hemorrhagic infarcts demonstrate foci of high signal intensity on T1-weighted images (Fig. 119.11). On T2-weighted images, the infarct usually appears as an area of low signal intensity, which is segmental rather than mass-like, though the signal intensity may be variable (Kim et al. 2007). Notably, the extent of the infarct may be larger depending on the severity of the etiology (Fig. 119.12). Gadolinium-enhanced T1-weighted MRI images, on the other hand, reveal rim enhancement with lack of internal enhancement (Cassidy et al. 2010; Kim et al. 2007; Fernández-Pérez et al. 2005). The management of choice is close follow-up with imaging, when segmental testicular infarction is suspected (Cassidy et al. 2010; Madaan et al. 2008).

Miscellanous Inflammatory Conditions

Acute Orchitis

Isolated bilateral orchitis is a rare phenomenon mostly occurring secondary to mumps or acquired immuno-deficiency syndrome. On US, an enlarged testis with diffuse, focal, or multifocal hypoechoic lesions and increased blood flow on color Doppler imaging can be detected (Oyen 2002).

Hidradenitis Suppurativa

Hidradenitis suppurativa is characterized by swollen, inflamed, and painful lesions in regions of the body containing apocrine glands, such as the axilla and groin (Kim et al. 2007). In cases with scrotal involvement of inguinal hidradenitis, US typically depicts scrotal skin thickening with a typically uninvolved underlying testis (Fig. 119.13a). On MRI, an area of high signal intensity on T2-weighted images representing edema and contrast-enhancement is

Fig. 119.13 Hidradenitis suppurativa. (**a**) Longitudinal color Doppler US image of a 57-year-old male patient suffering from a painful and tender groin demonstrates scrotal skin thickening with irregular, hypoechoic areas suggesting fluid collection. On T2-weighted MRI (**b**), the lesion appeared to have high signal intensity (*arrow*), confirming its fluid nature, and it showed marked enhancement on gadolinium-enhanced T1-weighted MRI image (**c**), consistent with the inflammatory change

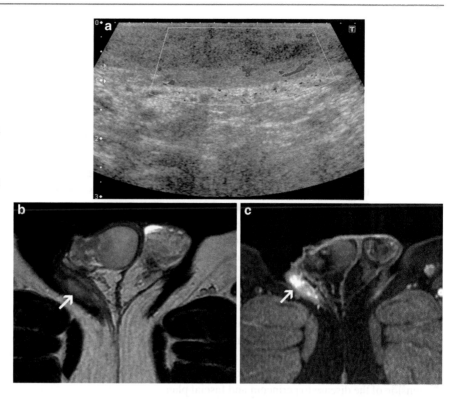

detected (Kim et al. 2007) (Fig. 119.13b, c). Furthermore, the imaging studies can sometimes demonstrate a complicating fistula or abscesses (Kim et al. 2007).

Cellulitis

Scrotal wall cellulitis with a swollen, tense, warm, and red testis usually occurs in obese, diabetic, or immunocompromised patients. The US features of the disease include increased scrotal wall thickness and hypoechoic areas with increased vascularity at color Doppler imaging (Fig. 119.14). Scrotal abscess may sometimes develop as a complication (Dogra 2003).

Fournier Gangrene

Fournier gangrene is polymicrobial necrotizing fasciitis of the perineum, which may rapidly extend to scrotal and lower abdominal skin (Dogra 2003). The entity is caused by the microorganisms passing through a point of entry and then spread through the perineal tissue planes (Uppot et al. 2003). Clinically, the disease presents with a sudden onset of perineal pain and swelling and has a high rate of mortality (Uppot et al. 2003). Therefore, an early diagnosis followed by prompt surgical and medical treatment is crucial. Imaging tools including conventional radiography,

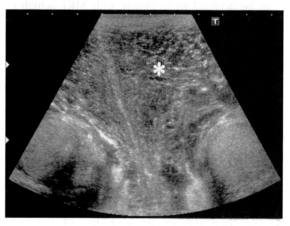

Fig. 119.14 Cellulitis. Transverse gray-scale US image in an immuncompromised patient shows marked increase in scrotal wall thickness with heterogeneous echogenicity and extensive hypoechoic areas (*asterisks*)

US, computed tomography (CT), and MRI may play a role in establishing the diagnosis in the presence of inconclusive clinical findings (Oktar et al. 2004; Rajan and Scharer 1998). The abdominal radiographs reveal soft-tissue edema and subcutaneous emphysema along the involved tissue planes (Rajan and Scharer 1998). US, on the other hand, depicts scrotal skin thickening with reverberation artifacts (Uppot et al. 2003). Most importantly, multiple, hyperechoic foci with dirty shadowing representing gas within the scrotal skin is the pathognomonic US finding (Rajan and Scharer 1998). The extratesticular localization of hyperechoic foci aids in differentiation from calcifications associated with several entities such as testicular microlithiasis, germ cell tumors, sarcoidosis, tuberculosis, or chronic infarct (Uppot et al. 2003). Owing to its separate blood supply, the testicle is usually not involved by the disease. Sonographically, gas located within the bowel lumen rather than the scrotal wall and extension of the course of the bowel within the peritoneal cavity are the distinctive features of scrotal bowel hernia, which should be taken into consideration for the differential diagnosis (Dogra 2003; Andipa et al. 2004). The main advantage provided by CT is that it can depict the extent of the soft tissue gas and can reveal the etiology such as perianal abscesses, incarcerated inguinal hernias, or fistulous tracts (Rajan and Scharer 1998). The technique can also show the fascial thickening and fat stranding of the involved areas. The extension of the disease to perineum and fascial planes can be depicted more clearly with MRI, which can assist in planning debridement (Oktar et al. 2004).

Miscellaneous Vascular Conditions

Varicocele

Scrotal pain or discomfort, worsening especially toward the end of the day is an usual presentation for idiopathic varicocele (Horstman 1997). An aching pain may occur with heavy lifting or prolonged standing implying gradual build up of pressure in the affected veins. The patients may present with the complaint of scrotal pain due to the stretching of the tunica albuginea after venous congestion, though most of them are asymptomatic and detected incidentally (Browne et al. 2005; Das et al. 1999). The pain may be worse in case thrombophelibitis develops in the affected veins.

Henoch-Schonlein Purpura Vasculitis

Henoch-Schönlein purpura, the most common systemic vasculitis in children, may manifest with painful scrotal swelling and ecchymosis (Clark and Kramer 1986; Caldamone et al. 1984). The involvement of the scrotum by the disease, which is responsible from 3% of all acute scrotum cases, may sometimes mimic testicular torsion clinically (Clark and Kramer 1986; Caldamone et al. 1984; Hara et al. 2004). Color Doppler US demonstrating normal or increased testicular blood flow may be helpful for an appropriate differentiation between the two entities, though associated edema of the scrotal wall may cause a diagnostic dilemma (Hara et al. 2004).

Thrombosis

In various conditions increasing the predisposition to stasis and thrombosis in internal spermatic or pampiniform plexus veins, such as longer course of the left spermatic vein and the "nutcracker phenomenon" representing the entrapment of the left renal vein between the superior mesenteric artery and the aorta, acute scrotal pain may be encountered. Recently, thrombosis of the renal vein has been reported to cause hemorrhagic infarction and necrosis of the testis probably due to a critical compression of the left testicular vein by the thrombosis leading to malperfusion of the testis (Maas et al. 2011). The typical color Doppler US finding is a thrombus material interrupting the luminal patency, usually appearing hyperechoic in the first few days and becomes hypoechoic with resolution in time (Turgut et al. 2008; Andipa et al. 2004). Furthermore, venous thrombosis can also be seen in severe inflammations like epididymo-orchitis and can cause testicular ischemia and infarct (Herbener 1996; Farriol et al. 2000). Importantly, the detection of reversal of flow during diastole by spectral Doppler evaluation in acute epididymo-orchitis implies venous infarction (Sanders et al. 1994).

Other Rare Causes

Acute Pancreatitis

Scrotal involvement is a rare complication of acute pancreatitis, which presents as unilateral or bilateral scrotal swelling and skin color change mimicking testicular torsion, epididymitis, and testicular tumor (Kim et al. 2011). The underlying mechanism is fat necrosis of scrotal soft tissues due to the destructive effect of pancreatic fluid caused by the accumulation of the pancreatic fluid (Kim et al. 2011) The differential diagnosis is critical because conservative management is sufficient for its treatment. Gray-scale and color Doppler US reveal imaging features associated with pancreatitis-related scrotal swelling (Choong 1996). Nevertheless, the most important clue for the diagnosis is that the testes are typically not affected in pancreatitis-related scrotal swelling as they are covered by the fibrous tunica albuginea and tunica vaginalis (Choong 1996). Abdominopelvic CT can usually show the scrotal extension of pancreatic inflammation (Kim et al. 2011).

Electrical Injury

Electrical injuries of the scrotum are rare and mostly associated with thermal injury resulting in burns. They result from the passage of an electric current through the body between points of entry and exit (Escudero-Nafs et al. 1990). Gray-scale US studies demonstrate infarction of the testis, whereas Doppler images reveal no flow in one or both testes (Deurdulian et al. 2007).

Vascular Injury

Rarely, blunt testicular trauma may cause an intratesticular pseudoaneurysm, appearing on gray-scale US as a round hypoechoic or anechoic lesion in the testis. Color Doppler US typically shows a mass demonstrating turbulent flow with a vascular neck producing a to-and-fro flow pattern (Deurdulian et al. 2007).

Pearls to Remember

- The primary goal for imaging in acute scrotum is to differentiate those warranting surgery from those who would be managed with a conservative approach.
- US is irreplaceable as the imaging method of choice for the evaluation of the scrotum on an emergency basis, which should include gray-scale, color, and spectral Doppler examination, as well as comparison of the affected hemiscrotal contents to those on the contralateral side.
- The lack of blood flow in the involved testis on color Doppler US in contrast with the normal flow in the contralateral testis is highly presumptive for testicular torsion, though arterial flow may not necessarily be absent for torsion to be present as is the case for incomplete torsion.
- US evaluation of the patients with torsion of testicular appendix may help exclude testicular torsion or epididymo-orchitis.

- Sonographic follow-up after medical treatment is crucial for focal testicular lesions presumed to be consistent with epididymo-orchitis because resolved lesions may help exclude tumor or infarction.

References

Anderson PA, Giacomantonio JM, Schwartz RD. Acute scrotal pain in children: prospective study of diagnosis and management. Can J Surg. 1989;32:29–32.

Andipa E, Liberopoulos K, Asvestis C. Magnetic resonance imaging and ultrasound evaluation of penile and testicular masses. World J Urol. 2004;22:382–91.

Angell JC. Torsion of the testicle. A plea for diagnosis. Lancet. 1963;1:19–21.

Baker LL, Hajek PC, Burkhard TK, Dicapua L, Landa HM, Leopold GR, Hesselink JR, Mattrey RF. MR imaging of the scrotum: pathologic conditions. Radiology. 1987;163:93–8.

Berman JM, Beidle TR, Kunberger LE, Letourneau JG. Sonographic evaluation of acute intrascrotal pathology. AJR Am J Roentgenol. 1996;166:857–61.

Bertolotto M, Derchi LE, Sidhu PS, Serafini G, Valentino M, Grenier N, Cova MA. Acute segmental testicular infarction at contrast-enhanced ultrasound: early features and changes during follow-up. AJR Am J Roentgenol. 2011;196:834–41.

Blaivas M, Sierzenski P, Lambert M. Emergency evaluation of patients presenting with acute scrotum using bedside ultrasonography. Acad Emerg Med. 2001;8:90–3.

Browne RF, Geoghegan T, Ahmed I, Torreggiani WC. Intratesticular varicocele. Australas Radiol. 2005;49:333–4.

Caldamone AA, Valvo JR, Altebarmakian VK, Rabinowitz R. Acute scrotal swelling in children. J Pediatr Surg. 1984;19:581–4.

Cass AS, Cass BP, Veerarghavan K. Immediate exploration of the unilateral acute scrotum in young male subjects. J Urol. 1980;124:829–32.

Cassar S, Bhatt S, Paltiel HJ, Dogra VS. Role of spectral Doppler sonography in the evaluation of partial testicular torsion. J Ultrasound Med. 2008;27:1629–38.

Cassidy FH, Ishioka KM, McMahon CJ, Chu P, Sakamoto K, Lee KS, Aganovic L. MR imaging of scrotal tumors and pseudotumors. Radiographics. 2010;30:665–83.

Cavusoglu YH, Karaman A, Karaman I, Erdogan D, Aslan MK, Varlikli O, Cakmak O. Acute scrotum- etiology and management. Indian J Pediatr. 2005;72:201–3.

Chin SC, Wu CJ, Chen A, Hsiao HS. Segmental hemorrhagic infarction of testis associated with epididymitis. J Clin Ultrasound. 1998;26:326–8.

Choong KK. Acute penoscrotal edema due to acute necrotizing pancreatitis. J Ultrasound Med. 1996;15:247–8.

Choyke PL. Dynamic contrast-enhanced MR imaging of the scrotum: reality check. Radiology. 2000;217:14–5.

Clark WR, Kramer SA. Henoch-Schönlein purpura and the acute scrotum. J Pediatr Surg. 1986;21:991–2.

Cokkinos DD, Antypa E, Tserotas P, Kratimenou E, Kyratzi E, Deligiannis I, Kachrimanis G, Piperopoulos PN. Emergency ultrasound of the scrotum: a review of the commonest pathologic conditions. Curr Probl Diagn Radiol. 2011;40:1–14.

Cook JL, Dewbury K. The changes seen on high resolution ultrasound in orchitis. Clin Radiol. 2000;55:13–8.

Das KM, Prasad K, Szmigielski W, Noorani N. Intra-testicular varicocele: evaluation using conventional and Doppler sonography. AJR Am J Roentgenol. 1999;173:1079–83.

Dattola P, Alberti A, Dattola A, Giannetto G, Basile G, Basile M. Inguino-crural hernias: preoperative diagnosis and postoperative follow-up by high-resolution ultrasonography. A personal experience. Ann Ital Chir. 2002;73:65–8.

Deurdulian C, Mittelstaedt CA, Chong WK, Fielding JR. US of acute scrotal trauma: optimal technique, imaging findings, and management. Radiographics. 2007;27:357–69.

Dibilio D, Serafini G, Gandolofo N, Derchi LE. Ultrasonographic findings in isolated torsion of the epididymis. J Ultrasound Med. 2006;25:417–9.

Doebler RW, Norburt AM. Localized testicular infarction masquerading as a testicular neoplasm. Urology. 1999;54:366.

Dogra V. Bell-clapper deformity. AJR Am J Roentgenol. 2003;180:1176–7.

Dogra V, Bhatt S. Acute painful scrotum. Radiol Clin North Am. 2004;42:349–63.

Dogra VS, Gottlieb RH, Rubens DJ, Liao L. Benign intratesticular cystic lesions: US features. Radiographics. 2001;21(Spec No):S273–81.

Dogra VS, Rubens DJ, Gottlieb RH, Bhatt S. Torsion and beyond: new twists in spectral Doppler evaluation of the scrotum. J Ultrasound Med. 2004;23:1077–85.

Dogra VS, Bhatt S, Rubens DJ. Sonographic evaluation of testicular torsion. Ultrasound Clin. 2006;1:55–66.

Donohue RE, Utley WL. Torsion of spermatic cord. Urology. 1978;11:184–90.

Elert A, Hegele A, Olbert P, Heidenreich A, Hofmann R. Isolated epididymal torsion in dissociation of testis-epididymis. Urologe A. 2002;41:364–5.

Escudero-Nafs FJ, Leiva-Oliva RM, Collado-Aromir F, Rabanal-Suirez F, De Molina-Nofiez JM. High-tension electrical burns: primary treatment of seventy patients. Ann MBC. 1990;3:1–7.

Farriol VG, Comella XP, Agromayor EG, Greixams XS, Martinez De La Torre IB. Gray-scale and power doppler sonographic appearances of acute inflammatory diseases of the scrotum. J Clin Ultrasound. 2000;28:67–72.

Favorito LA, Cavalcante AG, Costa WS. Anatomic aspects of epididymis and tunica vaginalis in patients with testicular torsion. Int Braz J Urol. 2004;30:420–4.

Feld R, Middleton WD. Recent advances in sonography of the testis and scrotum. Radiol Clin North Am. 1992;30:1033–51.

Fernández-Pérez GC, Tardáguila FM, Velasco M, Rivas C, Dos Santos J, Cambronero J, Trinidad C, San Miguel P. Radiologic findings of segmental testicular infarction. AJR Am J Roentgenol. 2005;184:1587–93.

Flanagan JJ, Fowler RC. Testicular infarction mimicking tumor on scrotal ultrasound: a potential pitfall. Clin Radiol. 1995;50:49–50.

Gorman B, Caroll BA. The scrotum. In: Rumack CM, Wilson SR, Charboneau JW, editors. Diagnostic ultrasound. 3rd ed. St Louis: Elsevier Mosby; 2005. p. 849–88.

Grainger AJ, Hide IG, Elliott ST. The ultrasound appearances of scrotal oedema. Eur J Ultrasound. 1998;8:33–7.

Hara Y, Tajiri T, Matsuura K, Hasegawa A. Acute scrotum caused by Henoch-Schönlein purpura. Int J Urol. 2004;11:578–80.

Herbener TE. Ultrasound in the assessment of the acute scrotum. J Clin Ultrasound. 1996;24:405–21.

Hörmann M, Balassy C, Philipp MO, Pumberger W. Imaging of the scrotum in children. Eur Radiol. 2004;14:974–83.

Horstman WG. Scrotal imaging. Urol Clin North Am. 1997;24:653–71.

Howlett DC, Marchbank ND, Sallomi DF. Pictorial review. Ultrasound of the testis. Clin Radiol. 2000;55:595–601.

Jee WH, Choe BY, Byun JY, Shinn KS, Hwang TK. Resistive index of the intrascrotal artery in scrotal inflammatory disease. Acta Radiol. 1997;38:1026–30.

Kadish HA, Bolte RG. A retrospective review of pediatric patients with epididymitis, testicular torsion, and torsion of testicular appendages. Pediatrics. 1998;102:73–6.

Karmazyn B, Steinberg R, Livne P, Kornreich L, Grozovski S, Schwarz M, Ziv N, Freud E. Duplex sonographic findings in children with torsion of the testicular appendages: overlap with epididymitis and epididymoorchitis. J Pediatr Surg. 2006;41:500–4.

Kass EJ, Lundak B. The acute scrotum. Pediatr Clin North Am. 1997;44:1251–66.

Kass E, Stone K, Cacciarelli A, Mitchell B. Do all children with an acute scrotum require exploration? J Urol. 1993;150:667–9.

Kim W, Rosen MA, Langer JE, Banner MP, Siegelman ES, Ramchandani P. US MR imaging correlation in pathologic conditions of the scrotum. Radiographics. 2007;27:1239–53.

Kim SB, Je BK, Lee SH, Cha SH. Scrotal swelling caused by acute necrotizing pancreatitis: CT diagnosis. Abdom Imaging. 2011;36:218–21.

Knight PJ, Vassy LE. The diagnosis and treatment of the acute scrotum in children and adolescents. Ann Surg. 1984;200:664–73.

Lee JC, Bhatt S, Dogra VS. Imaging of the epididymis. Ultrasound Q. 2008;24:3–16.

Lentini JF, Benson CB, Richie JP. Sonographic features of focal orchitis. J Ultrasound Med. 1989;8:361–5.

Liguori G, Bucci S, Zordani A, Benvenuto S, Ollandini G, Mazzon G, Bertolotto M, Cacciato F, Siracusano S, Trombetta C. Role of US in acute scrotal pain. World J Urol. 2011. doi:10.1007/s00345-011-0698-8.

Maas C, Müller-Hansen I, Flechsig H, Poets CF. Acute scrotum in a neonate caused by renal vein thrombosis. Arch Dis Child Fetal Neonatal Ed. 2011;96:149–50.

Madaan S, Joniau S, Klockaerts K, DeWever L, Lerut E, Oyen R, Van Poppel H. Segmental testicular infarction: conservative management is feasible and safe. Eur Urol. 2008;53:441–5.

Micallef M, Torreggiani WC, Hurley M, Dinsmore WW, Hogan B. The ultrasound investigation of scrotal swelling. Int J STD AIDS. 2000;11:297–302.

Middleton WD, Middleton MA, Dierks M, Keetch D, Dierks S. Sonographic prediction of viability in testicular torsion: preliminary observations. J Ultrasound Med. 1997;16:23–7.

Moschouris H, Stamatiou K, Lampropoulou E, Kalikis D, Matsaidonis D. Imaging of the acute scrotum: is there a place for contrast-enhanced ultrasonography? Int Braz J Urol. 2009;35:692–702.

Murphy FL, Fletcher L, Pease P. Early scrotal exploration in all cases is the investigation and intervention of choice in the acute paediatric scrotum. Pediatr Surg Int. 2006;22:413–6.

Muttarak M, Lojanapiwat B. The painful scrotum: an ultrasonographical approach to diagnosis. Singapore Med J. 2005;46:352–7.

Najmaldin A, Burge DM. Acute idiopathic scrotal oedema: incidence, manifestations and aetiology. Br J Surg. 1987;74:634–5.

Oktar SO, Yucel C, Ercan NT, Caplan D, Ozdemir H. Fournier's gangrene: US and MR imaging findings. Eur J Radiol Extra. 2004;50:81–7.

Oyen RH. Scrotal ultrasound. Eur Radiol. 2002;12:19–34.

Parenti GC, Feletti F, Brandini F, Palmarini D, Zago S, Ginevra A, Campioni P, Mannella P. Imaging of the scrotum: role of MRI. Radiol Med. 2009;114:414–24.

Prando D. Torsion of the spermatic cord: sonographic diagnosis. Ultrasound Q. 2002;18:41–57.

Prando D. Torsion of the spermatic cord: the main gray-scale and doppler sonographic signs. Abdom Imaging. 2009;34:648–61.

Rabinowitz R, Hulbert Jr WC. Acute scrotal swelling. Urol Clin North Am. 1995;22:101–5.

Ragheb D, Higgins JL. Ultrasonography of the scrotum: technique, anatomy, and pathologic entities. J Ultrasound Med. 2002;21:171–85.

Rajan DK, Scharer KA. Radiology of Fournier's gangrene. AJR Am J Roentgenol. 1998;170:163–8.

Sanders LM, Haber S, Dembner A, Aquino A. Significance of reversal of diastolic flow in the acute scrotum. J Ultrasound Med. 1994;13:137–9.

Sanelli PC, Burke BJ, Lee L. Color and spectral Doppler sonography of partial torsion of the spermatic cord. AJR Am J Roentgenol. 1999;172:49–51.

See WA, Mack LA, Krieger JN. Scrotal ultrasonography: a predictor of complicated epididymitis requiring orchiectomy. J Urol. 1988;139:55–6.

Shah J, Qureshi I, Ellis BW. Acute idiopathic scrotal oedema in an adult: a case report. Int J Clin Pract. 2004;58:1168–9.

Shteynshlyuger A, Freyle J. Familial testicular torsion in three consecutive generations of first-degree relatives. J Pediatr Urol. 2011;7(1):86–91.

Sica G, Teeger S. MR imaging of scrotal, testicular and penile diseases. Magn Reson Imaging Clin N Am. 1996;4:545–63.

Skoglund RW, McRoberts JW, Ragde H. Torsion of the spermatic cord: a review of the literature and an analysis of 70 new cases. J Urol. 1970;104:604–7.

Sriprasad S, Kooiman GG, Muir GH, Sidhu PS. Acute segmental testicular infarction: differentiation from tumour using high frequency colour Doppler ultrasound. Br J Radiol. 2001;74:965–7.

Terai A, Yoshimura K, Ichioka K, Ueda N, Utsunomiya N, Kohei N, Arai Y, Watanabe Y. Dynamic contrast-enhanced subtraction magnetic resonance imaging in diagnostics of testicular torsion. Urology. 2006;67:1278–82.

Trambert MA, Mattrey RF, Levine D, Berthoty DP. Subacute scrotal pain: evaluation of torsion versus epididymitis with MRI. Radiology. 1990;175:53–6.

Turgut AT, Olçücüoğlu E, Turan C, Kiliçoğlu B, Koşar P, Geyik PO, Koşar U, Dogra V. Preoperative ultrasonographic evaluation of testicular volume and blood flow in patients with inguinal hernias. J Ultrasound Med. 2007;26:1657–66.

Turgut AT, Bhatt S, Dogra VS. Acute painful scrotum. Ultrasound Clin. 2008;3:93–107.

Uppot RN, Levy HM, Patel PH. Case 54: Fournier gangrene. Radiology. 2003;226:115–7.

Varsamidis K, Varsamidou E, Mavropoulos G. Doppler ultrasonography in testicular tumors presenting with acute scrotal pain. Acta Radiol. 2001;42:230–3.

Venkatanarasimha N, Dubbins PA, Freeman SJ. MRI appearances of acute idiopathic scrotal oedema in an adult. Emerg Radiol. 2009;16:235–7.

Vijayaraghavan SB. Sonographic differential diagnosis of acute scrotum: real-time whirlpool sign, a key sign of torsion. J Ultrasound Med. 2006;25:563–74.

Watanabe Y. Scrotal imaging. Curr Opin Urol. 2002;12:149–53.

Watanabe Y, Dohke M, Ohkubo K, Ishimori T, Amoh Y, Okumura A, Oda K, Hayashi T, Dodo Y, Arai Y. Scrotal disorders: evaluation of testicular enhancement patterns at dynamic contrast-enhanced subtraction MR imaging. Radiology. 2000;217:219–27.

Watanabe Y, Nagayama M, Okumura A, Amoh Y, Suga T, Terai A, Dodo Y. MR imaging of testicular torsion: features of testicular hemorrhagic necrosis and clinical outcomes. J Magn Reson Imaging. 2007;26:100–8.

Williamson RC. Torsion of the testis and allied conditions. Br J Surg. 1976;63:465–76.

Woodward P, Sohaey R, O'Donoghue M, Green D. Tumors and tumor-like lesions of the testis: radiologic-pathologic correlation. Radiographics. 2002;22:189–216.

Yang DM, Lim JW, Kim JE, Kim JH, Cho H. Torsed appendix testis: gray scale and color Doppler sonographic findings compared with normal appendix testis. J Ultrasound Med. 2005;24:87–91.

Yang C, Song B, Tan J, Liu X, Wei GH. Testicular torsion in children: a 20-year retrospective study in a single institution. Scientific World J. 2011;11:362–8.

120

Scrotal Masses

Lorenzo E. Derchi and Michele Bertolotto

The role of radiology in the study of patients with scrotal masses is very important. Imaging, in fact, is used to confirm presence of the disease process, to evaluate its location and extent, and to assess its nature. These goals can be reached in many cases through careful analysis of imaging findings and correlation with clinical and laboratory tests.

This chapter will describe the appearances of the different mass lesions that can be encountered in the scrotum.

General Considerations

Identification of an abnormal lump at self-palpation is the most common way of presentation of scrotal masses. Less commonly, the patient may experience a change in the normal feeling of the testis or may experience pain, either dull or acute. Furthermore, nonpalpable nodules of the testis or of other scrotal structures can be detected as an incidental finding during imaging performed for indications others than presence of a palpable mass.

The primary goal of imaging is to identify whether a scrotal mass is actually a cancer of the testis. Testicular tumors are relatively rare, accounting for 1% of all malignant tumors in men, but are the most common malignancy in the 15–34 years group (Woodward et al. 2002).

US is commonly the first imaging study in these patients. It has to be stressed that a US study of the scrotum is a dynamic examination: simultaneous palpation of the scrotal content during the US study helps to correlate physical findings with the US images. This is especially useful in patients with small, mobile extratesticular masses that may be easily missed if a focused examination is not performed. Furthermore, a small loose body within the vaginal cavity may look as attached to the surface of the tunica vaginalis and may mimic a tumor; observing its movements during palpation may easily clarify its nature (Woodward et al. 2002, 2003; Hamm 1997; Dogra et al. 2003).

Although MR imaging allows good evaluation of the scrotum, it is not frequently needed to evaluate a scrotal mass given the high sensitivity of US in this field. There are, however, some indications for the use of this technique: in cases of discrepancies between US and clinical findings; when a diffuse, nonspecific change of testicular echogenicity is seen at US; when US findings are inconclusive; or when lesions containing fibrous tissue, fat, or hemorrhage are suspected (Muglia et al. 2002). It has to be noted that since the first papers dealing with MR imaging of the scrotum were published, the use of MR in this field is growing, and MR is now performed in almost 6% of cases to clarify US findings (Parenti et al. 2009).

Roles of Imaging

There are four questions which need to be answered in patients with a palpable scrotal mass:
- Is there really a mass?
- Is it intra- or extratesticular?
- Is it uni- or bilateral?
- Can we identify its nature?

L.E. Derchi (✉)
Department of Radiology, University of Genoa, Genoa, Italy

M. Bertolotto
Department of Radiology, University of Trieste, Trieste, Italy

B. Hamm, P. R. Ros (eds.), *Abdominal Imaging*, DOI 10.1007/978-3-642-13327-5_205,
© Springer-Verlag Berlin Heidelberg 2013

Fig. 120.1 Chronic, nonspecific epididymitis causing both diffuse enlargement of the epididymis (*arrowheads*) and a nodule at the tail (*arrows*). This nodule mimics an intratesticular mass. *T* testis

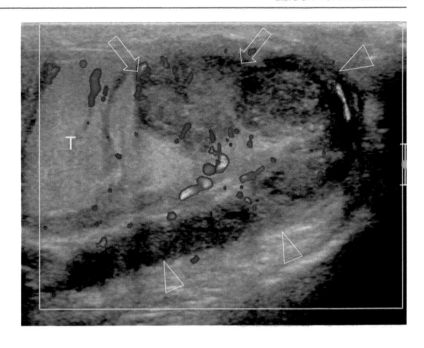

1. *Is there really a mass*? Enlargement of the scrotum from hydrocele or hernias is usually easily identified at physical examination. However, this can be difficult in some cases. US is almost 100% sensitive in detecting the presence of a scrotal mass. False-negative results are quite rare and may be due to presence of isoechoic testicular lesions or to presence of inguinal hernias containing fat, or to lipomatous tumors of the spermatic cord, that may be isoechogenic to surrounding subcutaneous fat.

2. *Is the mass intra- or extratesticular*? And where does it take origin? US is 98–100% sensitive in differentiating intra- versus extratesticular masses. Furthermore, it can identify in most cases whether it arises from the scrotal wall or from other scrotal tissues. Answering to this question is very important since most intratesticular masses are malignant and most extratesticular ones are benign. Simultaneous palpation and US imaging is particularly helpful to locate carefully a mass. Epididymal nodules can mimic a testicular lesion in rare cases; careful analysis of the shape of the whole epididymis, correlation with clinical history, and follow-up after therapy are helpful to clarify the diagnosis (Fig. 120.1).

3. *Is the mass unilateral or bilateral*? Up to 2% of seminomas and up to 38% of lymphomas may be bilateral, even simultaneously. Then, all imaging studies of the scrotum have always to be performed on both sides to determine the actual extent of a lesion.

4. *Can we identify its nature*? It must be stated that, unfortunately, in most cases, the answer is no. A histological diagnosis cannot be based on imaging findings alone. However, consideration of epidemiological, clinical, laboratory and imaging findings together can provide helpful diagnostic criteria.

Tumor markers (α-fetoprotein, human chorionic gonadotropin, and lactate dehydrogenase) are helpful in the diagnosis of solid testicular nodules. Increased α-fetoproteins are seen in yolk-sac tumors and in mixed tumors with yolk-sac elements; human chorionic gonadotropins elevate in lesions containing syncytiotrophoblasts. One or both of these markers are found increased in up to 80% of nonseminomatous germ cell tumors. Lactate dehydrogenase is a less specific marker that correlates with the bulk of the disease (Woodward et al. 2002).

Location of the mass is important since, as already said, most intratesticular masses are malignant, while the majority of extratesticular ones are benign (Woodward et al. 2003). Furthermore, correlation of mass location and structure helps to narrow the differential. A cystic extratesticular mass is usually an epididymal cyst, which is almost invariably benign.

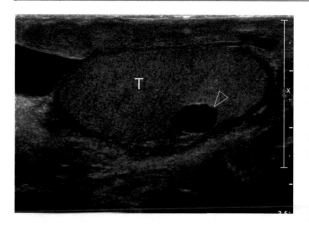

Fig. 120.2 Simple intratesticular cyst. The lesion (*arrowhead*) has regular margins and anechoic content, there is increased through transmission, and it is located close to the mediastinum testis. *T* testis

A cystic intratesticular nodule can be found in up to 10% of cases and can be classified as benign if it is purely cystic, with regular wall and increased through transmission at US, if it is localized close to the mediastinum testis (Fig. 120.2), or if it is at the tunica albuginea. A series of elongated, fluid-filled structures with thin walls at the mediastinum testis can be recognized as a dilated rete testis. When there are doubts at US on the presence of irregular walls or solid components within a cyst-like structure, MR imaging after contrast may be helpful. Solid lesions are more difficult to classify since most, whether intra- or extratesticular, have no special imaging features that help to identify their nature. The high sensitivity of modern equipment allows identification of color Doppler signals within most testicular nodules, either benign or malignant. Some truly avascular lesions exist, however, and this can be helpful to lower the probability of malignancy. Contrast-enhanced MRI seems able to differentiate seminomas from nonseminomatous testicular tumors: low signal intensity on T2-weighted images with septa enhancing more than tumor tissue after contrast suggests a diagnosis of seminoma, while marked heterogeneity both before and after contrast suggests nonseminomatous neoplasms (Tslili et al. 2007). Furthermore, MRI can provide high accuracy in local staging of the tumor through detection of involvement of the tunica albuginea, the spermatic cord, and the epididymis (Tsili et al. 2010).

Testicular Tumors

Tumors of the testis are classified in two categories:

- Germ cell tumors
- Non-germ cell tumors

The first ones arise from spermatogenic cells and are almost invariably malignant; the second ones arise from sex cords and stroma and are malignant in about 10% of cases only.

Germ Cell Tumors

Such lesions are the most common testicular neoplasms (Woodward et al. 2002). Up to 32–60% can present with more than one histological type within the mass and are classified as mixed lesions.

Seminomas are the most common germ cell tumor of the testis (up to 50% of all testicular neoplasms are seminomas, either pure or in mixed forms). Small lesions are typically hypoechoic at US and with homogeneous hypointense pattern at T2-weighted MR images. Larger lesions are usually lobulated, with hypoechoic nodules continuing one into another, divided by echogenic septa which, at MR images after contrast, enhance more than tumoral tissue. At color Doppler, vascular signals are present within the lesion, usually with irregularly shaped vessels (Fig. 120.3). Embryonal cell carcinomas are the second in frequency, being present in 87% of all mixed germ cell tumors. They have a more aggressive behavior than carcinoma and at imaging present with a nonspecific pattern, usually heterogeneous and with irregular borders (Fig. 120.4). Choriocarcinomas are rare, seen in less than 1% of pure tumors and in 8% of mixed lesions. They are very aggressive, and clinical symptoms are often due to metastases. Again, they have nonspecific pattern at imaging studies.

Yolk-sac tumors and teratomas are the most common testicular tumors in children, but they can be present in mixed tumors of adults. The first of these lesions can present with diffuse testicular infiltration, with quite subtle changes of echotexture of the involved testis. The second ones are usually heterogeneous, reflecting presence of tissues from different germ layers (mesoderm, endoderm, ectoderm), and often contain cystic-like or complex areas with thick walls and septa.

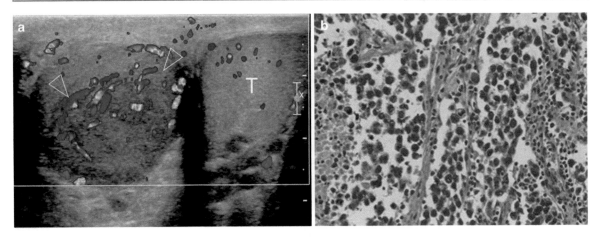

Fig. 120.3 Seminoma. (**a**) A palpable mass at the right testis was seen at color Doppler as a hypoechoic, homogeneous and hypervascularized lesion (*arrowheads*). (**b**) A seminoma was confirmed at histology. *T* Left testis

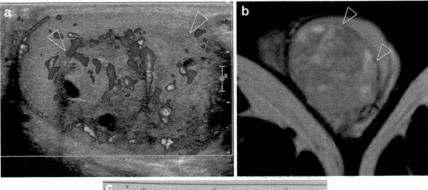

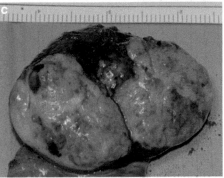

Fig. 120.4 Embryonal cell carcinoma. (**a**) Color Doppler shows large, heterogeneous, well-vascularized testicular mass (*arrowheads*). (**b**) At T2-weighted MR, the lesion (*arrowheads*) has heterogeneous signal intensity. (**c**) Macroscopic view confirms heterogeneity and presence of cystic areas within the tumor mass

Epidermoid cysts are benign germ cell lesions that often present with a typical US and MR pattern and can be correctly diagnosed preoperatively. They are true cysts containing laminated cheesy material with no malignant cells. Typical lesions present at US as well circumscribed, with hyperechoic (sometimes calcific) margins and laminated onion-skin internal echo pattern. At MR, they have well-defined outer margins and a target appearance, with low-intensity border and

internal content with high signal at both T1- and T2-weighted images. No internal flow is visible at color Doppler (Dogra et al. 2001) (Fig. 120.5). When such a lesion is suspected at imaging, testicular sparing surgery and intraoperative pathological analysis are suggested. It must be remembered that some epidermoid cysts have no characteristic pattern and that teratomas or other tumors may mimic such lesions. Care must be taken for possible signs of malignancy such as

Fig. 120.5 Epidermoid cyst presenting as a palpable nodule of the left testis. (**a**) Color Doppler US shows an avascular lesion (*arrowhead*), with a few calcifications within its walls and slightly hyperechoic internal content. (**b**) MR demonstrates a nodule with well-defined margins (*arrowheads*). (**c**) Gross appearance of the cyst, which has been opened after enucleation, showing its cheesy, laminated content

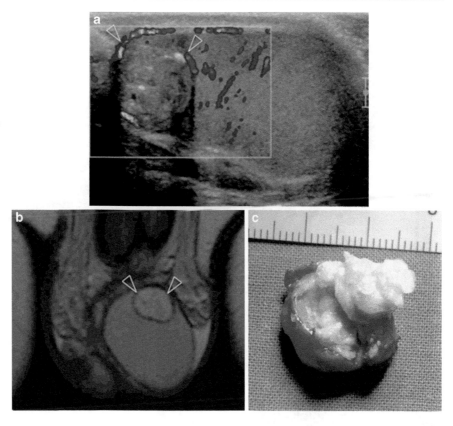

irregular borders or irregularities within the surrounding testicular parenchyma.

In rare cases, patients with metastatic germ cell tumors but with testes that are normal or even small at palpation can be encountered. A possible explanation to this phenomenon is necrosis and involution of a primary testicular germ cell tumor with high metabolic rate, which has outgrown its blood supply after it had already given origin to metastatic disease. These are called "burned-out" germ cell tumors. Imaging is very important in these patients to recognize small, nonpalpable testicular anomalies which indicate the testis as the primary site of disease. Small nodules, clusters of calcifications, or echogenic scars may be visible at US (Fig. 120.6). Enhancement after contrast injection in tissues surrounding such lesions can be demonstrated at MR (Fabre et al. 2004; Patel and Patel 2007).

Non-Germ Cell Neoplasms

They are far less common than germ cell tumors, but can comprise 10–30% of pediatric testicular neoplasms. Only 10% of such lesions are malignant. Leydig and Sertoli cell tumors are the most common; they may secrete hormones, and associated endocrinopathies (precocious virilization, gynecomastia, decreased libido) can be present clinically. Other, less common, tumors from testicular stroma are granulosa cell tumors, fibroma-thecoma, mixed cell stromal lesions, and mixed stromal cell-germ cell neoplasms.

Leydig cell tumors are the most common in this group (up to 3% of all testicular neoplasms). They arise from interstitial stroma and have been reported as nonspecific nodular lesions, with solid echotexture, either hyper- or hypoechogenic; cystic areas can be present. Internal vascular signals can be seen at color Doppler (Maizlin et al. 2004).

Sertoli cell tumors are less common (1% of all testicular tumors). They have been reported as hypoechoic at US, with hyperintensity at T2-weighted MR images. Internal vessels can be seen at color Doppler, and enhancement has been reported at postcontrast MR (Drevelengas et al. 1999). A subgroup of Sertoli cell tumors can show internal

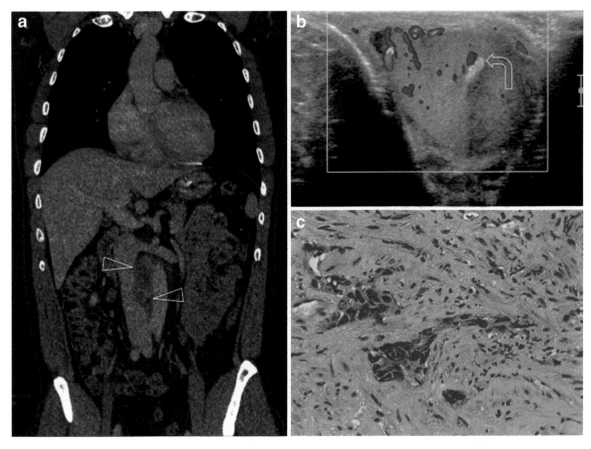

Fig. 120.6 "Burned-out" testicular neoplasm. (**a**) Enlarged ret-roperitoneal lymph nodes are seen at CT (*arrowheads*). (**b**) Testicular US demonstrates a small calcification with linear shape (*curved arrow*); a few vascular signals are close to the calcification. (**c**) A core-needle biopsy of the retroperitoneal nodes confirmed the diagnosis of germ cell tumor

calcifications and has been reported in association with Peutz-Jegher and Carney syndromes.

Lymphomas are the most common testicular tumor in men over 60 years. They may be primary or, more commonly, as testicular involvement in disseminated or recurrent disease. Two different forms have been described. Patients with diffuse lymphomatous involvement present with enlargement of the testis, which is markedly hypervascular; the vessels have a rectilinear course. Nodular involvement is seen as a testicular hypoechoic and hypervascular nodule. Also in these cases, however, vessels entering the nodule from adjacent normal parenchyma have a rectilinear course, without distortion from the mass, reflecting the infiltrative nature of the disease process (Fig. 120.7). Both types of lymphoma have a hypointense appearance at MR (Mazzu et al. 1995).

The Small, Indeterminate Testicular Mass

The widespread use of US for the evaluation of any scrotal problem leads to the discovery of small, asymptomatic nodular lesions whose nature cannot be identified basing on imaging and laboratory findings. Their prevalence has been reported from 0.21% to 1% of examined patients. Orchidectomy seems not justified in these cases, since these lesions are not always malignant tumors. Prevalence of malignancy, in fact, varies widely in reported series: from 0/10 cases (Carmignani et al. 2003) to 8/9 of operated subjects (Avci et al. 2008). In patients who have small, nonpalpable lesions (and have not increased tumor markers), targeted biopsy under intraoperative US guidance and simple enucleation if histology confirms their benign nature are recommended. Transscrotal biopsy of these lesions

Fig. 120.7 Testicular lymphoma, nodular type. (**a**) US shows a well-defined hypoechoic nodule (*arrowheads*) which, at surgery (**b**), has whitish appearance, with hemorrhagic area. (**c**) At color Doppler, the vessels which enter the nodule from adjacent normal parenchyma (*arrows*) are not distorted: the nodule does not cause mass effect on them. (**d**) Microscopy shows clear separation between normal (*at left*) and pathologic (*at right*) tissues, thus explaining the nodular appearance of the lesion; mononucleated cells in the involved part of the testis widen the spaces among the seminiferous tubules, but do not destroy them, thus demonstrating the infiltrative nature of the disease process

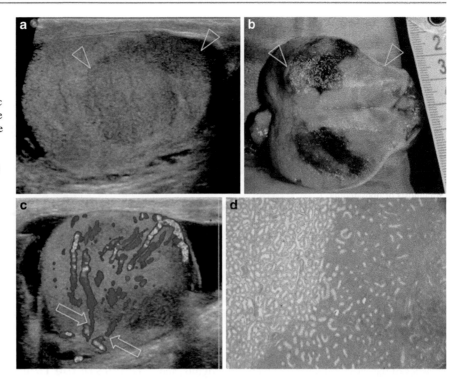

is not regarded as a possible option due to fear of "contamination" of the scrotal wall by possible tumor seeding along the needle path, consequent spread of tumor to inguinal lymph nodes, and worsening of patient's prognosis. Recently, however, core-needle biopsy to diagnose focal indeterminate testicular lesions has been suggested in four clinical scenarios: lesions with equivocal malignant US features, discrepancy between imaging and clinical findings, suspected lymphoproliferative disease, and atrophic testes, in which it is difficult to differentiate malignancy from heterogeneous testicular echogenicity (Soh et al. 2008). "Active" surveillance, with short-term follow-up US studies every 3 months, can be another choice; surgery is decided only for lesions that show interval growth. It has been suggested that demonstration at imaging of features indicating the benign nature of the disease process (such as lack of internal vascularization at contrast-enhanced studies or a "soft" consistency at elastography) can be used, together with lack of increased tumor marker, as a criterion to avoid surgery completely (Shah et al. 2010) or to decide for a follow-up program somewhat looser than that of "active" surveillance. Again, surgery is contemplated for lesions showing interval growth.

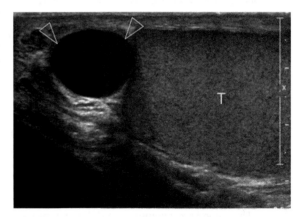

Fig. 120.8 Simple cyst of the epididymis seen at US as a fluid-filled nodule, with regular walls and increased through transmission (*arrowheads*), located within the epididymal head, cranial to the upper pole of the testis. *T* Testis

Extratesticular Masses

Extratesticular masses are most likely benign, with malignancies encountered in about 3% of cases. Most of these lesions are simple epididymal cysts, which are easily identified by US (Fig. 120.8). However, all

Fig. 120.9 Liposarcoma of the epididymis. The patient presented with a palpable, slightly tender, and growing scrotal mass caudal to the left testis. (**a**) US shows a heterogeneous lesion which was (**b**) hypervascular at color Doppler. (**c**) Macroscopic view of surgical specimen showing the close relationship of the mass with the testis. (**d**) Microscopy allowed the diagnosis of liposarcoma. *T* testis, *M* liposarcoma

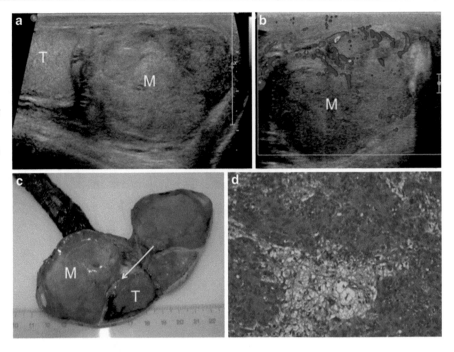

tissues of the scrotum (covering layers, epididymis, and spermatic cord) can give origin to mass lesions. In patients with solid nodules, imaging findings can usually identify the origin of the mass but, in most cases, cannot determine if it is benign or malignant (Woodward et al. 2003; Akbar et al. 2003; Lee et al. 2008).

Tumors of the Epididymis

Adenomatoid tumors are the most common neoplasms of the epididymis. They are benign and usually seen as solid, slightly hyperechoic nodules at US. At MR, they are nonspecific solid tumors with variable signal intensity. Rarely, cystic adenomatoid tumors can be encountered. The second most common epididymal tumors are leiomyomas, presenting as solid nodules with possible cysts and calcifications. Papillary cystadenoma of the epididymis are slowly growing tumors encountered in about 60% of patients with von Hippel-Lindau disease. They present at US with a variable appearance, either as solid nodules with internal cystic areas or as predominantly cystic lesions. Sporadic lesions can occur; presence of bilateral lesions is virtually pathognomonic of von Hippel–Lindau disease (Choyke et al. 1997). Malignant tumors of the epididymis are rare; they include sarcomas (Fig. 120.9), metastases, adenocarcinomas, and lymphomas.

Tumors of the Tunica Vaginalis

The tunica vaginalis, being lined by mesothelial cells, can give rise to mesotheliomas. They are almost invariably associated with hydrocele containing echogenic fluid and can be suspected when irregular thickening of the tunica, either focal or diffuse, and/or vegetating parietal nodules are seen. Fibrous pseudotumors of the tunica vaginalis are a benign fibroinflammatory reaction resulting in solitary or multiple nodular lesions. They are hypoechogenic at US, with nonspecific appearance. At MR, they are hypointense on both T1- and T2-weighted images, a finding which is diagnostic of their fibrous nature (Woodward et al. 2003; Garriga et al. 2009).

Tumors of the Spermatic Cord

Lipomas of the spermatic cord are the most common extratesticular scrotal masses. Most are hyperechoic at US and may be difficult to differentiate from adjacent subcutaneous fat. MR is often needed to evaluate the full extent of the disease process preoperatively. Differentiating a lipoma from a liposarcoma may be difficult on imaging ground alone; a liposarcoma may be suspected by a more heterogeneous internal structure, but excision is needed to establish the diagnosis. Rarely, other malignant extratesticular masses, such as rabdomyosarcomas, malignant fibrous histiocytomas, and undifferentiated sarcomas, can develop (Woodward et al. 2003; Akbar et al. 2003).

References

Akbar SA, Sayyed TA, Jafri SZ, et al. Multimodality imaging of paratesticular neoplasms and their rare mimics. Radiographics. 2003;23:1461–76.

Avci A, Erol B, Eken C, et al. Nine cases of nonpalpable testicular mass: an incidental finding in a large scale ultrasonographic survey. Int J Urol. 2008;15:833–6.

Carmignani L, Gadda F, Gazzano G, et al. High incidence of benign testicular neoplasms diagnosed by ultrasound. J Urol. 2003;170:1783–6.

Choyke PL, Glenn GM, Wagner JP, et al. Epididymal cystadenomas in von Hippel-Lindau disease. Urology. 1997;49:926–31.

Dogra VS, Gottlieb RH, Rubens DJ, et al. Testicular epidermoid cysts: sonographic features with histopathologic correlation. J Clin Ultrasound. 2001;29:192–6.

Dogra VS, Gottlieb RH, Oka M, et al. Sonography of the scrotum. Radiology. 2003;227:18–36.

Drevelengas A, Kalaitzoglou I, Destouni E, et al. Bilateral Sertoli cell tumor of the testis: MRI and sonographic appearance. Eur Radiol. 1999;9:1934.

Fabre E, Jira H, Izard V, et al. "Burned-out" primary testicular cancer. BJU Int. 2004;94:74–8.

Garriga V, Serrano A, Marin A, et al. US of the tunica vaginalis testis: anatomic relationships and pathologic conditions. Radiographics. 2009;29:2017–32.

Hamm B. Differential diagnosis of scrotal masses with ultrasound. Eur Radiol. 1997;7:668–79.

Lee JC, Bhatt S, Dogra VS. Imaging of the epididymis. Ultrasound Q. 2008;24:3–16.

Maizlin ZV, Belenky A, Kunichezky M, et al. Leydig cell tumors of the testis: gray scale and color Doppler sonographic appearance. J Ultrasound Med. 2004;23:959–64.

Mazzu D, Jeffrey Jr RB, Ralls PW. Lymphoma and leukemia involving the testicles: findings on gray-scale and color-Doppler sonography. AJR Am J Roentgenol. 1995;164:645–7.

Muglia V, Tucci Jr S, Elias Jr J, et al. Magnetic resonance imaging of scrotal diseases: when it makes the difference. Urology. 2002;59:419–23.

Parenti GC, Feletti F, Brandini F, et al. Imaging of the scrotum: role of MRI. Radiol Med. 2009;114:414–24.

Patel MD, Patel BM. Sonographic and magnetic resonance imaging appearance of a burned-out testicular germ cell neoplasm. J Ultrasound Med. 2007;26:143–6.

Shah A, Lung PF, Clarke JL, et al. New ultrasound techniques for imaging of the indeterminate testicular lesion may avoid surgery completely. Clin Radiol. 2010;65:496–7.

Soh E, Berman LH, Grant JW, et al. Ultrasound-guided core-needle biopsy of the testis for focal indeterminate intratesticular lesions. Eur Radiol. 2008;18:2990–6.

Tsili AC, Argyropoulou MI, Giannakis D, et al. MRI in the characterization and local staging of testicular neoplasms. AJR Am J Roentgenol. 2010;194:628–39.

Tslili AC, Tsampoulas C, Giannakopoulos X, et al. MRI in the histologic characterization of testicular neoplasms. AJR Am J Roentgenol. 2007;189:W331–7.

Woodward PJ, Sohaey R, O'Donoghue MJ, Green DE. From the archives of AFIP: tumors and tumorlike lesions of the testis: radiologic-pathologic correlation. Radiographics. 2002;22: 189–216.

Woodward PJ, Schwab CM, Sesterhenn IA. From the archives of AFIP: extratesticular scrotal masses: radiologic pathologic correlation. Radiographics. 2003;23:215–40.

Scrotal Trauma

121

Massimo Valentino, Michele Bertolotto, Sergio Murrone,
Mariangela Sabato, Lorenzo E. Derchi, and Cristina Rossi

Patient Management

Scrotal trauma accounts for less than 1% of all trauma-related injuries, because of the anatomic location and mobility of the scrotum (Cass and Luxenberg 1991). The peak occurrence of scrotal trauma is in the age range of 10–30 years (Wessells and Long 2006). Typically it results from direct injury due to sport injury, motor vehicle collision, or altercation (Deurdulian et al. 2007). Penetrating trauma is also possible, due to gunshot wounds, animal attacks, and self-mutilation. Postsurgical and thermal injuries are rare, but iatrogenic injuries resulting from complications of inguinal herniorrhaphy are quite common. The right testis is injured more often than the left one because of its greater propensity to be trapped against the pubis or inner thigh (Bhatt and Dogra 2008).

Patients with scrotal trauma usually present in emergency department, and rapid and accurate diagnosis is necessary to guide treatment and prevent loss of the testis.

Delay in diagnosis or inaccurate diagnosis may result in decreased fertility, delayed orchiectomy,

M. Valentino (✉) • M. Sabato
Emergency Radiology Unit, University Hospital of Parma, Parma, Italy

M. Bertolotto
Department of Radiology, University of Trieste, Trieste, Italy

S. Murrone
Radiology Unit, Hospital of Brindisi, Brindisi, Italy

L.E. Derchi
Department of Radiology, University of Genova, Genoa, Italy

C. Rossi
Radiology Unit, University Hospital of Parma, Parma, Italy

infection, ischemia or infarction, and atrophy (Djakovic et al. 2010; Chandra et al. 2007).

When a patient has scrotal trauma, a clinical assessment is made for acute scrotal pain, swelling, and bruising. The overlying skin is examined to determine the extent of its integrity and for sites of any entry and exit wounds. The testis and epididymis also are palpated, and a penile examination is performed by the physician.

After any necessary analysis is performed, the patient undergoes imaging with US unless there is scrotal avulsion (Morey et al. 2004).

Ultrasonography (US) is the first-line diagnostic tool for the evaluation of the testis in blunt scrotal trauma. It is commonly performed immediately, at the patient arrival, for the assessment of the scrotal contents, testicular integrity, and blood flow, as well as to visualize hematomas, other fluid collections, and foreign bodies.

The use of Magnetic Resonance Imaging (MRI) is claimed when US investigation is inconclusive or suspicious for neoplasm. MRI can be useful for the evaluation of the testis because of high soft-tissue contrast. It is able to have a better visualization of the tunica albuginea that appears as a dark signal intensity line on T2-weighted images (T2-WI) (Kim et al. 2009). MRI can also provide the stage of hematoma because of the known characteristic signal intensity, solving interpretation doubts with neoplasm (Parenti et al. 2009).

US Assessment

US is the first-line imaging test for scrotal trauma, and US findings are crucial in clinical decision making (Kaye et al. 2008; Buckley and McAninch 2006).

B. Hamm, P. R. Ros (eds.), *Abdominal Imaging*, DOI 10.1007/978-3-642-13327-5_207,
© Springer-Verlag Berlin Heidelberg 2013

US manifestations include fluid collections, testicular disruption, and vascular injury. A hydrocele, or fluid between the two layers of the tunica vaginalis, may hinder the clinical examination but aid US by providing an acoustic window.

Management of testicular trauma depends on testicular integrity and perfusion. If the testis is ruptured, emergent surgery can salvage the testis in 80–90% of cases (Buckley and McAninch 2006). The surgical approach varies with the type of trauma.

Blunt Injuries

Fluid Collection
Hydrocele

Hydrocele is an anechoic fluid collection that occurs in the space between the two layers of the tunica vaginalis (Fig. 121.1). Acquired hydroceles usually occur as a reaction to trauma. In trauma, hydroceles can have low-level echoes or fibrin strands (Woodward et al. 2003). Also rupture of the bulbous urethra may result in extravasation of urine into the scrotum, mimicking a hydrocele.

Hematoceles

Similar to hydrocele, hematocele is a complex collection that separates the visceral and parietal layers of the tunica vaginalis (Fig. 121.2). Like hematomas, acutely it is echogenic and becomes more complex and more hypoechoic with age. Subacute and chronic hematocele may contain fluid-fluid levels or low-level internal echoes (Dogra et al. 2003).

Intratesticular Hematoma

Intratesticular hematoma is a common occurrence in the traumatized scrotum and may manifest various features. It may range in size from small to large, and may or may not be associated with other testicular and extratesticular injuries.

The US appearance of a hematoma depends on the time that has passed between the occurrence of trauma and the US evaluation. Hyperacute and acute hematoma appears hypo- or hyperechoic to the surrounding testicular parenchyma or may have a diffusely heterogeneous appearance (Fig. 121.3). Chronic hematoma appears more hypo or anechoic and tends to decrease in size as it resolves. Color Doppler imaging helps differentiate such hematomas from tumors, which are

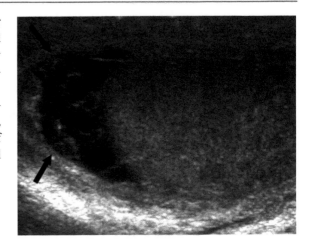

Fig. 121.1 Sagittal US image of the testis shows the presence of septate hydrocele (*black arrows*) in a patient with scrotal trauma

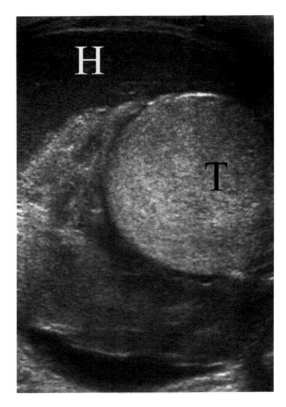

Fig. 121.2 Transverse US image of acute hematocele (*H*). The testis (*T*) shows normal echotexture

included in the differential diagnosis of intratesticular focal lesions (Kaye et al. 2008). Hematoma demonstrates an absence of vascularization (Fig. 121.4). A peripheral hyperemia is noted when it is superinfected.

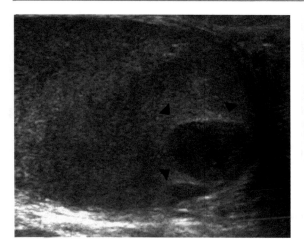

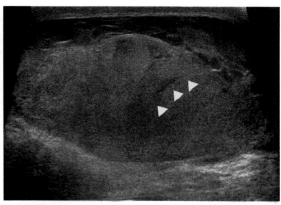

Fig. 121.5 Testicular fracture. Sagittal US image shows a diffuse heterogeneous echogenicity of the testicular parenchyma with a linear hypoechoic band that represents a testicular fracture (*arrowheads*)

Fig. 121.3 Intratesticular hematoma. Sagittal US image shows an ill-defined hypoechoic area (*arrowheads*) that represents the hematoma in the posterior part of the right testis

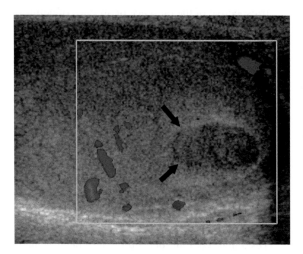

Fig. 121.4 Intratesticular hematoma (same case). Sagittal color Doppler US image demonstrates absence of flow in the area of hematoma

Small hematomas without any direct or indirect evidence of a testicular rupture are treated conservatively with clinical and US follow-up evaluation.

Follow-up US of all conservatively treated intratesticular hematomas until their resolution is essential, because of the high incidence rate of infection and necrosis, which may necessitate an orchiectomy. Another reason for continued follow-up is the fact that testicular tumors may be incidentally identified in patients with scrotal trauma and can be excluded if an intratesticular lesion shows progressive resolution (Blaivas and Brannam 2004). However, large intratesticular hematomas should be surgically explored and drained even in the absence of testis rupture, to reduce intratesticular pressure and ischemia, and resultant orchiectomy (Sung 2007).

Testicular Fracture

Testicular fracture refers to a break or discontinuity in the normal testicular parenchyma. A testicular fracture line is identified at US as a linear hypoechoic and avascular area within the testis, a finding that may or may not be associated with a tunica albuginea rupture (Fig. 121.5). A fracture line is rarely seen. Color Doppler imaging can help in identifying the fracture line and the presence of vascularity in the testicular parenchyma, indicative of its salvageability (Kaye et al. 2008).

Testicular Rupture

US plays a significant role in the early identification of a testicular rupture, allowing prompt surgical exploration and repair. Findings of a heterogeneous echotexture within the testis, testicular contour abnormality, and disruption of the tunica albuginea are considered sensitive and specific for the diagnosis of testicular rupture (Deurdulian et al. 2007; Bhatt and Dogra 2008; Buckley and McAninch 2006; Guichard et al. 2008) (Fig. 121.6). Buckley and McAninch demonstrated a sensitivity of 100% and a specificity of 93.5% for the diagnosis of testicular rupture on the basis of US findings of a heterogeneous echotexture and contour abnormality (Buckley and McAninch 2006). In addition, an absence of normal vascularity

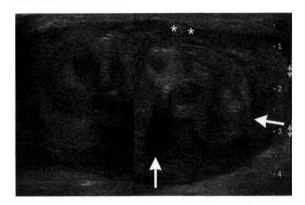

Fig. 121.6 Testicular rupture. Sagittal gray-scale US image of the left testis demonstrates an oblong testis with a heterogeneous echotexture and discontinuity in the tunica albuginea (*arrows*). The echogenic fluid surrounding the testis is consistent with a hematocele (*asterisk*)

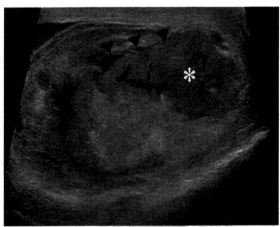

Fig. 121.8 Testicular rupture. Transverse US image of the testis shows a heterogeneous echotexture with discontinuity in the tunica albuginea and an intratesticular hematoma (*)

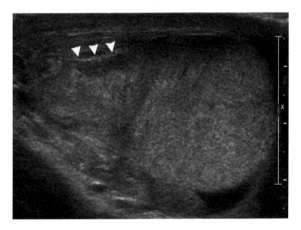

Fig. 121.7 Testicular rupture. Sagittal gray-scale US image demonstrates discontinuity in the tunica albuginea in the upper pole of the testis (*arrowheads*)

within the testis may help characterize a rupture. Then, the main US findings of testicular rupture are the following:

- *Disruption of the tunica albuginea* – At US, the normal tunica albuginea appears as two parallel hyperechoic layers outlining the testis. The demonstration at US of a discontinuity in the tunica albuginea in a patient with a clinical history of scrotal trauma supports the diagnosis of testicular rupture (Fig. 121.7). A large extratesticular hematocele may limit the capability of US for evaluating the tunica albuginea. In this case, surgical exploration should be performed in such patients,

irrespective of the presence or absence of definitive US signs of testicular rupture (Lee et al. 2008).

- *Contour abnormality of the testis* – Abnormality in the contour of the testis results from the extrusion of testicular parenchyma after disruption of the tunica albuginea (Dogra and Bhatt 2004; Bhatt et al. 2007). In the presence of a large extratesticular hematocele or large scrotal wall hematoma that may obscure a site of tunica disruption, an abnormality in the contour of the testis is consistent with rupture. US has a low accuracy for the diagnosis of testicular rupture on the basis of a finding of tunica disruption alone, with a reported sensitivity of 50% and specificity of 76% (Guichard et al. 2008). Testicular contour deformity and heterogeneous echotexture have been reported to increase the sensitivity and specificity of US for diagnosis of testicular rupture to 100% and 93.5% (Buckley and McAninch 2006).

- *Heterogeneous echotexture of the testis* – Heterogeneous echotexture and irregular testicular outline are associated with a tunica rupture. A heterogeneous echotexture of the testicular parenchyma, along with a contour abnormality of the testis, is considered highly sensitive and specific for the diagnosis of a testicular rupture (Bhatt and Dogra 2008; Kaye et al. 2008; Buckley and McAninch 2006) (Fig. 121.8). However, a heterogeneous echotexture also may be seen in the presence of intratesticular hematomas without a tunica albuginea rupture; therefore, it should not be considered indicative of testicular rupture unless it is accompanied by an observed tunica albuginea disruption or testicular contour irregularity (Jeffrey et al. 1983).

• Absence of vascularity in the testis – Color Doppler imaging is useful for the evaluation of traumatic injuries to the scrotum (Blaivas and Brannam 2004). Tunica albuginea rupture is almost always associated with a disruption of the tunica vasculosa because of the close apposition of the latter to the tunica albuginea. As a result, rupture of the testis results in a loss of vascularity to a portion or the

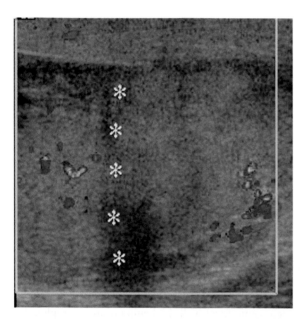

Fig. 121.9 Testicular rupture. Sagittal US color Doppler image shows a linear fracture in the middle testis (*asterisks*) with no flow in the inferior pole and extrusion of the testicular contents through the tunica albuginea

entirety of the testis, depending on the grade of injury (Deurdulian et al. 2007; Bhatt and Dogra 2008). The absence of vascularity in a focal area of the testis may be secondary to an intratesticular hematoma, which, if it is large, may require surgical evacuation (Fig. 121.9).

Testicular Dislocation

Testicular dislocation most commonly results from impact against the fuel tank in motorcycle accidents (Ječmenica et al. 2011). The possible sites of testicular dislocation are mainly in the inguinal canal, but other sites are also reported (Schwartz and Faerber 1994). In addition to US, computed tomography (CT) of the pelvis may be helpful for localizing a dislocated testis (Toranji and Barbaric 1994) (Fig. 121.10).

Delayed diagnosis of a dislocated testis and its tardy repositioning may lead to irreversible changes within the testis and may predispose it to malignant degeneration (Bromberg et al. 2003). A high index of suspicion combined with a careful physical examination and appropriate imaging are essential to avoid a delay in diagnosis.

Intratesticular Pseudoaneurysm

A pseudoaneurysm is a vascular leak that is surrounded and contained by a pseudocapsule. Intratesticular pseudoaneurysms are extremely rare (Pavlica and Barozzi 2001) and may result from either blunt or penetrating trauma. Gray-scale US demonstrates an anechoic area within the testis, which is filled by colors at color Doppler imaging (Fig. 121.11). Spectral Doppler at the neck of the pseudoaneurysmal sac reveals a to-and-fro flow pattern that is diagnostic of a pseudoaneurysm.

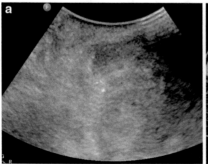
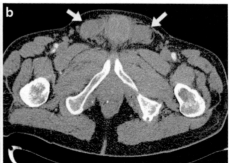
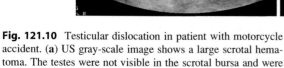

Fig. 121.10 Testicular dislocation in patient with motorcycle accident. (**a**) US gray-scale image shows a large scrotal hematoma. The testes were not visible in the scrotal bursa and were

found in the inguinal channels (not shown). (**b**) CT was performed because of the trauma and shows the position of the dislocated testes (*white arrows*)

Fig. 121.11 Testicular
rupture with pseudoaneurysm.
Gray-scale US demonstrates
an anechoic area within the
testis (**a**), which is filled by
colors at color Doppler
imaging (**b**)

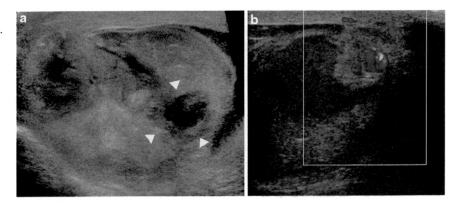

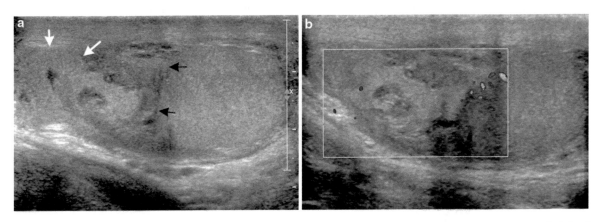

Fig. 121.12 Epididymal rupture. (**a**) US image shows a rupture of the upper pole of the testis (*black arrows*) with an ill-defined epididymis with heterogeneous echotexture (*white arrows*). (**b**) Color Doppler demonstrates absence of flow

Penetrating Injuries

The incidence of penetrating injuries to the scrotum has been on the rise over the years, paralleling with increasingly violent acts. They include gunshot injuries, stab wounds, and human or animal bites (Morey et al. 2004). Penetrating injuries range from a small insignificant hematocele to testicular rupture. The role of US in such cases is the same as in blunt trauma, which is to assess the severity of injuries in order to allow their appropriate management. Penetrating injuries secondary to animal bites, although rare, are potentially worrisome because they are associated with high risks of bacterial infection, tetanus, and rabies (Donovan and Kaplan 1989).

Scrotal Wall Hematoma

Scrotal wall hematoma is commonly associated with blunt trauma. It may be identified at US as an echogenic focal wall thickening or as a complex fluid collection within the wall, depending on the time that has passed between trauma and US examination. Scrotal wall hematomas usually resolve spontaneously or with conservative management, but those that are very large may require surgical evacuation.

Epididymal Fracture and Rupture

Epididymal injuries are usually seen in association with testicular injuries. The most commonly observed epididymal injury at US is traumatic epididymitis. Epididymal rupture is a common occurrence that is rarely diagnosed at US (Guichard et al. 2008). It is usually revealed during surgical exploration for testicular rupture or large hematoceles. An ill-defined epididymis with a heterogeneous echotexture and absence of blood flow (Fig. 121.12), in the presence of other intrascrotal injuries, should raise a suspicion of epididymal injury.

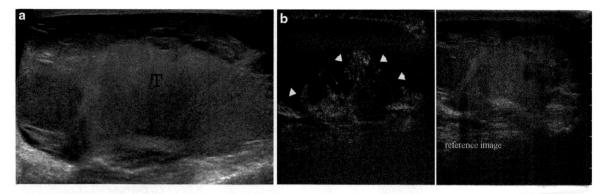

Fig. 121.13 Scrotal trauma. (**a**) Baseline US shows a nonhomogeneous testis (*T*) with extratesticular hematoma. (**b**) CEUS reveals a large hypoechoic hematoma within the testis with residual hyperechoic parenchyma (*arrows*). On the *right side* is reported the reference gray-scale image at low mechanical index

Unusual Complications and Findings

Scrotal trauma may be associated with acute epididymitis, epididymo-orchitis, and torsion. It has also been reported that 10–15% of testicular tumors are found incidentally at imaging after an episode of scrotal injury (Micallef et al. 2001).

Contrast-Enhanced Ultrasound (CEUS) in Traumatic Injuries

Contrast-enhanced ultrasound (CEUS) is a new tool for the sonographer. It can improve the depiction of parenchymal disorders on the basis of vascularity, helping in the differential diagnosis of focal lesions or traumatic changes (Moschouris et al. 2009; Valentino et al. 2011). In the testis, CEUS is able to demonstrate parenchymal vascularization, clearly depicting the fracture lines and the intratesticular hematoma, the interruption of the tunica albuginea, and the extratesticular hematoma (Fig. 121.13). It can assess exactly the amount of viable testis, allowing the urologist to decide when the partial salvage of the organ is a good solution (Hedayati et al. 2012). It can also be useful in the follow-up of nonoperative management, allowing a perfect evaluation of the amount of residual parenchyma of the patient.

MRI in Scrotal Trauma

US is a sensitive primary imaging modality of traumatic testicular lesions; however, the advent of MRI to

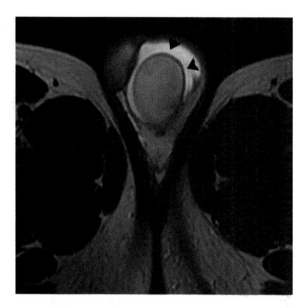

Fig. 121.14 MRI of normal testis. Axial T2-weighted MRI shows the intact tunica albuginea (*black arrowheads*). A moderate hydrocele is present

testicular lesions has improved the sensitivity of lesion characterization and localization.

MRI allows a better evaluation of integrity of the tunica albuginea. Tunica albuginea is well visualized on MRI as a dark signal intensity line on T2-weighted images (Kubik-Huch et al. 1999) (Fig. 121.14). Interruption of this dark signal intensity line is suggestive of testicular rupture (Kim et al. 2009) (Fig. 121.15).

Intratesticular hematoma may appear as hypoechoic lesion at US, giving a differential diagnosis with testicular neoplasm. MRI can resolve the doubt, because

Fig. 121.15 Testicular rupture. (**a**) Coronal T2-weighted MRI shows the fracture of the testis. Interruption of the dark signal intensity line of the tunica vaginalis (*arrows*) is consistent with rupture. (**b**) After contrast medium administration the rupture is well visualized

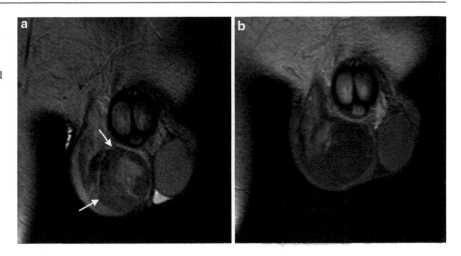

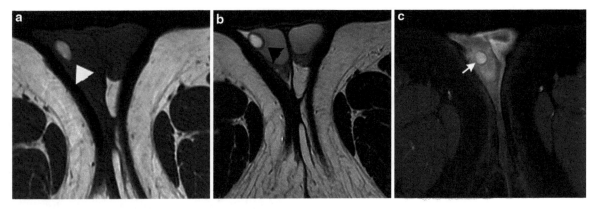

Fig. 121.16 Testicular hematoma. (**a**) Axial T1-weighted MRI shows hyperintensity of the lesion (*white arrowhead*) related to methemoglobin. (**b**) T2-weighted image shows the hyperintense lesion having a low-signal-intensity rim due to hemosiderin. (**c**) After contrast medium administration the lesion (*arrow*) does not show contrast uptake

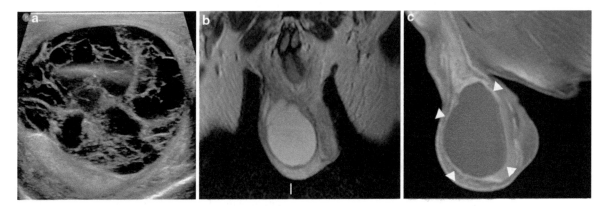

Fig. 121.17 Testicular hematoma. This patient presented at the emergency department for a swollen testis after trauma. US (**a**) showed a large ovoid cystic mass with multiple thin septa. Because of the uncertain diagnosis, an MRI was performed. The T2-weighted image (**b**) shows a mass with high intensity signal without enhancement after contrast medium administration (**c**). The diagnosis of hematoma was confirmed in the operating room

hematoma has T1 hyperintensity related to methemo-globin, and a characteristic hypointense perilesional rim on T2 related to the concentration of hemosiderin-laden macrophages (Fig. 121.16), whereas neoplasm appears hypointense on T1- and T2-weighted images, with contrast enhancement after contrast agent administration. MRI can also provide the stage of hematoma because of the known characteristic signal intensity of the evolutional change in combination with T1and T2 signals. In fact, in the hyperacute phase (4–6 h), hematoma has a high signal intensity on T2. In the acute phase (7–72 h), a central dark intensity appears in the high signal intensity background on T2; and in the late subacute phase (1–4 weeks), high signal intensity is seen on T2 and T1 (Osborn 1994).

In cases in which it is difficult to differentiate hematoma from abscess based on MRI and US, consideration may be given to follow-up MR studies to determine whether the signal characteristics follow those of degrading blood (Gupta et al. 2005) (Fig. 121.17).

The availability of MRI decreases its present value in clinical practice, but its outstanding accuracy makes it an interesting addition to the present diagnostic armamentarium.

Pearls to Remember

- Patient with scrotal trauma presents with acute swelling, pain, ecchymosis, lacerations, or skin loss. An adequate physical examination may often be difficult to obtain secondary to swelling. Therefore, imaging studies are often required to confirm diagnoses and evaluate the extent of injury.
- US provides a simple and rapid method to evaluate the scrotal contents and aids in distinguishing among the various pathologic entities.
- MRI can be a useful secondary imaging tool in limited conditions, especially in which US provides an inconclusive diagnosis.

References

Bhatt S, Dogra VS. Role of US in testicular and scrotal trauma. Radiographics. 2008;28:1617–29.

Bhatt S, Ghazale H, Dogra VS. Sonographic evaluation of scrotal and penile trauma. Ultrasound Clin. 2007;2:45–56.

Blaivas M, Brannam L. Testicular ultrasound. Emerg Med Clin North Am. 2004;22:723–48.

Bromberg W, Wong C, Kurek S, Salim A. Traumatic bilateral testicular dislocation. J Trauma. 2003;54:1009–11.

Buckley JC, McAninch JW. Use of ultrasonography for the diagnosis of testicular injuries in blunt scrotal trauma. J Urol. 2006;175:175–8.

Cass AS, Luxenberg M. Testicular trauma. Urology. 1991;37:528–30.

Chandra RV, Dowling RJ, Ulubasoglu M, Haxhimolla H, Costello AJ. Rational approach to diagnosis and management of blunt scrotal trauma. Urology. 2007;70:230–4.

Deurdulian C, Mittelstaedt CA, Chong WK, Fielding JR. US of acute scrotal trauma: optimal technique, imaging findings, and management. Radiographics. 2007;27:357–69.

Djakovic N, Plas E, Martínez-Piñeiro L, Santucci RA, Serafetinidis E, Turkeri LN, Hohenfellner M. Guidelines on urological trauma. Eur Urol. 2010;57:791–803.

Dogra V, Bhatt S. Acute painful scrotum. Radiol Clin North Am. 2004;42:349–63.

Dogra VS, Gottlieb RH, Oka M, Rubens DJ. Sonography of the scrotum. Radiology. 2003;227:18–36.

Donovan JF, Kaplan WE. The therapy of genital trauma by dog bite. J Urol. 1989;141:1163–5.

Guichard G, El Ammari J, Del Coro C, Cellarier D, Loock PY, Chabannes E, Bernardini S, Bittard H, Kleinclauss F. Accuracy of ultrasonography in diagnosis of testicular rupture after blunt scrotal trauma. Urology. 2008;71:52–6.

Gupta R, Alobaidi M, Jafri SZ, Bis K, Amendola M. Correlation of US and MRI findings of intratesticular and paratesticular lesions: from infants to adults. Curr Probl Diagn Radiol. 2005;34:35–45.

Hedayati V, Sellars ME, Sharma M, Sidhu PS. Contrast-enhanced ultrasound in testicular trauma: role in directing exploration, debridement and organ salvage. Br J Radiol. 2012;85:e65–8.

Ječmenica DS, Alempijević DM, Pavlekić S, Aleksandrić BV. Traumatic testicular displacement in motorcycle drivers. J Forensic Sci. 2011;56:541–3.

Jeffrey RB, Laing FC, Hricak H, McAninch JW. Sonography of testicular trauma. Am J Roentgenol. 1983;141:993–5.

Kaye JD, Shapiro EY, Levitt SB, Friedman SC, Gitlin J, Freyle J, Palmer LS. Parenchymal echo texture predicts testicular salvage after torsion: potential impact on the need for emergent exploration. J Urol. 2008;180:1733–6.

Kim SH, Park S, Choi SH, Jeong WK, Choi JH. The efficacy of magnetic resonance imaging for the diagnosis of testicular rupture: a prospective preliminary study. J Trauma. 2009;66:239–42.

Kubik-Huch RA, Hailemariam S, Hamm B. CT and MRI of the male genital tract: radiologic-pathologic correlation. Eur Radiol. 1999;9:16–28.

Lee SH, Bak CW, Choi MH, Lee HS, Lee MS, Yoon SJ. Trauma to male genital organs: a 10-year review of 156 patients, including 118 treated by surgery. BJU Int. 2008;101:211–5.

Micallef M, Ahmad I, Ramesh N, Hurley M, McInerney D. Ultrasound features of blunt testicular injury. Injury. 2001;32:23–6.

Morey AF, Metro MJ, Carney KJ, McAninch JW. Consensus on genitourinary trauma. BJU Int. 2004;94:507–15.

Moschouris H, Stamatiou K, Lampropoulou E, Kalikis D, Matsaidonis D. Imaging of the acute scrotum: is there a place for contrast-enhanced ultrasonography? Int Braz J Urol. 2009;35:692–702.

Osborn AG. Intracranial hemorrhage. In: Osborn AG, editor. Diagnostic neuroradiology. St. Louis: Mosby; 1994. p. 154–8.

Parenti GC, Feletti F, Brandini F, Palmarini D, Zago S, Ginevra A, Campioni P, Mannella P. Imaging of the scrotum: role of MRI. Radiol Med. 2009;114:414–24.

Pavlica P, Barozzi L. Imaging of the acute scrotum. Eur Radiol. 2001;11:220–8.

Schwartz SL, Faerber GJ. Dislocation of the testis as a delayed presentation of scrotal trauma. Urology. 1994;43:743–5.

Toranji S, Barbaric Z. Testicular dislocation. Abdom Imaging. 1994;19:379–80.

Valentino M, Bertolotto M, Derchi L, Bertaccini A, Pavlica P, Martorana G, Barozzi L. Role of contrast enhanced ultrasound in acute scrotal diseases. Eur Radiol. 2011;21:1831–40.

Wessells H, Long L. Penile and genital injuries. Urol Clin North Am. 2006;33:117–26.

Woodward PJ, Schwab CM, Sesterhenn IA. Extratesticular scrotal masses: radiologic-pathologic correlation. Radiographics. 2003;23:215–40.

Infertility (Including Varicocele)

122

Min Hoan Moon and Seung Hyup Kim

Infertility is defined as an inability to initiate a pregnancy in spite of unprotected intercourse of over 12 months. Infertility is caused by either male factors or female factors. Male factors are fully responsible for infertile couples in about 30% and, in another 20%, the male factors contribute to infertility along with female factors. Therefore, male factors are found in up to approximately 50% of infertile couples (Brugh and Lipshultz 2004). The evaluation of infertile men begins with a detailed medical history and a focused physical examination and then proceeds to appropriate laboratory tests including the semen analysis, the hormonal assays, the sperm function tests, and the genetic tests. Imaging studies can be used selectively as part of the comprehensive evaluation of male infertility for specific indications. In this chapter, we review the spectrum of diseases responsible for male infertility, discuss appropriate imaging modalities to be proven for specific clinical settings, and illustrate characteristic imaging features that permit specific diagnosis, with three main headings of obstruction in sperm passage, defect in sperm production, and impairment in sperm function.

M.H. Moon (✉)
Department of Radiology, Seoul Metropolitan Boramae Medical Center, Seoul National University, College of Medicine, Dongjak-Gu, Seoul, South Korea

S.H. Kim
Department of Radiology, Seoul National University Hospital, Seoul National University, College of Medicine, Chongno-gu, Seoul, South Korea

Obstruction in Sperm Passage

Infertile men with obstruction in sperm passage are usually presented with decreased sperm count (oligospermia or azoospermia) on the semen analysis. In such cases, the first step is to distinguish infertile men with defects in sperm production from those with obstruction in sperm passage. Scrotal US can be helpful in distinguishing defects in sperm production from obstruction in sperm passage (Moon et al. 2006). The presence of epididymal abnormalities depicted by scrotal US is more likely to be associated with obstruction in sperm passage than defects in sperm production and measured testis volume is higher in infertile men with obstruction in sperm passage than in those with defects in sperm production. If decreased sperm count is considered to be associated with obstruction in sperm passage, the next step is to identify the location of obstruction site. Obstructions can occur anywhere along the genital duct (epididymis, vas deferens, and ejaculatory duct) but proximal and distal genital duct obstruction account for most of obstruction in sperm passage. Scrotal US is used to demonstrate the pathologies causing proximal genital duct obstructions (e.g., chronic epididymitis) and transrectal US is performed to reveal the pathologies causing distal genital duct obstruction (e.g., congenital absence of the vas deferens or ejaculatory duct obstruction). The causes of genital duct obstruction are summarized in Table 122.1.

Pearls to Remember
- In infertile men with oligospermia or azoospermia, the first step is to distinguish infertile men with defects in sperm production from those with obstruction in sperm passage.

B. Hamm, P. R. Ros (eds.), *Abdominal Imaging*, DOI 10.1007/978-3-642-13327-5_211,
© Springer-Verlag Berlin Heidelberg 2013

Table 122.1 The causes for genital duct obstruction according to obstruction level

Obstruction level		Conditions	
Epididymis		Chronic epididymitis	
Vas deferens	Scrotal portion	Operation, trauma, iatrogenic	
	Inguinal portion	Operation, trauma, iatrogenic	
	Pelvic portion	Congenital absence of the vas deferens	
Ejaculatory duct		Ejaculatory duct obstruction	Inflammation associated
			Midline cysts associated

- If decreased sperm count is considered to be associated with obstruction in sperm passage, the next step is to identify the location of obstruction site. The combination of scrotal and transrectal US can be helpful in demonstrating most of pathologies causing obstruction in sperm passage.

Chronic Epididymitis

The epididymis consists of highly convoluted epididymal ducts that connect the seminiferous tubules to the vas deferens. Chronic epididymitis may affect male fertility through post-inflammatory obstruction of the epididymal ducts (Breeland et al. 1981). Scortal US is the procedure of choice in the evaluation of the proximal genital duct. On scrotal US, chronic epididymitis appears as focal or diffuse enlargement of the epididymis with heterogenous echogenicity (Fig. 122.1). Calcifications are often noted within the inflammatory mass. In addition, upstream dilatation of the epididymis (e.g., dilatation of the epididymal body in the case of chronic epididymitis of the epididymal tail) can be depicted on scrotal US. Because the determination of obstruction site may have important implications for selection of an appropriate treatment plan (Brugh and Lipshultz 2004; Kim and Lipshultz 1999), it is recommended to assess the possible obstruction site as well as the presence or absence of chronic epididymitis.

Pearls to Remember
- Scortal US is the procedure of choice in the evaluation of chronic epididymitis.
- Chronic epididymitis appears as focal or diffuse enlargement of the epididymis with heterogenous echogenicity on scrotal US, with upstream dilatation of the epididymis.

Congenital Absence of the Vas Deferens (CAVD)

CAVD can be divided into two groups according to their association with cystic fibrosis; the cases with mutation in cystic fibrosis transmembrane regulator gene (CFTR gene) and the cases without mutation in CFTR gene (Quinzii and Castellani 2000; Daudin et al. 2000). The former is the most common cause of obstructive azoospermia and usually presents as bilateral absence of the vas deferens without other clinical manifestations of cystic fibrosis. The presumed mechanism for absence of bilateral vas deferens is that the mutation in CFTR gene causes abnormal glycoprotein secretion from the epididymis, leads to subsequent obstruction in distal genital ducts, and results in progressive atrophy of the distal genital ducts (Tizzano et al. 1994). Transrectal US is the procedure of choice for demonstrating absence of bilateral vas deferens (Fig. 122.2). Due to the embryologic association, most of CAVD have associated seminal vesicle hypoplasia or agenesis. On the contrary to cystic fibrosis related CAVD, CAVD irrelevant to CFTR gene is a developmental anomaly of the Wolffian duct system, presenting as unilateral absence of the vas deferens associated with ipsilateral genitourinary anomaly such as renal agenesis or seminal vesicle cyst. CAVD irrelevant to CFTR gene is less responsible for male infertility than cystic fibrosis related CAVD because of its unilateral involvement of the genital duct.

Pearls to Remember
- Transrectal US is the procedure of choice in the evaluation of CAVD.
- Cystic fibrosis related CAVD is the most common cause of obstructive azoospermia and the absence of bilateral vas deferens is well demonstrated by using transrectal US.

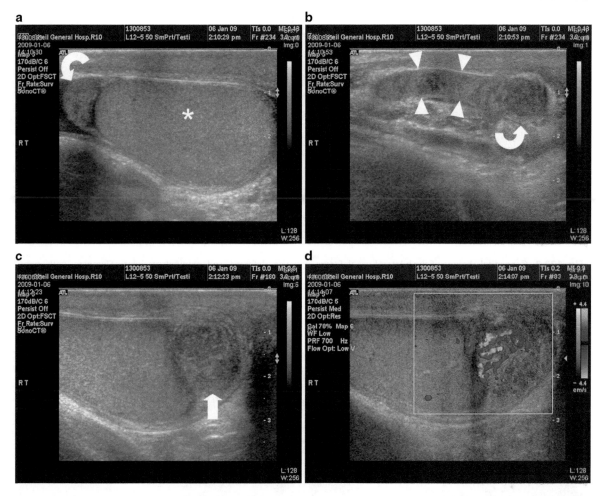

Fig. 122.1 Chronic epididymitis involving the epididymal tail in a 35-year-old man. (**a**) The testis (*asterisk*) and the epididymal head (*curved arrow*) seem to be normal on the longitudinal scan of the right scrotum. (**b**) In the right paratesticular area, dilated right epididymal body (*arrowheads*) is noted and the epididymal system begins to enlarge in the portion of the right epididymal tail (*curved arrow*). (**c**) On the longitudinal scan of the right scrotum, the right epididymal tail (*arrow*) forms an ill defined mass of heterogeneous echogenicity, suggestive of inflammatory mass. (**d**) Color Doppler US image shows prominent blood flow signal within the inflammatory mass involving the right epididymal tail

Ejaculatory Duct Obstruction: Inflammation Associated

Ejaculatory duct obstructions, a complication of seminal vesiculitis or prostatitis, are one of the important causes of male infertility. Traditionally, vasography was the gold standard for the diagnosis of ejaculatory duct obstruction, but its invasiveness with the potential risk of vasal scarring has narrowed its clinical use in the evaluation of ejaculatory duct obstruction. With the recent advance of transrectal US, transrectal US has become the most popular alternative to vasography because it is non-invasive and relatively inexpensive. On transrectal US, the diagnosis of ejaculatory duct obstruction is suggested by demonstrating ejaculatory duct cysts, echogenic lines along the course of the ejaculatory duct, or distension of the ejaculatory duct and/or seminal vesicle (Fig. 122.3). Although in theory, ejaculatory duct obstruction should result in the

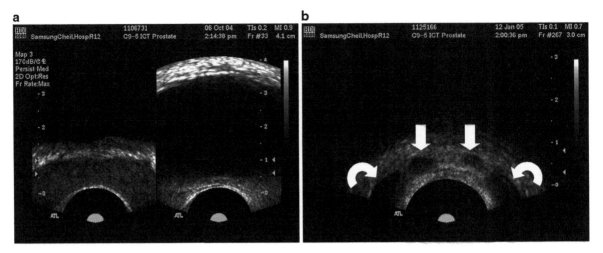

Fig. 122.2 Congenital absence of the bilateral vas deferens in a 36-year-old infertile man. The image acquired above the level of the prostate base (*right* in (**a**)) shows no demonstrable both vas deferens and seminal vesicles. Compare with normal transrectal US appearance of vas deferens (*arrows*) and seminal vesicle (*curved arrows*) in (**b**)

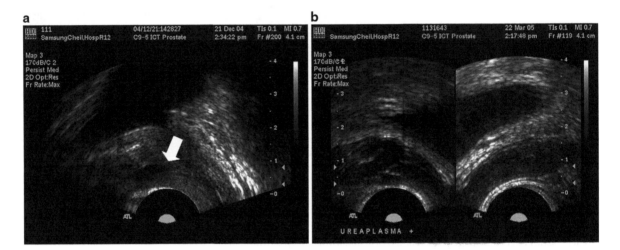

Fig. 122.3 US imaging findings of ejaculatory duct obstruction. (**a**) Longitudinal US image of the prostate gland shows luminal distension of the ejaculatory duct (*arrow*). The lumen of the ejaculatory duct is normally not demonstrated on transrectal US. (**b**) Seminal vesicle dilatation is another US imaging finding suggestive of ejaculatory duct obstruction. On oblique US image along the presumed long axis of both vas deferens, the right seminal vesicle is markedly dilated compared to the left side

dilatation of the seminal vesicle, it does not always occur in every patient because chronic epididymitis of atrophic change often goes with ejaculatory duct obstruction. Of notable, the transrectal US suggestion of ejaculatory duct obstruction should be done with caution because anatomical abnormalities, depicted by transrectal US, do not have consistent causal relationship with ejaculatory duct obstruction (Colpi et al. 1997; Purohit et al. 2004).

Pearls to Remember

- Transrectal US is the procedure of choice in the evaluation of inflammation-associated ejaculatory duct obstruction.
- Transrectal US diagnosis of ejaculatory duct obstruction is suggested by demonstrating ejaculatory duct cysts, echogenic lines along the course of the ejaculatory duct, or distension of the ejaculatory duct and/or seminal vesicle.

a

b

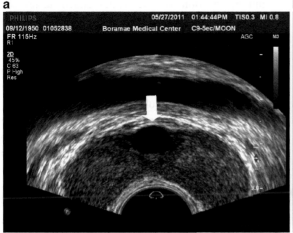

Fig. 122.4 A midline cyst in a 62-year-old man. A midline cyst appears as a round- or oval-shaped cyst (*arrow*) on the transverse scan of the prostate base (**a**) and as teardrop- or oval-shaped cysts (*curved arrow*) on the longitudinal scan (**b**) behind the verumontanum along the midline of the prostate gland

Ejaculatory Duct Obstruction: Midline Cysts

In infertile men with suspicion of ejaculatory duct obstruction, cystic lesions located along the midline of the prostate gland are commonly seen on transrectal US. Based on their embryologic origin, the cystic lesions can be classified into utricular cysts, Müllerian duct cysts, and ejaculatory duct cysts. Utricular cysts derive from a dilatation of the prostatic utricle and are often associated with other malformations, such as hypospadia or virilization defect (Hinman 1993). Unlike utricular cysts, Müllerian duct cysts, the embryologic remnants of the Müllerian duct, do not communicate with the prostatic urethra and are usually larger than utricular cysts. Ejaculatory duct cysts are of Wolffian duct origin and contain spermatozoa in their content. Ejaculatory duct cysts are the consequence of diverticulum formation from the obstruction of the ejaculatory duct, whereas both utricular cysts and Müllerian duct cysts may cause compression and displacement of the ejaculatory ducts, resulting in obstruction. However, transrectal US findings of those cystic lesions are similar irrespective of their embryologic origin and appear as teardrop- or oval-shaped cysts behind the verumontanum along the midline of the prostate gland (Fig. 122.4).

Pearls to Remember
- Based on embryologic origin, the midline cysts can be classified into utricular cysts, Müllerian duct cysts and ejaculatory duct cysts.

- Ejaculatory duct cysts are the result arising from the obstruction of the ejaculatory duct, whereas both utricular cysts and Müllerian duct cysts are etiology causing ejaculatory duct obstruction.

Defects in Sperm Production

Defects in sperm production can be divided into primary and secondary testicular failure (Table 122.2). Primary testicular failure results from end-organ failure, while secondary testicular failure results from hormonal imbalance of the hypothalamic-pituitary-gonadal axis. Initial endocrine evaluations help to distinguish primary testicular failure from secondary testicular failure. In the cases of primary testicular failure, endocrine evaluations show an elevated serum FSH level and a normal or low serum testosterone level. On the other hand, secondary testicular failure presents with low serum level of testosterone, LH, and FSH. Imaging studies are of limited value for evaluation of primary testicular failure. Small volume of both testes, irrespective of underlying etiologies, is the only imaging finding of primary testicular failure. The volume of the testis is usually measured by scrotal US. In contrast, for secondary testicular failure, a specific diagnosis can be made by cross-sectional imaging including CT or MR which can provide specific imaging features that, in association with clinical findings, allow a specific diagnosis to be made.

Table 122.2 The classification of defects in sperm production

Classification	Underlying pathology
Primary testicular failure	Y-chromosome microdeletion
	Klinefelter syndrome
	Cryptorchidism
	Viral or bacterial orchitis
Secondary testicular failure	Hemochromatosis
	Kallmann syndrome
	Hyperprolactinemia
	Congenital adrenal hyperplasia
	Androgen insensitivity syndrome

Pearls to Remember

- In primary testicular failure, small volume of both testes is the only imaging finding irrespective of underlying etiologies and the volume of the testis is usually measured by scrotal US.
- In secondary testicular failure, cross-sectional imaging including CT or MR can provide specific imaging features that allow a specific diagnosis to be made.

Primary Testicular Failure

A variety of underlying pathologies ranging from chromosomal abnormalities (numerical or structural) to congenital anomaly or infection can lead to primary testicular failure (Table 122.2). The two most common chromosomal abnormalities are Y-chromosome microdeletion and Klinefelter syndrome. Y-chromosome microdeletion is the defect of the genes on the long arm of the Y chromosome that are necessary for normal spermatogenesis and it accounts for 10–15% of infertile men with azoospermia or severe oligospermia. Klinefelter syndrome is the sex chromosome disorder (47, XXY) in which an extra X chromosome shortens the life span of the testicular germ cell, leading to azoospermia. Patients with this syndrome can present with the classic triad of small testes, azoospermia, and gynecomastia and Klinefelter syndrome can be found in up to 14% of infertile men with azoospermia (Rao and Rao 1977). Cryptorchidism is defined as failure of intraabdominal testes to descend into the scrotal sac and can lead to male infertility, especially in the cases of bilateral cryptorchidism. The inguinal canal (72%) is the most

common location of the undescended testes and followed by high scrotal (20%) and intraabdominal (8%) locations. As mentioned above, imaging studies are usually not helpful in making a specific diagnosis of primary testicular failure, except for cryptorchidism (Fig. 122.5). Instead, the role of imaging in the evaluation of primary testicular failure is to differentiate primary testicular failure from obstruction in sperm passage. Scrotal US can be helpful in distinguishing primary testicular failure from obstruction in sperm passage (Moon et al. 2006). On scrotal US, presence of epididymal abnormalities including tubular ectasia, tapering, absence, or inflammatory mass formation are more likely to be associated with obstruction in sperm passage than primary testicular failure (Fig. 122.6). Volume measurement of the testis is also helpful in distinguishing obstruction in sperm passage from primary testicular failure. Testis volumes can be measured by using the empiric formula of Lambert (1951): length * height * width * 0.71. According to our experience, testes with a volume of less than 10 ml are likely to have primary testicular failure, whereas those with a volume of more than 15 ml are likely to have obstruction in sperm passage. Intermediate-sized testis volume of 10–15 ml has the possibility of both primary testicular failure and obstruction in sperm passage.

Pearls to Remember

- Testes with a volume of less than 10 ml are likely to have primary testicular failure, whereas those with a volume of more than 15 ml are likely to have obstruction in sperm passage.
- Epididymal abnormalities including tubular ectasia, tapering, absence, or inflammatory mass formation is suggestive of obstruction in sperm passage.

Hemochromatosis

Hemochromatosis is a disorder of abnormal iron metabolism characterized by excess iron deposition in end organs that causes cellular damage and organ dysfunction. Hemochromatosis can be classified as primary (or genetic) hemochromatosis and secondary (or acquired) hemochromatosis. Primary hemochromatosis is an autosomal recessive disorder in which increase of intestinal iron absorption results in iron deposition in end organs whereas,

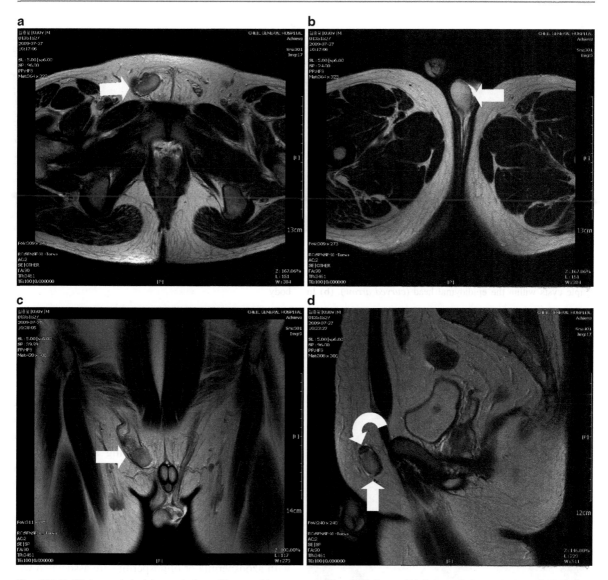

Fig. 122.5 Undescended right testis in a 30-year-old man. (**a, b**) T2-weighted axial images show undescended right testis (*arrow* in (**a**)) within the right inguinal canal. Note that the left testis (*arrow* in (**b**)) is normally located within the left scrotal sac. (**c, d**) Undescended right testis (*arrow* in (**c**) and (**d**)) is best expressed through coronal (**c**) and sagittal (**d**) T2-weighted images. Note the right epididymal head (*curved arrow* in (**d**)) of low signal intensity, just upper to the undescended right testis

in secondary hemochromatosis, iron deposition ensues from dietary iron overload, commonly in the form of repeated blood transfusion. Excess iron deposition in the pituitary gland affects male fertility in the form of hypogonadotropic hypogonadism (Siminoski et al. 1990; Bhansali 1992). MR is the most reliable imaging tool in the identification of iron deposition in the pituitary gland. Paramagnetic effect caused by iron deposition leads to signal loss of the pituitary gland on T2-weighted image (Fig. 122.7).

Pearls to Remember

- In the hemochromatosis, excess iron deposition in the anterior lobe of the pituitary gland leads to male infertility in the form of hypogonadotropic hypogonadism.
- Magnetic resonance imaging is the most reliable imaging tool in the diagnosis of hemochromatosis related infertility. Paramagnetic effect caused by iron deposition leads to signal loss of the pituitary gland on T2-weighted image.

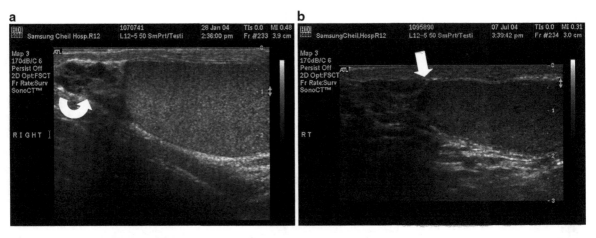

Fig. 122.6 Epididymal abnormalities suggestive of obstruction in sperm passage. (**a**) In a 30-year-old man proved to be CAVD patient, longitudinal US image of the right scrotum shows multiple cysts within the epididymal head (*curved arrow*). (**b**) In a 30-year-old man proved to be CAVD patient, longitudinal US image through the right paratesticular area shows abrupt narrowing (*arrow*) in the proximal portion of the epididymal body

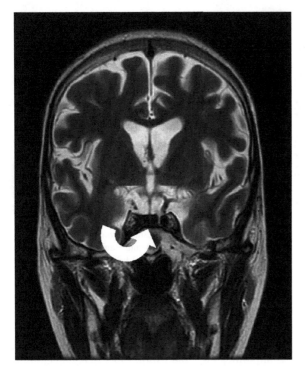

Fig. 122.7 Hemochromatosis in a 23-year-old man. Coronal T2-weighted image shows dark signal intensity (*curved arrow*) of the pituitary gland. Paramagnetic effect caused by iron deposition causes signal loss of the pituitary gland on T2-weighted image

Kallmann Syndrome

Idiopathic hypogonadotropic hypogonadism is defined as the cases in which abnormal synthesis and release of gonadotropin-releasing hormone lead to hypogonadism without underlying structural abnormalities. Kallmann syndrome is a subtype of idiopathic hypogonadotropic hypogonadism associated with anosmia and is the most common X-linked disorder in male infertility, with an incidence of 1 in 10,000–60,000 (Bick et al. 1992). The diagnosis of Kallmann syndrome is suspected when infertile men with azoospermia or oligospermia are associated with anosmia or hyposmia. The central to the imaging of Kallmann syndrome is to demonstrate the absence or hypoplasia of olfactory bulbs and tracts that can best be evaluated with MR (Fig. 122.8) (Yousem et al. 1996).

Pearls to Remember

- Kallmann syndrome is suspected when infertile men with azoospermia or oligospermia are associated with anosmia or hyposmia.
- The central to the imaging of infertile men suspected of Kallmann syndrome is to demonstrate the absence or hypoplasia of olfactory bulbs and tracts that can best be evaluated with MR.

Fig. 122.8 MR imaging of Kallmann syndrome. Coronal T2-weighted image (**a**) in a 28-year-old infertile man with anosmia shows absence of the olfactory tracts, suggesting the diagnosis of Kallmann syndrome. Compare with the normal olfactory tracts (*arrowheads* in (**b**)) obtained in a normal volunteer

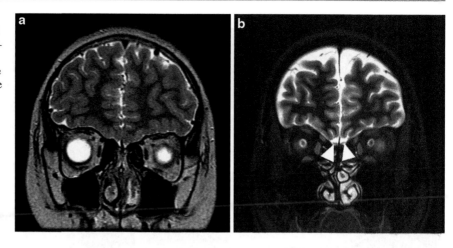

Fig. 122.9 Pituitary microadenoma in a 32-year-old man. (**a**) Prior to contrast material administration, mild convexity of the right portion of the pituitary gland is suspected but not definite on coronal T1-weighted image. (**b**) In the early phase of dynamic imaging, pituitary microadenoma (*arrow*) becomes apparent because pituitary microadenoma shows relatively weak enhancement compared to the normal pituitary gland

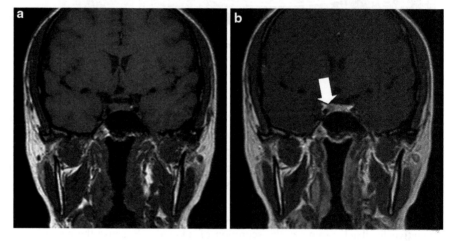

Hyperprolactinemia

The suppression of gonadotropin-releasing hormone induced by hyperprolactinemia can cause male infertility through a decrease in luteinizing hormone and follicle-stimulating hormone. Hyperprolactinemia can be suspected in infertile men with decreased libido, impotence, galactorrhea, or gynecomastia. The major cause of hyperprolactinemia is prolactin-producing pituitary adenoma. Pituitary macroadenomas can be easily identified on conventional MR. However, dynamic study with intravenous bolus injection of the contrast medium is needed for confidential assessment of pituitary microadenomas (Fig. 122.9). On dynamic MR, the normal pituitary gland and stalk have strong enhancement in the early phase acquired within 1 min after contrast injection, whereas microadenomas have relatively weak enhancement compared with the normal pituitary gland (Bartynski and Lin 1997).

Pearls to Remember

- Hyperprolactinemia can be suspected in infertile men with decreased libido, impotence, galactorrhea, or gynecomastia.
- The most common cause of hyperprolactinemia is prolactinomas that can be best evaluated with dynamic MR with intravenous bolus injection of the contrast medium.

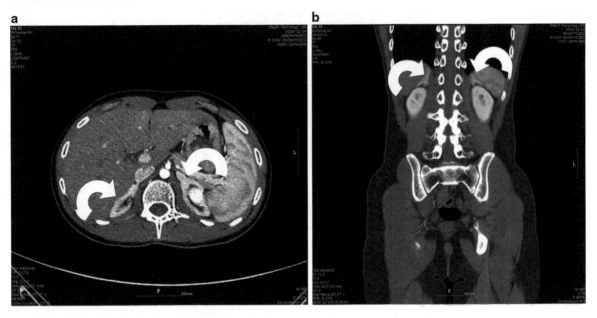

Fig. 122.10 Congenital adrenal hyperplasia in an 18-year-old man. Axial (**a**) and coronal (**b**) postcontrast CT scan show diffuse enlargement of both adrenal glands (*curved arrows*) with preservation of normal configuration

Congenital Adrenal Hyperplasia

Congenital adrenal hyperplasia is a group of autosomal recessive disorders with a deficiency of one of adrenocortical enzymes necessary for cortisol synthesis. More than 90% of cases result from a deficiency of 21-hydroxylase. The elevated ACTH level from loss of negative feedback promotes the secretion of adrenal androgens that inhibit the release of luteinizing hormone and follicle-stimulating hormone, leading to hypogonadotropic hypogonadism. Computed tomography is the primary imaging modality in the evaluation of the adrenal gland. Congenital adrenal hyperplasia appears as diffuse enlargement of both adrenal glands with preservation of normal configuration (Fig. 122.10) (Johnson et al. 2009). However, the presence of normal-sized adrenal glands does not exclude the diagnosis of congenital adrenal hyperplasia (Bryan et al. 1988).

Pearls to Remember

- Computed tomography is the primary imaging modality in the evaluation of the adrenal gland.
- Congenital adrenal hyperplasia appears as diffuse enlargement of both adrenal glands with preservation of normal configuration.

Androgen Insensitivity Syndrome

Androgen insensitivity (testicular feminization) syndrome is a rare syndrome that a lack of functional androgen receptor leads to an absence of Wolffian duct derivatives and development of a female phenotype (Coulam et al. 1984; Rutgers and Scully 1991). Because the patients with androgen insensitivity syndrome usually present as a female phenotype, the diagnosis is usually made in the work-up of women with amenorrhea. The role of imaging is to assess the internal genitalia and to provide clinician androgen insensitivity syndrome as a possible cause of amenorrhea. Imaging studies not only can demonstrate the absence of müllerian duct derivatives such as the uterus but also can show undescended testes in the inguinal canal or abdominal cavity (Fig. 122.11) (Gambino et al. 1992; Gale 1983).

Pearls to Remember

- Androgen insensitivity syndrome usually presents as a female phenotype without genital ambiguity.
- In women with amenorrhea, the absence of Müllerian duct derivatives and the presence of possible undescended testes suggest the diagnosis of androgen insensitivity syndrome.

Fig. 122.11 MR imaging of androgen insensitivity syndrome. (**a**) Coronal T2-weighted image shows both intraabdominal undescended testes (*arrows*) in the abdominal cavity. Note that the multiloculated cystic masses (*arrowheads*) adjacent to undescended testes are deformed epididymal structures. (**b**) On sagittal T2-weighted image, the uterus is absent and the vagina (*arrow*) ends as a blind pouch. Note that the external genitalia looks female.

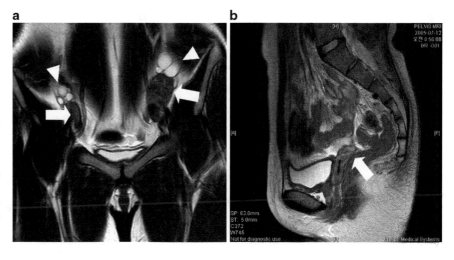

Impairments in Sperm Function

Infertile men with impairments in sperm function are generally presented with decreased sperm motility (asthenozoospermia) or abnormal sperm morphology (teratozoospermia). A variety of causes has been found to cause impairments in sperm function. Among these, imaging studies have role in the evaluation of varicocele and Kartagener syndrome.

Varicocele

Varicocele, abnormal dilatation of the pampiniform plexus, is the most common cause of male infertility, accounting for 40% of primary infertility and 45–80% of secondary infertility (Brugh and Lipshultz 2004; Brugh et al. 2003). It is uncertain how varicocele leads to male infertility. According to the most commonly accepted theory, varicoceles increase scrotal temperature and subsequent hyperthermia interferes with normal spermatogenesis, leading to decreased sperm count, decreased sperm motility, and abnormal sperm morphology (Takihara et al. 1991). Scrotal US is the primary imaging modality for identification of varicoceles. The presence of varicocele can be made by demonstrating anatomic and physiologic aspects of varicocele. On gray scale US, varicoceles appear as dilated tubular structures along the course of the spermatic cord.

The addition of Doppler US with the Valsalva maneuver confirms the diagnosis of varicocele by demonstrating prolonged, intense color flow signal within the dilated tubular structure on color Doppler evaluation and by showing retrograde filling of the dilated tubular structure on spectral Doppler interrogation (Fig. 122.12). However, it is noted that transient reflux during the Valsalva maneuver should not be mistaken for presence of varicoceles.

Pearls to Remember
- The use of color or pulsed Doppler US during the Valsalva maneuver confirms the diagnosis of varicocele by demonstrating prolonged color flow signal and retrograde filling of the dilated tubular structure along the spermatic cord.
- Transient reflux during the Valsalva maneuver should not be mistaken for presence of varicoceles.

Primary Ciliary Dyskinesia

Primary ciliary dyskinesia, also known as immotile ciliary syndrome, is a rare autosomal recessive disorder of ciliary dysfunction that causes upper and lower airway infection from impaired mucociliary clearance (Noone et al. 2004). In approximately half of cases, primary ciliary dyskinesia is associated with situs inversus. Kartagener syndrome is a subgroup of primary ciliary dyskinesia characterized by the clinical triad of sinusitis, bronchiectasis, and situs inversus.

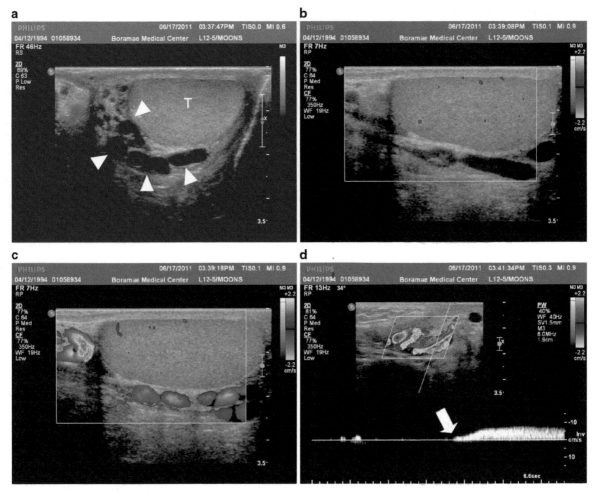

Fig. 122.12 Varicocele in an 18-year-old man. (**a**) Transverse US image of the left scrotum shows multiple anechoic tubular structures (*arrowheads*) in the paratesticular area. *T*, testis. (**b, c**) Color Doppler US images obtained on resting state (**b**) and during the Valsalva maneuver (**c**). Compared with resting state, intense color flow signal is noted within the dilated tubular structure during Valsalva maneuver. (**d**) Spectral Doppler interrogation shows a venous waveform with marked reflux during the Valsalva maneuver (*arrow*)

Because the tail of the sperm has a core structure identical to that of the cilia, primary ciliary dyskinesia affects male fertility in the form of asthenozoospermia (Afzelius 1979). Sinus and chest radiographs are sufficient to detect characteristic airway changes of primary ciliary dyskinesia such as sinusitis, bronchiectasis, and situs inversus (Fig. 122.13). High-resolution chest CT scan can be performed to detect early and subtle airway changes which can be missed by routine chest radiographs (Kennedy et al. 2007). The confirmation of immotile cilia syndrome is made by electron microscopic ultrastructural analysis of samples of nasal or airway mucosa acquired with minimally invasive techniques.

Pearls to Remember

- Primary ciliary dyskinesia can be suspected in infertile men with situs inversus.
- Sinus and chest radiographs can detect characteristic airway changes of primary ciliary dyskinesia such as sinusitis, bronchiectasis, and situs inversus.

Fig. 122.13 Kartagener syndrome in a 28-year-old woman. (**a**) Chest PA shows right-sided cardiac shadow, suggestive of dextrocardia and bronchovascular crowding (*asterisk*) of both lower lung fields, suggestive of associated bronchiectasis. Note that the stomach gas (*curved arrow*) is also seen in the right upper abdomen. (**b**) Waters Caldwell view obtained in a same patient reveals increased opacity (*asterisk*) in both maxillary sinus

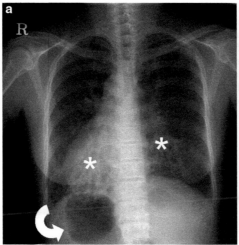
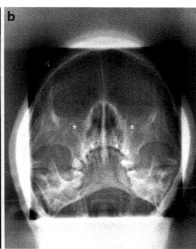

References

Afzelius BA. The immotile-cilia syndrome and other ciliary diseases. Int Rev Exp Path. 1979;19:1–43.

Bartynski WS, Lin L. Dynamic and conventional spin-echo MR of pituitary microlesions. AJNR Am J Neuroradiol. 1997;18:965–72.

Bhansali A, Banerjee PK, Dash S, Radotra B, Dash RJ. Pituitary and testicular involvement in primary haemochromatosis. A case report. J Assoc Physicians India. 1992;40(11):757–9.

Bick D, Franco B, Sherins RJ, Heye B, Pike L, Crawford J, et al. Brief report: intragenic deletion of the KALIG-1 gene in Kallmann's syndrome. N Engl J Med. 1992;326:1752–5.

Breeland E, Cohen MS, Warner RS, Leiter E. Epididymal obstruction in azoospermic males. Infertility. 1981;4(1): 49–66.

Brugh 3rd VM, Lipshultz LI. Male factor infertility: evaluation and management. Med Clin North Am. 2004;88(2):367–85.

Brugh VM, Matschke HM, Lipshultz LI. Male factor infertility. Endocrinol Metab Clin North Am. 2003;32:689–707.

Bryan PJ, Caldamone AA, Morrison SC, Yulish BS, Owens R. US findings in adrenogenital syndrome. J US Med. 1988;7:675–9.

Colpi GM, Negri L, Nappi RE, Chinea B. Is transrectal ultrasonography a reliable diagnostic approach in ejaculatory duct sub-obstruction? Hum Reprod. 1997;12:2186–91.

Coulam CB, Grahm 2nd ML, Spelsberg TC. Androgen insensitivity syndrome: gonadal androgen receptor activity. Am J Obstet Gynecol. 1984;150:531–3.

Daudin M, Bieth E, Bujan L, Massat G, Pontonnier F, Mieusset R. Congenital bilateral absence of the vas deferens: clinical characteristics, biological parameters, cystic fibrosis transmembrane conductance regulator gene mutations, and implications for genetic counseling. Fertil Steril. 2000;74: 1164–74.

Gale ME. Hermaphroditism demonstrated by computed tomography. Am J Roentgenol. 1983;141:99–100.

Gambino J, Caldwell B, Dietrich R, Walot I, Kangarloo H. Congenital disorders of sexual differentiation: MR findings. Am J Roentgenol. 1992;158:363–7.

Hinman Jr F. Prostate and urethral sphincters. Atlas of urosurgical anatomy. Philadelphia: WB Saunders; 1993. p. 345–88.

Johnson PT, Horton KM, Fishman EK. Adrenal imaging with MDCT: nonneoplastic disease. Am J Roentgenol. 2009;193:1128–35.

Kennedy MP, Noone PG, Leigh MW, Zariwala MA, Minnix SL, Knowles MR, Molina PL. High-resolution CT of patients with primary ciliary dyskinesia. AJR Am J Roentgenol. 2007;188(5):1232–8.

Kim ED, Lipshultz LI. Evaluation and imaging of the infertile male. Infert Reprod Med Clin North Am. 1999;10:377–409.

Lambert B. The frequency of mumps and of mumps orchitis. Acta Genet Stat Med. 1951;2(suppl 1):1–166.

Moon MH, Kim SH, Cho JY, Seo JT, Chun YK. Scrotal US for evaluation of infertile men with azoospermia. Radiology. 2006;239(1):168–73.

Noone PG, Leigh MW, Sannuti A, et al. Primary ciliary dyskinesia: diagnostic and phenotypic features. Am J Respir Crit Care Med. 2004;169:459–67.

Purohit RS, Wu DS, Shinohara K, Turek PJ. A prospective comparison of 3 diagnostic methods to evaluate ejaculatory duct obstruction. J Urol. 2004;171:232–6.

Quinzii C, Castellani C. The cystic fibrosis transmembrane regulator gene and male infertility. J Endocrinol Invest. 2000;23:684–9.

Rao MM, Rao DM. Cytogenetic studies in primary infertility. Fertil Steril. 1977;28(2):209–10.

Rutgers JL, Scully RE. The androgen insensitivity syndrome (testicular feminization): a clinico-pathologic study of 43 cases. Int J Gynecol Pathol. 1991;10:126–44.

Siminoski K, D'Costa M, Walfish PG. Hypogonadotropic hypogonadism in idiopathic hemochromatosis: evidence for combined hypothalamic and pituitary involvement. J Endocrinol Invest. 1990;13(10):849–53.

Takihara H, Sakatoku J, Cockett AT. The pathophysiology of varicocele in male infertility. Fertil Steril. 1991;55:861–8.

Tizzano EF, Silver MM, Chitayat D, Benichou JC, Buchwald M. Differential cellular expression of cystic fibrosis transmembrane regulator in human reproductive tissues. Clues for the infertility in patients with cystic fibrosis. Am J Pathol. 1994;144(5):906–14.

Yousem DM, Geckle RJ, Bilker W, McKeown DA, Doty RL. MR evaluation of patients with congenital hyposmia or anosmia. Am J Roentgenol. 1996;166:439–43.

Disorders of Erectile Function

123

Paul S. Sidhu and C. Jason Wilkins

Introduction

The definition of erectile dysfunction (ED) is the inability to attain or maintain a penile erection of sufficient quality to allow for satisfactory sexual activity (NIH Consensus Conference 1993). The Massachusetts Male Aging Study, observing men aged 40–70 years, found that 35% of men reported moderate or complete erectile dysfunction and up to 52% of men had experienced ED at some stage (Feldman et al. 1994). Severity and prevalence increase with age, with an estimated 20–30 million men in the USA affected by ED (Benet and Melman 1995). There are many reasons for the onset of ED, including vascular causes, some of which can be treatable. Ultrasonography (US) plays an important role in the evaluation of penile pathology, and the assessment of ED, as US provides a truly dynamic investigation through all the phases of an erectile response, in real-time circumstances denied to other imaging techniques such as magnetic resonance. High-frequency "small parts" linear transducers allow interrogation of the gray-scale anatomy and vascular components of the normal and diseased penis. Images can be obtained with few artifacts, in a noninvasive manner and without exposure to ionizing radiation.

The use of US in the evaluation of ED was established in 1985 (Lue et al. 1985), following the discovery that the intra-cavernosal injection of a vasoactive agent produces an erection in the absence of sexual arousal. More recently, the introduction of effective oral therapies such as Sildenafil, a phosphodiesterase type 5 (PDE-5) inhibitor, has revolutionized the management of ED and with it the role of US assessment. This has resulted in a decline in the use of a stimulated US examination; a "trial" of a PDE-5 inhibitor serves as the initial diagnostic test. If the patient responds to the medication, this confirms the adequacy of penile arterial inflow and veno-occlusive erectile mechanisms and eliminates the need for further testing.

However, US examination will still remain useful; many patients benefit psychologically from a normal result and an US examination may be important prior to revascularization surgery following penile trauma and to document vascularity prior to surgery for Peyronie's disease (Golijanin et al. 2007). The patients who do not respond to a PDE-5 inhibitor will still undergo US.

Normal Anatomy and Ultrasound Appearances

An appreciation of the anatomy of the penis is important. The penis is comprised of three cylindrical structures of erectile tissue. These are the two dorsal corpora cavernosa and a ventral corpus spongiosum containing the penile urethra. The spongiosum is smaller proximally but expands distally to form the glans penis (Fig. 123.1). The corpora cavernosa contain multiple smooth muscle and endothelial-lined sinusoidal cells which is distensible and essential to the erectile process. A fibrous capsule, the tunica albuginea, invests the corpora cavernosa, with a thinner layer covering the corpus spongiosum

P.S. Sidhu (✉) • C.J. Wilkins
Department of Radiology, King's College London,
King's College Hospital, London, UK

B. Hamm, P. R. Ros (eds.), *Abdominal Imaging*, DOI 10.1007/978-3-642-13327-5_210,
© Springer-Verlag Berlin Heidelberg 2013

Fig. 123.1 Anatomical drawing of the structures of the normal penis

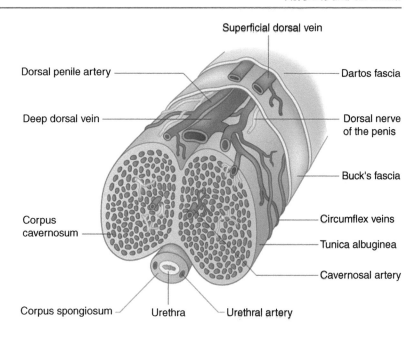

Dorsal penile artery

Deep dorsal vein

Corpus cavernosum

Corpus spongiosum

Superficial dorsal vein

Dartos fascia

Dorsal nerve of the penis

Buck's fascia

Circumflex veins

Tunica albuginea

Cavernosal artery

Urethra

Urethral artery

(Williams et al. 1989). The tunica albuginea provides rigidity to the erectile tissue and also functions as the veno-occlusive mechanism. Beneath the skin are two layers of fascia enveloping the shaft of the penis: the superficial dartos fascia and the deeper Buck's fascia, which covers the corpora cavernosa and corpus spongiosum and attaches posteriorly to the suspensory ligaments of the penis (Bella et al. 2008). The arterial supply to the penis is via the internal pudendal artery (a branch of the anterior division of the internal iliac artery), which divides into terminal branches, the dorsal penile artery (supplying the glans penis), the cavernosal artery (supplying the corpora cavernosa), and the bulbar artery (supplying the bulb and the corpus spongiosum) (Fig. 123.2). The cavernosal arteries are the main contributors to erectile function. Anatomical variations of the cavernosal arteries are common, an important consideration for the US examination. The cavernosal arteries have numerous helicine branches which supply the sinusoids. Perforations in the intra-cavernosal septum allow communication of blood supply across the midline, which is important when one cavernosal artery is occluded. Emissary veins pierce the tunica albuginea, and drain into the deep dorsal vein via the spongiosal, circumflex, and cavernosal veins (Wilkins and Sidhu 2006).

Ultrasonography identifies the paired corpora cavernosa, the cavernosal arteries, the tunica albuginea, and the corpus spongiosum (Fig. 123.3). The corpora cavernosa are of intermediate reflectivity while the corpus spongiosum is of slightly higher reflectivity. Buck's fascia and the tunica albuginea are indistinguishable as they surround the corpora and appear as a thin reflective envelope (<2 mm thick), while Buck's fascia is visible as a separate high reflectivity line overlying the corpus spongiosum. The highly reflective walls of the cavernosal arteries are usually readily identified at the base of the penis and will be identified as two parallel high reflective lines on longitudinal imaging (Fig. 123.4). The normal urethra is identified if distended and this will only occur if the patient presses on the glans penis and attempts micturition.

Erectile Function

Penile erection is the consequence of complex pathway of neurovascular events triggered by a combination of psychological and hormonal factors. Sexual stimulation results in the release of neuro-transmitters that cause relaxation of the smooth muscle of the arteries supplying erectile tissue, with resulting several-fold

Fig. 123.2 Arterial supply to the penis

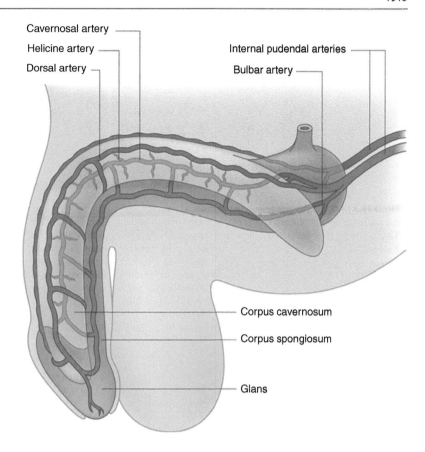

Cavernosal artery

Helicine artery

Dorsal artery

Internal pudendal arteries

Bulbar artery

Corpus cavernosum

Corpus spongiosum

Glans

increase in sinusoid compliance, rapid filling with blood and expansion of the sinusoids with penile erection the outcome.

Physiology of the Erectile Process

The flaccid penis demonstrates high resting tone of the smooth muscle and sinusoids, with low volume inflow (manifesting a high-resistance pattern on the US spectral Doppler waveform trace), and low volume outflow. With the onset of penile erection, there is relaxation of the smooth muscle of the sinusoids and elevation of arterial input. This increased cavernosal artery blood flow causes sinusoidal filling and distension of the corpora cavernosa against the noncompliant tunica albuginea. The rise in intra-tunica pressure compresses the sub-tunica venous plexuses between the trabecula and tunica albuginea, which partially occludes venous drainage from the penis and results

in tumescence. Complete occlusion of venous outflow is achieved during sexual activity by compression of the engorged corpora cavernosa at their base by contraction of the ischio-cavernosal muscles. This final stage results in rigidity.

Erectile Dysfunction

Erectile dysfunction is the result of a failure of this process and may be due to a wide number of reasons: neurogenic, psychogenic, vascular (arterial or venous) or as the result of disruption of the tunica albuginea, posttraumatic or due to Peyronie's disease. Other factors may play a role; for example patient medication, systemic disorders such as diabetes mellitus with multifactorial causes often encountered. Indeed ED may be the first manifestation of a number of diseases, such as coronary artery disease, hyperlipidemia, diabetes mellitus, hypertension, pituitary tumors, and pelvic malignancies.

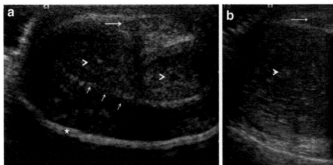

Fig. 123.3 (a) A transverse gray-scale ultrasound view through the flaccid penis with the transducer placed on the dorsal aspect. The paired medium-level echo corpora cavernosa demonstrate a central rounded low reflective area (*arrowheads*) representing the cavernosal arteries. The corpora spongiosum (*long arrow*) is of slightly higher echogenicity, smaller, and contains the urethra. The corpora cavernosa are enveloped in the tunica albuginea (*short arrows*), a thin echogenic structure. Subcutaneous tissue surrounds the penile structures with the skin of the penile shaft (*asterisk*) seen as a thick echogenic structure. (**b**) A transverse gray-scale ultrasound view through the erect penis with the transducer placed on the dorsal aspect. The cavernosal arteries (*arrowheads*) are more clearly defined, surrounded by distended sinusoids. The corpora spongiosum (*long arrow*) remains relatively echogenic and non-distended

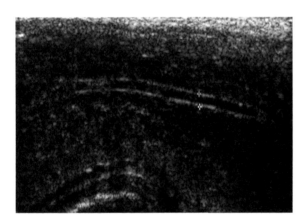

Fig. 123.4 A longitudinal gray-scale image of the cavernosal artery (between *cursors*) in the erect penis with echogenic walls clearly demonstrated. The artery becomes prominent during the erectile process but diameter measurements are not reliable for the assessment of erectile response

Stimulated Color Doppler Ultrasound (CDUS)

Pharmacological Agents

Prostaglandin E1 (PGE-1) is commonly used for pharmacological stimulation of the erectile process. PGE-1 is a safe drug when administered intra-cavernosally with a small risk of priapism (less than 1%) (Gontero et al. 2004). Other agents such as papaverine, the second most commonly used stimulant, has an incidence of iatrogenic priapism of 18% (Lomas and Jarow 1992) and has now been superseded by PGE-1. A combination of three drugs PGE-1, papaverine, and phentolamine (alpha-lytic agent that produces smooth muscle relaxation), known as "Trimix," is also used but complications are more frequent (Govier et al. 1995). The normal dosage of PGE-1 is between 5 and 20 mcg, but most commonly 20 mcg is administered at the outset of the test, to avoid a repeat injection which is uncomfortable for the patient, although this may result in a higher incidence of priapism. The examination is significantly shortened with the single dose method. Patients should be fully informed of the risks of priapism and given appropriate advice. Patients should be instructed to seek treatment if they have an erection lasting greater than 4 h. Direct access to an on-site urology opinion to ensure prompt treatment should be available.

During stimulated CDUS, absence of cavernosal artery flow or absent diastolic flow was thought to be highly specific in predicting priapism, but experience suggests that absence of diastolic flow is a frequent occurrence in the "normal" responder, and is not a harbinger of priapism (Cormio et al. 1998).

Technique

The stimulated CDUS examination should ideally be performed with a chaperone, in a setting that offers patient privacy with little possibility of interruption. Many patients are intimidated by more than one operator, and it is acceptable to perform this examination single-handed. Anxiety interferes with the examination as the associated catecholamine-induced increase in vascular tone reduces the sensitivity of the CDUS examination. The entire examination may last up to 30 min, with frequent US examinations to document the spectral Doppler waveform identified in a cavernosal artery, using a high-frequency linear array transducer with a small footprint. Intracavernosal injection of PGE-1 is performed with a small gauge needle (typically 30-G); ideally the injection site is between the proximal and mid-thirds of the shaft at the dorsolateral aspect of the penis (vasoactive substance will diffuse to the contralateral side). Following injection of the vasoactive substance the angle-corrected velocity of either the left or the right cavernosal artery is recorded at 5 min intervals from baseline (Govier et al. 1995). Tumescence and rigidity, assessed subjectively, are documented. Color Doppler ultrasound of the cavernosal arteries should be performed with the transducer positioned at the base of the penis on the dorsal surface, although some examiners prefer the ventral approach. The angle for Doppler analysis needs to be optimized (<60°) with box-steering, angle correction and orientation of the transducer essential to ensure reproducible, valid measurements. Measurement of the peak systolic velocity (PSV) and the end diastolic velocity (EDV) are most reproducible at the base of penis where the angle of the cavernosal vessel is not parallel with the transducer (Golijanin et al. 2007) and this area should be repeatedly sampled during the examination (Kim et al. 1994) (Fig. 123.5).

Baseline Imaging

Gray-scale US is performed in longitudinal and transverse planes with the penis held by the patient in the anatomical position (dorsal view) and a detailed US examination of the penis undertaken. Abnormalities such as fibrotic plaque disease (Peyronie's disease), focal cavernosal fibrosis, arterial calcification, or tunica

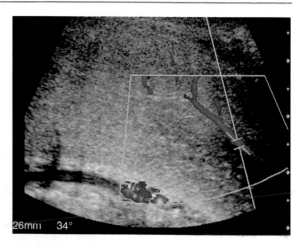

Fig. 123.5 A longitudinal color Doppler ultrasound image of the cavernosal artery in the erect penis. The Doppler gate is placed over the color Doppler signal at the base of the penis, with the Doppler angle corrected to <60° (34° in this patient). The base of the penis is the most suitable position to repeatedly measure velocities accurately

disruption may be seen. The cavernosal arteries range in diameter from 0.3 to 0.5 mm in the flaccid state. Using the color Doppler mode and the spectral Doppler gate, the PSV of the cavernosal artery in the flaccid penis is measured and recorded. In normal patients, the PSV is 10–15 cm/s, but on some occasions may be difficult to detect. The baseline examination provides only limited information for the study (Fig. 123.6).

Normal Response

Normally maximal arterial engorgement occurs early in tumescence. Cavernosal artery variations such as bifurcation, duplication, and a common origin are often seen (Jarrow et al. 1993). Cross-communications between left and right cavernosal arteries are frequent (Bertolotto et al. 2008a). Arterial anomalies could lead to a misinterpretation of the PSV assessment and if there is asymmetry of the cavernosal arteries, this should be documented and both arteries sampled during the course of the assessment. Focal arterial stenosis and arterial wall calcifications in patients with diabetes mellitus may be encountered. The full length of the cavernosal arteries should be imaged on color Doppler US to exclude distal stenosis and arterial anomalies. The helicine arteries are not visible in the flaccid penis but become apparent during the onset of erection and branch in a radial

Fig. 123.6 A longitudinal color Doppler ultrasound image of the cavernosal artery in the flaccid penis. The normal unstimulated spectral Doppler waveform may be difficult to demonstrate. The normal configuration is a rapid upstroke in systole, a narrow systolic peak and rapid descent in diastole, often with flow reversal. The peak systolic velocity in this patient is measured at 17.1 cm/s

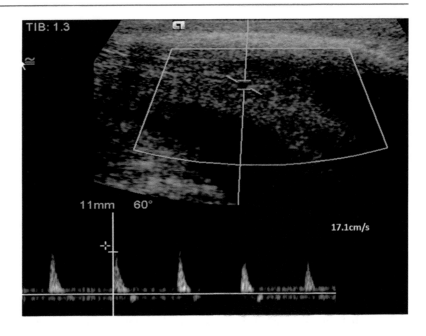

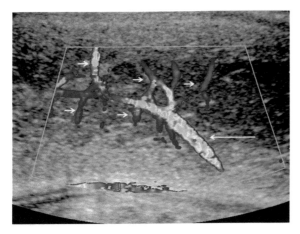

Fig. 123.7 A longitudinal color Doppler ultrasound image of the cavernosal artery (*long arrow*) in the erect penis. The helicine branches (*short arrows*) become prominent as the penis responds to the stimulation of the vasoactive drug

direction from the cavernosal arteries (Fig. 123.7). During the course of tumescence, erection and full rigidity the helicine arteries become less visible as progressive venous occlusion leads to a reduction and cessation of arterial inflow (Bertolotto et al. 2008a).

Pharmacologically induced erection follows a sequence of changes on CDUS in patients without ED and progresses through the following stages (Schwartz et al. 1989):

Phase 0: The dorsal arteries of the penis are more clearly identified than the cavernosal arteries in the pre-injection stage. The normal spectral waveform is monophasic with a high-resistance pattern showing minimal or no diastolic flow (Fig. 123.6).

Following pharmaco-stimulation, marking the onset of erection, these subsequent phases are recognized:

Phase 1: The systolic and diastolic flow increase resulting in continuous flow throughout the arterial cycle. In normal men, the PSV is >35 cm/s and the peak EDV is >8 cm/s (Fig. 123.8).

Phase 2: As pressure increases within the corpora cavernosa there is a decrease in the diastolic flow with the development of tumescence.

Phase 3: Corresponds to no diastolic flow.

Phase 4: Characterized by reversal of diastolic flow and represents full erection (Fig. 123.9).

Phase 5: The final stage of rigidity, usually not seen in clinical practice, shows a decrease in systolic velocities, which may approach zero (Schwartz et al. 1989). This is followed by detumescence and return to the baseline appearances.

This sequence of events has a variable time course. During the pharmacologically induced erection US assessment of the spectral Doppler waveform is performed, normally at 5 min intervals for a total of 20–30 min, depending on the response (Chiou et al. 1999). The cavernosal arteries increase

Fig. 123.8 A longitudinal color Doppler ultrasound image of the cavernosal artery in the course of a normal response to the vasoactive drug. At 10 min following intra-cavernosal injection, the peak systolic velocity is measured at 42.0 cm/s and the end diastolic velocity measured at 5.3 cm/s. A dicrotic notch (*arrow*) accompanies the narrowing of the systolic upstroke and the presence of forward flow in diastole as the penis engorges

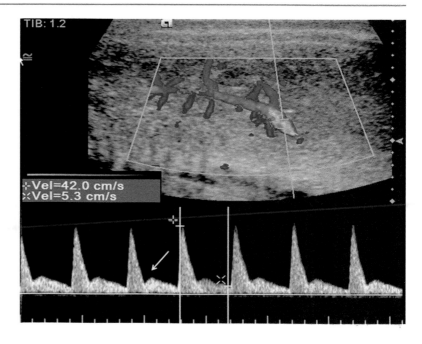

Fig. 123.9 A longitudinal color Doppler ultrasound image of the cavernosal artery in the course of a normal response to the vasoactive drug. At 20 min there is flow reversal in diastole (*arrow*), measured at −27.9 cm/s indicating a fully functional veno-occlusive mechanism. The peak systolic velocity is measured at 141.5 cm/s and indicates a normal arterial inflow

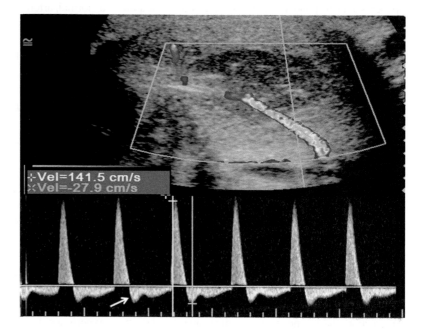

in diameter from 0.3 to 0.5 mm in the flaccid state to 1.0–1.2 mm during erection (Fig. 123.4), but this measurement is inaccurate and is not often recorded (Bertolotto et al. 2008a; Virag 1982; Montague et al. 2003).

Arteriogenic Erectile Dysfunction

Arteriogenic ED is less common, occurring predominantly in the older man with existing risk factors for arteriosclerosis such as a smoking history, diabetes

Fig. 123.10 A longitudinal color Doppler ultrasound image of the cavernosal artery in the course of an abnormal response to the vasoactive drug. The image obtained at 20 min following intra-cavernosal injection demonstrates a peak systolic velocity measured at 25.9 cm/s, below the threshold for arterial integrity (>35 cm/s) and an end diastolic velocity of 4.0 cm/s

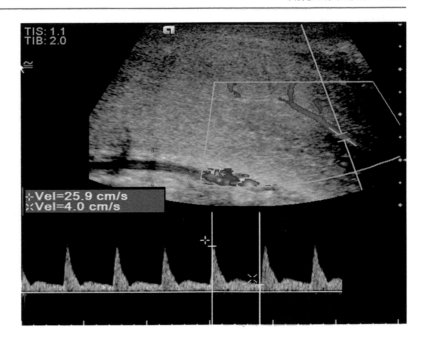

mellitus, and hypertension. It is often this group of patients that respond to Sildenafil, and do not require a dynamic ED study. The PSV of the cavernosal artery following injection of vasoactive agents is the most accurate indicator of arterial disease; a PSV of ≥35 cm/s is unequivocally normal, while a PSV of <25 cm/s specifies arterial insufficiency (Benson et al. 1993). Intermediate values are not specific and again use of Sildenafil is often beneficial (Fig. 123.10). Arteriogenic ED can be recognized by measuring the PSV in the flaccid penis, with a value of <10 cm/s in the non-erect penis being 96% sensitive and 92% specific in the diagnosis according to one study (Roy et al. 2000). The diameter change of the cavernosal artery during the erectile process may provide some information: In normal patients, the vessel increases in size by 75–100%, and in patients with arteriogenic erectile dysfunction this figure is <75% (Chiou et al. 1999). However, the increase in the baseline diameter following pharmacological stimulation does not correlate with either the measured PSV or clinical grading of erection, and it is not routine to measure arterial diameters (Patel and Lees 1995).

Veno-Occlusive Erectile Dysfunction

Ultrasound may only be used to identify veno-occlusive dysfunction in patients with a normal arterial inflow; patients with arteriogenic ED may also have venous ED but this is masked. Having established a normal arterial response with a PSV >35 cm/s, an EDV of >5 cm/s is usually accepted as the level above which a venous leak is present (Quam et al. 1989; Bassiouny and Levine 1991), although a cutoff of 7 cm/s is also quoted (Patel et al. 1993) (Fig. 123.11). The resistive index (RI) may be used as an alternative measure for the diagnosis; an RI of <0.8 with a normal PSV is regarded as diagnostic of venous leak (Kassouf and Carrier 2003), whereas an RI of 1.0 is normal. In young patients with good arterial input, reversal of EDV should normally be seen and it may be appropriate to lower the EDV threshold in this group; the inversion of the diastolic flow indicates a normal veno-occlusive mechanism and other causes of ED should be sought.

Anxiety-Related Venous Leak

The dynamic CDUS examination for ED is a difficult experience for most men, and there is likely to be considerable anxiety associated with the procedure. This may interfere with normal mechanisms of the erectile process, due to elevation of adrenergic tone, and may be responsible for a false positive result for venous leak (Gontero et al. 2004). Elevated levels of adrenaline prevent complete relaxation of the corpora cavernosa smooth muscle resulting in failure of the normal veno-occlusive mechanism. This is seen as forward

Fig. 123.11 A longitudinal color Doppler ultrasound image of the cavernosal artery in the course of an abnormal response to the vasoactive drug. The image obtained at 20 min following intra-cavernosal injection demonstrates a peak systolic velocity approaching 100 cm/s (*short arrow*) with an end diastolic velocity approaching 15 cm/s (*long arrow*). This is indicative of a venous leak as a cause of the erectile dysfunction in this patient (The X-axis is calibrated in m/s)

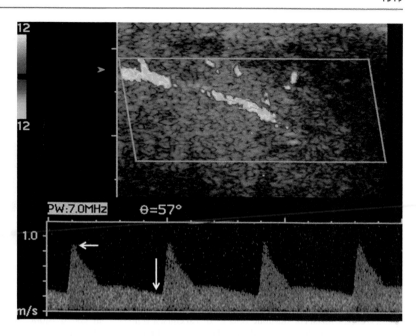

flow in the cavernosal artery throughout and is indistinguishable from a positive finding of venous incompetence. A subgroup of patients, normally the young and anxious, with features of venous incompetence following PGE-1 stimulation, may undergo administration of an intra-cavernosal injection of phentolamine, an alpha-adrenoreceptor antagonist. Phentolamine is safe at an intra-cavernosal dose of 2 mg with no significant impact on systemic blood pressure. Aversa et al. (Aversa et al. 1996) found that phentolamine normalized erectile response in 77% (20/26) of patients where PGE-1 diagnosed a venous leak (Fig. 123.12) and furthermore, phentolamine led to a significant increase in erection grade, PSV and a decrease in EDV (Aversa et al. 1996). This has been replicated in a further study (Gontero et al. 2004) although not subsequently by a further group (Arafa et al. 2007). The marked reduction in false positive results suggests that intra-cavernosal phentolamine is necessary before a venous leak can be diagnosed in the younger patient.

Further Imaging and Treatment

The diagnosis of venous incompetence on US requires normal arterial inflow; further imaging may be required in mixed etiology of ED requiring dynamic infusion cavernosometry and cavernosography, as well as diagnostic or therapeutic arteriography. Dynamic infusion cavernosometry and cavernosography remain the diagnostic reference standard for the diagnosis of venous leak, as this technique measures outflow resistance without the need for adequate arterial inflow and also will map the sites of incompetence (Lue et al. 1986). Following a CDUS diagnosis of venous leak, cavernosography is usually required if surgical venous ligation is planned. Surgical intervention for venous leak has a limited success rate and its effects may be short lived, but is a relatively minor surgical procedure and may, for the young patient, provide a temporary improvement in symptoms. An alternative treatment is coil embolization via a direct approach using a draining vein (Fowlis et al. 1994). Surgical procedures for the treatment of venous leaks have poor long-term clinical outcomes. The use of arterial reconstructive surgery is indicated only in a small group of patients with new onset focal arterial occlusion with few or no features of systemic vascular disease (Montague et al. 2003, 2005).

Specific Local Conditions That Cause Erectile Dysfunction

Peyronie's Disease

Peyronie's disease is a benign localized connective tissue disorder that affects the tunica albuginea resulting in fibrous thickening and calcification, affecting 3.2% of

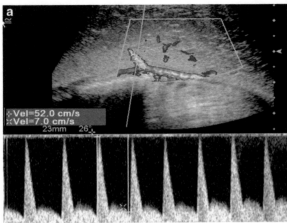
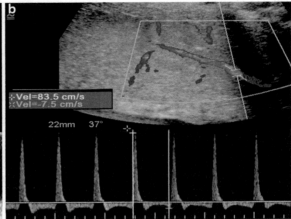

Fig. 123.12 (a) A longitudinal color Doppler ultrasound image of the cavernosal artery in the course of an abnormal response to the vasoactive drug. The image obtained at 20 min following intra-cavernosal injection demonstrates a peak systolic velocity of 52.0 cm/s with an end diastolic velocity of 7.0 cm/s, a venous leak by definition. (**b**) A longitudinal color Doppler ultrasound image of the cavernosal artery in the course of an abnormal response to the vasoactive drug, and the subsequent administration of intra-cavernosal phentolamine (2 mg). The image obtained at 5 min following intra-cavernosal injection of phentolamine demonstrates a peak systolic velocity of 83.5 cm/s with an end diastolic velocity of −7.5 cm/s; a normal study by definition

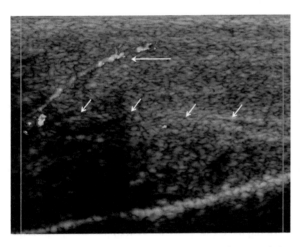
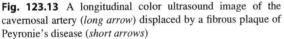
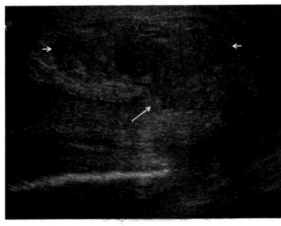

Fig. 123.13 A longitudinal color ultrasound image of the cavernosal artery (*long arrow*) displaced by a fibrous plaque of Peyronie's disease (*short arrows*)

Fig. 123.14 A longitudinal gray-scale ultrasound image of a penile fracture. A subcutaneous hematoma is present (between *small arrows*) arising from a defect in the tunica albuginea (*long arrow*). This is a surgical emergency and the defect in the tunica should be promptly repaired to avoid erectile dysfunction

men with incidence highest in the 40–60 year old (Schwarzer et al. 2001). Peyronie's disease may be associated with Dupuytren's contracture. Fibrotic plaque formation results from vascular inflammation but the etiology is controversial, although evidence does not corroborate the long-held belief that trauma is a primary cause (Zargooshi 2000). Peyronie's disease most commonly presents with dorsal curvature of the penis with other malformations including penile shortening, bottle-neck deformities (due to annular plaques), and indentations also occurring. Erectile dysfunction is a common association found in 20–40% and may be multifactorial, with vascular reasons the most common; distortion of the tunica albuginea may cause a venous

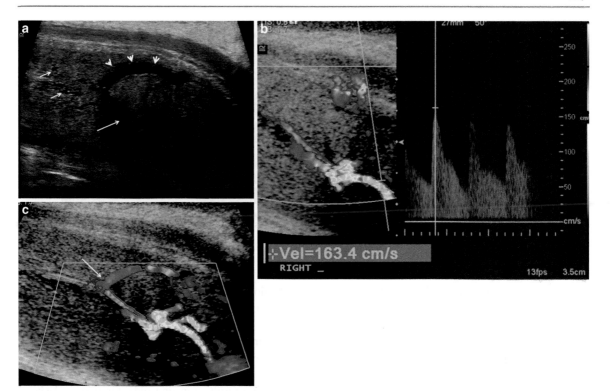

Fig. 123.15 (a) A longitudinal gray-scale ultrasound image of a posttraumatic fistula. There is an intra-cavernosal hematoma (*long arrow*) with evidence of sinusoidal engorgement (*short arrows*) and a tubular structure (*arrowheads*) which is a prominent draining vein. (b) The peak systolic velocity of the cavernosal artery is measured at 163.4 cm/s, indicating high-flow priapism. (c) The color Doppler ultrasound image demonstrates the arteriovenous fistula that has developed as a consequence of the trauma (*arrow*)

leak (Weidner et al. 1997) or plaque may encase the cavernosal arteries and cause arterial dysfunction (Bertolotto et al. 2002). There is an increased incidence of arterial and mixed vascular abnormalities (Kadioglu et al. 2000). Color Doppler US examination is important prior to corrective surgery, to ascertain the course of the cavernosal arteries in relation to plaques (Levine and Coogan 1996) (Fig. 123.13).

Penile Trauma

A penile fracture results from blunt trauma causing rupture of the tunica albuginea of the corpus cavernosum. Blunt trauma to the flaccid penis will rarely result in a fracture, but often results in extra-tunica or cavernosal hematoma formation. A penile fracture occurs as a result of compression of the erect penile shaft against the pubic symphysis during sexual intercourse. Presentation is usually acute with a history of pain, swelling, and sudden loss of tumescence

during intercourse (Zargooshi 2000). Ultrasound in the acute setting identifies defects in the tunica albuginea and allows assessment of the extent of acute hematoma formation (Fig. 123.14). Urethral injury may be present in up to 20% of cases (Fergany et al. 1999). Rupture of the tunica albuginea is a surgical emergency requiring immediate exploration and repair of the defect, as delay in treatment significantly increases the risk of long-term sequelae, particularly ED (El Bahnasawy and Gomha 2000). Erectile dysfunction is most often due to impairment of the veno-occlusive mechanism (Gontero et al. 2000).

Priapism

Priapism is defined as an erection that is maintained in the absence of sexual stimulation (Mihmanli and Kantarci 2007; Keoghane et al. 2002). There are two main categories of priapism: non-ischemic and ischemic priapism, with a further type described as

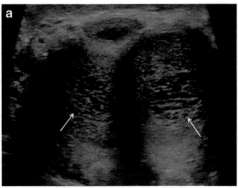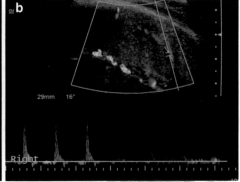

Fig. 123.16 (**a**) A transverse gray-scale ultrasound image of low-flow priapism. There is engorgement of both corpora cavernosa (*arrows*). (**b**) The spectral Doppler waveform demonstrates a sharp systolic upstroke, narrow systolic peak, and no forward flow in diastole typical of a high-resistance pattern seen in low-flow priapism

"stuttering" or recurrent priapism which occurs during sleep and persists on waking, often seen in sickle cell disease (Muneer et al. 2008). The diagnosis of priapism remains clinical and relies on the history, examination, and analysis of blood aspirated from the corpora cavernosa. Ultrasound may provide clinically useful information in some cases (Bertolotto et al. 2008b). The differentiation between ischemic and non-ischemic priapism is important; ischemic priapism is a surgical emergency and requires prompt treatment with aspiration and surgical shunting.

Non-Ischemic Priapism

Non-ischemic, high-flow, or posttraumatic priapism is a manifestation of damage to the cavernosal arteries with the development of arterio-cavernous fistulas (Mihmanli and Kantarci 2007). These patients give a history of perineal or genital trauma and present with prolonged painless, nonrigid tumescence from the time of injury. Cavernous blood is arterial and oxygenated. Gray-scale US will demonstrate a hypo-echoic intra-cavernosal abnormality, normally a hematoma, in the vicinity of the damaged artery (Bertolotto et al. 2008b). The cavernosal artery PSV is elevated with high forward diastolic flow at spectral Doppler US examination (Fig. 123.15). The draining veins are prominent and may exhibit arterialized waveforms in the presence of an arterio-sinusoidal fistula, which may also be directly visualized (Wilkins et al. 2003; Bertolotto and Mucelli 2004). Elective arterial embolization of the internal pudendal or cavernosal artery is the ideal management of non-ischemic arterial priapism, allowing selective ablation of the feeding artery and preserving erectile function (Walker et al. 1990; Kang et al. 1998).

Ischemic Priapism

Ischemic or low-flow priapism is essentially a compartment syndrome caused by veno-occlusive problems resulting in sinusoidal thrombosis. Ischemic priapism presents with a painful, rigid erection of the corpora cavernosa but a soft glans. This is a urological emergency that requires prompt treatment, with diagnosis usually made on clinical examination. Aspiration of the cavernosal blood is both therapeutic and diagnostic, confirmed by the presence of deoxygenated blood and a low pH. If untreated for >24 h severe cellular damage occurs and there may be penile necrosis. Long-term corporal fibrosis with concomitant loss of erectile function may ensue. Imaging is not normally performed prior to therapeutic intervention. On gray-scale imaging there is engorgement of the cavernosal sinusoids of variable echogenicity depending on the degree of sinusoidal thrombosis (Fig. 123.16). Color Doppler US demonstrates a low or absent diastolic flow with variable, usually not high, arterial inflow consistent with a high-resistance vascular bed (Wilkins et al. 2003).

References

Arafa M, Eid H, Shamloul R. Significance of phentolamine redosing during prostaglandin E1 penile color Doppler ultrasonography in diagnosis of vascular erectile dysfunction. Int J Urol. 2007;14:467–77.

Aversa A, Rocchietti-March M, Caprio M, Giannini D, Isidori A, Fabbri A. Anxiety-induced failure in erectile response to intracorporeal prostaglandin-E1 in non-organic male impotence: a new diagnostic approach. Int J Androl. 1996;19:307–13.

Bassiouny HS, Levine LA. Penile duplex sonography in the diagnosis of venogenic impotence. J Vasc Surg. 1991;13:75–82.

Bella AJ, Brant WO, Lue TF. Penile anatomy. In: Bertolotto M, editor. Color Doppler US of the penis. 1st ed. Berlin: Springer; 2008. p. 11–4.

Benet AE, Melman A. The epidemiology of erectile dysfunction. Urol Clin North Am. 1995;22:699–709.

Benson CB, Aruny JE, Vickers MA. Correlation of duplex sonography with arteriography in patients with erectile dysfunction. AJR Am J Roentgenol. 1993;160:71–3.

Bertolotto M, Mucelli RP. Nonpenetrating penile traumas: sonographic and Doppler features. AJR Am J Roentgenol. 2004;183:1085–9.

Bertolotto M, de Stefani S, Martinoli C, Quaia E, Buttazzi L. Color Doppler appearance of penile cavernosal-spongiosal communications in patients with severe Peyronie's disease. Eur Radiol. 2002;12:2525–31.

Bertolotto M, Lissiani A, Pizzolato R, Fute MD. US anatomy of the penis: common findings and anatomical variations. In: Bertolotto M, editor. Color Doppler US of the penis. 1st ed. Berlin: Springer; 2008a. p. 25–38.

Bertolotto M, Mucelli FP, Liguori G, Sanabor D. Imaging priapism: the diagnostic role of color Doppler US. In: Color Doppler US of the penis. 1st ed. Berlin/New York: Springer; 2008b. p. 79–88.

Chiou RK, Alberts GL, Pomeroy BD, Anderson JC, Carlson LK, Anderson JR, et al. Study of cavernosal arterial anatomy using color and power Doppler sonography: impact on hemodynamic parameter measurement. J Urol. 1999;162:358–60.

Cormio L, Bettocchi C, Ricapito V, Zizzi V, Traficante A, Selvaggi FP. Resistance index as a prognostic factor for prolonged erection after penile dynamic colour Doppler ultrasonography. Eur Urol. 1998;33:94–7.

El Bahnasawy MS, Gomha MA. Penile fractures: the successful outcome of immediate surgical intervention. Int J Impot Res. 2000;12:273–7.

Feldman HA, Goldstein I, Hatzichristou DG, Krane RJ, McKinlay JB. Impotence and its medical and psychosocial correlates: results of the Massachusetts male aging study. J Urol. 1994;151:54–61.

Fergany AF, Angermeier KW, Montague DK. Review of Cleveland clinic experience with penile fracture. Urology. 1999;54:352–5.

Fowlis GA, Sidhu PS, Jager HR, Agarwal S, Jackson JE, Zafar F, et al. Preliminary report: combined surgical and radiological penile vein occlusion for the management of impotence caused by venous-sinusoidal incompetence. Br J Urol. 1994;74:492–6.

Golijanin D, Singer E, Davis R, Bhatt S, Seftel AD, Dogra VS. Doppler evaluation of erectile dysfunction – part 1. Int J Impot Res. 2007;19:37–42.

Gontero P, Sidhu PS, Muir GH. Penile fracture repair: assessment of early results and complications using color Doppler ultrasound. Int J Impot Res. 2000;12:125–9.

Gontero P, Sriprasad S, Wilkins CJ, Donaldson N, Muir GH, Sidhu PS. Phentolamine re-dosing during penile dynamic colour Doppler ultrasound: a practical method to abolish a false diagnosis of venous leakage in patients with erectile dysfunction. Br J Radiol. 2004;77:922–6.

Govier FE, Asase D, Hefty TR, McClure RD, Pritchett TR, Weissman RM. Timing of penile color flow duplex ultrasonography using a triple drug mixture. J Urol. 1995;153:1472–5.

Jarrow JP, Pugh VW, Routh WD, Dyer RB. Comparison of penile duplex ultrasonography to pudendal arteriography. Variant penile arterial anatomy affects interpretation of duplex ultrasonography. Invest Radiol. 1993;28:806–10.

Kadioglu A, Tefekli A, Erol H, Cayan S, Kandirali E. Color Doppler ultrasound assessment of penile vascular system in men with Peyronie's disease. Int J Impot Res. 2000;12:263–7.

Kang BC, Lee DY, Byun JY, Baek SY, Lee SW, Kim KW. Post-traumatic arterial priapism: colour Doppler examination and superselective arterial embolization. Clin Radiol. 1998;53:830–4.

Kassouf W, Carrier S. A comparison of the international index of erectile function and erectile dysfunction studies. BJU Int. 2003;91:667–9.

Keoghane SR, Sullivan ME, Miller MA. The aetiology, pathogenesis and management of priapism. BJU Int. 2002;90:149–54.

Kim SH, Paick JS, Lee SE, Choi BI, Yeon KM, Han MC. Doppler sonography of deep cavernosal artery of the penis: variation of peak systolic velocity according to sampling location. J Ultrasound Med. 1994;13:591–4.

Levine LA, Coogan CL. Penile vascular assessment using color duplex sonography in men with Peyronie's disease. J Urol. 1996;155:1270–3.

Lomas GM, Jarow JP. Risk factors for papaverine-induced priapism. J Urol. 1992;147:1280–1.

Lue TF, Hricak H, Marich KW, Tanagho EA. Vasculogenic impotence evaluated by high-resolution ultrasonography and pulsed Doppler spectrum analysis. Radiology. 1985;155:777–81.

Lue TF, Hricak H, Schmidt RA, Tanagho EA. Functional evaluation of penile veins by cavernosgraphy in papaverine-induced erection. J Urol. 1986;135:479–82.

Mihmanli I, Kantarci M. Erectile dysfunction. Semin Ultrasound CT MRI. 2007;28:274–86.

Montague DK, Jarow J, Broderick GA, Dmochowski RR, Heaton JP, Lue TF, et al. American urological association guideline on the management of priapism. J Urol. 2003;170:1318–24.

Montague DK, Jarow JP, Broderick GA, Dmochowski RR, Heaton JP, Lue TF, et al. Chapter 1: the management of erectile dysfunction: an AUA update. J Urol. 2005;174:230–9.

Muneer A, Minhas S, Arya M, Ralph DJ. Stuttering priapism–a review of the therapeutic options. Int J Clin Pract. 2008;62:1265–70.

NIH Consensus Conference. NIH consensus conference. Impotence. NIH consensus development panel on impotence. JAMA. 1993;270:83–90.

Patel U, Lees WR. Penile sonography. In: Solibiati L, Rizzatto G, editors. Ultrasound of superficial structures. 1st ed. London: Churchill Livingstone; 1995. p. 229–42.

Patel U, Amin Z, Friedman E, Vale J, Kirby RW, Lees WR. Colour flow and spectral Doppler imaging after papaverine-induced penile erection in 220 impotent men: study of temporal patterns and the importance of repeated sampling, velocity asymmetry and vascular anomalies. Clin Radiol. 1993;48:18–24.

Quam JP, King BF, James EM, Lewis RW, Brakke DM, Ilstrup DM, et al. Duplex and color Doppler sonographic evaluation of vasculogenic impotence. AJR Am J Roentgenol. 1989;153:1141–7.

Roy C, Saussine C, Tuchmann C, Castel E, Lang H, Jacqmin D. Duplex Doppler sonography of the flaccid penis: potential role in the evaluation of impotence. J Clin Ultrasound. 2000;28:290–4.

Schwartz AN, Wang KY, Mack LA, Lowe M, Berger RE, Cyr DR, et al. Evaluation of normal erectile function with color flow Doppler sonography. AJR Am J Roentgenol. 1989;153:1155–60.

Schwarzer U, Sommer F, Klotz T, Braun M, Reifenrath B, Englemann U. The prevalance of Peyronie's disease: results of a large survey. BJU Int. 2001;88:727–30.

Virag R. Intracavernous injection of papaverine for erectile failure. Lancet. 1982;2(8304):938.

Walker TG, Grant PW, Goldstein I, Krane RJ, Greenfield AJ. "High-flow" priapism: treatment with superselective transcatheter embolization. Radiology. 1990;174:1053–4.

Weidner W, Schroeder-Printzen I, Weiske WH, Vosshenrich R. Sexual dysfunction in Peyronie's disease; an analysis of 222 patients without previous local plaque therapy. J Urol. 1997;157:325–8.

Wilkins CJ, Sidhu PS. Diseases of the penis with functional evaluation. In: Baxter GM, Sidhu PS, editors. Ultrasound of the urogenital system. 1st ed. Stuttgart: Thieme; 2006. p. 181–92.

Wilkins CJ, Sriprasad S, Sidhu PS. Colour Doppler ultrasound of the penis. Clin Radiol. 2003;58:514–23.

Williams PL, Warwick R, Dyson M, Bannister LH. Splanchnology. In: Williams PL, Warwick R, Dyson M, Bannister LH, editors. Gray's anatomy. 37th ed. London: Churchill Livingstone; 1989, p. 1432–3.

Zargooshi J. Penile fracture in Kermanshah, Iran: report of 172 cases. J Urol. 2000;164:364–6.

Penile Lumps

Michele Bertolotto, Massimo Valentino, William Toscano,
Giovanni Serafini, and Lorenzo E. Derchi

Introduction

Penile lumps are commonly encountered in urologist's surgery. Most of patients actually have Peyronie's disease, but differential diagnosis is needed with a wide series of other benign and malignant pathologies. Patients are usually given a preliminary diagnosis based on history, onset of symptoms, and physical examination; imaging is often required to confirm the diagnosis, or for staging purpose.

Penile Cysts

A variety of cystic lumps can be recognized in the penis, either congenital or acquired. Diagnosis of most of them is straightforward based on clinical appearance. Imaging can be indicated especially in large lesions, to confirm diagnosis and to assess the relationships with the adjacent structures.

M. Bertolotto (✉) • W. Toscano
Department of Radiology, University of Trieste, Trieste, Italy

M. Valentino
Emergency Radiology Unit, University Hospital of Parma, Parma, Italy

G. Serafini
Department of Radiology, S. Corona Hospital, Pietra Ligure, Italy

L.E. Derchi
Department of Radiology, University of Genova, Genova, Italy

Cysts of the Median Raphe

These cysts are relatively common in newborns, but occasionally are identified also in adults. They are due to midline-developmental disorders of the urethral groove with entrapment of epithelial cells during fusion of the genital folds. Cysts of the median raphe contain clear mucinous fluid. They are usually in foreskin or glans, but can be anywhere in the ventral aspect of the penis from the anus to the urinary meatus (Otsuka and Terauchi 1990).

Epidermoid and Dermoid Cysts

Epidermoid cysts are uncommon lumps composed of keratin producing epithelium located either on the dorsum of the penis or, less frequently, on the ventral aspect of the shaft. They appear as firm, oval, or lobulated nodules of variable size.

Dermoid cysts are extremely rare in the penis with only few cases reported in the literature. They are lined by an epidermis with fully mature epidermal appendages. Hair follicles containing hairs are often present. The dermis can contain sebaceous, eccrine, and apocrine glands.

Sebaceous Cysts

Sebaceous cysts are found most commonly in the scrotum, but can be found on the penile shaft as well. They are formed by an abnormal sac of retained excretion from the sebaceous follicles and appear as tender, painless flesh-colored or whitish-yellow lumps underneath the skin.

B. Hamm, P. R. Ros (eds.), *Abdominal Imaging*, DOI 10.1007/978-3-642-13327-5_208,
© Springer-Verlag Berlin Heidelberg 2013

Penile Inflammation

Cellulitis is an inflammation of the connective tissue underlying the penile skin. Balanitis and balanoposthitis are inflammation of the glans penis and prepuce. While these pathologies have a poor clinical and radiological relevance, infection of the corpora cavernosa can be a serious life-threatening complication.

Impaired immune response and cavernous tissue ischemia represent predisposing factors for severe infection. Diabetic patients, in particular, may develop penile infections following self-administration of intracavernosal drug injection and after surgical maneuvers or prosthesis implantation. Penile abscesses usually result as a complication of an advanced or untreated superficial balanitis or cellulitis, from infection of the corpora cavernosa, or following a systemic infection with lymphatic or hematogenous dissemination.

Thrombosis and Thrombophlebitis of the Dorsal Veins

Thrombosis of the dorsal veins can be associated with thrombophilia, can follow vigorous intercourse or self-stimulation, or be associated to pelvic malignancy which reduces penile blood outflow. This pathological condition, however, may also present spontaneously in patients without known risk factors. Clinically, patients present with a rod-like induration of the dorsal aspect of the shaft which is usually painless in patients with non-complicated thrombosis, while it is painful in those with thrombophlebitis. Fever is another sign suggestive for thrombophlebitis.

Sclerosing Lymphangitis of the Penis

Sclerosing lymphangitis of the penis is a rare, usually painless condition involving the distal lymphatics that is characterized by a firm, cord-like lump which almost encircles the penis in the coronal sulcus. It is most commonly associated with vigorous sexual activity, but it is also seen with infections including gonorrhea, syphilis, chlamydia, and herpes.

Penile Fibrosis

Localized corporeal fibrosis may follow trauma or cavernosal drug injection (Chew et al. 1997). It often presents as a firm lump at palpation. Increased penile consistency is often present also in patients with diffuse fibrosis which, however, is not always palpable. Fibrosis localized at the corporal crura can develop in equestrians, long-distance bikers, and racing cyclists following repeated microtraumas. Diffuse fibrotic changes may follow ischemic priapism and cavernosal tissue inflammation as well (El-Bahnasawy et al. 2002).

Primary Tumors

Penile cancer usually presents clinically with an area of induration or a warty exophytic growth. Histologically, it is a squamous cell carcinoma in 95% of cases. Diagnosis of tumor is suspected based on clinical presentation and physical examination, and confirmed with biopsy. Imaging is indicated for staging purposes. Glans is the most common location (48%), followed by prepuce (21%), glans and prepuce (9%), coronal sulcus (6%), and shaft (<2%). Penile cancer is uncommon in the western world but represents a significant health problem in developing countries. The highest incidence rates are seen in Africa, Asia, and in areas of Brazil, where it accounts for 10–20% of all malignancies in men.

Urethral cancer is a rare disease most often observed during the seventh decade (Wasserman 2000). It is usually a squamous cell carcinoma, less often a transitional cell carcinoma. Sporadic cases of lymphoma, melanoma, and neuroendocrine tumors have been reported.

The most frequent benign tumor of the penis is hemangioma of the glans which typically presents as a superficial reddish spot barely visible at imaging. Giant cavernous hemangioma is rare. It may involve the entire glans and a variable portion of the corpora cavernosa, scrotum, and perineum.

Secondary Tumors

Metastatic cancer to the penis is uncommon and is usually encountered in patients with a known malignancy in an advanced stage. Primary sources are prostate, bladder, lung tumors, malignant melanoma, colon, and kidney tumors.

Invasion of the corpora cavernosa by tumor tissue usually presents clinically with a painful lump or induration, either circumscribed or diffuse. Diagnosis is based on history and clinics.

Patient Management

When a patient seeks medical attention for a penile lump, either painful or painless, clinical assessment is of foremost importance. An important part of the history involves asking how long is it the lump appeared, if it appeared after an incidental or sexual trauma, whether it is stable in size, and if it changed location or orientation.

Cysts, Inflammation, Thrombosis, and Sclerosing Lymphangitis

Therapy of penile cysts consists in the surgical removal. Infected cyst may require oral antibiotics or other treatment before excision. Before the operation, imaging is indicated especially in patients with large, rapidly growing cysts to confirm the nature of the lesion and to assess the relationships with adjacent organs.

Cellulitis, balanitis, and thrombophlebitis can be treated successfully with antibiotics. Cavernositis and abscesses, on the contrary, often require aggressive treatment with antibiotics, corporotomy, debridement, and placement of intracorporeal irrigation and suction drains. Acute purulent cavernositis often fails to respond to conservative therapy, and requires penile amputation. In case of recovery cavernosal fibrosis usually develops producing irreversible erectile dysfunction.

Thrombosis of the dorsal veins is usually treated with fibrinolytics and anticoagulation, associated with discontinuance of sexual activity.

Sclerosing lymphangitis is usually self-limited, lasting only a few weeks, and conservative management is indicated. Patient should refrain from vigorous sexual activity until the lesion disappears. Surgical removal is indicated in rare cases in which there are persistent symptoms.

Penile Fibrosis

Differential diagnosis between cavernosal tissue fibrosis and other causes of penile induration is clinically relevant because fibrosis constitutes an end-organ failure. Oral medications are ineffective in these patients, as well as surgery for veno-occlusive or arteriogenic dysfunction. Also, prosthesis implantation may be technically difficult.

Biopsy is the most accurate method to establish cavernosal fibrosis, but it is very invasive and not well accepted as a routine preoperative procedure. Imaging features are often characteristic enough to guide the appropriate treatment of the patient.

Primary and Secondary Tumors

Treatment options for small penile cancers of the foreskin can be circumcision, Mohs micrographic surgery, laser ablation, and radiation therapy. Tumors involving the glans and the distal shaft are best managed by partial penectomy. For bulky proximal tumors involving the base of the penis total penectomy is necessary.

Because of the aggressive nature of the disease, conservative surgery should only be offered to highly selected patients with urethral cancer. Patients with low-stage distal urethral lesion and a normal proximal urethra are offered partial penectomy. Involvement of the corpus spongiosum or corpora cavernosa may be a contraindication to this procedure. Patients who are not candidates for partial penectomy because of the location or size of the disease are treated with radical penectomy, with or without en bloc resection of the scrotum, anterior pubis, and cystoprostatectomy.

Diagnosis of penile metastases is based on history and clinical appearance. Biopsy can be useful to confirm diagnosis and to distinguish metastases from primary malignancies or other causes of penile induration. Imaging is confirmatory and can be useful to evaluate the local extent of the disease. Therapy has only a palliative purpose.

Appropriateness of Different Imaging Modalities

Knowledge of the different clinical situations that may present with painful penile induration is necessary to guide interpretation of imaging features. Patient history and a basic clinical investigation enclosing penile inspection and palpation should be performed by the radiologist as well because it is of great help in

Fig. 124.1 Penile cysts.
(**a**) Median raphe cyst (*)
showing anechoic content.
(**b**) Sebaceous cyst (*)
presenting with
homogeneously echogenic
content. (**c**) Epidermoid cyst
(*) presenting as an echogenic
mass containing hypoechoic
foci (*arrowheads*)

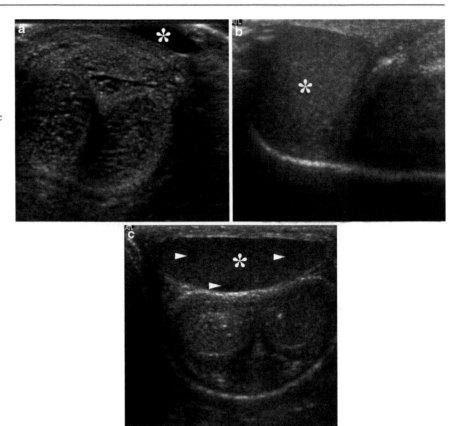

selecting the best imaging modality, examination technique, and to seek clinically relevant information which may produce a shift in the management of the patient.

Cysts

Cysts of the median raphe appear at ultrasound with anechoic content. Sebaceous cysts are homogeneously hypoechoic or relatively echogenic. Epidermoid cysts are relatively echogenic with hypoechoic foci and may contain calcifications (Bertolotto et al. 2008b) (Fig. 124.1).

Color signal is lacking in all cysts at Doppler interrogation. Infected cysts, however, may present with increased vascularity of the surrounding soft tissues.

At magnetic resonance imaging cysts are well-circumscribed masses lacking contrast enhancement. Median raphe and sebaceous cysts present with low signal intensity on T1-weighted images and high signal intensity on T2-weighted images. Epidermoid cysts present with signal intensity similar or higher compared to muscle on T1-weighted images while signal intensity is high on T2-weighted images (Fig. 124.2). Irregular low signal intensity areas are recognized on both T1- and T2-weighted images (Bertolotto et al. 2008b).

Inflammation

In patients with severe penile inflammation imaging may have a role to rule out involvement of the corpora cavernosa and abscess formation (Bertolotto et al. 2009). Cavernositis presents at ultrasound with markedly increased vascularity of the cavernosal bodies (Fig. 124.3). Cavernosal tissue edema presents with increased echogenicity, while abscesses present as hypoechoic collections with corpuscolated content, internal debris, or even gas. Abscesses are avascular (Fig. 124.4), while the surrounding tissues usually

Fig. 124.2 Epidermoid cyst of the penis. (**a**) Axial T2-weighted image showing a high signal intensity lesion with irregular low signal intensity foci. (**b**) Axial T1-weighted image showing a higher signal intensity mass compared to muscle (*M*) with lower signal intensity foci

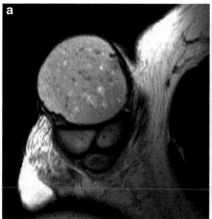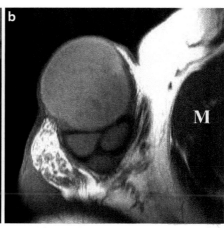

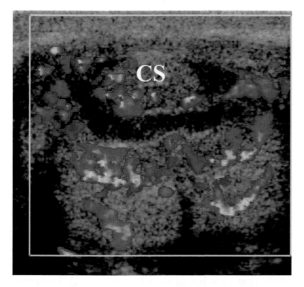

Fig. 124.3 Cavernositis. Axial color Doppler image showing hypervascularity of the corpora cavernosa and of the corpus spongiosum. A small fluid collection surrounds the corpus spongiosum (*CS*)

present with inflammatory hyperemia at color Doppler interrogation (Bertolotto et al. 2009). CT (Fig. 124.4) and magnetic resonance imaging (Fig. 124.5) have a role to evaluate the extent of the disease to the perineum, abdominal wall, fascial planes, and buttocks. As occurs elsewhere in the body, penile abscesses present at CT as fluid collections, sometime containing air bubbles, with edema in the adjacent fat and wall hyperemia after contrast administration. At MR imaging they present with intermediate-to-low

signal intensity on T1-weighted images, and high signal intensity on T2-weighted images, with rim enhancement after gadolinium injection (Kickuth et al. 2001).

Thrombosis of the Dorsal Vein and Sclerosing Lymphangitis of the Penis

Penile venous thrombosis presents with noncompressible echogenic material within the dorsal vein, isolated or spreading over the circumflex veins (Fig. 124.6). Signal is lacking at color Doppler interrogation (Bertolotto et al. 2008b).

Diagnosis of sclerosing lymphangitis of the penis is based on typical clinical presentation of a cord-like lump which encircles the penis in the coronal sulcus. Ultrasonography confirms the diagnosis showing a dilated serpiginous structure with anechoic content (Fig. 124.7) resembling rosary beads (Bertolotto et al. 2008b). No color signals are appreciable at Doppler interrogation.

Fibrosis

Focal fibrotic changes within the corpora cavernosa present at ultrasound as hyperechogenic areas or nodules with variable attenuation of the ultrasound beam (Fig. 124.8) (Bertolotto et al. 2008a). Calcifications are occasionally present. Magnetic resonance imaging is at least as effective as ultrasonography in evaluation of

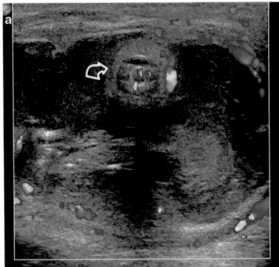

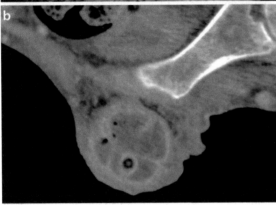

Fig. 124.4 Penile abscesses. (a) Axial US scan showing the cavernous tissue at the base of the penis replaced by avascular content with mixed echogenicity consistent with abscess formation. The corpus spongiosum (*curved arrow*) and the tissues surrounding the abscess are hypervascularized at color Doppler interrogation. Hyperechoic spots within the abscess suggest presence of air bubbles. (b) Contrast-enhanced CT confirms abscess with air bubbles replacing the cavernous tissue at the base of the penis

fibrous changes in the corpora cavernosa, with the advantage of panoramic view and better contrast resolution. Severe and diffuse fibrotic changes appear as areas of low signal intensity on T1-weighted and T2-weighted images prevailing around the cavernosal arteries (Fig. 124.9) with poor enhancement after intravenous gadolinium administration (Bertolotto et al. 2008a).

Primary Tumors

Imaging for local staging of penile cancer requires intracavernosal PGE1 injection (Bertolotto et al. 2005; Kayes et al. 2007). When the penis becomes turgid and the shaft enlarges, the tunica albuginea straightens and thins out, and evaluation of the relationships between the tumor and the surrounding structures improves. Unfortunately, many patients with penile cancer are old men with preexisting erectile dysfunction in whom artificial erection cannot be obtained even following intracavernosal injection of large quantities of vasoactive drugs.

Ultrasonography is more accurate than clinical examination for measuring the local extension of penile cancer (Agrawal et al. 2000; Lont et al. 2003). The tumor usually presents with variable echogenicity and poor vascularization, which may increase in inflamed tumors. Obvious infiltration of the corpora cavernosa appears as an interruption of the thin echogenic interface of the tunica albuginea (Fig. 124.10). In patients with initial infiltration, however, the tunica albuginea may be not interrupted, but appears in contact with the lesion, focally thickened and with decreased echogenicity (Bertolotto et al. 2005).

MR imaging is the gold standard modality for staging primary penile malignancies (Singh et al. 2005; Kayes et al. 2007; Singh et al. 2007). It allows a more accurate local staging of penile cancer compared to ultrasound due to the excellent depiction of the tunica albuginea on all sequences, with the possibility to detect even small interruption. Different imaging protocols can be used. In general, when the tumor is small, superficial coils may be used to obtain a better spatial resolution. In patients with larger tumors more panoramic phased array coils are preferred. At least axial T1-weighted images with fat suppression and T2-weighted images on two orthogonal planes should be produced. If gadolinium is administered, fat-saturated T1-weighted images should be obtained on the three planes before and after contrast administration. In addition, axial T1-weighted images of the pelvis should be obtained to look for inguinal and obturator lymphadenopathy.

Penile tumor is usually hypointense to corpora on T2-weighted images, and hypointense or isointense relative to the corpora on T1-weighted images

Fig. 124.5 Penile abscesses. Coronal T1-weighted (**a**), T2-weighted (**b**), and gadolinium-enhanced T1-weighted images (**c**) showing the cavernous tissue at the base of the penis (*curved arrows*) replaced by content with intermediate signal intensity on T1-weighted image (**a**) and high signal intensity on T2-weighted image (**b**). The lesion lacks vascularization on gadolinium-enhanced T1-weighted image (**c**) while the surrounding tissues are hyperemic. Intralesional signal-void spots on all sequences are consistent with air

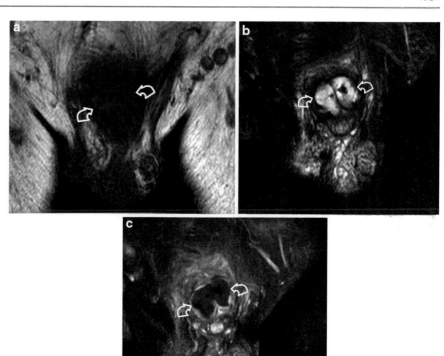

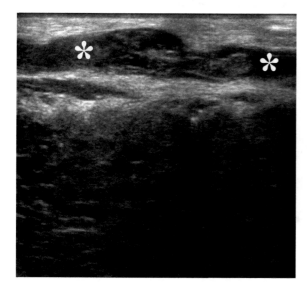

Fig. 124.6 Thrombosis of the deep dorsal vein. Patient presenting with a rod-like painless induration on the dorsal aspect of the penis. There was no history of penile trauma or inflammation. Longitudinal US scan with the probe on the dorsal aspect of the penis showing echogenic material within the deep dorsal vein (*)

(Pretorius et al. 2001; Vossough et al. 2002). Contrast enhancement after gadolinium administration is variable. In the clinical practice the higher contrast resolution between the tumor, corpora and the tunica albuginea is obtained on T2-weighted images and local staging of the disease is best accomplished using these sequences (Fig. 124.11). Injection of contrast material is often not necessary.

In advanced penile cancers CT has a role in identification of pathological nodes and of distant metastatic deposits. It is also indicated in patients with lymphoma to check for presence of other localizations of the disease.

Ultrasound and MR appearance of benign and malignant penile tumors different from squamous cell carcinoma is usually nonspecific, with the exception of giant cavernous hemangioma, which appears at ultrasound as a heterogeneously echogenic mass with multiple hypoechoic lacunae, sometimes containing phleboliths (Serafini et al. 2008). No vascularization is usually appreciable at color

Fig. 124.7 Sclerosing lymphangitis of the penis. (**a**) Photograph showing a cord-like lump encircling the penis in the coronal sulcus. The lump was painless and firm at palpation. (**b**) Axial US scan showing an anechoic elongated structure (*arrowheads*) in the coronal sulcus lacking vascularization at color Doppler interrogation (not shown)

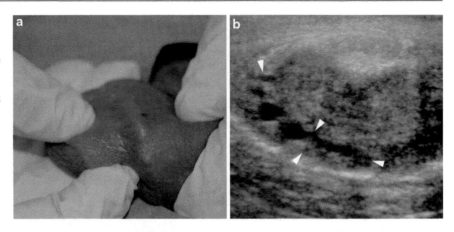

Fig. 124.8 Posttraumatic circumscribed cavernosal fibrosis. (**a**) Longitudinal US scan showing a strongly attenuating echogenic scar (*arrowheads*) within the corpus cavernosum. (**b**) T2-weighted sagittal image showing low signal intensity fibrotic tissue (*arrowhead*)

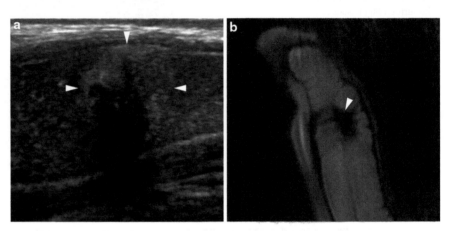

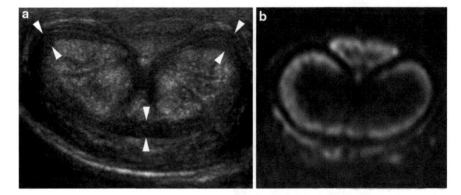

Fig. 124.9 Diffuse penile fibrosis following prolonged ischemic priapism. (**a**) Axial US scan showing hyperechogenic tissue on both corpora cavernosa. Only a thin sub-albugineal portion of normally appearing cavernosal tissue is visible (*arrowheads*). (**b**) Axial T2-weighted MR image showing low signal intensity tissue within the corpora cavernosa surrounded by a thin rim of normally appearing, hyperintense cavernous tissue

Doppler interrogation. At MR imaging cavernous hemangioma presents with high signal intensity on T2-weighted images (Kim et al. 1991). This technique is especially indicated in large hemangiomas spreading in the scrotal wall, in the perineum and involving the penile bodies.

Urethral Cancer

Urethral tumors present at urethrography as irregular narrowing of the urethral lumen. Retrograde urethrography is best suited to evaluate anterior urethral lesions while voiding urethrography best depicts posterior urethral tumors (Pavlica et al. 2003a, b;

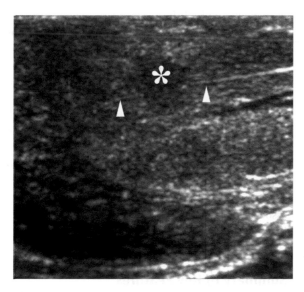

Fig. 124.10 Squamous cell carcinoma of the penis. Local staging. Focal infiltration (*) of the corpus cavernosum presenting as an interruption of the echogenic line of the tunica albuginea (*arrowheads*) (Reprinted with permission from: Serafini G, Bertolotto M, et al. (2008). Penile Tumors: US Features. In: Color Doppler US of the penis. M. Bertolotto (ed.). Berlin Heidelberg, Springer-Verlag: 115–124)

Kawashima et al. 2004). Using modern equipment tumors of the anterior urethra can be investigated with ultrasound as well, provided that the urethral lumen is distended with saline or gel (Nash et al. 1995; Pavlica et al. 2003a, b). The posterior portion of the penile urethra can be investigated using linear high-frequency endorectal probes (Pavlica et al. 2003a, b).

Urethral carcinoma appears at ultrasound as a hypo- to isoechoic, irregularly marginated lesion. Ultrasound is able to identify the mass and the associated urethral stricture. It can also detect tumor spreading into the surrounding periurethral tissue, in particular, infiltration of the cavernosal bodies (Fig. 124.12).

Major indications of CT scan in patients with urethral malignancies are evaluation of nodal disease and identification of pulmonary, cerebral, liver, adrenal, and other abdominal metastases. Compared to MR imaging local staging is limited by the lower contrast resolution.

With its multiplanar capability and high tissue contrast, MR imaging is widely used for local staging of urethral cancer (Pavlica et al. 2003a, b; Kawashima et al. 2004; Kim et al. 2007). Tumor infiltration of the penile bodies and of the other periurethral tissues can be investigated. MR imaging is especially useful for those tumors that invade the root of the penis for which a comprehensive physical examination is often limited. At MR imaging, urethral cancer is seen as a soft-tissue mass along the course of the urethra with similar or lower signal intensity on T1-weighted images, and

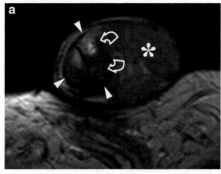
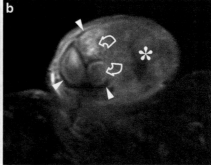
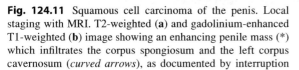

Fig. 124.11 Squamous cell carcinoma of the penis. Local staging with MRI. T2-weighted (**a**) and gadolinium-enhanced T1-weighted (**b**) image showing an enhancing penile mass (*) which infiltrates the corpus spongiosum and the left corpus cavernosum (*curved arrows*), as documented by interruption of the low signal intensity line of the tunica albuginea (*arrowheads*). Gadolinium-enhanced T1-weighted image does not add significantly to T2-weighted image for tumor staging in this patient

lower signal intensity on T2-weighted images compared to the corpus spongiosum (Kawashima et al. 2004; Kim et al. 2007). Tumor enhancement is variable. Sometimes tumor tissue shows high signal intensity on T2-weighted images due to associated inflammation.

Secondary Tumors

Penile metastases can present with nodular deposits or direct infiltration on the penile shaft by adjacent

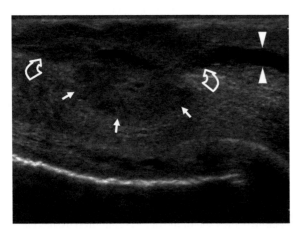

Fig. 124.12 Carcinoma of the penile urethra infiltrating the corpora cavernosa. Sonourethrography in the sagittal scan. The sonogram shows the lesion (*curved arrows*) replacing the corpus spongiosum, and causing irregular narrowing of the urethral lumen (*arrowheads*). The corpora cavernosa are widely infiltrated by the mass (*small arrows*)

primary malignancies. At ultrasound, hematogenous or lymphatic metastases usually present with cavernosal and spongiosal nodules of variable echogenicity and vascularization (Fig. 124.13). Metastatic involvement from adjacent organs can present with multiple nodules or with diffuse infiltration on the penile shaft. Infiltration of the tunica albuginea is detected as interruption of the echogenic linear interface surrounding the corpora (Bertolotto et al. 2005). In patients with diffuse secondary involvement of the shaft or with isoechogenic metastases, the lesions may be barely visible except for mild alteration of the penile echotexture, diffuse or focal infiltration of the tunica albuginea, or irregular bulking of the shaft (Fig. 124.14).

At MR imaging penile metastases may present with discrete enhancing nodules of low signal intensity on both T1- and T2-weighted images (Fig. 124.13) or with diffuse infiltration of the shaft. Focal or widespread infiltration of the tunica albuginea is identified as tumor tissue growth replacing the normal cavernous tissue, associated with interruption of the low signal intensity line of the tunica albuginea (Bertolotto et al. 2009).

Summary of Key Features

When a penile lump is identified history and physical examination usually allow a preliminary diagnosis.

With the exclusion of primary penile malignancies ultrasound is the imaging modality of choice to

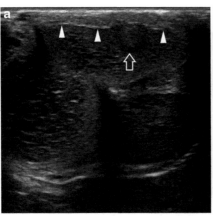
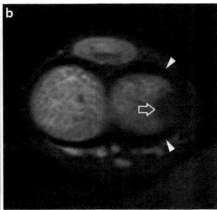
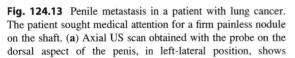

Fig. 124.13 Penile metastasis in a patient with lung cancer. The patient sought medical attention for a firm painless nodule on the shaft. (**a**) Axial US scan obtained with the probe on the dorsal aspect of the penis, in left-lateral position, shows a slightly hypoechoic nodule in the corpus cavernosum (*arrow*) bulging the tunica albuginea (*arrowheads*). (**b**) T2-weighted axial MR image shows the lesion in the left corpus cavernosum (*arrow*) infiltrating the tunica albuginea (*arrowheads*)

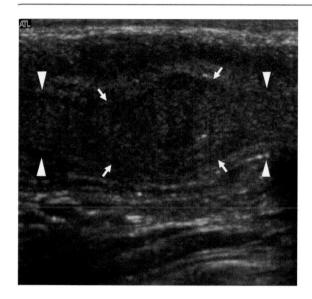

Fig. 124.14 Penile metastasis in a patient with advanced bladder cancer. Longitudinal US scan showing a barely visible isoechoic metastatic nodule (*arrows*) bulging the corpus cavernosum (*arrowheads*)

evaluate penile lumps. MR imaging is a problem solving technique.

In patients with penile inflammation ultrasound is able to indentify abscess formation and involvement of the erectile bodies. CT and MR imaging are indicated in severe inflammatory processes to evaluate the extension of the disease.

Penile tumor is a histological diagnosis. Imaging is indicated for staging. For this purpose, MR imaging is preferred because compared to ultrasound it is more panoramic and provides a better tissue contrast resolution.

References

Agrawal A, Pai D, et al. Clinical and sonographic findings in carcinoma of the penis. J Clin Ultrasound. 2000;28(8):399–406.

Bertolotto M, Serafini G, et al. Primary and secondary malignancies of the penis: ultrasound features. Abdom Imaging. 2005;30(1):108–12.

Bertolotto M, Martingano P, et al. Penile scar and fibrosis. Springer-Verlag: Color Doppler US of the Penis. M. Bertolotto. Berlin Heidelberg; 2008a. p. 153–62.

Bertolotto M, Pavlica P, et al. Miscellaneous benign diseases. Springer-Verlag: Color Doppler US of the Penis. M. Bertolotto. Berlin Heidelberg; 2008b. p. 175–82.

Bertolotto M, Pavlica P, et al. Painful penile induration: imaging findings and management. Radiographics. 2009;29(7):477–93.

Chew KK, Stuckey BG, et al. Penile fibrosis in intracavernosal prostaglandin E1 injection therapy for erectile dysfunction. Int J Impot Res. 1997;9(4):225–9 discussion 229–230.

El-Bahnasawy MS, Dawood A, et al. Low-flow priapism: risk factors for erectile dysfunction. BJU Int. 2002;89(3):285–90.

Kawashima A, Sandler CM, et al. Imaging of urethral disease: a pictorial review. Radiographics. 2004;24 Suppl 1:S195–216.

Kayes O, Minhas S, et al. The role of magnetic resonance imaging in the local staging of penile cancer. Eur Urol. 2007;51(5):1313–8. discussion 1318–1319.

Kickuth R, Adams S, et al. Magnetic resonance imaging in the diagnosis of Fournier's gangrene. Eur Radiol. 2001;11(5):787–90.

Kim SH, Lee SE, et al. Penile hemangioma: US and MR imaging demonstration. Urol Radiol. 1991;13(2):126–8.

Kim B, Kawashima A, et al. Imaging of the male urethra. Semin Ultrasound CT MR. 2007;28(4):258–73.

Lont AP, Besnard AP, et al. A comparison of physical examination and imaging in determining the extent of primary penile carcinoma. BJU Int. 2003;91(6):493–5.

Nash PA, McAninch JW, et al. Sono-urethrography in the evaluation of anterior urethral strictures. J Urol. 1995;154(1):72–6.

Otsuka T, Terauchi M. Cysts of the genito-perineal raphe: a study of 160 reported cases. Jap J Plast Reconstruct Surg. 1990;33:777–83.

Pavlica P, Barozzi L, et al. Imaging of male urethra. Eur Radiol. 2003a;13(7):1583–96.

Pavlica P, Menchi I, et al. New imaging of the anterior male urethra. Abdom Imaging. 2003b;28(2):180–6.

Pretorius ES, Siegelman ES, et al. MR imaging of the penis. Radiographics. 2001; Spec No S283–98; discussion S298–89.

Serafini G, Bertolotto M, et al. Penile tumors: US features. Springer-Verlag: Color Doppler US of the Penis. M. Bertolotto. Berlin Heidelberg; 2008. p. 115–24.

Singh AK, Saokar A, et al. Imaging of penile neoplasms. Radiographics. 2005;25(6):1629–38.

Singh AK, Gonzalez-Torrez P, et al. Imaging of penile neoplasm. Semin Ultrasound CT MR. 2007;28(4):287–96.

Vossough A, Pretorius ES, et al. Magnetic resonance imaging of the penis. Abdom Imaging. 2002;27(6):640–59.

Wasserman NF. Urethral neoplasms. In: Pollack H, McClennan B, editors. Clinical urography, vol. 2. Philadelphia; Saunders; 2000. p. 1699–715.

Michele Bertolotto, Massimo Valentino, Marco Cavallaro,
Giovanni Serafini, and Lorenzo E. Derchi

Introduction

Injury may result from penetrating and non-penetrating traumas to the erect or to the flaccid penis, and from acute bending of the erect shaft. Subcutaneous or intracorporeal hematomas, tunical disruption, and urethral lesions may result. The spectrum of injuries resulting from traumas to the flaccid and to the erect penis is different, since the possibility to bend, the degree of motility, and position of the organ differ substantially.

With the exception of those produced during sexual foreplay penetrating injuries to the penis usually occur while flaccid and severity is variable depending on whether the skin, the urethra, or the erectile tissues are involved. The most common of them are self-inflicted in mentally deranged patients, or inflicted by a second part. Other relatively common injuries are iatrogenic, following cavernosal injection of vasoactive drugs and inappropriate surgical or circumcision maneuvers. Penetrating injuries can also result from farm and war accidents, gunshot wounds, animal or human bites. Zipper injuries are rare and often not significant.

M. Bertolotto (✉) • M. Cavallaro
Department of Radiology, University of Trieste, Trieste, Italy

M. Valentino
Emergency Radiology Unit, University Hospital of Parma,
Parma, Italy

G. Serafini
Department of Radiology, S. Corona Hospital,
Pietra Ligure, Italy

L.E. Derchi
Department of Radiology, University of Genova, Genoa, Italy

Blunt traumas to the flaccid and to the erect penis may result from a variety of accidents or may be produced during intercourse.

Injuries to the Flaccid Penis

The flaccid penis is much less frequently injured than other parts of the body since it is mobile and largely protected by its position. It can be wounded, however, as a result of various events including self-mutilation, road or work accidents, gunshot wounds, burns, and sexual foreplay. A blunt trauma to the flaccid penis usually does not lead to albugineal disruption. Most of injuries are disruption of the superficial veins and extratunical and cavernosal hematomas. Immediate treatment consists in catheterization, ice packs, and anti-inflammatory agents. It is mandatory to exclude cavernosal artery disruption, which presents clinically with high-flow priapism.

Injuries to the Erect Penis

The erect penis has limited bending capability, reduced mobility, and elasticity, and is therefore more susceptible to injury compared to the flaccid penis. Several lesions should be considered including intra-albugineal and extraalbugineal hematomas, isolated septal hematoma, rupture of the suspensory ligament, disruption of the dorsal and cavernosal vessels, and penile fracture. The latter requires surgical repair to reduce the incidence of penile deformity and erectile dysfunction.

B. Hamm, P. R. Ros (eds.), *Abdominal Imaging*, DOI 10.1007/978-3-642-13327-5_212,
© Springer-Verlag Berlin Heidelberg 2013

Penile Fracture

Penile fracture usually occurs during vigorous sexual intercourse when the rigid penis slips out of the vagina and is misdirected against the partner's pubic bone or perineum. This trauma causes a sudden rise of the intracorporeal pressure resulting in further distention of the already thinned tunica albuginea of the erect penis, thereby causing it to tear. Rupture of the tunica albuginea may be monolateral or bilateral, usually associated to disruption of the cavernous tissue below it. Besides occurring during intercourse, penile fracture can follow self-inflicted abnormal downward bending of the erect penis to achieve detumescence. Other reported causes are rare. They include rolling over in bed with an erect penis, direct blunt injury, and injury secondary to a bite during sexual foreplay.

History and clinical presentation of penile fracture is usually characteristic. During the acute bending of the erect penis the patient experiences a sharp pain and hears a cracking or popping sound followed by rapid detumescence, penile swelling, and deformity.

Vascular Injuries

Rupture of the dorsal vessels usually manifests with penile swelling due to hematoma and ecchymosis. It may mimic clinically penile fracture, but deformation and immediate detumescence usually do not occur because the tunica albuginea is intact. Venous injury is relatively more frequent than arterial injuries. Rupture of small venous collaterals is more common that injury of the main branches. The characteristics of the associated hematoma depend on the site of vascular disruption and on the integrity of the Buck's fascia. Rupture of the deep dorsal vessels below an intact Buck's fascia produces a hematoma confined to the shaft, while if the superficial vessels are torn, or if the Buck's fascia is injured, a butterfly hematoma develops involving the scrotum, pubis, and anterior perineum.

Posttraumatic thrombosis of the deep dorsal vein can follow vigorous intercourse or self-stimulation. Clinically the patients present with a rod-like painless induration of the dorsal aspect of the shaft.

Isolated Rupture of the Penile Septum

Injury to the erect penis may produce a circumscribed disruption of the septum with formation of an isolated septal hematoma (Brant et al. 2007). History usually reports an episode of penile bending during vigorous intercourse or masturbation associated with pain and a snapping sensation. Contrary to penile fracture, in isolated rupture of the septum immediate detumescence of the penis does not usually follow the traumatic episode. Patients with isolated rupture of the penile septum usually seek for medical attention complaining of painful intercourse, mild erectile dysfunction, and penile curvature or shortening.

Injury to the Suspensory Ligament

The suspensory ligament anchors the penis to the symphysis pubis. When the ligament is intact the erect penis assumes a position of approximately 30° to the anterior abdominal wall and is stable enough to allow coitus. Rupture of the suspensory ligament can occur when the erect penis is forcibly displaced toward the feet. The shaft remains unstable; it does not assume the normal position during erection and tends to slip out of the vagina. Diagnosis of rupture of the suspensory ligament is made by history and by palpation of a gap between the base of the shaft of the penis and the symphysis pubis. An abnormal angle is noted during erection.

Posttraumatic Erectile Dysfunction

Patients with vertebral, pelvic, or perineal injuries and patients undergoing extensive pelvic surgery can present with posttraumatic erectile dysfunction.

Trauma-related neurogenic impotence can result from spinal cord injury or isolated damage to the penile nerves. Doppler ultrasound findings may be normal in these patients or may show exaggerated response to vasoactive agents.

Posttraumatic arterial insufficiency is due to vascular lesions which characteristically involve the distal portion of the internal pudendal arteries at the level of the urogenital diaphragm and the proximal portion of the penile arteries.

Patient Management

Following the EUA (European Urology Association) guidelines on urological trauma (Djakovic et al. 2009), surgical exploration and conservative debridement of necrotic tissue is recommended in severe penetrating injuries. Nonoperative management is recommended in small superficial injuries with intact Buck's fascia. Skin graft is used in case of extensive loss of penile shaft skin.

Injuries resulting from blunt trauma can be managed conservatively if the tunica albuginea is intact (Koifman et al. 2010). In these cases, nonsteroidal analgesics and ice packs are recommended. Blood aspiration under ultrasound guidance is recommended in patients with isolated septal hematoma to prevent fibrotic changes which can cause penile shortening and focal lack of rigidity (Brant et al. 2007).

Some urologists consider surgical intervention in large extraalbugineal hematomas to avoid abscess formation, even though the tunica albuginea is intact (Zaman et al. 2005).

In penile fracture early surgical repair is recommended. Several approaches have been proposed. In case of a single defect of one corpus cavernosum, some urologists perform direct incision over the lesion with minimal dissection. Most urologists, however, prefer a circumcising type incision in all cases, with complete degloving of the skin of the penile shaft. This approach allows an excellent exposure of both corpora cavernosa and urethra and it is very helpful in case of bilateral rupture with or without associated urethral injury. If urethral injury is present, treatment depends on the site and extent of the rupture.

Rupture of the suspensory ligament usually does not require treatment. If the patient complains for an abnormal angulation of the penis during erection a simple suture of the ligament through a suprapubic access can be performed.

Rupture of the dorsal vessels of the penis usually does not require treatment. Posttraumatic thrombosis of the deep dorsal vein is usually treated with fibrinolytics and anticoagulation, associated with discontinuance of sexual activity. The best treatment for cavernosal artery tear presenting with high-flow priapism still remains controversial. Most of groups recommend superselective embolization of the torn artery.

The aim of penile revascularization surgery is to restore penile vascular supply in patients with posttraumatic arterial insufficiency. Indication is limited to a very selected group of young, otherwise healthy, not vasculopathic patients with established posttraumatic vascular injury. Prosthesis implantation can be considered in the other patients who developed posttraumatic erectile dysfunction unresponsive to oral medications and cavernosal prostaglandin injection.

Appropriateness of Different Imaging Modalities

The appropriateness of imaging in patients with penile traumas is debated among the urologists. While in many medical centers imaging evaluation is routinely performed during the clinical work-up of the patient to differentiate between the surgical and the nonsurgical penile lesions, some urologists claim operation for the majority of the patients, irrespective of whether the tunica albuginea is disrupted or not (Zaman et al. 2005; Wessells and Long 2006). This different view is due in part from the fact that imaging penile traumas requires adequate equipment and an operator with a specific skill in this field. It is not always the case of an emergency setting.

Ultrasonography is the first imaging modality in patients with penile trauma (Bertolotto and Pozzi Mucelli 2004). The nature and extent of the different injuries can be fully evaluated in most of cases. Magnetic resonance imaging (MRI) is a problem-solving technique. Compared to ultrasound, advantages are panoramicity and excellent tissue contrast. Because high cost and restricted availability, however, MRI is not currently considered a routine part of the evaluation of penile trauma. Retrograde urethrography is indicated to rule out associated urethral injury. Other imaging modalities such as X-ray, CT, angiography, and cavernosography are seldom indicated.

Penetrating Injuries

Diagnosis of penetrating injuries to the penis is usually straightforward. Retrograde uretrography and sonourethrography can be used to assess integrity of the urethra (Bertolotto et al. 2005). In patients with

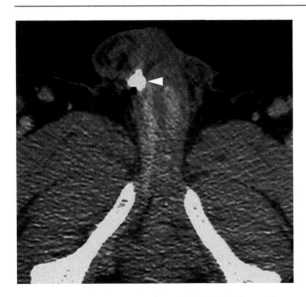

Fig. 125.1 Gunshot wound to the penis. Axial CT image showing a bullet (*arrowhead*) retained within the right corpus cavernosum

genital gunshot wounds to the genitalia plain X-ray, ultrasound, and CT (Fig. 125.1) have a role to identify hematomas, localize bullets and other foreign bodies retained within the penis, assess their relationship with the penile bodies, and guide retrieval (Bertolotto et al. 2008). Color Doppler interrogation of cavernosal arteries allows evaluation of associated vascular injuries (Bertolotto et al. 2008). Also associated cavernositis and abscess formation can be evaluated.

Penile Fracture

Several imaging techniques can be used to evaluate patients with penile fracture looking for presence of the albugineal tear, associated hematomas, and injuries to the penile vessels and the urethra.

Ultrasound

Use of ultrasound in patients with clinically suspected penile fracture is questionable among urologists, because early investigations missed a considerable number of lesions. Ultrasound technology, however, changed significantly in the last years. When modern ultrasound equipment and high-frequency, broadband probes are used by a skilled operator ultrasonography is now able to differentiate penile fracture from the other penile injuries which do not require surgical

management. The tear is identified as an interruption of the thin echogenic line of the tunica albuginea (Bertolotto and Pozzi Mucelli 2004; Bertolotto et al. 2005, 2008; Bhatt et al. 2005).

Besides identification of the albugineal tear, ultrasound is able to evaluate associated hematomas (Bertolotto and Pozzi Mucelli 2004) (Fig. 125.2). Cavernosal artery injuries can be detected at color Doppler interrogation (Fig. 125.3). High-flow priapism does not develop in patients with penile fracture because of blood leakage from the albugineal tear (Bertolotto et al. 2008).

As with other imaging modalities, associated urethral injuries are identified with difficulty at ultrasound (Bhatt et al. 2005). In absence of external penetrating traumas an indirect signs of urethral disruption is presence of air in the cavernosal bodies (Bertolotto and Pozzi Mucelli 2004) or in the corpus spongiosum (Fig. 125.4). Sonourethrography may help identify interruption of the urethral wall (Bhatt et al. 2005; Berna-Mestre and Berna-Serna 2009), but retrograde X-ray urethrography is still indicated.

MRI

Compared to ultrasound, the integrity of the tunica albuginea is best evaluated with MRI due to the higher contrast resolution between the tunica albuginea, the cavernosal bodies, and the surrounding tissues. MRI allows accurate evaluation of the size, location, and orientation of the albugineal tear (Choi et al. 2000; Abolyosr et al. 2005). The key finding for the diagnosis of fracture is recognition of an interruption of the low-signal-intensity line of the tunica albuginea, which is well seen on both T1- and T2-weighted images. In our experience, albugineal tear is best identified on T2-weighted sequences (Figs. 125.2, 125.5), and noncontrast MRI is sufficient in almost all cases. Signal intensity of associated cavernosal and extraalbugineal hematomas, however, vary with time and may present with low signal intensity on T2-weighted images (Fig. 125.5). In this case, contrast differences between the tunica albuginea and the adjacent hematoma reduces, the hematoma may mimic the intact tunica albuginea, and small fractures may be overlooked (Uder et al. 2002; Kirkham et al. 2008). When visualization of the tunica albuginea is reduced on T2-weighted images disruption is best seen on T1-weighted images obtained before and after contrast administration.

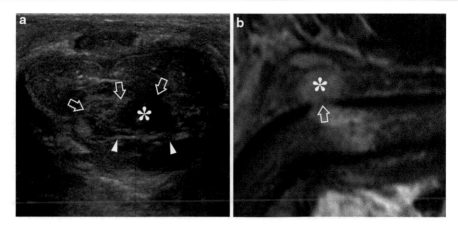

Fig. 125.2 Penile fracture at the base of the penis with rupture of the dorsal aspect of both corpora cavernosa. (**a**) Axial scan showing a large albugineal tear (*open arrows*) as an interruption of the thin echogenic line of the tunica albuginea. An associated hematoma is recognized below (*) and above the Buck's fascia (*arrowheads*). (**b**) Sagittal T2-weighted MR image confirms discontinuity (*open arrow*) of the low-signal-intensity tunica albuginea and the associated hematoma (*)

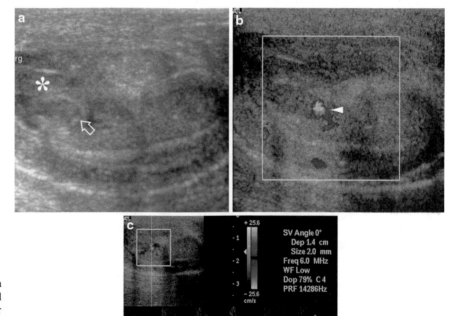

Fig. 125.3 Penile fracture with rupture of the right cavernosal artery. (**a**) Axial scan showing a large albugineal tear (*open arrow*) of the right corpus cavernosum and associated extraalbugineal hematoma (*). (**b**) Axial color Doppler image showing color blush (*arrowhead*) within the right corpus cavernosum consistent with cavernosal artery tear. (**c**) Duplex Doppler interrogation of the torn cavernosal artery shows high velocity turbulent flows

Preliminary investigation suggests that MRI performs better than ultrasound in identification of associated urethral injury (Choi et al. 2000; Turpin et al. 2008), but current data are limited.

Cavernosography

Cavernosography has been used in the past to identify cavernosal tissue tear, with extravasation from the corpora considered to be diagnostic

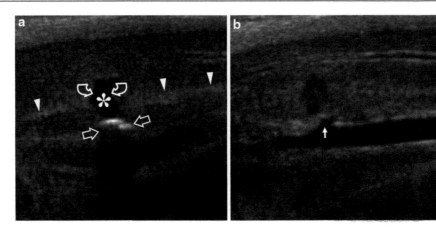

Fig. 125.4 Penile fracture with associated rupture of the corpus spongiosum and of the urethra. (**a**) Longitudinal US scan performed with the probe on the dorsal aspect of the penis showing a ventral tear of the corpora cavernosa (*curved arrows*) as an interruption of the thin echogenic line of the tunica albuginea (*arrowheads*). A dorsal tear of the corpus spongiosum is associated (*open arrows*) containing air. There is a small hematoma (*) at the level of the fracture involving both the cavernosal and the spongiosal tissue. (**b**) Sonourethrography of the same patient showing the interruption of the urethral lumen (*small arrow*)

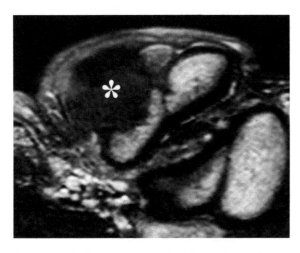

Fig. 125.5 Penile fracture. T2-weighted axial image showing rupture of the right corpus cavernosum as an interruption of the low-signal-intensity line of the tunica albuginea. The associated hematoma (*) has low-signal intensity consistent with presence of deoxyhemoglobin and other products of blood denaturation

(Mydlo et al. 1998). This procedure, however, is invasive and not currently recommended preoperatively. False-negative results may occur when clotting obliterates the corporeal defect, or in case of small tears presenting with minimal or no extravasation. Several urologists still use cavernosography during the operation. Potential risks include infection, priapism, contrast reaction, and cavernosal fibrosis from extravasated contrast medium.

Hematomas

Extraalbugineal hematomas and ecchymosis result from rupture of the dorsal vessels or their branches. Cavernosal hematomas are often bilateral. They can result from crushing of the penile crura against the pelvic bones. Cavernosal artery tear presenting with high-flow priapism may be associated. When the tunica albuginea is intact hematomas and ecchymosis can be managed conservatively. Their differentiation from penile fracture is therefore important. Ultrasound and MRI appearance vary with the age of the lesion.

Ultrasound

Early after the trauma hematomas appear as hyperechoic or complex masses which become more cystic with time (Fig. 125.6) (Bhatt et al. 2005). Isolated septal hematoma presents at ultrasound (Fig. 125.7) as a well-defined cystic-like area in the septal region (Brant et al. 2007). Aspiration under ultrasound guidance is recommended to prevent circumscribed septal fibrosis, penile shortening, or focal lack of rigidity.

MRI

At MRI hyperacute hematomas present with relatively low signal intensity on T1-weighted images and high signal intensity on T2-weighted images.

Fig. 125.6 Penile hematomas with intact tunica albuginea. (**a**) Superficial hematoma. (**b**) Intracavernosal hematoma (*)

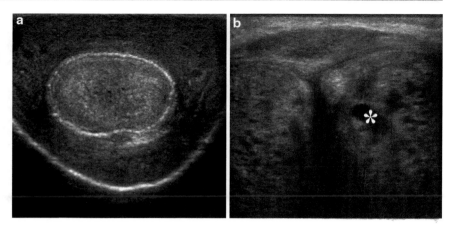

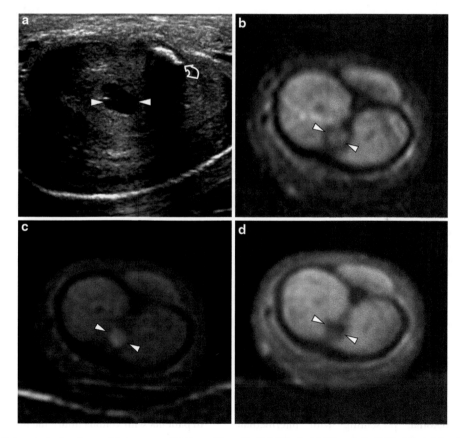

Fig. 125.7 Subacute isolated septal hematoma. Patient with already known Peyronie's disease presenting after having experienced acute penile pain and snapping sensation during intercourse 10 days before. The patient sought medical attention because of appearance of a small penile lump in the midshaft. (**a**) Grey-scale US shows a ventral calcific plaque (*curved arrow*) and an anechoic, slightly corpuscolated lesion in the penile septum (*arrowheads*) consistent with isolated septal hematoma.

(**b–d**) MRI. Axial T2-weighted (**b**), T1-weighted (**c**), and contrast-enhanced T1-weighted (**d**) images. MRI confirms US diagnosis of isolated septal hematoma showing a small lesion in the penile septum (*arrowheads*) with high signal intensity on T2-weighted (**b**) and T1-weighted (**c**) images, consistent with presence of blood products, lacking enhancement after paramagnetic contrast medium administration (**d**)

Fig. 125.8 MRI appearance of extraalbugineal hematomas. T1-weighted (**a**) and T2-weighted (**b**) images showing a relatively high signal intensity lesion (*) consistent with subacute hematoma below the Buck's fascia (*curved arrow*). The tunica albuginea (*arrowheads*) is intact. A superficial ecchymosis is associated (*small arrows*) with lower T1 and higher T2 signal intensity, suggesting acute bleeding

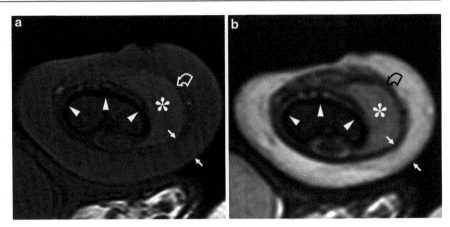

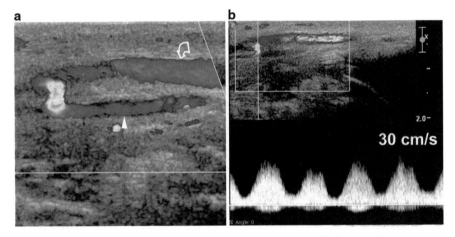

Fig. 125.9 Posttraumatic superficial arteriovenous communication. The patient experienced pain and a snapping sensation during vigorous intercourse, followed by appearance of a small localized pulsatile swelling on the shaft. There was no loss in penile rigidity. (**a**) Color Doppler US shows a communication between a superficial artery (*arrowhead*) and vein (*curved arrow*). (**b**) Duplex Doppler interrogation of the fistula documents relatively high velocity (30 cm/s), turbulent flow

Then, deoxyhemoglobin is formed and signal on T2-weighted images reduces. Conversion of deoxyhemoglobin to methemoglobin results in high signal intensity on T1 weighted images (Figs. 125.2, 125.5, 125.7, 125.8) (Abolyosr et al. 2005; Turpin et al. 2008). A hemosiderin rim is eventually present in chronic hematoma, presenting with intermediate signal intensity on T1-weighted images and low signal intensity on T2-weighted images. In general, penile hematomas are best demonstrated on T2-weighted images. When they are isointense relative to the erectile bodies on T2-weighted images they are better seen after contrast material administration (Uder et al. 2002; Kirkham et al. 2008).

Isolated Vascular Injuries

Cavernosal artery disruption presents clinically with high-flow priapism (Bertolotto et al. 2003). Imaging appearance is described in a dedicated chapter of this book.

In patients with venous injury the torn veins usually collapse and are not visible directly at imaging (Bertolotto and Pozzi Mucelli 2004). Only the associated hematomas are identified. Venous thrombosis presents with non-compressible echogenic material within the dorsal vein, isolated or spreading over the circumflex veins. Signal is lacking at color Doppler interrogation (Bhatt et al. 2005).

In posttraumatic arteriovenous fistulas (Fig. 125. 9) Doppler interrogation reveals high velocity, low resistance arterial flows and high velocity, turbulent venous flows (Bertolotto and Pozzi Mucelli 2004; Bertolotto et al. 2005).

Injury to the Suspensory Ligament

Imaging is usually not required in patients with rupture of the suspensory ligament. Ultrasonography is able to document the gap between the pubis and the penile shaft and associated hematomas of the soft tissues (Bertolotto and Pozzi Mucelli 2004). At MRI rupture appears on T2-weighted images as a disruption of the normally well-defined low-signal-intensity strands of the ligament (Kirkham et al. 2008).

Posttraumatic Erectile Dysfunction

The integrity of the arterial vascular supply to the penis can be assessed by Doppler interrogation of the cavernosal arteries. A peak systolic velocity of 25 cm/s or less after prostaglandin E1 intracavernosal injection reflects arterial insufficiency. Further investigation is warranted only in patients undergoing penile revascularization. In these patients patency and symmetry of the dorsal arteries and presence of cavernosal-to-dorsal arterial communications should be investigated. The course and caliber of hypogastric arteries should be evaluated as well. Angiography or CT-angiography are indicated to assess abnormalities of pelvic vessels (Bertolotto et al. 2005).

Summary of Key Features

In patients with penile traumas the most important differential diagnosis is between penile fracture, which requires surgery, and injuries in which the tunica albuginea is intact, that can be managed conservatively.

Imaging has a controversial role in the clinical management of patients with penile traumas. Ultrasound and MR imaging are able to identify rupture of the tunica albuginea and are therefore useful to guide the management of the patient.

Ultrasound can provide in most of cases all clinically relevant information for the differential diagnosis of traumatic injuries to the penis, but requires high-end ultrasound equipment, high-frequency probes, and adequate operator's skill on this specific field.

Compared to ultrasound MRI is more panoramic and has an increased contrast-tissue resolution. Its availability, however, is limited for use in emergency.

References

Abolyosr A, Moneim AE, et al. The management of penile fracture based on clinical and magnetic resonance imaging findings. BJU Int. 2005;96(3):373–7.

Berna-Mestre JD, Berna-Serna JD. Anterior urethral trauma: role of sonourethrography. Emerg Radiol. 2009;16(5):391–4.

Bertolotto M, Pozzi Mucelli R. Nonpenetrating penile traumas: sonographic and Doppler features. AJR Am J Roentgenol. 2004;183(4):1085–9.

Bertolotto M, Quaia E, et al. Color Doppler imaging of posttraumatic priapism before and after selective embolization. Radiographics. 2003;23(2):495–503.

Bertolotto M, Calderan L, et al. Imaging of penile traumas–therapeutic implications. Eur Radiol. 2005;15(12):2475–82.

Bertolotto M, Privitera C, et al. US evaluation of patients with penile traumas. In: Bertolotto M, editor. Color Doppler US of the penis. Berlin/Heidelberg: Springer; 2008. p. 95–106.

Bhatt S, Kocakoc E, et al. Sonographic evaluation of penile trauma. J Ultrasound Med. 2005;24(7):993–1000; quiz 1001.

Brant WO, Bella AJ, et al. Isolated septal fibrosis or hematoma–atypical Peyronie's disease? J Urol. 2007;177(1):179–82; discussion 183.

Choi MH, Kim B, et al. MR imaging of acute penile fracture. Radiographics. 2000;20(5):1397–405.

Djakovic N, Plas E, et al. Guidelines on urological trauma; 2009. p. 1–84.

Kirkham AP, Illing RO, et al. MR imaging of nonmalignant penile lesions. Radiographics. 2008;28(3):837–53.

Koifman L, Barros R, et al. Penile fracture: diagnosis, treatment and outcomes of 150 patients. Urology. 2010;76(6):1488–92.

Mydlo JH, Hayyeri M, et al. Urethrography and cavernosography imaging in a small series of penile fractures: a comparison with surgical findings. Urology. 1998;51(4):616–9.

Turpin F, Hoa D, et al. MRI of the post-traumatic penis. J Radiol. 2008;89(3 Pt 1):303–10.

Uder M, Gohl D, et al. MRI of penile fracture: diagnosis and therapeutic follow-up. Eur Radiol. 2002;12(1):113–20.

Wessells H, Long L. Penile and genital injuries. Urol Clin North Am. 2006;33(1):117–26.

Zaman ZR, Kommu SS, et al. The management of penile fracture based on clinical and magnetic resonance imaging findings. BJU Int. 2005;96(9):1423–4.

Peyronie's Disease

Pietro Pavlica, Massimo Valentino, Michele Bertolotto,
Libero Barozzi, and Lorenzo E. Derchi

Introduction

Peyronie's disease (PD) is a benign disease of the penis
of unknown cause. First fully described almost
300 years ago by François de La Peyronie, although
"nodus penis" has been already described centuries
before by Fallopius and Vesalius (Fornara and
Gerbershagen 2004). Peyronie's disease is defined as
an acquired disorder of the tunica albuginea with the
development of a plaque of fibrous tissue, associated
with progressive penile bending and shortening. Pain
on erection can be the first symptom of the disease in
about 10–15% of the patients. As the result of progressive penile deformity, difficulties of penetration can
develop with impairment of erectile capacity.

P. Pavlica (✉)
Department of Radiology, Villalba Hospital, Bologna, Italy

M. Valentino
Emergency Radiology Unit, University Hospital of Parma,
Parma, Italy

M. Bertolotto
Department of Radiology, University of Trieste, Trieste, Italy

L. Barozzi
Emergency, Surgery and Transplants, Department – Radiology
Unit – S. Orsola-Malpighi, University Hospital, Bologna, Italy

L.E. Derchi
Department of Radiology, University of Genova, Genoa, Italy

Epidemiology and Incidence

The contemporary state of knowledge of the epidemiology of PD is unknown, and there are only two
population-based cross-sectional studies that analyzed
the incidence and prevalence of this disease. Lindsay
et al. (1991) analyzing Mayo Clinic centralized medical records calculated the age-adjusted incidence rate
of 27.7 per 100, 000 men per year and a prevalence of
388.8 (0.39%) per 100, 000 of population. Mean
patient age at diagnosis was 53 years (range
18–83 year) and the highest incidence was observed
in men 50–59 years of age.

In Europe, a population cross-section study was
performed by Sommer et al. (2002) who reported an
incidence of 3.2% with a progressive increase in prevalence with the age up to 6.5% in patients greater than
70 year old. They found a statistically significant relationship between PD and diabetes (18.3% vs 6%) and
the use of β-blockers (22.5% vs. 14.2%), but no relationship with other comorbidities such as heart insufficiency, atherosclerosis, chronic drug therapies, lower
urinary tract symptoms (LUTS), urologic surgery,
drinking, and smoking.

In the literature, case series are more frequently
reported and the epidemiologic data on PD incidence
are extremely variable (Kadioglu et al. 2007). A rate of
0.3–0.7% in all male patients attending one urological
facility was reported in 1968 by Ludvik et al. In an
autopsy series of 100 patients, Smith (1969) reported
a histological evidence of fibrosis in the tunica
albuginea in 23% of men, who had no history of
symptoms of PD.

In some more recent studies, Mulhall et al. (2004)
reported the results of the prevalence of PD in 534 men

B. Hamm, P. R. Ros (eds.), *Abdominal Imaging*, DOI 10.1007/978-3-642-13327-5_209,
© Springer-Verlag Berlin Heidelberg 2013

presenting for prostate cancer screening. Penile plaques on physical examination were detected in 8.9% of patients, with a mean age of 68.2 year. The prevalence of PD based on age group was 2.8% for those 40–49 year, 8.6% for patients 50–59 year, 9.7% for those 60–69 year, and 10.95 for those 70–79 year. Hypertension and diabetes were statistically associated to PD, while chronic coronary disease and hyperlipemia did not show any statistical correlation.

La Pera et al. (2001) on the base of a questionnaire administered to 10 centers throughout Italy revealed a prevalence of 7.1% for PD, and it varied in different age groups, with a higher prevalence in older men. It varies from 55 in the 50–54 years of age to 9.1% in the 65–69 year group.

Natural History

The most diffuse opinion is that PD is a progressive disease, but many studies have shown that gradual spontaneous resolution has been observed in 13% of the patients (Gelbard et al. 1990) while stable disease was seen in 47%. It worsened only in 40% (Gelbard et al. 1990) and 30.2% (Kadioglu et al. 2002) with progression of the deformity. Men with stable disease followed for 8.4 months without any treatment were 66.7%. Clinical features that are against spontaneous resolution are the duration of the disease at presentation greater than 2 years, plaque calcifications, curvature greater than 45°, and associated Dupuytren' contracture.

Regarding curvature and extension of the fibrotic plaques, Lania et al. (2004) described a tendency to stabilize in patients older than 50 years. Surgery is more frequently necessary in younger men when progression is more common and surgical solution is necessary for maintaining a normal sexual activity.

Etiology

The pathogenesis of PD is poorly understood and is considered to be the result of reported microvascular injuries of the tunica albuginea. Different causative factors including genetic predisposition, trauma, and tissue ischemia have a role in the pathogenesis of PD. It is widely recognized that micro-traumas leading to the bleeding within the tunica albuginea, the accumulation

of fibrin, and the migration of inflammatory cells into the injured area induce upregulation of cytokine and growth factors and excess increase in the matrix protein which in combination result in the development of a plaque. The most accepted theory of the origin of PD is trauma acute and/or chronic during intercourse. This leads to delamination of the tunica albuginea and small hemorrhage. Subsequent fibrosis with excessive collagen deposition is responsible for decreased elasticity and shortening of the tunica albuginea. Over time, calcifications can develop into the rich collagen depositions, which are typical for PD.

Histologic studies have shown an increase collagen with higher ratio of Type III collagen to Type I, than in normal tunica albuginea (Akkus et al. 1997). There is an increase number of inflammatory cells in the early phase of the disease, followed by fibroblasts proliferation (Fig. 126.1). In chronic disease, calcifications may be detected in up to 35% of cases.

Most frequently the plaques develop on the dorsal aspect of the penis, but may extend beyond the palpable lesion and intersect the ventral aspect of the albuginea and/or the intercavernosal septum (Fig. 126.2) (Brant et al. 2007). Normally elastic fibers of the albuginea are replaced by inelastic collagen-rich tissue, with deviation and loss of length of the penis. The focal loss of elasticity of the tunica albuginea may compromise the normal veno-occlusive mechanism of erection and thus leads to venous leak and erectile dysfunction (Hellestrom 2003).

Clinical Evaluation

Patients with PD usually complain one or more signs or symptoms including curvature in 50–100%, palpable penile plaque in 78–100%, painful erection in 20–70%, and decreased erectile function in 20–54% (Usta et al. 2004; Kadioglu et al. 2002; Schwarzer et al. 2001).

Occasionally individual patients complain of losing penile length in flaccid and more evident in erect penile condition. Men presenting with PD have slightly shorter penile length compared to patients with other pathologies (ED; prostate and bladder disease). Penile length nomogram can be used in clinical practice (Mondaini et al. 2002). The clinical evaluation is usually performed in the flaccid state which allows to detect the number, site, and size of the plaques. Penile curvature and penile length are evaluated after an

Fig. 126.1 Drawing of the pathogenesis of the plaque at the level of the tunica albuginea. Tunical injuries lead to initial tunical micro-hemorrhage (*1*) with subsequent increase in inflammatory cells and fibroblast activation (*2*), which leads to excessive collagen deposition and development of a fibrotic plaque (*3*). It involves the tunica and can extend to the adjacent cavernosal tissue

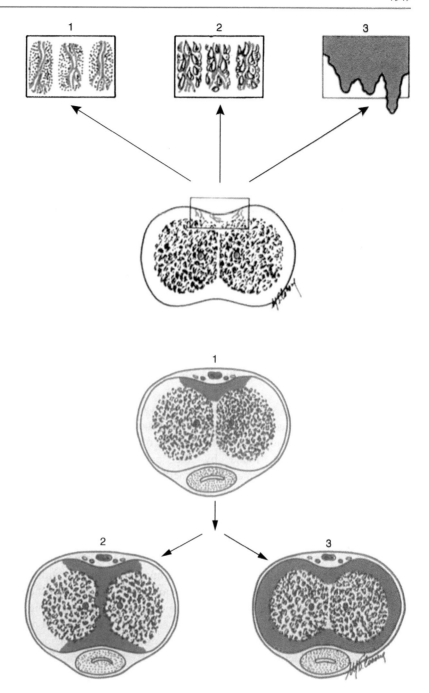

Fig. 126.2 Diagram of the most frequent evolution of the plaque in Peyronie's disease. Initially, the lesion is located on the dorsal aspect of the penis (*1*). It can extend to the septum and the ventral face of the albuginea (*2*). Complex plaques extend to the lateral surfaces of the penis and produce an annular constriction with hourglass deformity associated to reduced distension of the erectile tissue (*3*)

artificial erection is induced by a pharmacologic intracorporeal vasoactive drug injection (Fig. 126.3). Penile deformity is assessed during maximum penile rigidity, and a goniometer can be used to measure the degree of curvature. The center of the goniometer is positioned over the point of maximum curvature and the limb positioned along the shaft proximal to and distal to this point (Moskovic et al. 2011).

Erectile function of the patient should be considered to establish the psychological consequence of the PD and patient's quality of life. Vascular evaluation of erectile function is important for planning the therapy

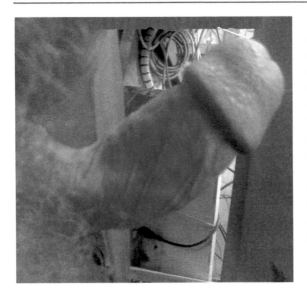

Fig. 126.3 Photography of the penis after artificial erection. Evident hourglass deformity with dorsal curvature of the penis due to a dorsal plaque

in men with PD who are not able to achieve sexual intercourse.

Associated disorders such as diabetes, cardiovascular disease, smoking, and genitourinary disease should be recorded. It is helpful to have photographs of the erect penis taken at home by the patients (autophotography) or performed in the facility if an erection is induced (Moskovic et al. 2011).

Imaging

Ultrasonography with color-Doppler and MR imaging performed in advanced tumescence or erection, after pharmacologic stimulation, are the imaging modalities employed in the clinical practice to confirm the clinical diagnosis, evaluate the extension of the disease, and to assess associated erectile dysfunction.

Ultrasonography

Penile ultrasound is performed with gray-scale sonography using a high-frequency linear probe (7.5–13 MHz) after 10–20 μg of prostaglandin E1 injection into the corpora cavernosa. The higher dose is employed in patients that refer erectile dysfunction (Bertolotto et al. 2005).

With the penis in erection, transverse and longitudinal scans of the penis are performed, starting from the base. Using real-time spatial compounding and adaptive image-processing techniques, it is recommended to reduce artifacts and enhance margins of the examined anatomical structures, to improve visualization of tissue conspicuity, and to increase diagnostic confidence in the evaluation of the tunica albuginea thickness and analyze tissue structure.

After plaque assessment with gray-scale imaging, color-Doppler is performed to analyze the vascular response and the spectra at the level of both cavernosal arteries. Anatomical variations, arterial vascular communications, and leakage pathways along the penile shaft should be explored with particular attention to arterial and venous vessels at the level of PD plaques or in the neighbouring sites.

Recently, the use of sonoelastography has been used to assess the extension and the stiffness of the fibrotic plaques.

Gray-scale Ultrasonography

Penile ultrasonography has emerged as a valuable extension of the clinical examination in patients presenting with symptoms of PD. Sonography permits noninvasive, objective, and detailed analysis of the penis anatomy and allows to define disease severity, monitor disease evaluation, and assess the response to medical therapy, that can be missed with clinical evaluation (Breyer et al. 2010).

Tunical thickening, septal thickening, subalbugineal fibrosis, and penile calcifications must be measured along the penis. The tunica albuginea of patients with PD shows focal areas of thickening and increased echogenicity, compared to normal adjacent albuginea (Fig. 126.4). The normal albuginea thickness in erect penis is of 0.6 mm, and when it results in 1 mm or more, it is to be considered pathologic. To increase the measurements accuracy, zooming the suspected area can be particularly useful (Fig. 126.5) (Bertolotto 2008).

In a small group of patients (about 5–10%) with PD do not show focal plaques, but a diffuser thickening of the tunica albuginea. This is commonly observed in cases with evident penile shortening and deformity, associated to ED in men with long-standing history of the disease.

The plaques are usually isoechoic or slightly hyperechoic depending on their thickness and of US

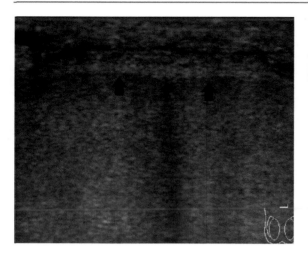

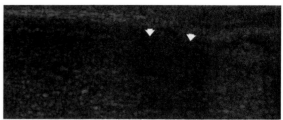

Fig. 126.6 Interruption of the tunica albuginea with a hypoechoic plaque (*arrows*) in a patient with pain during erection but no palpable lump, expression of a lesion in the early phase. Sonography in longitudinal scan on the dorsal surface

Fig. 126.4 Dorsal plaque in Peyronie's disease (*arrows*). Sonography of the dorsal surface of the penis in transverse scan. The albuginea is thickened and slightly hyperechoic

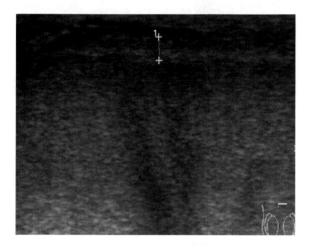

Fig. 126.5 Dorsal plaque in longitudinal scanning. Zooming the image increases the measurement accuracy of the thickness of the plaque

beam characteristics. In our experience, hypoechoic plaques have been observed only in the early phase (Fig. 126.6). Hypoechoic areas can be due to incorrect insonation or to acoustic artifacts as acoustic shadowing or high attenuation of the ultrasound beam.

Plaque size, location, number, and thickness are much better evaluated in erection or good tumescence. More often they are located on the dorsal aspect of the penis, with extension to the lateral or ventral surface (Fig. 126.7). Less frequently, they are found only at the level of the septum (Fig. 126.8) or on the ventral

surface (Fig. 126.9). The progression of the plaque can produce hourglass deformity, with an annular circumferential course with reduced distension of the cavernosal tissue compared to normal proximal and distal regions of the penis.

US has a superior accuracy compared to clinical examination in the detection and definition of the plaques and has a high sensitivity in the identification of calcifications (Fig. 126.10). Acoustic shadowing is typical of all calcifications and their size is inferior to that of the plaques because they are surrounded by non-calcified fibrotic tissue (Fig. 126.11).

Penile septum involvement is commonly associated with pain during erection, and this localization of PD usually contraindicates plaque removal with grafting. The involved septum loses its normal septate ultrasonography features and is replaced by hyperechoic inhomogeneous tissue extending into the surrounded cavernosal tissue, with fuzzy margins. Sometimes small calcifications can be observed or plaque enhancement of the cavernosal arteries.

Color-Doppler Sonography

Color-Power-Doppler imaging and spectral Doppler interrogation of the cavernosal arteries are mandatory before planning a medical or surgical therapy in patients with PD. They show a higher incidence of venous leakage than age-matched control men (Kadioglu et al. 2000). As underlined by Montorsi et al. (1994), the venules draining the corpora cavernosa are no more passively compressed in the area adjacent to the plaque with consequent widespread venous occlusive dysfunction or in localized venous leakage at the level of the fibrotic plaque (Fig. 126.12). In patients with plaque-related leakage

Fig. 126.7 Dorsal Peyronie's plaque extending to the lateral surfaces in transverse scan (**a**) and longitudinal scan (**b**). The albuginea is thickened and hyperechoic and is associated with reduced distension of the underlying erectile tissue

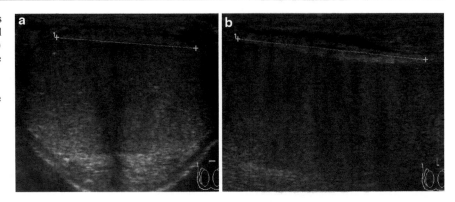

Fig. 126.8 Peyronie's disease with isolated septal plaque (*arrows*) which appears as a rounded hyperechoic area in the center of the penis (**a**). In longitudinal scan, performed on the lateral surface of the penis, the septal plaque appears as a longitudinal hyperechoic stripe (**b**)

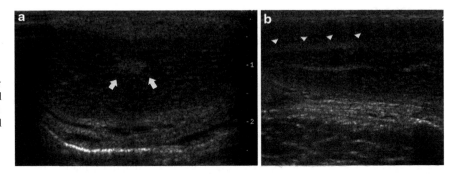

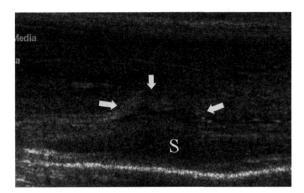

Fig. 126.9 Ventral plaque at the level of the penile's midshaft. The plaque developed dorsally (*arrows*) to the corpus spongiosum (*S*) which is stretched

abnormal cavernosal waveform are identified at Color Imaging adjacent to the plaque.

Doppler spectral studies have shown that in patients with severe PD, cavernosal-spongiosal communications near the plaque remain patent with high systolic peak velocity and lower resistive index, compared to normal cavernosal-spongiosal communications, supporting the hypothesis of arterial blood leakage through these vessels (Bertolotto et al. 2002). Although the majority of patients with PD claiming ED show a venous leakage, arterial inflow dysfunction must be explored. Arterial insufficiency was detected in 30–35% of patients with PD. Sometimes plaque enhancement of the cavernosal arteries has been observed with secondary arteriogenic erectile dysfunction.

Sonoelastography

Elastography is based on the fact that tissue compression produces strain within the tissue and the strain is lower in harder tissue than in soft. It is well known that many diseases lead to a change of tissue hardness (so-called elasticity). The imaging reconstruction of tissue elasticity provides additional information which can be applied for the detection and/or staging of disease.

Some preliminary studies demonstrate the feasibility and accuracy of sonoelastography in detection and visualization of plaques of PD. The improvement is valuable particularly in septal plaques which are

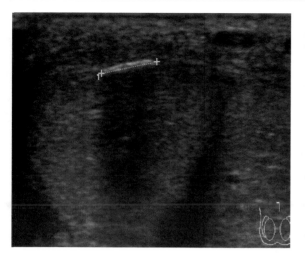

Fig. 126.10 Calcified dorsal plaque, at the level of the right corpus cavernosum. The size is easily measured with the electronic calipers

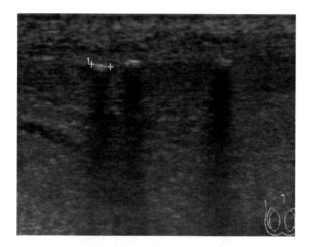

Fig. 126.11 Multiple tiny calcifications in a dorsal plaque surrounded by noncalcified fibrotic tissue

difficult to assess by palpation and by palpation and with conventional sonography with conventional sonography. Plaque extension comparisons showed higher grade lesions, underestimated by B-mode sonography (Pinggera et al. 2007).

Magnetic Resonance Imaging

First experiences on the use of MR imaging in patients with PD are 20 years old (Hricak 1991; Helweg et al. 1992). The clinical results have shown that MR

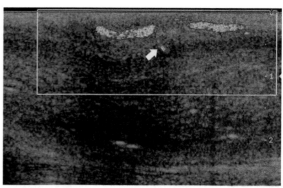

Fig. 126.12 Plaque-related venous leakage. Color-Doppler ultrasound in longitudinal scan. An emissary vein passing through the plaque (*arrow*)

imaging is at least as sensitive as sonography in the assessment of the site and extension of the plaques. It is also more sensitive than gray-scale ultrasound in the detection of Peyronie's lesion at the penile base (Hauch et al. 2003) and is very useful in the follow-up of patients undergoing medical treatment as an objective method to evaluate therapeutic response.

Technique

Appropriate patient positioning and correct scanning sequences are mandatory to obtain diagnostic information. The evaluation should always be performed after intercavernosal injection of vasoactive drugs. The injection should be performed about 20 min before starting the MR scanning so that a maximal rigidity can be obtained. A folded towel is placed between the patient's legs to elevate the penis and scrotum, the erect penis is dorsiflexed against the lower abdominal wall and taped in that position to reduce organ motion during the scanning procedure (Barozzi et al. 1994). Surface coil with a small field of view is preferred so that detailed images can be obtained. A high matrix and thin sections are used to increase the contrast and spatial resolution. The scanning is performed in three planes so that sagittal, transversal, and coronal images are obtained, allowing the complete documentation of the penile surface. T1-weighted and T2 weighted sequences are used, and gadolinium contrast injection is rarely used in clinical practice.

Imaging Analysis

Normal corpora cavernosa shows an intermediate signal intensity on T1-weighted images and a high signal

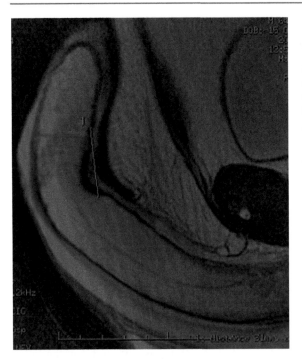

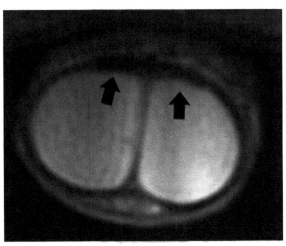

Fig. 126.14 Typical dorsal plaque with dorsal thickening of the albuginea on transverse T2-weighted MR image (*arrows*)

Fig. 126.13 Dorsal Peyronie's plaque with dorsal curvature of the penis. MR imaging with T2 weighted sequence, in sagittal scan. The plaque appears as a hypointense thickening of the dorsal albuginea

intensity on T2-weighted images. The hyperintensity in T2 images is particularly evident in erect penis. The tunica albuginea is hypointense in all sequences, and appears as a thin black line around the corpora cavernosa (Pretorius et al. 2001).

Peyronie's plaques appear in T1- and T2-weighted images as focal (Fig. 126.13) or diffuse thickening of the dorsal albuginea (Fig. 126.14), with low signal intensity. Sometimes the plaques have a nodular aspect and are associated to fibrotic stripes due to the extension of the disease into the corpora cavernosa (Fig. 126.15). The albuginea's thickening can extend to the lateral surface (Fig. 126.16) or sometimes to the ventral surface of the penis (Fig. 126.17); these localizations are better documented with transversal scans. Septal plaques can be connected to a dorsal plaque or can be isolated and are well documented in coronal and transversal scans (Fig. 126.18). MR imaging has a low sensitivity in the detection of calcifications inside the plaque.

The use of gadolinium contrast media in PD is still controversial. Several authors (Andresen et al. 1998) have reported a contrast enhancement of the plaque in

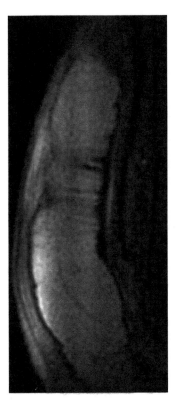

Fig. 126.15 Long dorsal plaque with extensions into the septum. T2 MR imaging in sagittal plane. The albuginea is thickened with reduced extension of the erectile penis which shows a dorsal curvature

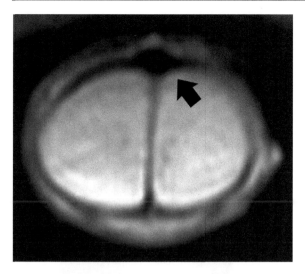

Fig. 126.16 Localized dorsal midline plaque with initial extension to the right side on transverse T2-weighted MR image. The corpora cavernosa are distended and appear hyperintense, while the albuginea is hypointense with focal area of thickening (*arrow*)

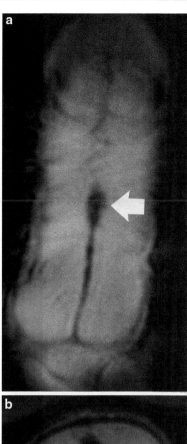

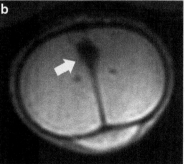

Fig. 126.18 Septal plaque studied with MRI with T2-weighted sequences in coronal scan (**a**) and in axial scan (**b**). The plaque is small and appears as a well-defined hypointense nodule in the middle of the septum (*arrow*)

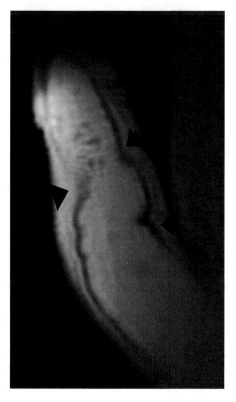

Fig. 126.17 Multiple plaques with deformity and shortening of the distal part of the penis (*arrows*). MR imaging in sagittal plane performed before surgical planning

cases of active inflammation, with no enhancement in stable lesion. This procedure could theoretically be useful as a prognostic criterium and to guide an appropriate medical therapeutic strategy. Other investigators have found no correlation between contrast enhancement and activity or pain (Vosshenrich et al. 1995), and the utility of the method requires well-conducted randomized studies.

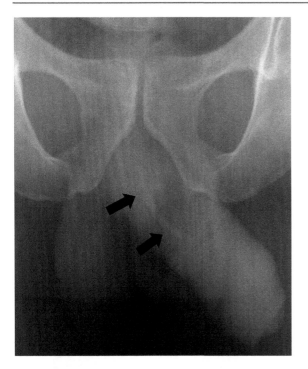

Fig. 126.19 Conventional radiography of the penis with a linear calcified Peyronie's plaque (*arrows*)

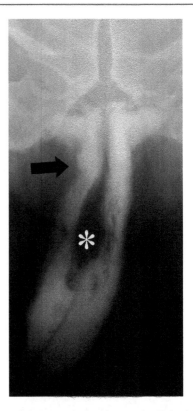

Fig. 126.20 Cavernosography after contrast injection into the corpus cavernosum. Deformity of the penis with a large septal plaque (*) and surface plaques at the level of the proximal penis (*arrow*). There is no venous leakage observed at the base of the penis

Other Imaging Modalities

Andresen et al. (1998) compared the performance of different imaging methods like X-ray mammography technique, computed tomography (CT), sonography, and MR imaging, with the conclusion that sonography is the first-line method for diagnosis.

Conventional radiography and CT are able to detect calcifications in the plaques, but they are not able to identify non-calcified plaques (Fig. 126.19).

Before the extensive introduction of ultrasound in the assessment of patients with PD, cavernosography was the imaging procedure commonly used in planning surgical procedures. Cavernosography allows to obtain objective information on the deformity of the penis and define the site and extension of the plaques (Fig. 126.20). At the same time, it is possible to observe the presence of abnormal venous drainage that can be diffuse or localized at the level or near the plaque. This procedure that is painful is no longer used to assess men with PD, but its use is limited to evaluate the site of venous leakage in patients with ED due to veno-occlusive disease.

Patient Management

The ideal management of Peyronie's disease is not defined and extensively debated. This is the consequence of the limited knowledge of its etiology and causative results. There are no randomized, double-blind, placebo-controlled studies that attest the benefits of different treatments used in the clinical practice. Many clinical reports attest the limited benefits that each has to offer (Kumar and Nehra 2009).

Medical therapy is usually the first-line approach, and its aim is to relieve the pain usually present in the initial stages of PD and possibly minimize the extension of the plaque and the deformity. This initial medical therapy may last for a period of time ranging from 6 to 18 months.

Current oral systemic therapies include vitamin E, alone or in combination with propionyl-L-carnitine, potassium para aminobenzoate (PABA), colchicine, and tamoxifen. The results are variable, and the results are more evident in the initial acute stage of the disease.

Intralesional therapies with direct injections into the plaque are one of the most commonly used minimally invasive treatments. Many agents in varying combinations have been uses with generally good results. Verapamil, collagnenase, and interferons are the most frequently employed. Only one study provided level 1 evidence of improvement in plaque size and penile curvature using intralesional injections of interferon.

Verapamil can be used transdermally with iontophoresis showing significant benefits. Complete resolution of pain was observed in 87% of patients and decreased curvature in 78% of men after therapy.

Collagenase local injections are associated with an 80% incidence of adverse events, even if the results are promising.

The efficacy of extracorporeal shock wave therapy (ESWT) is debated, but the results are contradictory. A statistically significant reduction of penile curvature in 47% of patients is reported.

Local radiotherapy is rarely used in the management of PD, and there is a complete lack of consensus on the approach, dose, and duration of the treatment. There is still a need for well-designed randomized studies in order to define the role of radiotherapy in the treatment of the disease.

Surgical therapy for PD has the objective to straighten the penile's curvature and to restore the erectile function. Preserving the penile length and girth are very important to preserve sexual validity (Tornehl et al. 2004). Currently, the most used surgical procedures include tunical plication, graft interposition, or use of prosthetic devices. Tunical placation is associated with a shortening of the penis and is recommended only in men in whom the postsurgical length is expected to be adequate and the patient has a good baseline erectile function.

There is an increasing trend to use autologous graft material that is commercially available and avoids donor site complications from autologous tissue.

The conclusion is that there is no defined therapy in patients with PD. The results of existing strategies have shown variable results. For acute stage, medical or local injective therapies are used that limit the progression of the disease, without evident regression of existing plaques or curvature. Surgical treatment is proposed in patients with established plaques and curvature with significant rates of success and patient satisfaction.

Appropriateness of Different Imaging Modalities

Knowledge of the different clinical aspects of PD is the initial step in patients presenting with penile pain, focal or multiple palpable induration associated to progressive penile curvature. Patient history and clinical investigation associated to penile inspection and palpation should be performed before any imaging procedure because it is mandatory in selecting the best imaging modality, examination technique, and to guide the interpretation of the images obtained (Smith et al. 2009).

The imaging results are used in the management strategies and to inform the patient of the different treatment options.

Sonography has the advantages compared to other imaging techniques because it has a 100% sensitivity in detecting calcified plaques and a high spatial resolution that allows even non-calcified plaques detection. It is the initial modality to investigate patients with clinically evident PD or to identify lesions nonpalpable or located in the septum. US examination must be performed in advanced tumescence or erection induced pharmacologically. Sonography is easy to perform, has no negative side effects but requires up-to-date technology to measure the exact plaque size and thickness. It is also the simplest tool for following patients under medical, local, or surgical therapy (Prando 2009).

MRI is less frequently used in clinical practice and is still a limited and expensive modality, not suitable for follow-up. The panoramic depiction of the penis and the high contrast resolution are the main advantages of the method, but it requires an accurate methodology in performing the scanning images. The use of gadolinium-DPTA does define the activity of the plaque, showing the contrast enhancement in and around the plaque needs more extensive studies.

Future developments include sonoelastography, MR diffusion, and elastography.

Summary of Key Features

When a Peyronie's disease is suspected or clinically identified, history and physical examination usually allow a definite diagnosis. The precise definition of the size and number of the plaques is sometimes challenging and related to the physician experience.

Ultrasound is the imaging modality of choice to evaluate PD patients before treatment and in the follow-up. MR imaging is a problem-solving technique and can be used in the evaluation of therapeutic results in clinical research. In this period of cost containment, sonography with color-Doppler technique provides the best cost-effectiveness compared to MR imaging.

A simple diagnostic algorithm in the clinical evaluation of patients with Peyronie's disease can be proposed.

Diagnostic Algorithm

Patient and Partner History
- Medical, sexual, and psychosocial history
- History of penile trauma and pain
- Length of time of plaque/deformity/curvature
- Stability of plaque/deformity/curvature
- Prior therapies (including herbals/vitamins/laser/surgery)
- Rule out: ejaculatory or orgasmic dysfunction
- Endocrinological and laboratory evaluation

Physical Examination
- Complete genitourinary examination
- Palpable penile plaque (location, size, severity)
- Penile stretch, length, sensation, pain

Morphologic and Vascular Evaluation in the Erect State
- Photography in erection
- Ultrasonography
- Plaque evaluation and penile deformity (location, size, severity)
- Penile color-Doppler ultrasonography
- Magnetic resonance imaging in erection

References

Akkus E, Carrier S, Baba K, Hsu GL, Padma-Nathan H, Nunes L, Lue TF. Structural alterations in tunica albuginea of the penis: impact of Peyronie's disease, ageing and impotence. Brit J Urol. 1997;79:47–53.

Andresen R, Wegner HEH, Miller K, Banzer D. Imaging modalities in Peyronie's disease. Eur Urol. 1998;34:128–35.

Barozzi L, Pavlica P, Balzani E, et al. Ecografia e risonanza magnetica del pene. Parte I: anatomia. Radiol Med. 1994;87:814–21.

Bertolotto M. Color-Doppler US of the Penis. Berlin/New York: Springer; 2008.

Bertolotto M, de Stefani S, Martinoli C, Quaia E, Buttazzi L. Color Doppler appearance of penile cavernosal-spongiosal communications in patients with severe Peyronie's disease. Eur Radiol. 2002;12:2525–31.

Bertolotto M, Gasparini C, Calderan L, Lissiani A, Cova MA. L'eco-color Doppler penieno: stato dell'arte. Giornale Italiano di Ecografia. 2005;8:113–27.

Brant WO, Bella AJ, Garcia MM, et al. Isolated septal fibrosis or hematoma – atypical Peyronie's disease? J Urol. 2007;177:179–82.

Breyer BN, Shindel AW, Huang YC, Eisenberg ML, Weiss DA, Lue TF, Smith JF. Are sonographic characteristics associated with progression to surgery in men with Peyronie's disease? J Urol. 2010;183:1484–8.

Fornara P, Gerbershagen HP. Ultrasound in patients affected with Peyronie's disease. Word J Urol. 2004;22:365–7.

Gelbard MK, Dorey F, James K. The natural history of Peyronie's disease. J Urol. 1990;144:1376–9.

Hauck EW, Hackstein N, Vosshenrich R, et al. Diagnostic value of magnetic resonance imaging in Peyrinie’s disease-a comparison both with palpation and ultrasound in the evaluation of plaque formation. Eur Urol. 2003;43:293–98.

Hellestrom WJG. History, epidemiology and clinical presentation of Peyronie's disease. Int J Impot Res. 2003;15(supp 15):S91–2.

Helweg G, Judmaier W, Buchberger W, et al. Peyronie's disease: MR findings in 28 patients. Am J Roentgenol. 1992;158:1261–4.

Hricak H. The penis and male urethra. In: Hricak H, Carrington BM, editors. MRI of the pelvis. London: Martin Duritz; 1991. p. 383–415.

Kadioglu A, Sanli O. Epidemiology of Peyronie's disease. In: Levine LA, editor. Peyronie's disease. A guide to clinical management. Humana Press Inc, Totowa, NJ. 2007. pp. 9–18.

Kadioglu A, Tefekli A, Erol B, et al. Color Doppler ultrasound assessment of penile vascular system in men with Peyronie's disease. Int J Impot Res. 2000;12:263–7.

Kadioglu A, Tefekli A, Erol B, Oktar T, Tunc M, Tellaloglu S. A retrospective review of 307 men with Peyronies disease. J Urol. 2002;168:1075–9.

Kumar R, Nehra A. Surgical and minimally invasive treatments for Peyronie's disease. Curr Opin Urol. 2009;19:589–94.

La Pera G, Pescatori ES, Calabrese M, et al. Peyronie's disease: prevalence and association with cigarette smoking. A multicenter population-based study in men aged 50–69 years. Eur Urol. 2001;40:525–30.

Lania C, Grasso M, Franzoso F, Blanso S, Rigatti P. Peyronie's disease, natural history. J Urol. 2004;171(Suppl 4):331.

Lindsay MB, Sehain DM, Grambasch P, Benson RC, Beard M, Kurkland T. The incidence of Peyronie's disease in Rochester, Minnnesota, 1950 through 1984. J Urol. 1991;146:1007–8.

Ludvik W, Wasserburger K. Die Radiumbehandlung der induratio penis plastica. Z Urol Nephrol. 1968;61:319–25.

Mondaini N, Ponchietti R, Gontero P, et al. Penile length is normal in most men seeking penile lengthening procedures. Int J Impot Res. 2002;14:283–6.

Montorsi F, Guazzoni G, Bergamaschi F, Consonni P, Rigatti P, Pizzini G, Miani A. Vascular abnormalities in Payronie's disease: the role of color Doppler sonography. J Urol. 1994;151:373–5.

Moskovic DJ, Alex B, Choi JM, Nelson CJ, Mulhall JP. Defining predictors of response to intralesional verapamil injection therapy for Peyronie's disease. BJU Int. 2011;101:1–5.

Mulhall JP, Creech SD, Boorjian SA, et al. Subjective and objective analysisi of the prevalence of Peyronies disease in a population presenting for prostate cancer. J Urol. 2004;171:2350–3.

Pinggera GM, Pallwein L, Aigner F, Frauscher F, Mitterberger M, Leonhartsberger N, Strasser H, Bartsch G (2007) Assessment of Peyronie's disease by sonoelastography: preliminary

results. American Urological Association Annual Meeting, Anaheim, USA

Prando D. New sonographic aspects of Peyronie's disease. J Ultrasound Med. 2009;28:217.

Pretorius ES, Siegelman ES, Ramchandani P, Banner MP. MR imaging of the penis. Radiographics. 2001;21:283–98.

Schwarzer U, Sommer F, Klotz T, Braun M, Reifenrath B, Engelmann U. The prevalence of Peyronie's disease: results of a large survey. BJU Int. 2001;88:727.

Smith BH. Subclinical Peyronie's disease. Am J Pathol. 1969;52:385–90.

Smith JF, Brant WD, Fradedt V, et al. Penile sonographic and clinical characteristics in men with Peyronie's disease. J Sex Med. 2009;6:2858.

Sommer F, Schwarzer U, Wassmer G, et al. Epidemiology of Peyronie's disease. Int J Impot Res. 2002;14:379–83.

Tornehl CK, Carson CC. Surgical alternatives for treating Peyronie's disease. BJU Intl. 2004;94:774–83.

Usta MF, Bivalacqua TJ, Tokatli Z, Rivera F, Gulkesen KH, Sikka SC, Hellstrom WJG. Stratification of penile vascular pathologies in patients with Peyronie's disease and in men with erectile dysfunction according to age: a comparative study. J Urol. 2004;172:259–62.

Vosshenrich R, Schroeder-Printzen I, Weider W, et al. Value of magnetic resonance imaging in patients with penile induration (Peyronie's disease). J Urol. 1995;153:1122–5.

Urethra

Ullrich G. Mueller-Lisse and Ulrike L. Mueller-Lisse

Introduction

The male urethra may be subdivided into the anterior and posterior urethra. Starting at the bladder neck, the posterior urethra is lined with transitional epithelium and consists of the prostatic urethra and the membranous urethra. The prostatic urethra is characterized by the orifices of numerous prostatic ductules and by the verumontanum or seminal collicle at its posterior aspect. The latter represents a small mound that carries the orifices of the ejaculatory ducts at its lateral aspects and the prostatic utricle as a blindly ending diverticulum in its center. The membranous urethra crosses through the urogenital diaphragm, to connect the intracorporal part of the urethra to the extracorporal or anterior part. The anterior urethra, in turn, is lined with squamous cell epithelium and completely surrounded by the corpus spongiosum. It divides into the bulbous urethra and the pendulous urethra. The bulbous urethra is characterized by its covering by the bulbocavernosus muscle inferiorly, and by the openings of the bulbourethral or Cowper's gland ducts. Cowper's glands are up to 4.5 cm long. In addition, numerous small lacunar Littre's glands open into the anterior urethra. At the distal end of the urethra, close to its orifice, the navicular fossa represents a bulbus dilation of about 1 cm in length (Barbaric 1994).

As in the male urethra, the female urethra extends caudal from the trigonum of the urinary bladder, with respective continuity of the smooth muscle coating. However, the typical three-layered aspect of smooth muscle coating of the trigonum is replaced by a single layer of smooth muscle whose orientation is circular in the male urethra and longitudinal in the female urethra at the level of the bladder neck and acts as an internal sphincter. Further caudal, at the level of the urogenital diaphragm, the external sphincter is composed of striated muscle of the pelvic floor, including the Mm. transversi perinei profundus and superficialis muscles and the M. Levator ani muscles, and of the mixed smooth and striated muscular bundles of the M. Sphincter urethrae (Palmtag et al. 2007). In women, both the transitional cell epithelium of the urethra and the vaginal epithelium, and the respective subepithelial connective tissues are estrogen dependent. Estrogen deficiency in postmenopausal women causes local blood perfusion deficits and consecutive atrophy of those tissue layers. Urinary symptoms include stress incontinence, urge incontinence, and recurrent urinary tract infection (Palmtag et al. 2007).

Depending on the specific clinical traditions and current standards of care, radiological imaging of the urethra may fall into one or both of the medical subspecialties, urology and radiology. With the increasing application of endoscopic imaging methods by urologists, however, alternatives to radiological imaging are at hand.

This chapter introduces radiological imaging techniques and findings in congenital anomalies and normal variants, trauma, inflammatory and infectious diseases, benign neoplasms, and malignant neoplasms of the urethra.

U.G. Mueller-Lisse (✉)
Department of Clinical Radiology, University of Munich Hospitals, Munich, Germany

U.L. Mueller-Lisse
Department of Urology, University of Munich Hospitals, Muenchen, Germany

B. Hamm, P. R. Ros (eds.), *Abdominal Imaging*, DOI 10.1007/978-3-642-13327-5_234,
© Springer-Verlag Berlin Heidelberg 2013

Technique

Conventional Radiography of the Urethra

Radiology of the urethra is still based on retrograde urethrography (RUG) and voiding cystourethrography (VCUG), which demonstrate the urethral lumen in both "still" morphologic and "movie-like" dynamic images. RUG in particular appears to be best suited for delineating luminal abnormalities of the urethra and thus is commonly applied as the primary imaging modality for patients with various urethral disorders, such as trauma, inflammation, and stricture (Kim et al. 2007). However, those conventional radiography studies are limited in demonstrating involvement of adjacent structures in pathological alterations (Ryu and Kim 2001).

Retrograde Urethrography

RUG is considered to represent the primary imaging modality for evaluating anterior urethral anatomy and pathology, particularly including traumatic injury, inflammatory and post-inflammatory disease, and urinary stricture of the male urethra (Kawashima et al. 2004; Pavlica et al. 2003). Barbaric (1994) describes RUG with a small (10F) Foley catheter which is purged of air and inserted into the distal urethra such that the balloon of the catheter is placed in the navicular fossa and inflated to secure position. The position of the Foley catheter may be additionally secured by a clamp. Sterile, diluted contrast media (about 30%) is then applied either by drip infusion or by hand injection with a syringe. Conventional radiographic images and/or spot films at fluoroscopy are then obtained with the patient supine and in 35–45° oblique position. RUG should not be performed immediately after cystoscopy or other transurethral endoscopy, since small mucosal lacerations may lead to contrast extravasation into the corpus spongiosum, with the possible consequence of septic infection. Prophylactic antibiotic treatment may be necessary (Barbaric 1994).

Voiding Cysturethrography

VCUG is frequently used to detect bladder neck pathology, postsurgical stenosis, and neoplasms in the posterior urethra, and to evaluate urethral diverticula in women (Kawashima et al. 2004; Pavlica

et al. 2003). In patients with neuromuscular bladder dysfunction, functional aspects of the bladder neck and posterior urethra can be studied by means of VCUG (Pavlica et al. 2003). Barbaric (1994) describes VCUG as an antegrade urethrography during which contrast-enhanced urine is being voided from the urinary bladder to distend the urethra. Conventional radiographic images and/or spot films at fluoroscopy are obtained during voiding. At VCUG, the normal anterior urethra does not distend to the degree found at RUG. However, particularly for functional examination of the posterior urethra in the presence of obstruction, VCUG demonstrates both the level and the degree of obstruction (Barbaric 1994). Fernbach and coworkers (2000) describe VCUG in children with prenatally diagnosed hydronephrosis, urinary tract infections, and voiding abnormalities as an imaging procedure that can be performed with many variations. Variations are designed to optimize visualization of disease and minimize radiation exposure. They include in their description of VCUG an assessment of the spine and pelvis, of masses or opaque calculi, of urethral appearance, of bladder capacity, contour, and emptying capability, and of the presence and grade of urinary reflux. Images should be obtained at different times and states of bladder filling, including anteroposterior imaging of the bladder at early filling, and steep oblique images centered on the ureterovesical junction at complete bladder filling. In case of vesicoureteral reflux, the ipsilateral renal fossa can be imaged prior to voiding. Bladder refilling is recommended when voiding volume is smaller than expected, and voiding around the catheter is also recommended. Imaging of the urethra at VCUG usually includes one anteroposterior image in girls, while the entire urethra has to be demonstrated in boys. Steep oblique imaging is recommended to this end. At the conclusion of voiding, each renal fossa should be imaged to detect reflux missed at fluoroscopy and other anomalies (Fernbach et al. 2000). Artificial outflow obstruction may be created by means of a clamp, to improve urethral distension during VCUG (Barbaric 1994). Videourodynamic examination includes conventional radiographic imaging and simultaneous measurement of bladder and urethral pressure. It is considered to be the most precise modality available for diagnosing complex incontinence and voiding disorders (McGuire et al. 1996).

Double-Balloon Urethrography

Double-balloon catheter urethrography is another conventional radiography modality to evaluate urethral diverticula in women (Ryu and Kim 2001). Both the proximal and the distal end of the female urethra are covered and closed with the two inflated balloons of the double-balloon catheter whose lumen is previously cleared from air or gas. Sterile, diluted contrast media is then instilled and enters the urethra through side holes of the catheter in between the two balloons. Contrast media distends the urethra, eventually opening the neck of a diverticulum. The diverticulum can thus be located, and the respective length and width of the diverticulum and its neck can be determined.

Cross-Sectional Imaging of the Urethra

Cross-sectional imaging modalities play an increasing role in the assessment of periurethral structures and their respective involvement in urethral disease processes.

Sonourethrography

Sonourethrography of the anterior urethra, after distension of the urethral lumen with sterile saline solution, allows for the study of urethral mucosa and periurethral spongy tissue, which may be involved in urethral strictures, diverticula, trauma, and tumors (Pavlica et al. 2003). Sonourethrography of the posterior urethra currently serves in the assessment of the thickness and length of bulbar urethral stricture, whether in post-inflammatory, posttraumatic or neoplastic disease. In the bulbar urethra, sonourethrography measures stricture length more accurately than RUG (Morey and McAninch 2000; Pavlica et al. 2003). Voiding sonourethrography may be an adjunct or alternative method to assess functional aspects of the posterior urethra (Pavlica et al. 2003). Sonourethrography demonstrates spongiofibrosis with decreased urethral distensibility during retrograde instillation of saline solution. After severe trauma, sonourethrography may show posterior shadowing of the urethra. Sonourethrography of complex or postoperatively recurrent anterior strictures may demonstrate complicating features, such as calculi, urethral hair, false passages, or stent encrustation. Sonourethrography is considered to be more accurate than RUG in measuring stricture length throughout the anterior urethra. (Morey and McAninch 1996, 2000).

Magnetic Resonance Imaging

Magnetic resonance imaging (MRI) may be applied to the anterior urethra, particularly after instillation of sterile saline solution, to study urethral mucosa and periurethral spongy tissue, which can be involved in urethral pathologies such as strictures, diverticula, trauma, and tumors (Pavlica et al. 2003). In the posterior urethra, MRI evaluates bulbar urethral stricture in men and urethral diverticula in women. MRI may demonstrate such urethral diverticula that are not seen at VCUG, RUG, or double-balloon catheter study (Ryu and Kim 2001). MRI is an accurate modality in the local staging of urethral tumors (Kawashima et al. 2004; Ryu and Kim 2001). In patients with congenital anomalies, MRI evaluates internal organs in cases of intersex anomalies or complex genitourinary anomalies. MRI demonstrates inflammatory periurethral infiltration or periurethral abscesses and sinus tracts. MRI is an adjunct modality in cases of urethral trauma, to assess the presence and extent of anterior or posterior urethral injury and predict the occurrence of complications (Ryu and Kim 2001). In female patients, MRI with endovaginal application of a small loop coil that is covered by an inflatable balloon which, in turn, is mounted on a short stalk that carries the connecting cables, appears to be a very reliable diagnostic test in the detection and characterization of various urethral pathologic conditions, such as congenital anomalies, diverticula, urethritis, and benign and malignant neoplasms (Elsayes et al. 2006). High-resolution multiplanar MRI with combined phased-array pelvic and endovaginal coils appears to demonstrate female urethral anatomy in greater detail than female pelvic ultrasonography (Prasad et al. 2005). MRI of the male urethra can be performed during voiding, or with retrograde injection of saline or jelly through the urethral meatus, to improve visualization of urethral luminal abnormalities (Kim et al. 2007).

Computed Tomography

Computed tomography (CT) does not play an immediate role in the imaging evaluation of the urethra, although multidetector CT (MDCT) voiding urethrography may demonstrate the urethra during micturition (Chou et al. 2008). However, CT serves to investigate surrounding structures and their involvement in disease processes affecting the urethra, or affection of the urethra by disease spreading from different organs, particularly in the pelvis. Thus, CT is predominantly being applied in locoregional and distant tumor staging of patients suffering from malignant neoplastic disease of the pelvis and pelvic floor that may involve the urethra, and in cases of traumatic injury to the pelvis (Kim et al. 2007).

Virtual Endoscopy and Endoscopic Image Processing

Various computer algorithms generate 3-D images based on information inherent in either helical CT or MRI data sets. Virtual Endoscopy (VE) simulates conventional endoscopy that allows for endoluminal navigation through hollow organs. In cases of endoluminal stenosis or obstruction, VE permits virtual endoluminal navigation both cranial and caudal to the stenotic segment of the urinary tract. VE of the urethra could help to examine urethral strictures noninvasively. While different clinical studies have demonstrated the diagnostic utility of virtual cystoscopy in the detection of bladder tumors, published experience in VE of the renal pelvis, ureter and urethra is currently scarce (Kagadis et al. 2006). While helical CT and MRI data sets may be used to generate 3-D images, panoramic and 3-D images may also be created by computer processing from digital video images obtained at conventional endoscopy and laparoscopy which address common shortcomings, such as narrow field of view, lack of depth information, and discontinuous imaging information (Igarashi et al. 2009).

Congenital Anomalies and Normal Variants

In infancy, congenital anomalies of the lower urinary tract are a significant cause of morbidity (Berrocal et al. 2002). Lower urinary tract obstruction, as a sequel to congenital anomaly, affects about 2.2 per 10,000 births. The most common anomalies include posterior urethral valves (64%) and/or urethral atresia (39%). In the fetus, those conditions are associated with high morbidity and mortality, particularly due to progressive renal failure and oligohydramnion, and hence fetal pulmonary hypoplasia (Lissauer et al. 2007). Clinical investigation is oftentimes

supported by radiologic examinations of urinary tract anomalies. However, special care needs to be taken to avoid inconvenience or unnecessary radiation exposure to the patient or delay of surgical corrections. Ultrasonography is oftentimes the initial imaging modality applied in pediatric patients to diagnose structural anomaly when urologic disorders are suspected. In the presence of upper urinary tract dilation, voiding cysturethrography (VCUG) determines the presence and extent of vesicoureteral reflux or other causes of urinary tract dilation (Berrocal et al. 2002). Congenital anomalies of the urethra may require different imaging approaches, depending on the specific clinical presentation and clinical questions involved.

Posterior Urethral Valves

The precise embryologic and anatomic origins of posterior urethral valves remain undefined. While pertinent literature is abundant in theories regarding the origin of posterior urethral valves, only a limited number of reports on the anatomy of posterior urethral valves that is based on reproducible scientific techniques such as histopathology (Krishnan et al. 2006). Posterior urethral valves represent flaps of urethral mucosa that protrude into the urethral lumen and interfere with normal urine flow. Moderate to severe outflow obstruction is oftentimes associated with a large or unstable, potentially trabeculated bladder, dilated ureters, vesicourethral reflux, and, possibly hydronephrotic or dysplastic kidneys. Barbaric (1994 distinguishes three types of posterior urethral valves, including mucosal flaps with infracollicular fusion (Plicae colliculi) that create a narrow passage, an infracollicular mucosal web with a narrow central opening, and a third, probably nonexistent type. Although many of the findings are demonstrated by ultrasonography, VCUG is the imaging method to establish posterior urethral valves and their sequels. Primary treatment consists of endoscopic fulguration; however, temporary or even permanent urinary diversion may become necessary (Barbaric 1994).

Anterior Urethral Valves

Anterior urethral valves are less common than posterior urethral valves. However, they may represent a severe diagnostic problem when VCUG does not adequately demonstrate the entire urethra, such that the point of obstruction may be missed when it is far distal. Anterior urethral valves may be difficult to differentiate from wide-mouthed diverticulum of the anterior urethra (Barbaric 1994).

Congenital Diverticulum

Wide-mouthed diverticulum of the anterior urethra is a congenital anomaly that presents with diverticular outpouching. When located at the dorsal side of the anterior urethra, this kind of diverticulum is also being referred to as Lacuna magna. The anterior or distal flap of the neck of the anterior urethral diverticulum may impede normal urine flow and cause bladder outflow obstruction. In the posterior urethra, the prostatic utricle may develop into a diverticulum. Other types of urethral diverticula are usually acquired rather than congenital (Barbaric 1994).

Congenital Strictures

Congenital urethral strictures may cause significant bladder outflow obstructions. They are usually short and web-like, and are relatively simple to remove operatively (Barbaric 1994).

Urethral Duplication

Urethral duplication is a rare congenital anomaly which is part of the spectrum of caudal duplication anomalies. Barbaric (1994) describes three different types of urethral duplication, with type 1 demonstrating complete duplication of the entire urethra, from the bladder or bladder neck to the meatus, with parallel course of the two urethras, type 2 showing with a common bladder neck and posterior urethra and duplication starting external to the symphysis pubis, with parallel course of the two urethras, and type 3 featuring duplication at or immediately distal to the bulbar urethra, with the second urethral channel pointing caudal toward the perineum (Barbaric 1994). Urethral duplication may be associated with bladder duplication, either in the coronal or in the sagittal plane. Bae and coworkers (2005) report findings in a 7-year-old boy with complete duplication of the bladder and urethra in the coronal plane, without any other associated congenital anomalies. Alfadhel and coworkers (2009) describe findings at prenatal ultrasonography and MRI in a boy with postnatal clinical and surgical findings confirming duplication of bladder, urethra, and bowel from distal ileum to rectum.

Meatal Stenosis

The length of meatal stenosis needs to be determined to plan treatment. At RUG and VCUG, it is important to include the distal end and navicular fossa of the urethra in order to demonstrate or rule out meatal stenosis. Meatal stenosis is a potential cause of bladder outflow obstruction and its sequels (Barbaric 1994).

Megalourethra

Megalourethra demonstrates with an abnormally wide and elongated urethra. The underlying disorder is partial or complete absence of the corpus spongiosum, which supports and shapes the urethra (Barbaric 1994).

Hypospadia

Hypospadia is a congenital defect of the distal urethra, with the urethra opening not in its usual location at the meatus in the center of the Glans penis, but at the caudal side of the penis, exiting through the corpus spongiosum. Unless associated with other anomalies, particularly those which would cause bladder outflow obstruction, radiologic imaging is usually not required for the diagnosis.

Epispadia

Epispadia is a congenital defect of midline closure that is characterized by a pathologic opening of the urethra pointing cranial, toward the symphysis pubis. Epispadia does not involve the body of the bladder or the hindgut. However, epispadia affects the urethra and may involve the bladder neck. Functionally, epispadia is considered to be the least severe defect of the epispadia-exstrophy complex of lower midline closure defects. However, the spectrum of severity is wide and may include urinary continence if the epispadia reaches far enough proximal to affect the urinary sphincter (Grady and Mitchell 2002). The diagnosis of epispadia is usually clinical, and radiologic imaging serves as an adjunct to identify associated anomalies.

Anomalies Deemed to Be Acquired

Cowper's Syringocele

The bulbourethral or Cowper's glands open toward the bulbous urethra with their ducts. Cowper's syringocele has been described as a rare, cystic or diverticular dilation of the bulbourethral ducts (Barbaric 1994; Melquist et al. 2010). Based on the configuration of the orifice of the affected bulbourethral duct to the urethra, Cowper's syringocele may be described as open or closed. Open syringocele may be characterized clinically by post-void dribbling, hematuria, or urethral discharge. Closed syringocele may be associated with obstructive symptoms. Clinically, those symptoms are shared by many serious urologic conditions, such that differential diagnosis is critical. Radiologic imaging includes ultrasonography, RUG, and/or VCUG. Endoscopy, MRI, and CT may be useful as adjunct modalities to clear the differential diagnosis. Once established, conservative observation may be recommended. However, when symptoms persist, Cowper's syringocele is usually treated with endoscopic marsupialization, unless contraindicated (Melquist et al. 2010).

Female Urethral Diverticulum

Female urethral diverticulum is a rare pathologic entity which likely originates from the periurethral glands, may demonstrate with a variety of chronic or recurrent symptoms involving the lower urinary tract, including frequency and dysuria, alguria, stress urinary incontinence, and infection. Vaginal examination may reveal an anterior mass (Arzoz Fábregas et al. 2004; Chou et al. 2008; Prasad et al. 2005; Rovner 2007; Tembely et al. 2008). Repetitive treatment with antibiotics and urethral dilatation often fails to resolve the clinical problem. Definitive treatment usually requires surgical excision to provide relief (Lee and Fynes 2005).

Surgical treatment options include transvaginal diverticulectomy and transurethral diverticulectomy with the Sachse urethrotome (Arzoz Fábregas et al. 2004).

In women with urethral diverticula, urethrography provides information on luminal abnormalities of the urethra (Chou et al. 2008; Prasad et al. 2005). Double-balloon catheter urethrography is another conventional radiography modality to evaluate urethral diverticula in women (Ryu and Kim 2001). Multidetector CT voiding urethrography demonstrates both the urethra and the diverticulum and diverticular orifice during micturition. Both 2- and 3-D reformatted CT images can be obtained. Interactive virtual urethroscopy simulates endoscopic visualization of the intraluminal anatomy and the diverticular orifice (Chou et al. 2008). Both ultrasonography and MRI with surface or endoluminal coils may demonstrate the number of diverticula and their respective location, size, configuration, and possible contents. In addition, cross-sectional imaging may identify the position of the neck of the diverticulum for surgical planning. As a differential diagnosis, periurethral cysts do not communicate with the urethra, such that they can often be differentiated from urethral diverticula at endocavitary MRI (Chou et al. 2008; Prasad et al. 2005).

Male Urethral Diverticulum

Barbaric (1994) describes acquired male urethral diverticula resulting from infected and abscessed glands of Littre in the anterior urethra in chronic urethritis. Kawakami and coworkers (1995) report on an acquired diverticulum of the male anterior urethra in a 67-year-old man with Pott's paralysis, due to tuberculous spondylitis, and recurrent urinary tract infection deemed to result from urine collection applying a condom penile sheath. Imaging included RUG, VCUG, and MRI as well as urethroscopy. The diverticulectomy specimen revealed squamous epithelium and fibrous connective tissue in the wall (Kawakami et al. 1995).

Urinary Incontinence

Urinary incontinence (UI) is a very common condition which causes significant psychosocial and hygienic problems in the aging female population (Macura and Genadry 2008). While clinical history, including standardized symptom and quality-of-life questionnaires, and physical examination play pivotal roles in the assessment of female urinary incontinence, various modalities are applied to assess and measure types and degrees of underlying pathology. While there is no single definitive test for the diagnosis of intrinsic urethral sphincteric deficiency, multiple tests should be employed to reach a consensus for the diagnosis. Understanding the limitations and variability of the specific studies and the respective equipment utilized should help to standardize the approach to assessing the extent of urethral dysfunction (Betson et al. 2003). The purpose of imaging procedures is to investigate correlations between morphology and function of both the bladder and urethra, and to detect concomitant defects of the pelvic floor. However, definitive studies comparing different diagnostic options and their respective impact on patient management and outcome are still lacking (Novara and Artibani 2006). Also, the various diagnostic tests that have been described in attempts to accurately and comprehensively assess urethral function suffer from a lack of standardization or from inconsistencies in quoted reference values (Betson et al. 2003).

Traditionally, modalities evaluating female urinary incontinence include urodynamic analysis, cystourethroscopy, cystourethrography, and ultrasonography (Macura et al. 2006). Ultrasonography has also been applied to follow up on treatment for female urinary incontinence, e.g., injection therapy with bulking agents (Poon et al. 2005).

Although its role is considered to be minor in female urinary incontinence, high-resolution MRI visualizes both anatomy and function of the female urethra and demonstrates the urethral sphincter and supporting ligaments. MRI thus may contribute to the assessment of intrinsic urethral sphincter deficiency, urethral hypermobility, and defects of urethral support ligaments. Abnormalities visualized include a small urethral sphincter, with foreshortening or thinning of the sphincter muscle, bladder neck insufficiency, as demonstrated by funneling at the bladder neck, distortion or disruption of periurethral support ligaments and vaginal attachments, cystocele, abnormal vaginal shape, enlarged retropubic space, increased vesicourethral angle, asymmetric pubococcygeus muscles, and defects within the levator ani muscle (Macura et al. 2006; Macura and Genadry 2008).

Neurogenic Lower Urinary Tract Disorders

When local reasons are excluded in patients suffering from lower urinary tract symptoms, nervous system disorders need to be considered in the differential diagnosis. Nervous system structures involved in the control of the lower urinary tract are usually categorized by means of a neuroanatomical classification system as being suprapontine, pontine, spinal, or sacral. In addition to clinical assessment, imaging and laboratory tests, neurophysiologic studies, including electromyography, cortical and lumbar somatosensory evoked potential (SEP), and motor evoked potential (MEP) examinations may be useful (Podnar 2007).

Trauma

Traumatic lesions to the urethra may be caused by blunt force or by penetrating objects in the course of accidents, or by invasive surgical measures, such as catheterization, prostatectomy, or sling operations for urinary obstruction or urinary continence or by foreign bodies deliberately introduced into the urethra. Diagnostic clarification of the exact location and nature of urethral injury requires high-quality imaging studies by specialists in the field (Pinggera et al. 2005).

In patients who have suffered either blunt or penetrating abdominal or pelvic trauma, or polytrauma, multiorgan injury is common and frequently involves the genitourinary tract. Since covers all solid and hollow organs of the abdomen and pelvis, including the upper and lower urinary tract, contrast-enhanced CT is currently considered to be the primary imaging technique to evaluate trauma patients, (Ingram et al. 2008; Ramchandani and Buckler 2009). In trauma affecting the pelvis, urethral injury is a common complication which may lead to significant long-term morbidity if it remains undiagnosed. The posterior urethra, which is close to the pubic rami and the puboprostatic ligaments, is particularly vulnerable in pelvic trauma (Ingram et al. 2008). Certain types of pelvic fractures are associated with an increased risk of urethral injury. Recognition of these fractures by timely radiologic imaging facilitates the early diagnosis of urethral injury and ensures that serious long-term sequelae are minimized (Kommu et al. 2007).

Urethral injury is better assessed and classified by means of urethrography than by CT, such that the traditional imaging modalities of RUG, VCUG, and cystography remain useful both in the initial evaluation and in the follow-up of trauma to the urinary bladder and urethra (Ali et al. 2003; Ingram et al. 2008; Ramchandani and Buckler 2009). Complete urethral imaging is required in the initial evaluation after pelvic or urethral trauma because insertion of a transurethral bladder catheter may exacerbate existing urethral injury, e.g., by turning a partial urethral tear into a complete urethral transection. Urethrography after pelvic trauma may be particularly challenging when the patient is immobilized or when a surgical fixation device or indwelling urethral catheter is present (Ingram et al. 2008).

The management approach to urethral trauma remains controversial (Kommu et al. 2007). The specific surgical techniques applied and the timing of reconstructive procedures will depend on the cause and nature of urethral injury (Pinggera et al. 2005). While urethral trauma secondary to either penetrating gunshot wounds or penile fracture requires immediate surgical exploration and repair (Kommu et al. 2007), definitive surgical intervention is not generally recommended in most lesions resulting from accidents, especially when lesions are located in the posterior urethra (Pinggera et al. 2005). However, primary realignment of the urethra by means of a combined antegrade and retrograde endoscopic approach can be considered as a surgical management option to restore urethral continuity early in highly selected cases of complete anterior and posterior urethral disruption (Kommu et al. 2007). Any treatment algorithm should strive to assure an adequate quality of life and to prevent postsurgical complications, such as, e.g., incontinence, impotence, recurrent urinary tract infection, which, in turn, would necessitate multiple subsequent operations (Pinggera et al. 2005).

Blunt Urethral Trauma

Blunt external trauma is the most common cause of injury to the lower urinary tract. While minor injury often heals uneventfully with catheter drainage, penetrating trauma is best treated with primary repair.

However, while urethral disruption may be safely and effectively treated with delayed reconstruction in the majority of cases, minimally invasive immediate realignment represents an alternative (Morey et al. 1999). Since the management approach to blunt urethral trauma remains controversial, and definitive surgery is not generally recommended, particularly when lesions affect the posterior urethra (Kommu et al. 2007; Pinggera et al. 2005), an anatomically based classification system for blunt urethral injury that may help in the management approach appears to be valuable.

Goldman and coworkers (1997) have proposed a simple classification system that is both comprehensive and anatomically consistent. The classification includes aspects of both the older surgical classification that simply divides urethral injuries anatomically into anterior and posterior, and the Colapinto and McCallum classification (Goldman et al. 1997). The classification proposed by Goldman and coworkers (1997) comprises the following common types of blunt urethral injuries.

Type I Posterior urethra intact but stretched (Colapinto and McCallum type I)

Type II Partial or complete pure posterior injury with tear of membranous urethra above the urogenital diaphragm (Colapinto and McCallum type II)

Type III Partial or complete combined anterior and posterior urethral injury with disruption of the urogenital diaphragm (Colapinto and McCallum type III)

Type IV Bladder neck injury with extension into the urethra

Type IVA Injury of the base of the bladder with periurethral extravasation simulating a true type IV urethral injury

Type V Partial or complete pure anterior urethral injury

Goldman and coworkers (1997) suggest that their classification system should permit comparison of various management or treatment modalities at various institutions if it were universally adopted.

Ali and coworkers (2003) studied CT scans of patients with both pelvic fractures and urethrography-proved posterior urethral injury, and of patients with similar pelvic fractures but without urethral injury to establish CT signs associated with different types of posterior urethral injury. They report that the following CT findings are more frequently present in patients with pelvic fractures and associated urethral injuries than in patients with uncomplicated pelvic fractures (Ali et al. 2003).

- Distortion or obscuration of the urogenital diaphragm fat plane
- Hematoma of the ischiocavernosus muscle
- Distortion or obscuration of the prostatic contour
- Distortion or obscuration of the bulbocavernosus muscle
- Hematoma of the obturator internus muscle

When compared with the classification system proposed by Goldman and coworkers (1997), Ali and coworkers (2003) suggest that the following CT findings are specifically associated with certain types of urethral injury.

Type I Elevation of the prostatic apex

Type II Extravasation of urinary tract contrast material above the urogenital diaphragm

Type III Extravasation of urinary tract contrast material below the urogenital diaphragm

Type IV/IVa Extraperitoneal bladder rupture and periurethral extravasation of contrast material

This attempt (Ali et al. 2003) to translate the urography-based anatomical classification system for blunt urethral trauma (Goldman et al. 1997) into associated CT findings may be particularly helpful when a CT scan is the first imaging procedure applied in a trauma patient with signs of blunt pelvic and/or abdominal injury. It appears, though, that additional CT scans will have to be acquired in the excretory phase after intravenous administration of contrast media to apply the translated classification system, since portal venous phase images, as usually obtained, would not suffice to investigate the patency of the urinary tract.

Pelvic MRI and sonourethrography are no first-line imaging procedures in cases of blunt pelvic or abdominal trauma potentially affecting the urethra, but represent important ancillary modalities for patients who require complex urethral reconstruction (Morey et al. 1999).

Posttraumatic Urethral Stricture

Posttraumatic urethral stricture oftentimes can be attributed to one of two major groups of underlying reasons. One includes iatrogenic injury, which may relate in particular to transurethral resection of the prostate or to stricture and stenosis at the anastomosis site after radical prostatectomy in the male urethra. The other includes pelvic trauma with associated urethral transection or urethral tear.

In strictures and injuries of the urethra, imaging includes both retrograde and antegrade urethrography studies (Dobry and Danuser 2009). Dynamic RUG is considered to be the initial imaging test for suspected urethral stricture, because it is easy to perform and detects clinically relevant strictures either involving the anterior urethra or extending into the membranous urethra. Other imaging modalities, including antegrade imaging of the bladder and urethra, sonourethrography, and MRI, represent adjunct means to visualize the extent of disease and to assist in guiding reconstruction (Gallentine and Morey 2002).

In cases of complete urethral stricture, RUG fails to demonstrate the superior extension. Since suprapubic catheterization will almost always be performed under these circumstances, combined RUG and suprapubic cystography may clarify the extent of the lesion (Barbaric 1994). Postoperatively, after urethral repair, VCUG is appropriate to evaluate complete healing and success of repair (Gallentine and Morey 2002).

Sonourethrography, with 2-D and 3-D image acquisition options, is a relatively simple modality that does not require radiation exposure and demonstrates and measures the extent of urethral strictures (Morey and McAninch 1996, 2000). Sonourethrography provides a dynamic, precise assessment of anterior urethral strictures which may be applied in men with known symptomatic strictures which require operative therapy. Sonourethrography measures more accurately the length of short bulbar strictures than RUG and it therefore helps to determine whether to excise a stricture or to place a graft. Assessment of lesion diameter in long or complex strictures by means of sonourethrography may be helpful in determining flap width or in identifying focal urethral segments to be excised (Gallentine and Morey 2002).

MDCT, with multiplanar 2-D reformatting and, possibly, 3-D displays, performed in the excretory phase after intravenous administration of contrast media, possibly accompanied by retrograde administration of contrasting agents into the anterior urethra, may also be applied to demonstrate the stricture or tear.

T2-weighted or fluid-weighted MRI or T1-weighted MRI performed in the excretory phase after intravenous administration of contrast media, with multiplanar 2-D images or virtual 3-D displays, may alternatively be applied to demonstrate the presence and extent of urethral stricture (Barbaric 1994; Kim et al. 2007). Posttraumatic MRI visualizes altered or distorted pelvic anatomy which is frequently associated with traumatic posterior urethral strictures. MRI may help to decide if a transperineal or a transpubic approach is best suited for reconstruction of the posterior urethra. MRI tasks include locating the prostate and determining the length of the defect in the prostatic and membranous urethra (Gallentine and Morey 2002).

False Urethral Passages

False passages often result from instrumentation in patients with urethral strictures or obstructions. False passages created inadvertently may end blindly, but they may also reenter the bladder. They may bring about a diverticular outpouching (Barbaric 1994).

Traumatic Diverticulum

Urethral diverticula may be acquired as a complication of urethral instrumentation, urethral surgery, or prolonged application of an external urethral anti-incontinence clamp (Barbaric 1994).

Fracture of the Penis

Fracture of the penis is a rare traumatic entity which is mostly acquired by young adults during sexual intercourse (Agarwal et al. 2009; Grima et al. 2006; Martínez Portillo et al. 2003). It includes rupture of the tunica albuginea and corpus cavernosum and may extend to the urethra in some cases (Grima et al. 2006; Martínez Portillo et al. 2003). In a case series including 17 patients with fracture of the penis, Agarwal and coworkers (2009) report corpus-cavernosum tears in 15 patients and urethral injury in four of those patients at surgical exploration.

Penile fracture is considered to be a serious urological disorder. Although controversy exists between surgical and conservative treatment of penile fracture, many authors agree that penile fracture usually demands elective surgical management (Grima et al. 2006; Martínez Portillo et al. 2003). Arguments for immediate surgical repair include that it offers complete recovery for patients with fracture of the penis in most cases, even in the presence of urethral injury, and that it is associated with shorter hospitalization, less morbidity, and an early return to sexual activity when compared with other clinical management options (Martínez Portillo et al. 2003). Elective surgery includes evacuation of the subcutaneous hematoma and suturing of the tear in the tunica albuginea (Grima et al. 2006).

Possible complications of and significant morbidity associated with penile fracture include erectile dysfunction up to complete loss of erectile function, painful erection, deviation of the erect penis, development of plaques resembling those of Peyronie's disease, urethro-cavernous or urethro-cutaneous fistulation, and dysuria secondary to urethral stricture (Grima et al. 2006; Martínez Portillo et al. 2003).

Authors agree that clinical history and physical examination should be obtained in all patients suspected of suffering from penile fracture. While investigating urinary status is recommended by some (Martínez Portillo et al. 2003), others state that evaluation beyond clinical history and physical examination is not necessary (Agarwal et al. 2009). The role of imaging procedures in patients with penile fracture remains controversial. Agarwal and coworkers (2009) argue that radiological examinations did not influence clinical management in any of their patients, although RUG was highly sensitive and accurate in detecting urethral injury and sonourethrography was highly specific but not sensitive for detecting a cavernosal tear. Grima and coworkers (2006) claim that ultrasonography, cavernography, or MRI of the penis can be performed to determine the exact site of the fracture. Martínez Portillo and coworkers (2003) state that imaging procedures, such as ultrasonography or cavernosography, determine the location, extent, and severity of rupture in the tunica albuginea, which takes foremost priority for the correct choice of treatment.

Urine Leaks and Urinomas

Urine leaks, whether emanating from the kidney, ureter, bladder, or urethra, most commonly result from trauma. Treatment may be conservative or surgical. Conservative management has been advocated for extraperitoneal urinary bladder rupture and type 1 urethral injury according to the classification by Goldman and coworkers (1997; Titton et al. 2003). Urine leaks that require more extensive, may be managed safely and effectively with image-guided intervention applying combinations of percutaneous urinoma drainage catheters, percutaneous nephrostomy catheters, ureteral stents, and bladder drainage systems (Titton et al. 2003).

Radiologic imaging determines the presence, extent, and potential cause of urine leaks. The most important radiologic studies to this end include RUG, CT with imaging in the excretory phase after intravenous administration of contrast media, and CT cystography. Excretory urography, antegrade and retrograde pyelography, renal scintigraphy, and image-guided needle aspiration of fluid collections represent complementary second-line examinations (Titton et al. 2003).

Urinomas may be initially occult. Missed or infected urinomas may lead to complications such as abscess formation and electrolyte imbalance if left undiagnosed or inappropriately managed (Titton et al. 2003). Image-guided drainage procedures should be considered as a minimally invasive alternative to surgical management. In the appropriate setting, image-guided interventional radiologic management options may reduce complications associated with urinoma and limit or eliminate the need for urologic surgery (Titton et al. 2003).

Inflammatory and Infectious Diseases

While uncomplicated urethritis as such may not require imaging procedures for its diagnosis and treatment, complications of urethritis, particularly inflammatory urethral stricture, involve radiologic imaging both for diagnosis and follow-up.

Inflammatory Urethral Stricture

Inflammatory urethral stricture oftentimes results from untreated or inadequately treated infection of the periurethral glands of Littre around the anterior urethra, particularly from gonococcal infection. Scars in periurethral tissues cause partial obstruction of the distal urethra, and increased pressure proximal to the obstruction induce mucosal injury and secondary stricture. Secondary infection may be a sequel that results in the formation of diverticula, abscesses, fistulas, and other lesions. Inflammatory stricture is very rare in the posterior urethra. Uncommon causes include infection with tuberculosis or schistosomiasis. Inflammatory narrowing of the posterior urethra may be found as a sequel of prostatitis with inflammatory edema of the prostate (Barbaric 1994).

Inflammatory urethral strictures may be localized or diffuse, and skip lesions with intercalated segments of normal urethra have to be anticipated. When localized to the bulbous urethra, inflammatory urethral stricture may be misdiagnosed as a functional state of the normal external sphincter, although the latter is located more cranial, at the level of the urogenital diaphragm and the membranous part of the posterior urethra (Barbaric 1994).

Inflammatory urethral strictures may be hard or soft, depending on the degree of submucosal or periurethral scarring. In the presence of soft strictures, the urethra may be quite distensible. This feature is particularly important when soft stricture occurs at or extends into the external sphincter region, because treatment needs to be adapted to the specific extent and location of the stricture (Barbaric 1994).

In strictures partially obstructing the urethra, urethrography and urethroscopy identify the respective location and length of the stricture (Barbaric 1994). Fibrosis of the corpus spongiosum as a complication or sequel of urethritis evades diagnosis by means of urethrography and urethroscopy. While Barbaric (1994) describes spongiography as an invasive radiologic procedure that involves injection of sterile, nonionic, iodinated contrast media into the Glans penis and demonstration of fibrosis in the corpus spongiosum as an interruption or sparing of contrast enhancement within the corpus spongiosum, that procedure has probably been outdated by modern cross-sectional imaging modalities, including ultrasonography, sonourethrography, and MRI. The latter may also serve to detect, localize, and measure the extent of sequels or complications of urethritis, such as diverticula, abscesses, fistulas, and other lesions. Comparison between urethrography, sonourethrography, and MRI in the detection, localization, and determination of length of urethral strictures is discussed above, in the section on "Posttraumatic Urethral Stricture."

Benign Neoplasms

In all, benign urethral neoplasms are rare entities that may be either congenital or acquired after birth.

Prostatic Urethral Polyp

Prostatic urethral polyps are rare, epithelialized polypoid tumors with a fibrovascular core that may feature a stalk connecting them to the normal urethra. They are located in the posterior urethra, at the verumontanum or seminal collicle, or at the bladder neck. Prostatic urethral polyps may cause bladder outflow obstruction. They may be detected in childhood or in adulthood, by means of RUG, VCUG, excretory urography, endoscopy, CT, or MRI (Barbaric 1994; Li et al. 2003).

Leiomyoma of the Urethra

Leiomyomas are histologically benign tumors that originate from smooth muscle cells and usually affect the uterus, being found in approximately 20–30% of women older than 35 years of age. However, leiomyomas may occur in nearly any anatomic site, with rare but typical locations in the genitourinary tract involving the vulva, ovaries, urethra, and urinary bladder. Unusual patterns of growth or distribution may be found, including metastatic, intravenous, retroperitoneal, parasitic, or disseminated intraperitoneal leiomyomatosis. While synchronous findings of uterine leiomyoma or a history of previous hysterectomy for primary uterine leiomyoma may be indicative, some manifestations of extrauterine leiomyoma may mimic malignancy, such that serious diagnostic errors may result (Fasih et al. 2008).

Cornella and coworkers (1997) present a case series of 23 women with extrauterine leiomyomas affecting the urinary bladder and/or the urethra. In the majority of their patients, leiomyomas of the bladder and urethra were asymptomatic and nonobstructive. Those leiomyomas were incidentally detected at surgery performed for other reasons. However, two of their 23 patients presented with pain, and 10 had palpable masses at physical examination (Cornella et al. 1997). Pain and pollakisuria were the presenting features in two of three female patients with leiomyoma of the urinary bladder that was detected by means of pelvic MRI and cystoscopy in the case series reported by Ishida and coworkers (2003).

Cornella and coworkers (1997) suggest to delay definitive treatment of asymptomatic, nonobstructive, and nonproblematic leiomyomas and follow up with ultrasonography, cystoscopy, and biopsy. Karadag and coworkers (2010) report a case of leiomyoma developing within a female urethral diverticulum that was not detected by traditional diagnostic methods, including VCUG. Fasih and coworkers (2008), however, advocate ultrasonography, CT, and MRI as being the most useful radiologic imaging modalities for the detection of extrauterine leiomyomas.

Malignant Neoplasms

Malignant neoplasms of the urethra are rare pathologic entities (Miller and Karnes 2008). Among the primary urethral malignancies, squamous cell carcinoma is the most common. It usually occurs in patients with previously diagnosed strictures and often involves the bulbous urethra. Transitional cell carcinoma may be found in the posterior urethra. Other primary malignant entities within the urethra include adenocarcinoma, glandular carcinoma, undifferentiated carcinoma, sarcoma, and melanoma (Barbaric 1994; Miller and Karnes 2008; Mostofi et al. 1992). Primary periurethral malignant lymphoma, surrounding the female urethra, has been reported (Shimizu et al. 1997). Primary carcinoma of Cowper's glands is an extremely rare pathologic entity. Metastases to the urethra are also rare and are most commonly due to malignant melanoma (Barbaric 1994).

Urethral hemorrhage is a common presentation in malignant urethral lesions (Barbaric 1994). Pollakisuria, dysuria, bladder outflow obstruction, and incomplete voiding or acute urinary retention may be other presenting features (Seki et al. 2001; Ouzaid et al. 2010; Yamaguchi et al. 2003). Vaginal examination may reveal a mass palpable through the anterior vaginal wall (Hayashi et al. 2009). Endoscopy of the urethra and bladder may fail to demonstrate the urethral tumor (Kamoto et al. 1993).

Although excretory urography may demonstrate urethral tumor as a filling defect of the bladder, and ultrasonography and CT may show a pelvic mass and extreme thickening of the urethral wall (Hayashi et al. 2009; Seki et al. 2001), most authors agree that MRI reveals the mass within or around the urethra and determines tumor extension. However, while MRI may help to distinguish between fibromuscular tumor, which most often demonstrates with low signal at T2 weighted imaging is potentially benign, and potentially malignant neoplastic disease, which most often shows with bright signal at T2-weighted imaging (Barbaric 1994), imaging features do not distinguish between histological subtypes of malignant urethral lesions, and biopsy is necessary for detailed pathologic analysis (Prasad et al. 2005). Whole-body CT supports staging of lymphadenopathy and distant metastasis (Imamura et al. 1998).

Appropriate Utilization of Imaging Resources and Management of Patients

- Radiology of the urethra predominantly involves retrograde urethrography (RUG) and voiding cystourethrography (VCUG), which demonstrate the urethral lumen in both "still" morphologic and "movie-like" dynamic images.
- RUG evaluates anterior urethral anatomy and pathology, particularly in traumatic injury, inflammatory and post-inflammatory disease, and male urethral stricture.
- VCUG detects bladder neck pathology, post-surgical stenosis, and neoplasm of the posterior urethra, and evaluates female urethral diverticula.
- Sonourethrography of the anterior urethra investigates urethral mucosa and periurethral spongy tissue in urethral strictures, diverticula, trauma, and tumors.
- Sonourethrography of the posterior urethra measures the thickness and length of bulbar urethral stricture, whether in post-inflammatory, posttraumatic, or neoplastic disease.
- Magnetic resonance imaging (MRI) of the anterior urethra investigates urethral mucosa and periurethral spongy tissue in urethral strictures, diverticula, trauma, and tumors.

- MRI of the posterior urethra evaluates bulbar urethral stricture in men and urethral diverticula in women, particularly when urethral diverticula are not seen at VCUG, RUG, or double-balloon catheter examination.
- MRI is an accurate modality in the local staging of urethral tumors.
- MRI evaluates internal organs in cases of complex congenital genitourinary anomalies or intersex anomalies.
- CT is predominantly being applied in cases of traumatic injury to the pelvis or in locoregional and distant tumor staging of patients suffering from malignant neoplastic disease of the pelvis and pelvic floor that may involve the urethra.

Summary of Key Features/"Pearls to Remember"

- The female urethra is rather short; the state of its inner lining is hormone dependent.
- The male urethra may be subdivided into the posterior urethra, from the bladder neck to the urogenital diaphragm, and the anterior urethra, from below the urogenital diaphragm to the meatus.
- Congenital anomalies of the lower urinary tract are a significant cause of morbidity and even mortality in infancy when undetected. The most common congenital anomalies include posterior urethral valves and urethral atresia.
- Urinary incontinence is a very common condition in the aging female population that requires multiple tests to reach a consensus for the diagnosis.
- Urethral trauma may be caused by blunt force, by penetrating objects, or by foreign bodies deliberately introduced into the urethra. High-quality imaging studies determine the exact location and nature of urethral injury prior to definitive treatment.
- Blunt urethral trauma can be classified anatomically according to Goldman and coworkers when conventional radiography studies are applied or according to Ali and coworkers when CT studies are applied.
- Urethral stricture is a common pathologic entity whose origin may be traumatic, post-inflammatory or postinfectious, or neoplastic. RUG and VCUG

are traditional first-line imaging studies; sonourethrography and MRI are supportive imaging modalities.

- Urine leaks and urinomas and their respective complications are usually investigated by means of RUG and contrast-enhanced CT with imaging in the excretory phase.

- Benign and malignant neoplastic disease of the urethra is rare. Various imaging tests are applied for the diagnosis and staging. Biopsy is required to obtain a definitive diagnosis of the underlying pathology.

References

Agarwal MM, Singh SK, Sharma DK, Ranjan P, Kumar S, Chandramohan V, Gupta N, Acharya NC, Bhalla V, Mavuduru R, Mandal AK. Fracture of the penis: a radiological or clinical diagnosis? A case series and literature review. Can J Urol. 2009;16(2):4568–75.

Alfadhel M, Pugash D, Robinson AJ, Murphy JJ, Senger C, Afshar K, Armstrong L. Pre- and postnatal findings in a boy with duplication of the bladder and intestine: report and review. Am J Med Genet A. 2009;149A(12):2795–802.

Ali M, Safriel Y, Sclafani SJ, Schulze R. CT signs of urethral injury. Radiographics. 2003;23(4):951–63. discussion 963–6.

Arzoz Fábregas M, Ibarz Servio L, Areal Calama J, Saladié Roig JM. Female urethra diverticula. Arch Esp Urol. 2004;57(4):381–8 [Article in Spanish].

Bae KS, Jeon SH, Lee SJ, Lee CH, Chang SG, Lim JW, Kim JI. Complete duplication of bladder and urethra in coronal plane with no other anomalies: case report with review of the literature. Urology. 2005;65(2):388.

Barbaric ZL. Chapter 22, Male urethra and seminal tract. In: Principles of genitourinary radiology. 2nd ed. New York: Thieme Medical; 1994. p. 426–42.

Berrocal T, López-Pereira P, Arjonilla A, Gutiérrez J. Anomalies of the distal ureter, bladder, and urethra in children: embryologic, radiologic, and pathologic features. Radiographics. 2002;22(5):1139–64.

Betson LH, Siddiqui G, Bhatia NN. Intrinsic urethral sphincteric deficiency: critical analysis of various diagnostic modalities. Curr Opin Obstet Gynecol. 2003;15(5):411–7.

Chou CP, Levenson RB, Elsayes KM, Lin YH, Fu TY, Chiu YS, Huang JS, Pan HB. Imaging of female urethral diverticulum: an update. Radiographics. 2008;28(7):1917–30.

Cornella JL, Larson TR, Lee RA, Magrina JF, Kammerer-Doak D. Leiomyoma of the female urethra and bladder: report of twenty-three patients and review of the literature. Am J Obstet Gynecol. 1997;176(6):1278–85.

Dobry E, Danuser H. Imaging of the kidney and the urinary tract. Ther Umsch. 2009;66(1):39–42 [Article in German].

Elsayes KM, Mukundan G, Narra VR, Abou El Abbass HA, Prasad SR, Brown JJ. Endovaginal magnetic resonance imaging of the female urethra. J Comput Assist Tomogr. 2006;30(1):1–6.

Fasih N, Prasad Shanbhogue AK, Macdonald DB, Fraser-Hill MA, Papadatos D, Kielar AZ, Doherty GP, Walsh C, McInnes M, Atri M. Leiomyomas beyond the uterus: unusual locations, rare manifestations. Radiographics. 2008;28(7):1931–48.

Fernbach SK, Feinstein KA, Schmidt MB. Pediatric voiding cystourethrography: a pictorial guide. Radiographics. 2000;20(1):155–68. discussion 168–71.

Gallentine ML, Morey AF. Imaging of the male urethra for stricture disease. Urol Clin North Am. 2002;29(2):361–72.

Goldman SM, Sandler CM, Corriere Jr JN, McGuire EJ. Blunt urethral trauma: a unified, anatomical mechanical classification. J Urol. 1997;157(1):85–9.

Grady RW, Mitchell ME. Management of epispadias. Urol Clin North Am. 2002;29(2):349–60. vi.

Grima F, Paparel P, Devonec M, Perrin P, Caillot JL, Ruffion A. Management of corpus cavernosum trauma. Prog Urol. 2006;16(1):12–8 [Article in French].

Hayashi T, Ujike T, Yamamoto Y, Kamoto A, Nin M, Nishimura K, Miyoshi S, Kawano K. Female urethral adenocarcinoma with urinary retention: a case report. Hinyokika Kiyo. 2009;55(7):429–32 [Article in Japanese].

Igarashi T, Suzuki H, Naya Y. Computer-based endoscopic image-processing technology for endourology and laparoscopic surgery. Int J Urol. 2009;16(6):533–43.

Imamura M, Ohmori K, Nishimura K. A case of clear cell adenocarcinoma of the female urethra. Hinyokika Kiyo. 1998;44(4):289–92 [Article in Japanese].

Ingram MD, Watson SG, Skippage PL, Patel U. Urethral injuries after pelvic trauma: evaluation with urethrography. Radiographics. 2008;28(6):1631–43.

Ishida K, Yuhara K, Kanimoto Y. Leiomyoma of the urinary bladder: report of three cases. Hinyokika Kiyo. 2003;49(11):671–4 [Article in Japanese].

Kagadis GC, Siablis D, Liatsikos EN, Petsas T, Nikifordis GC. Virtual endoscopy of the urinary tract. Asian J Androl. 2006;8(1):31–8.

Kamoto T, Noguchi T, Okabe T, Takai I, Matsumoto M. A case of clear cell adenocarcinoma of the female urethra. Hinyokika Kiyo. 1993;39(10):965–9 [Article in Japanese].

Karadag D, Caglar O, Haliloglu AH, Ataoglu O. Leiomyoma in a female urethral diverticulum. Jpn J Radiol. 2010;28(5):369–71.

Kawakami T, Arai Y, Okada Y, Tomoyoshi T. A case of urethral diverticulum in a male paraplegic patient. Hinyokika Kiyo. 1995;41(11):887–90 [Article in Japanese].

Kawashima A, Sandler CM, Wasserman NF, LeRoy AJ, King Jr BF, Goldman SM. Imaging of urethral disease: a pictorial review. Radiographics. 2004;24(Suppl 1):S195–216.

Kim B, Kawashima A, LeRoy AJ. Imaging of the male urethra. Semin Ultrasound CT MR. 2007;28(4):258–73.

Kommu SS, Illahi I, Mumtaz F. Patterns of urethral injury and immediate management. Curr Opin Urol. 2007;17(6):383–9.

Krishnan A, de Souza A, Konijeti R, Baskin LS. The anatomy and embryology of posterior urethral valves. J Urol. 2006;175(4):1214–20.

Lee JW, Fynes MM. Female urethral diverticula. Best Pract Res Clin Obstet Gynaecol. 2005;19(6):875–93.

Li H, Sugimura K, Boku M, Kaji Y, Tachibana M, Kamidono S. MR findings of prostatic urethral polyp in an adult. Eur Radiol. 2003;13(Suppl 6):L105–8.

Lissauer D, Morris RK, Kilby MD. Fetal lower urinary tract obstruction. Semin Fetal Neonatal Med. 2007;12(6):464–70.

Macura KJ, Genadry RR. Female urinary incontinence: pathophysiology, methods of evaluation and role of MR imaging. Abdom Imaging. 2008;33(3):371–80.

Macura KJ, Genadry RR, Bluemke DA. MR imaging of the female urethra and supporting ligaments in assessment of urinary incontinence: spectrum of abnormalities. Radiographics. 2006;26(4):1135–49.

Martínez Portillo FJ, Seif C, Braun PM, Spahn M, Alken P, Jünemann KP. Penile fractures: controversy of surgical vs. conservative treatment. Aktuelle Urol. 2003;34(1):33–6 [Article in German].

McGuire EJ, Cespedes RD, Cross CA, O'Connell HE. Videourodynamic studies. Urol Clin North Am. 1996;23(2):309–21.

Melquist J, Sharma V, Sciullo D, McCaffrey H, Khan SA. Current diagnosis and management of syringocele: a review. Int Braz J Urol. 2010;36(1):3–9.

Miller J, Karnes RJ. Primary clear-cell adenocarcinoma of the proximal female urethra: case report and review of the literature. Clin Genitourin Cancer. 2008;6(2):131–3.

Morey AF, McAninch JW. Ultrasound evaluation of the male urethra for assessment of urethral stricture. J Clin Ultrasound. 1996;24(8):473–9.

Morey AF, McAninch JW. Sonographic staging of anterior urethral strictures. J Urol. 2000;163(4):1070–5.

Morey AF, Hernandez J, McAninch JW. Reconstructive surgery for trauma of the lower urinary tract. Urol Clin North Am. 1999;26(1):49–60. viii.

Mostofi FK, Davis Jr CJ, Sesterhenn IA. Carcinoma of the male and female urethra. Urol Clin North Am. 1992;19(2):347–58.

Novara G, Artibani W. Imaging for urinary incontinence: a contemporary perspective. Curr Opin Urol. 2006;16(4):219–23.

Ouzaid I, Hermieu JF, Dominique S, Fernandez P, Choudat L, Ravery V. Management of adenocarcinoma of the female urethra: case report and brief review. Can J Urol. 2010;17(5):5404–7.

Palmtag H, Goepel M, Heidler H. Chapter 1, Grundlagen. In: Urodynamik. 2nd ed. Heidelberg: Springer Medizin; 2007. p. 3–58.

Pavlica P, Barozzi L, Menchi I. Imaging of male urethra. Eur Radiol. 2003;13(7):1583–96.

Pinggera GM, Rehder P, Bartsch G, Gozzi C. Urethral trauma. Urologe A. 2005;44(8):883–97 [Article in German].

Podnar S. Neurophysiology of the neurogenic lower urinary tract disorders. Clin Neurophysiol. 2007;118(7):1423–37.

Poon CI, Zimmern PE, Wilson TS, Defreitas GA, Foreman MR. Three-dimensional ultrasonography to assess long-term durability of periurethral collagen in women with stress urinary incontinence due to intrinsic sphincter deficiency. Urology. 2005;65(1):60–4.

Prasad SR, Menias CO, Narra VR, Middleton WD, Mukundan G, Samadi N, Heiken JP, Siegel CL. Cross-sectional imaging of the female urethra: technique and results. Radiographics. 2005;25(3):749–61.

Ramchandani P, Buckler PM. Imaging of genitourinary trauma. AJR Am J Roentgenol. 2009;192(6):1514–23.

Rovner ES. Urethral diverticula: a review and an update. Neurourol Urodyn. 2007;26(7):972–7.

Ryu J, Kim B. MR imaging of the male and female urethra. Radiographics. 2001;21(5):1169–85.

Seki H, Ukimura S, Mizutani Y, Kawauchi A, Nakao M, Miki T. A case of primary adenocarcinoma of the female urethra. Hinyokika Kiyo. 2001;47(7):509–12 [Article in Japanese].

Shimizu Y, Ogawa O, Terachi T, Okada Y, Yoshida O. A case of primary urethral lymphoma presenting as a huge mass surrounding the female urethra. Hinyokika Kiyo. 1997;43(3):229–32.

Tembely A, Cissé MC, Doumbia D, Sanogo Z, Cissé M, Samassékou A, Ouattara K. The diverticulum of the female urethra. Clinical aspects, paracliniques and therapeutiques. In connection with ten cases. Le Mali Méd. 2008;23(4):5–10 [Article in French].

Titton RL, Gervais DA, Hahn PF, Harisinghani MG, Arellano RS, Mueller PR. Urine leaks and urinomas: diagnosis and imaging-guided intervention. Radiographics. 2003;23(5):1133–47.

Yamaguchi Y, Miyagawa Y, Tsujimura A, Nonomura N, Matsumiya K, Okuyama A, Koyama M, Tsujimoto Y, Aozasa K, Hanafusa T, Miura H. A case of clear cell adenocarcinoma of the female urethra. Hinyokika Kiyo. 2003;49(10):627–30 [Article in Japanese].

Section XV

Ovary and Adnexa

Anju Sahdev

Introduction

Imaging plays an integral and diverse role in the investigation and management of patients with gynecological disorders. Noninvasive imaging techniques offer the gynecologist important additional information as an adjunct to clinical examination. The imaging modalities discussed in this chapter are ultrasound (US), computed tomography (CT), magnetic resonance imaging (MRI), and positron emission tomography (PET). Strengths and limitations of these different techniques and their optimal application in assessment of ovarian and adnexal lesions will be highlighted.

Ultrasound

The most frequently used imaging technique to evaluate the ovaries and adnexa is ultrasound. At present ultrasound is the preferred method of evaluation of the female pelvis due to its ease of availability, lack of radiation, and relative cost-effectiveness. It is often the first and only imaging modality used to demonstrate gynecological anatomy and to evaluate physiological and pathological changes. There are a variety of

A. Sahdev (✉)
Department of Radiology, St Bartholomew's Hospital, Barts and The London NHS Trust and Queen Mary's School of Medicine and Dentistry, London, UK

Department of Diagnostic Imaging, King George V wing, St Bartholomew's Hospital, London, UK

approaches that can be used for ultrasound evaluation of adnexa. These include transabdominal (TAUS), transvaginal (TVUS), transrectal (TRUS), or transperineal approaches.

Transabdominal Ultrasound

Transabdominal ultrasound is performed with a full bladder which acts as an acoustic window to visualize pelvic organs. This utilizes 3.5–5 MHz curvilinear or linear transducers to provide a global, large field of view of the pelvis, particularly the upper pelvis (Fig. 128.1). It is useful to interrogate the bladder, abnormal bowel loops, and pelvic side wall for enlarged nodal disease in patients with adnexal masses. Transabdominal ultrasound directs TVUS and images should be acquired to document longitudinal and transverse uterine size and the relationship between the uterus and any adnexal pathology. In patients with superficial ovaries lying high within the pelvis or lower abdomen, TAUS may allow better visualization and evaluation of the ovaries than TVUS. Pedunculated lesions, particularly leiomyomas arising from the uterine fundus, are best seen on TAUS and may be missed on TVUS due to its small field of view (Fig. 128.2). The true fundal anatomy is best seen on TAUS, an important point in patients being investigated for congenital anomalies (Andolf and Jörgensen 1990; Mendelson et al. 1988). The advantages of TAUS are summarized in Table 128.1. In patients unable or unwilling to undergo TVUS, TAUS can provide limited but adequate anatomical detail of the uterus and ovaries. This is particularly

B. Hamm, P. R. Ros (eds.), *Abdominal Imaging*, DOI 10.1007/978-3-642-13327-5_134,
© Springer-Verlag Berlin Heidelberg 2013

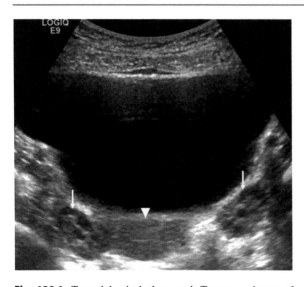

Fig. 128.1 Transabdominal ultrasound: Transverse image of the pelvis in a 46-year-old woman. The image shows a normal transverse section of the uterine fundus (*arrowhead*). Both ovaries are well demonstrated in the ovarian fossae with benign functional follicles (*arrows*)

Table 128.1 The additional value of TAUS in evaluation of the pelvis

Allows evaluation of the bladder	Identifies focal masses e.g., endometriotic deposits
	Bladder wall thickening and identification of significant residual volumes
	Identification of bladder or ureteric calculi causing pelvic pain
Measurement and assessment of uterine size and orientation	Provides accurate longitudinal axis of the uterus and gives the true uterine and cervical orientation
Identification of uterine fundal lesions	Pedunculated leiomyomas may lie beyond the view of TVUS or the true connection to the uterus may be missed
	In congenital malformations, TAUS provides the best coronal view of the uterus
Identifies large pelvic masses that are too large for TVUS detection or evaluation	Very large masses, particularly fat-rich dermoids may appear as pelvic fat rather than a focal mass on TVUS
Identifies ovaries lying high within the pelvis out of reach for TVUS evaluation	Ovarian masses and ectopic pregnancies may be missed on TVUS alone
Allows identification of non-gynecological causes of pelvic pain	Appendicitis, diverticulitis, ureteric/bladder calculi, pelvic lymphadenopathy etc.

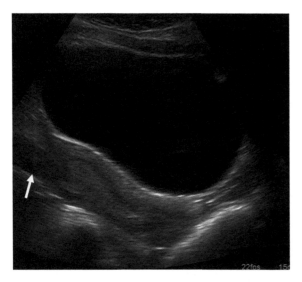

Fig. 128.2 Transabdominal ultrasound: Longitudinal image of the uterus showing a subserosal fibroid (*arrow*) arising from the fundus. This was best demonstrated on TAUS and poorly seen on TVUS

true for children, patients not sexually active or patients who have undergone radiotherapy or vaginal surgery which makes TVUS difficult due to vaginal stenosis.

Transvaginal Ultrasound

Transvaginal ultrasound is the mainstay of gynecological ultrasound. It has a wide range of applications when investigating gynecological pathologies. It provides accurate estimation of endometrial thickness in patients with postmenopausal bleeding detecting benign or malignant endometrial masses, exquisite detail of ovarian follicles and their physiological development, ovarian stroma, and adnexal masses (Figs. 128.3, 128.4, 128.5). It provides detailed assessment of small ovarian cysts and has a high sensitivity for detecting ovarian malignancy. TVUS can be performed in pre- and postmenopausal women with equal effectiveness (Coleman et al. 1988). Prior to the scan, the procedure should be explained to the patient in detail and verbal consent should be obtained. It is advisable for male operators to have an escort in the examination room. TVUS is performed using small endocavity transducers introduced into the vaginal

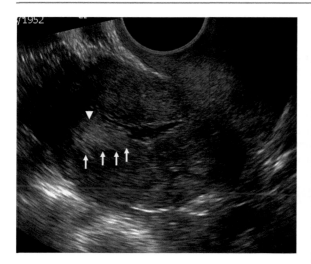

Fig. 128.3 Transvaginal ultrasound of the pelvis: Midline longitudinal image of the uterus showing the endometrial cavity. A hyperechoic endometrial mass is seen in the fundal endometrium (*arrowhead*). The mass has irregular borders and extends into the underlying myometrium (*arrows*). Histological resection confirmed a grade 2 endometrioid endometrial carcinoma

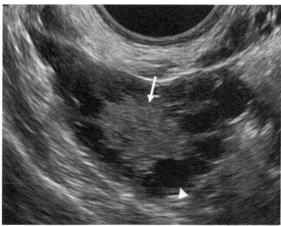

Fig. 128.5 Transvaginal scan of the pelvis: Polycystic ovary with hyperechoic enlarged stroma. The functional follicles are distributed along the periphery (*arrow*) of the ovary forming the "string of pearls" sign (*arrowhead*)

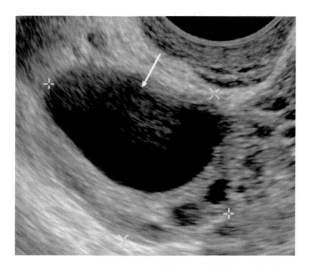

Fig. 128.4 Transvaginal ultrasound of the pelvis: The right ovary showing a preovulatory dominant follicle on day 12 of the menstrual cycle (*arrow*). The follicle has no perceptible wall, no internal architecture and no internal or wall Doppler flow in keeping with a benign cyst

cavity, covered with a condom containing acoustic jelly and secured with a rubber band to avoid cross-infection. After each examination, the probe must be cleaned with a disinfectant. To aid patient comfort, the bladder must be empty at the time of TVUS and a soft lumbar support or lateral knee supports can be used.

In postmenopausal women, generous use of acoustic jelly is recommended to reduce discomfort due to vaginal dryness.

TVUS utilizes high-frequency (5–12 MHz) curved linear-array transducers with a small field of view (a few centimeters only) that provide high-resolution images. These high-resolution images are achieved partly by proximity of adnexal structures to the high-frequency transducers, due to optimal line density and a high send-and-receive element ratio in transvaginal transducers. The ultrasound beam orientation should be checked by touching the probe surface prior to the transducer being placed in to the vaginal cavity. Usually, vaginal probes have a notch or groove indicating the "up side." When images are obtained with the apex of the image at the top of the screen, the long axis of the transducer corresponds to patients' sagittal plane. In this plane the urinary bladder should appear at the upper left corner of the image. Small degrees of rotation and gentle lateral sweep in the longitudinal plane will provide the whole longitudinal uterine axis. Rotating the transducer counterclockwise by 90° provides the transverse plane. In this plane, patients' right side should be on the left of the screen. Confirmation of the sides allows correct placement of detected adnexal pathology. In anteverted uteri, withdrawing the transducer to mid-vagina will allow the best depiction of transverse uterine plane. As routine, the entire endometrium, myometrium, and both adnexae should be evaluated in two planes.

Table 128.2 Normal physiological appearances of the ovaries

	Phase	Normal appearance	Supplementary features
Premenopausal	Follicular phase (day 0–14)	Multiple follicles (5–15) develop along the peripheral cortex of the ovary. Varying sizes and thin walled	In areas of follicular development, intraovarian Doppler flow is demonstrated
	Ovulation (day 14)	Dominant follicle between 2–4 cm (average 2.5 cm) in size releases the ovum	Hemorrhagic changes may be seen in the cyst along with pelvic free fluid
	Secretory phase (day 15–28)	The dominant follicle develops a thick wall and forms the corpus luteum secreting progesterone	The corpus luteum has the typical "ring of fire" appearance with circumferential, low-impedance flow
		If no pregnancy occurs, the corpus luteum involutes into the stroma	
Postmenopausal	*Without HRT*	No follicular function. May continue to have small <1 cm simple follicles numbering less than 5	In the absence of follicular activity, little or no intraovarian Doppler flow is seen

The adnexa lie between lateral margins of the uterus and pelvic side wall. They are composed of the paired ovaries, fallopian tubes, broad and round ligaments, and uterine and ovarian vessels. Normal ovaries may vary considerably in their location. In young nulliparous women, ovaries usually lie in the ovarian fossae. These can be found by identifying the transverse plane of the uterus, sweeping laterally toward the pelvic side wall up to the iliac vessels. The ovarian fossae are bordered by the external iliac vessels laterally, the internal iliac vessels and ureters posteriorly, and the uterus medially. In cases of difficulty, the internal iliac vessels can be used as a guide, the ovaries usually lie medial to the vein. Other sites where the ovaries may "hide" include the Pouch of Douglas, adjacent to the cervix or the uterine fundus. In retroverted uteri the ovaries may lie anterior to the uterus. In parous women ovaries can lie high in the pelvis or in the abdomen, where they were displaced during pregnancy to accommodate the gravid uterus. Abdominal palpation can be helpful in displacing bowel in difficult cases and also assess mobility of pelvic organs in suspected adhesions. Normal ovaries are oval in shape and their size is measured as a volume. This is acquired by multiplying 0.5 to the 3 orthogonal dimensions of the ovary. In prepubertal (<12 years) females, the mean ovarian volume is less than 1 ml and in childbearing age, the normal mean ovarian volume is between 5 and 14 ml. In postmenopausal women, ovaries involute, become follicular and mean volume should be no more than 8 ml (Fig. 128.5). In premenopausal women, a size discrepancy between the two ovaries is a common finding and has no clinical significance. However in postmenopausal women, the ovaries should be of similar size and ovaries greater than twice the volume of their counterpart are abnormal. The normal physiological cyclical appearances of the ovaries are summarized in Table 128.2.

Normal fallopian tubes are not identified on TVUS. However, dilated fallopian tubes resulting in hydrosalpinges, pyo-or hematosalpinges may be seen in the adnexa. The fallopian tube patency may be assessed by contrast studies in the form of conventional or US hysterosalpingograms (Fig. 128.6). In patients undergoing investigations for pelvic pain, special examination of pelvic adnexal vascularity is recommended. Pelvic congestion syndrome is a common cause for protracted pelvic pain thought to be due to ovarian vein incompetence resulting in retrograde ovarian vein flow and pelvic varices. The normal ovarian vein diameter is less than 5 mm. The uterine fundal arcuate veins drain into ovarian plexus while arcuate veins from the uterine body drain to parametrial plexus and then into internal iliac veins.

Doppler Evaluation

Doppler evaluation of the ovaries should be included in all routine transvaginal gynecological ultrasound examinations. It is performed with the same TVUS transducers and allows assessment of blood flow and waveforms which is helpful in evaluating several pelvic pathologies. The Doppler trace or waveform varies with the size of vessels interrogated. The larger vessels have a more uniform, lower velocity flow while smaller intraparenchymal vessels have more turbulent flow with higher range and mean velocities.

The smallest sample volume is used and the vessel course is visualized. The Doppler angle is set between 20° and 60° along the vessel course for optimal acquisition of Doppler wave form. Calculations of the vessel impedance should be acquired. Vessel impedance is assessed using resistive index (peak systolic minus diastolic divided by systolic) or pulsatility index (peak systolic minus diastolic divided by the mean). In normal ovarian arterioles, there is a muscular wall which regulates parenchymal perfusion, with a typically high pulsatility and lack of diastolic notch. Doppler waveforms may also help distinguish between benign and malignant adnexal masses. Malignant vessels typically have a haphazard arrangement, lack normal muscular wall, and have high diastolic flow and

velocities. Therefore, benign lesions have a PI greater than 1.0 (high impedance flow), flow in the periphery only, a diastolic notch in the wave form, peripheral distribution of vessels, and low vessel density. Malignant lesions have a PI less than 1.0 (low impedance flow), flow in the center and periphery of the lesion, high vessels density, and absent diastolic notch (Figs. 128.7 and 128.8) (Fleischer and Emerson 1993).

In patients with chronic pelvic pain, its role in pelvic congestion syndrome has been discussed above. In acute pelvic pain, Doppler is useful in diagnosis of ovarian torsion and inflammatory disease. The ovary has dual arterial supply from the adnexal branch of the uterine artery and directly from the ovarian artery. In torsion, the ovary is massively enlarged

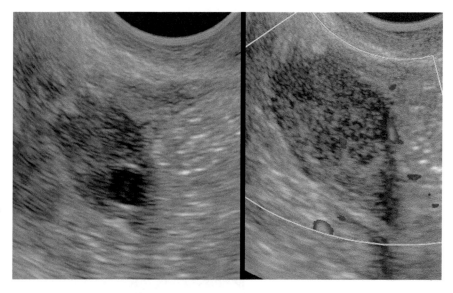

Fig. 128.6 Transvaginal ultrasound of the pelvis: Postmenopausal ovary showing small, solid ovary with a single follicle only. The stroma is uniformly hypoechoic and there is a reduction of vascular Doppler flow in the central stroma

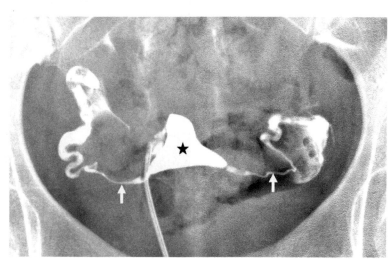

Fig. 128.7 Hysterosalpingogram to assess tubal patency: Transvaginal contrast instilled into the endometrial cavity opacifies a normal endometrial cavity (*asterisk*) and normal fallopian tubes bilaterally (*arrows*)

with hyperechoic edematous stromal engorgement. The ovarian follicles are pushed to the periphery (Fig. 128.9). There is a high impedance pattern or absent arterial flow. There is impeded venous return with resultant stromal enlargement, hemorrhagic changes, and ultimately gangrene. However, in chronic intermittent torsion, the arterial waveforms may be highly variable. There may be arterial collaterization, arterial flow may be seen in capsular arteries but not intraovarian vessels or there may be non-pulsatile arterial flow mimicking venous flow (Fleischer and Emerson 1993). Associated with ovarian torsion may be a fusiform structure created by a hematosalpinx representing an associated tubal torsion.

As US is a dynamic examination, it should ideally be reported immediately by the performing operator to minimize errors. The US reports should be simple and structured. Undoubtedly, the more experienced the performer, the more precise the report. However, by following a structured reporting system, even new operators can deliver a good pelvic evaluation for clinicians. A suggested reporting format, modified

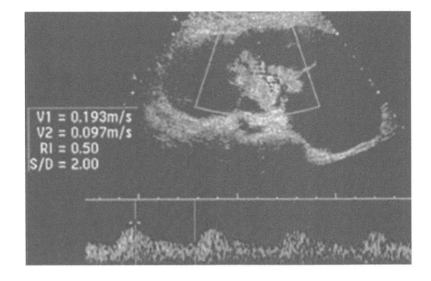

Fig. 128.8 Transvaginal ultrasound of the pelvis: Doppler trace from a solid-cystic adnexal mass. The mass shows central flow within a solid vegetation. The trace has a high diastolic flow, low resistive index of 0.45, features typical of a malignant mass

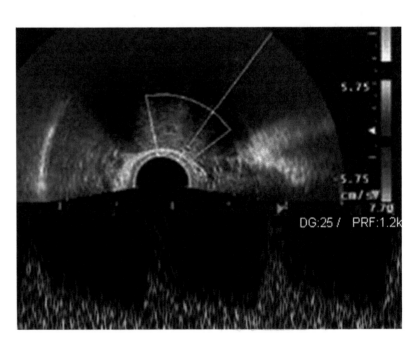

Fig. 128.9 Transvaginal ultrasound of the pelvis: Benign ovarian fibroma. The Doppler trace from a confirmed fibroma shows low diastolic flow and a high resistive index of 0.9

from the United Kingdom Association of Sonographers and the College of Radiographers Guidelines for Professional Working Standards: Ultrasound practice is summarized in Table 128.3 United Kingdom Association of Sonographers (2008).

Computed Tomography (CT)

Although ultrasound and MRI are the modalities of choice for detailed investigation of the female pelvis, in selected patients, CT may be used. The inherent tissue contrast on CT does not always permit distinction of normal from abnormal pelvic tissues, and anatomical resolution is also limited when compared

Table 128.3 Recommended standard pelvic US report

Uterus	Position
	Shape
	Size
	Appearance of the myometrium, myometrial masses if present
	Endometrial thickness
Ovaries	Size
	Shape
	Follicular pattern and internal echo pattern
	Stromal echogenicity
Adnexae	Masses if present and size
Pouch of Douglas	Presence of free fluid or masses
Pelvic side wall	Nodal disease if present, presence of varices or dilated ovarian veins

to US and MRI. Its main role is to identify disease beyond the pelvis in peritoneal surfaces, serosa, omentum, and upper abdominal viscera (Fig. 128.10). The diagnostic performance of CT and MRI is comparable for detection of nodal disease as both rely on morphological increase in nodal size for detection of nodal metastases. In acutely unwell patients and patients unable to undergo MRI, CT may provide limited information in pelvic disease (Fig. 128.11). Non-gynecological diseases, such as appendicitis, diverticulitis, or renal tract calculi causing pelvic pain, are easily demonstrated on CT. When tissue diagnosis is required or for treatment of acute pelvic abscesses, CT is the imaging modality of choice to guide percutaneous biopsy and drainage.

The tissue contrast of pelvic structures can be improved by use of oral and intravenous contrast media. Oral contrast medium outlines the lumen of bowel allowing better separation of normal bowel from adnexal pathology, mesenteric, serosal, or peritoneal disease, useful in assessment of disseminated ovarian or endometrial cancer (Figs. 128.10 and 128.12). Oral administration of 1,000 ml of a dilute gastrograffin solution, 40–60 min prior to the CT examination will allow luminal opacification of small and large bowels. Intravenous contrast media is administered usually into a large peripheral vein, commonly in the antecubital fossa, at variable rates. The most frequently used regimen is injection of 100 ml of iodinated contrast media at the rate of 3–4 ml/s followed by image acquisition, 60 s after commencement of contrast injection. This is taken up by pelvic vessels, uterus, and its suspensory ligaments, adnexae,

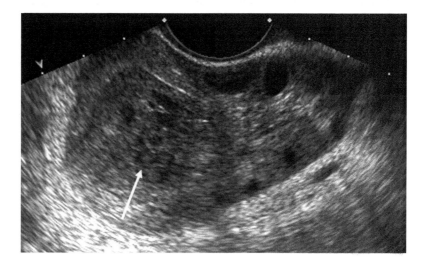

Fig. 128.10 Transvaginal ultrasound of the pelvis: Surgically confirmed ovarian torsion. 36-year-old woman presenting with acute pelvic pain. The TVUS shows an enlarged ovary with marked expansion of the stroma and peripheral displacement of the ovarian follicles.
A hemorrhagic focus is also noted in the ovary (*arrow*). No intraovarian vascular flow was present

Fig. 128.11 Coronal reconstruction of axial CT with oral and intravenous contrast enhancement: 56-year-old woman with serous papillary adenocarcinoma of the ovary. The CT shows extensive disease in the upper abdomen; *A* – left subdiaphragmatic disease, *B* – disease in the gastrosplenic ligament, *C* – peri-hepatic subcapsular disease, *D* – disease in Morrison's pouch, *E* – right paracolic gutter, and *F* – bilateral adnexal malignant masses

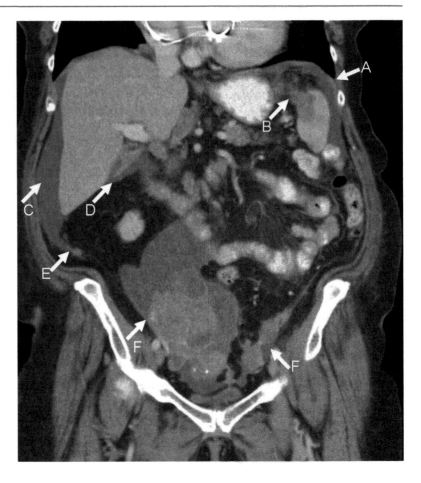

the vaginal, bowel, and bladder walls. Viable soft tissue in adnexal masses will also enhance following intravenous contrast media (Fig. 128.13). Although the vagina may be outlined by insertion of a vaginal tampon, this is rarely necessary in modern CT. Spasmolytics are also no longer routinely indicated. On CT, normal ovaries can only be identified positively after administration of intravenous contrast media. The detection of low-attenuation, nonenhancing ovarian follicles in the ovarian fossae identifies the ovaries. The identification of normal ovaries is particularly difficult in thin patients with little pelvic fat. In such cases, the ovarian veins can be traced from the IVC or renal vein to the adnexa, where they lead to the ovaries (Fig. 128.13). The adnexal para-uterine vascular plexus is seen as serpiginous structures enhancing as much as or more than the myometrium. The adnexal ligaments on CT and MRI are only well seen in the presence of ascites which outlines the round, broad, cardinal, and uterosacral ligaments (Fig. 128.14).

The major disadvantage of CT is a significant radiation burden, CT accounting for the largest proportion of medical radiation exposure in the Western world. Direct radiation exposure of the female pelvis is to be avoided as the ovaries are among the most radiation-sensitive organs. For this reason and for its better tissue characterization, MRI has superseded CT in evaluation of female pelvis. Intravenous iodine-based contrast agents are nephrotoxic particularly in patients in renal failure, where they are usually avoided except under particular circumstances. In patients presenting with acute renal dysfunction, due to pelvic pathologies that are obstructing the ureters, intravenous contrast media which improves the diagnostic ability of CT, cannot be administered. Therefore increasingly, the role of CT is diminishing in characterizing primary adnexal diseases. It continues to be the modality of choice in staging and surveillance of ovarian and endometrial cancer by detecting extra-ovarian and extra-pelvic disease.

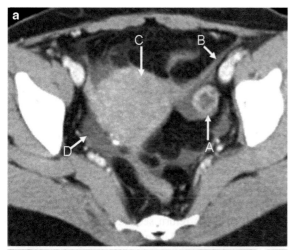

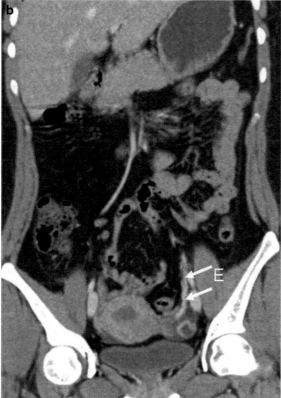

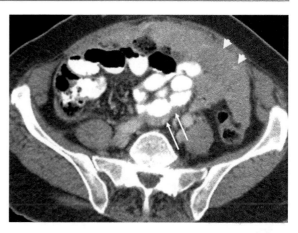

Fig. 128.13 Intravenous contrast-enhanced CT of the abdomen and pelvis from a 65-year-old woman undergoing staging for suspected ovarian cancer: CT demonstrates a thick infra-colic omental cake (*arrowheads*) which was biopsied to obtain confirmation of ovarian cancer. Oral contrast in small bowel loops enhances the detection of serosal disease (*arrows*) which would otherwise have blended with the bowel wall

Fig. 128.12 Intravenous contrast-enhanced CT of the abdomen and pelvis from a 27-year-old woman with acute pelvic pain: (**a**) Axial image of the normal pelvis demonstrating: *A* – rim enhancement of a corpus luteal cyst within the left ovary, *B* – enhancement of the round ligament, *C* – normal enhancement of the myometrium, *D* – normal right ovary with mild enhancement of normal ovarian stroma surrounding multiple normal ovarian follicles. (**b**) Coronal reconstruction demonstrating the distal left ovarian vein arising from the ovarian pedicle (*E*)

Magnetic Resonance Imaging (MRI)

The exquisite anatomical ability to detect early pathologies and the lack of radiation burden makes MRI an adjunct to US in imaging gynecological diseases. The role of MRI in gynecological disease is continuously evolving. It provides detailed anatomical information of pelvic organs. On high-resolution images, MRI delineates ovarian, endometrial, and cervical pathologies better than TVUS. It has a natural high contrast between tissues allowing MRI to accurately separate fat, blood, and fluid. This ability makes MRI ideally suited for characterization of adnexal masses. Table 128.4 summarizes the signal intensities of common adnexal tissues on MR imaging. Its multiplanar imaging abilities were an advantage but this importance has diminished with the advent of multidetector CT. MRI has no known in vivo adverse effects on embryonal, fetal tissues or ovaries, allowing diagnostic imaging during pregnancy for placental, adnexal, and fetal disorders (Fig. 128.15). The main disadvantages of MRI include longer imaging times than US and CT, less widespread availability and a need for specialist training in image acquisition and interpretation. The combination of long imaging period in a closed space and noise generated by loud radiofrequency pulses can result in claustrophobia in adults and studies are

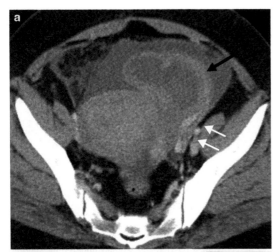

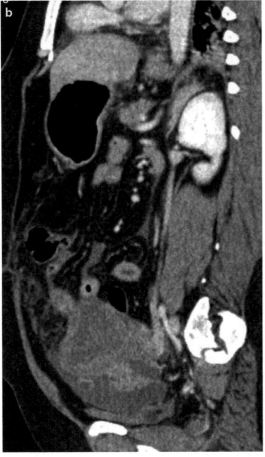

Table 128.4 MR signal intensities of common adnexal tissues

Tissue	T1 signal	T2 signal	T1 with fat saturation
Blood	high	Variable according to age of blood	Very high
Fat	high	High	Very low
Fibrous tissue	Low	Low	Intermediate
Mucin	high	high	low

difficult for children to tolerate without sedation or general anesthetic. During pregnancy, supine or prone MR imaging may not be possible due to impaired venous return secondary to compression of the IVC by the gravid uterus. The performance of MRI is also highly protocol and technique dependent. To achieve reproducibility and to obtain the optimum performance of MRI, acquisition technique has to be meticulous. High-resolution images are crucial in the detection of subtle disease like small endometriotic deposits in deep pelvic endometriosis or small papillary projections in adnexal masses that distinguish malignant from benign masses (Fig. 128.16). Recommended image sequences and techniques based on the United Kingdom Royal College of Radiologists' recommendations and the authors' institutional experience are summarized in Table 128.5 (The Royal College of Radiologists 2009).

Conventional pelvic MR images are acquired in the supine position, with pelvic or cardiac phase array surface coils. However in patients with mild claustrophobia, prone images acquired with the patients head outside the MR tunnel can be very successful. Oral spasmolytics are routinely used in the author's institution to minimize bowel peristaltic artifacts. MRI contrast agents have an established role in imaging gynecological disorders (Yamashita et al. 1995). These are paramagnetic molecules used to improve the natural contrast between soft tissue structures. The most frequently used group of contrast agents are gadolinium-based intravascular blood pool agents which remain in the intravascular compartment. Gadolinium agents can assess tissue perfusion and provide information about capillary permeability. The blood pool properties make them suitable for angiography. Angiography of pelvic vessels is useful for assessment of fibroid vascularity, investigation of chronic pelvic pain, and tumor perfusion. Gadolinium allergy and previous or ongoing history of nephrogenic systemic

Fig. 128.14 Ovarian carcinoma. (**a**) Axial CT with oral and intravenous contrast enhancement. (**b**) Coronal oblique reconstruction of axial CT. A large left solid-cystic adnexal mass is demonstrated (*black arrow*). This is likely to be ovarian in origin as the left ovarian vein (*white arrows*) extends into the mass. The mass was resected and confirmed an ovarian carcinoma of the left ovary

Fig. 128.15 Axial T2-weighted images of the pelvis in a 72-year-old woman with known serous adenocarcinoma of the ovary. There is extensive ascites in the pelvis which allows the visualization of the round (*A*) and lateral (*B*) ligaments of the uterus. Multiple peritoneal metastatic nodules (*white arrows*) are also well seen due to the ascites

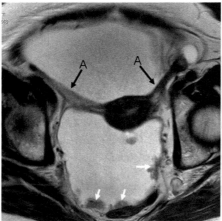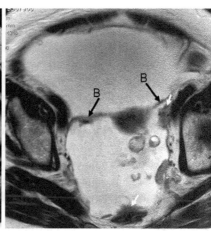

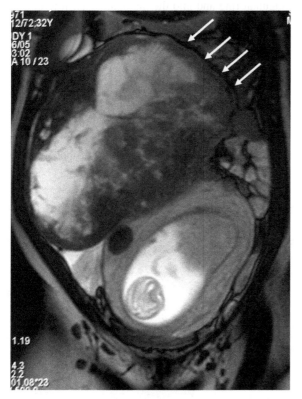

Fig. 128.16 Coronal T2-weighted image of a 32-year-old pregnant woman with an ultrasound detected solid-cystic adnexal mass on the dating scan. The large right sided solid-cystic mass is demonstrated (*arrows*). This has a background of very low T2 signal intensity with central high T2 signal intensity. The appearances are typical for cystic degeneration in a subserosal fibroid

Table 128.5 Safety of MRI

Absolute contraindication	Relative contraindication
Metallic intraocular foreign bodies	First trimester of pregnancy
Non-MRI-compatible cerebral aneurysm clips	Joint prostheses are generally acceptable but may cause susceptibility artifacts in the images and patients may experience discomfort due to heating of metallic prosthesis
Non-MRI-compatible cardiac pacemakers	
Non-MRI-compatible neurostimulator devices or cochlear implants	
Patients with metallic surgical clips up to 6 weeks after surgery	

are absolute contraindications in clinical use (Kuo et al. 2007). Relative contraindications for gadolinium use include pregnancy, lactation, hepatorenal syndrome, chronic hepatic disease, previous anaphylaxis to gadolinium, and significant renal impairment with an eGFR below 30.

Diffusion-weighted imaging (DWI) is a relatively new inclusion in gynecological MR imaging. This constitutes MRI sequences that use Brownian motion of proton molecules to evaluate different tissues. Brownian motion of protons is reduced with increasing cellular density/cell membranes and increasing extracellular macromolecules. This reduction of motion is seen as increasing signal intensity on diffusion-weighted images. The degree of proton motion can be quantified by the apparent diffusion coefficient (ADC value). DWI is used in association with routine MRI sequences to improve the overall performance of MRI (Namimoto et al. 2009).

On MRI, normal ovaries can be identified best on T2-weighted images between the uterine cornu and the pelvic side wall. On T1-weighted images, the ovaries have a homogenous intermediate T1 signal intensity.

The ovaries lie in the hollow between the origins of the internal and external iliac arteries. These may be found more superiorly if previously displaced by a gravid uterus, fibroids, or pelvic surgery. In premenopausal women, ovarian stroma has intermediate T2 signal intensity but may demonstrate high T2 signal intensity varying with menstrual phase. The ovaries are easily identified by the presence of multiple follicles of high T2 signal intensity. Following administration of gadolinium, ovarian stroma enhances avidly but less than myometrium. In postmenopausal women, ovaries contain very few, if any, follicles and the stroma has intermediate T2 signal intensity with little enhancement after gadolinium administration (Figs. 128.17 and 128.18). Common normal variations include polycystic ovaries, hemorrhagic functional follicles, and corpus luteal cysts. In polycystic ovaries, follicles are arranged in a peripheral distribution, the stroma is hypertrophied, of high T2 signal intensity with an overall increase in ovarian size. Normal follicles have a thin rim with enhancement. In contrast, corpus luteal cysts demonstrate a thick enhancing rim reflecting an increase in vascularity. These cysts are often hemorrhagic with a high T1 signal intensity. Dominant follicles (2–3 cm in size) may also undergo hemorrhage and alter their uniform high T2 signal intensity.

Depending on the time of hemorrhage, areas of high T1, high or low T2 signal intensity with "layering" may be seen in the cysts but without a thick enhancing rim (Fig. 128.19).

Normal fallopian tubes are not seen on MRI or TVUS. Lateral to the uterus there is a prominent uterine and parametrial vascular plexus. These are seen as very high T2, low T1 signal intensity serpiginous structures. In the normal state, flow through these vessels is slow and hence seen as high T2 signal intensity. In states of high flow, signal voids are seen on both T2 and T1 signal intensity (Fig. 128.20). Most of the support ligaments of the uterus are well demonstrated on MRI. The round ligament is seen as a low T2 signal intensity cord projecting anteriorly from the cornu toward the internal inguinal ring and into the inguinal canal. It terminates inserting diffusely into the mons pubis. The lateral uterine and cervical ligaments (cardinal ligaments) and uterosacral ligaments are seen as strands of low T2 signal intensity anchoring the uterine body and cervix to the lateral pelvic wall and sacrum, respectively. Strands of uterosacral ligaments also merge into the perirectal fascia (Fig. 128.14). The broad ligament is a peritoneal reflection encompassing the round ligament, fallopian tubes, and venous plexus but cannot be seen as a distinct structure on MRI.

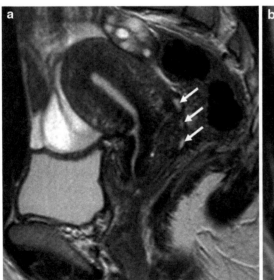 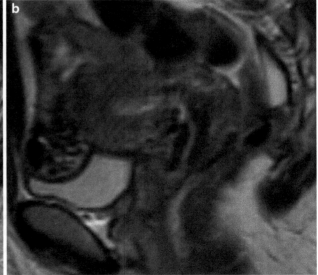

Fig. 128.17 (a) Sagittal T2-weighted image from a 33-year-old woman with known endometriosis. Small high T2 signal intensity endometriotic deposits (*arrows*) are seen along the posterior surface of the uterus. The identification of these deposits requires high resolution MRI. (b) sagittal T2-weighted image of the pelvis from the same patient but as the image is not high resolution, the small endometriotic deposits cannot be seen. This case emphasizes the need for appropriate protocols in MRI to avoid misdiagnosis

Within the pouch of Douglas, free peritoneal fluid is a common finding in premenopausal women. The amount varies with the menstrual cycle and peaks in the secretory phase. In the normal state, no associated enhancement of the peritoneum is seen after gadolinium administration. However in diffuse endometriosis, inflammatory and malignant diseases, there may be enhancement of the peritoneum along with an increase in the amount of pelvic free fluid.

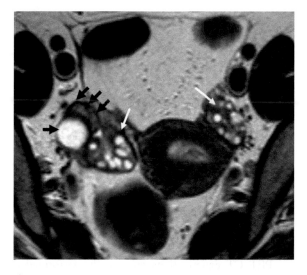

Fig. 128.18 Axial T2-weighted image of normal adult ovaries. Both ovaries (*white arrows*) contain normal small high T2 signal intensity follicles. The central stroma has intermediate to high signal intensity. In the right ovary, there is a dominant follicle (*black arrow*) which illustrates the "beak sign." Normal ovarian stroma is stretched over the follicle (*black arrows*) forming the "beak" over the follicle. This sign is useful to confirm an ovarian origin of a cyst distinguishing it from para-ovarian and inclusion adnexal cysts

PET CT

PET CT is infrequently used as a primary imaging modality in the evaluation of the adnexa. However in patients with a high likelihood of a malignant mass, primary or secondary PET CT is useful to confirm ovarian and extra-ovarian disease. For characterization of adnexal masses, PET CT has an improved specificity when compared to TVUS but a lower sensitivity. In a study of 50 patients, Castellucci et al. showed a PETCT and TVUS had a sensitivity, specificity, NPV, PPV, and accuracy of 87%, 100%, 81%, 100%, and 92% for PET CT, respectively, compared with 90%, 61%, 78%, 80%, and 80%, respectively, for TVUS (Castellucci et al. 2007). More recent studies report much lower sensitivities and specificities of 58% and 76%, respectively, for FDG PET; 92% and 60% respectively for US; 83% and 84%, respectively, for MR imaging. The false positive lesions arise due to normal functional ovarian uptake of FDG, pelvic inflammatory disease, and endometriosis (Fig. 128.21). False negative results are due to

Fig. 128.19 Axial oblique T2-weighted image in a 78-year-old woman with a large endometrial carcinoma (*black arrow*). The axial oblique orientation demonstrates small, solid, afollicular ovaries (*white arrows*). Histology following hysterectomy and bilateral salpingo-oophorectomy confirmed normal post menopausal ovaries

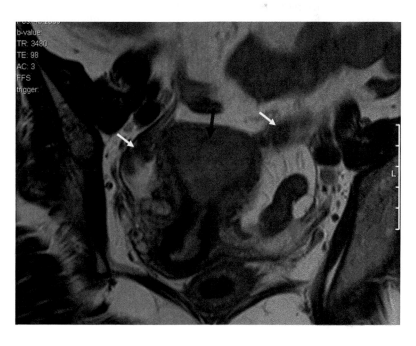

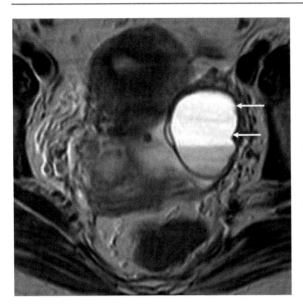

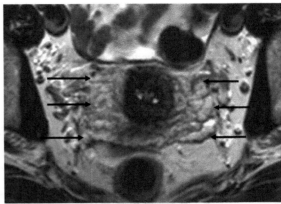

Fig. 128.21 Axial T2-weighted image showing a prominent para-cervical and para-uterine plexus (*arrows*) with high signal intensity and no flow voids indicating a normal state of slow flow within the plexus

Fig. 128.20 Axial T2-weighted image showing a left adnexal cyst with smooth, thin walls and no internal septa or nodules. The internal signal intensity has a "stained glass" or "shaded" appearance (*arrows*). This is caused by degradation and precipitation of blood products with serous high signal fluid in the anterior part of the cyst and denser lower signal intensity material in the posterior or dependent part of the cyst

stage 1 or low-grade adenocarcinomas and borderline tumors of the ovary (Rieber et al. 2001; Fenchel et al. 2002). MRI therefore remains the modality of choice in characterizing lesions deemed indeterminate on TVUS.

The main strength of PET CT is detection of CT occult peritoneal disease resulting in improved lesion detection and accuracy when staging ovarian carcinoma. PET CT is playing an expanding role in treatment planning and follow-up of patients with ovarian cancer. For predicting correct stage, addition of PET to contrast-enhanced CT has been shown to improve accuracy from 89% to 94% when compared to operative surgical findings (Kitajima et al. 2008). Combined with CT, it is the most accurate technique to evaluate suspected recurrent ovarian cancer. A meta-analysis comparing techniques for detection of recurrence determined that PET CT (sensitivity, 91%; specificity, 88%) performed better than CT (sensitivity, 79%; specificity, 84%) or MRI (sensitivity, 75%; specificity, 78%) (Gu et al. 2009). The technique is limited in its ability to detect lesions smaller than 10 mm leading to a false negative rate between 10% and 20%.

Misregistration of PET and CT images particularly in bowel can lead to false positive interpretation of serosal disease.

PET CT examinations are usually performed on integrated scanners that include multidetector CT and a PET system. Patients are fasted for 4–6 h prior to imaging. The blood glucose level should be below 10 mmol/l before injection of 370–740 MBq of FDG administered according to patient body weight. After 1 h, attenuation correction CT is acquired from skull base to mid-thigh for anatomic localization of FDG. PET images are acquired in 2D and fused with the CT images for visual evaluation and measurements. If clinically required, a diagnostic post-contrast CT can be added, imaging the neck, chest, abdomen, and pelvis. In premenopausal women, FDG uptake by the ovaries and endometrium varies with the menstrual cycle. Ovarian FDG uptake occurs in the luteal phase seen as a smooth rounded or ovoid focus of FDG which can be correlated to the ovary on the CT. In postmenopausal women, any ovarian FDG uptake is pathological.

References

Andolf E, Jörgensen C. A prospective comparison of transabdominal and transvaginal ultrasound with surgical findings in gynecologic disease. J Ultrasound Med. 1990;9(2):71–5.

Castellucci P, Perrone AM, Picchio M, Ghi T, Farsad M, Nanni C, et al. Diagnostic accuracy of 18 F-FDG PET/CT in characterizing ovarian lesions and staging ovarian cancer: correlation with transvaginal ultrasonography, computed tomography, and histology. Nucl Med Commun. 2007;28(8):589–95.

Coleman BG, Arger PH, Grumbach K, Menard MK, Mintz MC, Allen KS, Arenson RL, Lamon KA. Transvaginal and transabdominal sonography: prospective comparison. Radiology. 1988;168(3):639–43.

Fenchel S, Grab D, Nuessle K, et al. Asymptomatic adnexal masses: correlation of FDG PET and histopathologic findings. Radiology. 2002;223:780–8.

Fleischer A, Emerson D. Colour Doppler sonography in obstetrics and gynaecology. New York: Churchill-Livingstone; 1993.

Gu P, Pan LL, Wu SQ, Sun L, Huang G. CA 125, PET alone, PET-CT, CT and MRI in diagnosing recurrent ovarian carcinoma: a systematic review and meta-analysis. Eur J Radiol. 2009;71:164–74.

Kitajima K, Murakami K, Yamasaki E, et al. Diagnostic accuracy of integrated FDG-PET/contrast-enhanced CT in staging ovarian cancer: comparison with enhanced CT. Eur J Nucl Med Mol Imaging. 2008;35:1912–20.

Kuo PH, Kanal E, Abu-Alfa AK, Cowper SE. Gadolinium-based MR contrast agents and nephrogenic systemic fibrosis1. Radiology. 2007;242:647–9.

Mendelson EB, Bohm-Velez M, Joseph N, Neiman HL. Gynecologic imaging: comparison of transabdominal and transvaginal sonography. Radiology. 1988;166(2):321–4.

Namimoto T, Awai K, Nakaura T, Yanaga Y, Hirai T, Yamashita Y. Role of diffusion-weighted imaging in the diagnosis of gynecological diseases. Eur Radiol. 2009; 19(3):745–60.

The Royal College of Radiologists (2009) Recommendations for cross-sectional imaging in cancer management. Issue 2.1. www.rcr.ac.uk/docs/oncology/pdf/Cross_Sectional_Imaging_12.pdf. Accessed 28 Feb 2011.

Rieber A, Nussle K, Stohr I, et al. Preoperative diagnosis of ovarian tumors with MR imaging: comparison with transvaginal sonography, positron emission tomography, and histologic findings. AJR. 2001;177:123–9.

United Kingdom Association of Sonographers (2008) Guidelines for professional working standards. Ultrasound practice. http://www.bmus.org/policies-guides/SoR-Professional-Working-Standards-guidelines.pdf. Accessed 23 Feb 2011.

Yamashita Y, Torashima M, Hatanaka Y, Harada M, Higashida Y, Takahashi M, Mizutani H, Tashiro H, Iwamasa J, Miyazaki K, et al. Adnexal masses: accuracy of characterization with transvaginal US and precontrast and postcontrast MR imaging. Radiology. 1995;194(2):557–65.

Inflammatory and Infectious Diseases

Matthias Meissnitzer and Rosemarie Forstner

Pelvic inflammation continues to pose a challenge because of diversity in clinical presentation, occurrence in up to 10% of women in fertile age, and resulting implications in public health in the acute setting and due to long-term sequelae (Livengood 2011). Pelvic inflammatory disease (PID) refers to infection of the upper genital tract due to ascension from the vagina, and is typically found in sexually active females. PID has to be discriminated from infections of the genital organs in the postpuerperal period and from hematogenous spread. Furthermore pelvic inflammation may result secondary to inflammatory pelvic processes including diverticulitis, appendicitis, Crohn's disease, and pelvic surgery. Although pain and tenderness are the most consistent clinical features, symptoms are often atypical, and in 20% of patients with PID, laboratory signs of inflammation or fever are missing (Quiroz 1999). The role of imaging in suspected pelvic inflammatory disease is to rule out non-gynecological causes of pelvic inflammation, to confirm the diagnosis of PID in advanced cases, particularly to diagnose tubo-ovarian abscess formation and its complications, and to perform abscess drainage.

Pelvic Inflammatory Disease

Clinical Background

PID is defined as infection of the upper genital tract involving uterus, fallopian tubes, ovary, and pelvic peritoneum. It is most typically associated with sexually transmitted diseases, specifically with *Neisseria gonorrhoeae* and *Chlamydia trachomatis*, although 30–40% are polymicrobial (Livengood 2011). Furthermore, surgical and diagnostic procedures, e.g., abortion, hysteroscopy, curettage, hysterosalpingography, or tubal inflation bear a higher risk of PID. IUD presents only a higher risk in the immediate phase after implantation and in long indwelling (Livengood 2011). Central to these conditions is the loss of the normal function of the mucus in the cervical canal as protective barrier which gives rise to infection of the upper genital tract with subsequent development of salpingitis and eventually of tubo-ovarian abscess (TOA). Long-term sequelae of PID include chronic pelvic pain, infertility, and an estimated 4–10× increased risk of ectopic pregnancy (Ghiatas 2004). Ten to thirty percent of patients with PID may develop

M. Meissnitzer (✉) • R. Forstner
Department of Radiology, Landeskrankenhaus Salzburg,
Paracelsus Medical University, Salzburg, Austria

B. Hamm, P. R. Ros (eds.), *Abdominal Imaging*, DOI 10.1007/978-3-642-13327-5_137,
© Springer-Verlag Berlin Heidelberg 2013

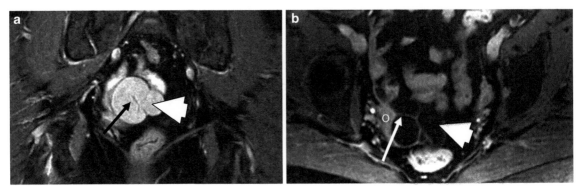

Fig. 129.1 Hydrosalpinx: coronal T2FS (**a**) and contrast-enhanced transaxial T1FS MRI (**b**). Typical finding of hydrosalpinx (*arrowhead*) demonstrating a fluid-filled tubular right adnexal structure with incomplete septations (*arrow*) and thin walls. Ovary (*O*)

Fritz-Hugh–Curtis syndrome which is characterized as pain in the right upper quadrant due to perihepatitis affecting the right anterior lower liver surface (Kim et al. 2009b).

Early PID

Imaging Findings

In early PID, subtle findings including enlargement of an ovary and loss of its cortico-medullary differentiation may be the only imaging findings on US. In oophoritis, stromal edema may result in a polycystic ovarian appearance. Associated findings include edema of pelvic fat planes, endometritis resulting in fluid in the endometrial canal, and nonspecific free fluid in the cul-de-sac (am et al. 2002).

Advanced PID

Pyo-Hydrosalpinx

Clinical Background

The hallmark of PID is salpingitis which results from occlusion typically at the fimbrial end and in endoluminal fluid retention. The dilated fallopian tube is visualized as a fluid-filled, c- or s-shaped, sausage-like, or in more advanced cases as a bowel-like tubular structure. It arises from the uterine fundus and extends toward the ovary (Ghattamaneni et al. 2009). Although tubal dilatation may occur as an

isolated finding, it is most commonly associated with PID. In the acute stage the tube is filled with pus, which may resorb and be finally transformed into hydrosalpinx (Kim et al. 2009a).

Imaging Findings

Incomplete septal folds ("interdigitating sepations") are highly specific of tubal dilatation and are best demonstrated by multiplanar imaging (Fig. 129.1) (Ghattamaneni et al. 2009). Pyosalpinx is characterized by enhancing and thickened walls and in variable findings of the endoluminal fluid. MRI is superior to CT and US in characterization of pus. However, often pyosalpinx cannot be reliably differentiated from hydrosalpinx (Kim et al. 2009a). In MRI, pus has variable SI on T1 and T2WI. A typical finding of pus is amorphous or geographic shading on T2WI. Fine non-enhancing strands presenting synechiae may also be present (Ghattamaneni et al. 2009). Secondary signs of active inflammation include mesh-like stranding of adjacent pelvic fat and engorgement of ovarian pedicle (Ghattamaneni et al. 2009).

Tubo-Ovarian Abscess

Clinical Background

TOA represents late complication of PID, typically resulting from progression of salpingitis into the ovarian parenchyma with ovarian disintegration and suppuration. Rarely, ovarian abscesses originate from bacterial stromal invasion by hematogenous or lymphatic route. TOA can present as a frank abscess or an

Fig. 129.2 Tubo-ovarian abscess: transaxial contrast-enhanced CT shows a complex adnexal mass with cystic areas (*). The waist sign (*black arrows*) and surrounding inflammatory fatty reaction (*white arrow*) are typical features of an inflammatory adnexal process. Bladder (*B*), uterus (*U*)

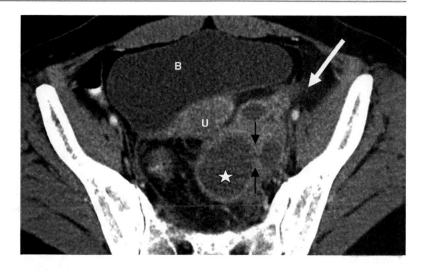

inflammatory mass including the dilated fallopian tube that is inseparable from the adjacent ovary, the "tubo-ovarian complex" (Quiroz 1999). Untreated ovarian abscesses may rupture and result in sepsis. Tubo-ovarian abscess in postmenopausal age is rare and may be associated with diabetes. However, tubal obstruction resulting from cancer should be considered (Rodriguez-de Valesques et al. 1995).

Imaging Findings

TOA presents as uni- or more often bilateral complex cystic adnexal masses with enhancing, uniformly thick walls and internal septations. Identification of tubal involvement (beak sign and waist sign) facilitates establishing the diagnosis of an inflammatory process (Fig. 129.2) (Ghattamaneni et al. 2009). Furthermore, signs of peritonitis, including mesh- or lace-like stranding of pelvic fat, thickening of ovarian and uterine ligaments, and enhancement of subperitoneal structures are other findings supporting the diagnosis of an inflammatory process. In contrast to other abdominal abscesses, internal gas is only rarely seen in TOA (Callen 1979). Complications of TOA include hydronephrosis, bowel obstruction, and fistula formation.

Differential Diagnosis

Characteristics for differentiation of TOA/pyosalpinx from complex neoplastic adnexal masses include the waist and peak signs that result from convolution of

tubular structures (Ghattamaneni et al. 2009). In secondary abscesses (e.g., after pregnancy, gynecologic surgery, or bowel perforation), predefined pelvic structures including broad ligaments, pelvic wall and peritoneal recesses, or bowel form abscess boundaries (Osborne 1986). Tubal dilatation may also be associated with other conditions, such as adhesions and fallopian tube cancer. Hematosalpinx which is found in endometriosis, tubal pregnancy, and in ovarian torsion is characterized by high SI on T1 and T1FS (Rezvani and Shaaban 2011). Endometrioma usually can be easily differentiated from TOA by hemorrhagic cystic lesions on T1WI and only mild enhancement of a sometimes thick capsule. Furthermore, shading with sedimentation is a typical finding only seen in endometrioma and not in pus (Ghattamaneni et al. 2009).

Uncommon Manifestations of Pelvic Infections

Actinomycosis

Clinical Background

Actinomycosis is a chronic suppurative and granulomatous infection caused by *Actinomyces israelii*. Actinomycosis of the female genital organs is rare and may affect endometrium, fallopian tubes, and one or both ovaries. Due to its predominantly solid morphology and the invasive growth, it mimics ovarian cancer. Typical macroscopical features include multiple abscess formations, abundant granulation tissue, and fibrosis.

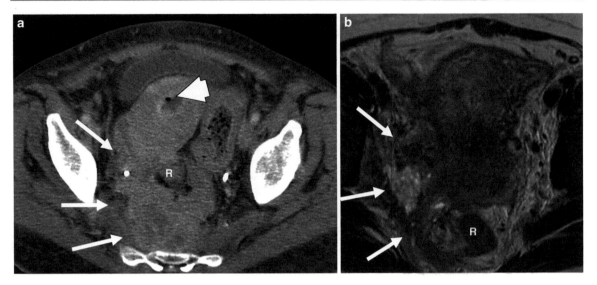

Fig. 129.3 Actinomycosis: transaxial contrast-enhanced CT (**a**) and T2WI (**b**) demonstrate an infiltrative pelvic mass (*arrows*) with extension along the pelvic sidewall into the perirectal space. In both modalities, it displays inhomogeneous predominantly solid morphology with some liquid areas. The rectum (*R*) is displaced anteriorly. Air and fluid is seen (*arrow head*) within the endometrial cavity (**a**) (Courtesy of Dr. JA Spencer, Leeds)

The association with IUD is under debate, but it is more commonly found in women with an IUD in place for more than 3 years (Schmidt 1982).

Imaging Findings

TOA from actinomycosis include predominantly solid adnexal masses with some cystic areas. On MRI, they display heterogeneous SI on T2WI and small rim-enhancing lesions. Solid elements representing fibrous structures display low SI on T2 and contrast enhancement (Kim et al. 2004). A typical feature suggestive of actinomycosis is local invasive growth with linear enhancing lesions infiltrating perirectal space and cul-de-sac disregarding tissue planes (Fig. 129.3). Furthermore, hydronephrosis and rectosigmoid invasion are common findings.

Tuberculosis

Clinical Background

Tuberculosis affecting the genital tract is rare and may originate from hematogenous or peritoneal dissemination. In one series, endometrium (72%) and fallopian tubes (34%) were most commonly involved, with ovaries only affected in 13% (Namavar et al. 2001).

Imaging Findings

Tuberculous TOA include uni- or bilateral adnexal masses with irregular, serrated, or nodular inner abscess walls. Other findings suggesting tuberculous TOA include loculated fluid collections with internal septations in pelvis or cul-de-sac and necrotic lymph nodes (Kim et al. 2004). In peritoneal tuberculosis, ovarian involvement is usually minimal and tuberculous peritonitis mimics peritoneal carcinomatosis (Kim et al. 2004). Serum-CA 125 levels are elevated in both entities. In the typical clinical setting, image-guided biopsy may assist in establishing the definitive diagnosis (Spencer et al. 2010).

Postpartum Pelvic Infections

Clinical Background

Postpartum infection refers to fever (>38°C) and tenderness in the postpartum period except for the first 24 h after delivery. Immediately after birth, mild postpartal fever is common and usually resolves, particularly after vaginal delivery (Chen 2011). Endometritis is the leading cause of puerperal infection; alternative pathologies include postsurgical wound infections or hematomas, urinary tract infections, deep venous thrombosis, and septic ovarian vein phlebitis (Rooholamini et al. 1993).

Endometritis refers to polymicrobial infection developing during day 2–10 after delivery (Chen 2011). It is reported in 1–3% of births, and it is more common (up to 20%) after cesarean section (Chen 2011). Infection of pregnancy endometrium may progress to myometrium and parametria, and subsequently cause pelvic peritonitis, or rarely septic pelvic phlebitis.

Imaging Findings

Imaging findings include widening of the endometrial cavity of >2 cm in anteroposterior (AP) diameter, often with fluid–fluid levels (Rooholamini et al. 1993). The cavity wall may display variable findings from smooth well-defined borders to irregular delineation, with an overlap between normal and pathologic features. Normally air within the endometrial cavity is consistent with endometritis. However, it may present a normal finding after vaginal delivery and persist for up to 3 weeks (Wachsberg and Kurtz 1992).

Postpartum pelvic abscesses may result from superinfection of uterine and periuterine hematomas. *Tubo-ovarian abscess* after delivery presents a late sequelae of endometritis and is typically found more than 3 weeks after delivery (Rooholamini et al. 1993).

Pearls to remember	
Mild PID	-Normal findings -Polycystic-like ovary -Fluid in ovarian fossa -Edema of fat planes
Advanced PID	-Dilatation of fallopian tube -Complex adnexal mass with tubal elements -Thickening of tubes due to salpingitis and signs of pelvic inflammation
Actinomycosis	-Adnexal mass with locally invasive growth -Long indwelling IUD
Tuberculosis	-Pelvic abscess with irregular walls -Necrotic lymph nodes -Pelvic tuberculous peritonitis resembles peritoneal carcinomatosis

Appropriateness of Different Imaging Modalities

Sonography is the first-line imaging modality in assessing pelvic inflammation. Complementary cross-sectional imaging, preferably MRI is performed to evaluate advanced cases of PID or to exclude other causes of pelvic inflammations. Due to problems of availability in the acute setting, or when a non-gynecological etiology is suspected, CT is a good alternative.

References

Callen PW. Computed tomographic evaluation of abdominal and pelvic abscesses. Radiology. 1979;131:171–5.

Chen KT. Postpartum endometritis. 2011. http://www.uptodate.com. Accessed 11 May 2011.

Ghattamaneni S, Bhuskute N, Weston MJ, et al. Discriminative MRI features of fallopian tube masses. Clin Radiol. 2009;64:815–35.

Ghiatas AA. The spectrum of pelvic inflammatory disease. Euro Radiol. 2004;14:184–92.

Kim SH, Kim SH, Yang DM, et al. Unusual causes of tubo-ovarian abscess. CT and MR imaging findings. Radio-Graphics. 2004;24:1575–89.

Kim MY, Rha ES, Oh SN, et al. MR findings of hydrosalpinx: a comprehensive review. RadioGrahics. 2009a;29:495–507.

Kim JY, Kim Y, Jeong WK, et al. Perihepatitis with pelvic inflammatory disease on MDCT: characteristic findings and relevance to PID. Abdom Imaging. 2009b;34:737–42.

Livengood CH. Pathogenesis and risk factors of PID. 2011. http://www.uptodate.com

Namavar JB, Parsanezhad ME, Ghane-Shirazi R. Female genital tuberculosis and infertility. Int J Gynaecol Obstet. 2001;75:269–71.

Osborne NG. Tubo-ovarian abscess: pathogenesis and management. J Natl Med Assoc. 1986;78:937–51.

Quiroz FA. Pelvic inflammatory disease. Appl Radiol. 1999;28:30–5.

Rezvani M, Shaaban AM. Fallopian tube disease in the nonpregnant patient. Radiographics. 2011;31:527–48.

Rodriguez-de Valesques A, Yoder CI, Velasquez PA, et al. Imaging effects of diabetes on the genitourinary system. Radiographics. 1995;15:1051–68.

Rooholamini S, Au AH, Hansen GC, et al. Imaging of pregnancy related complications. RadioGraphics. 1993;13:753–70.

Sam JW, Jacobs JE, Birnbaum BA. Spectrum of CT findings in acute pyogenic pelvic inflammatory disease. Radiographics. 2002;22:1327–34.

Schmidt WA. IUD's, inflammation and infection: assessment after two decades of IUD use. Hum Pathol. 1982;13:878–81.

Spencer JA, Weston JM, Saidi S, et al. Clinical utility of image-guided peritoneal and omental biopsy. Nat Rev Clin Oncol. 2010;7:623–31.

Wachsberg RH, Kurtz A. Gas within the endometrial cavity at postpartum US: a normal finding after spontaneous vaginal delivery. Radiology. 1992;183:431–3.

Anju Sahdev

Introduction and Definition

The adnexa adjoin the uterus and contain the ovaries, fallopian tubes, associated vessels, support ligaments and connective tissue. Pathology in the adnexa may also arise from the uterus, bowel, bladder, retroperitoneum, nerves or peritoneal metastatic deposits from another site particularly breast, stomach or colon. Processes that lead to development of adnexal masses include congenital masses, functional cysts, haemorrhagic lesions, neoplastic masses or inflammatory diseases. As treatment options will vary considerably depending on the etiology of the mass, accurate diagnosis is of paramount importance.

Prevalence/Incidence

The reported prevalence varies widely depending upon the population studied, modality used and selection criteria employed. In a random sample of 335 asymptomatic women who underwent TVUS aged 25–40 years the prevalence of an adnexal lesion defined as a cyst greater than 2.5 cm in size or a cyst with solid parts regardless of size was 7.8%. Of these lesions 82% had resolved in 3 months (Borgfeldt and Andolf 1999). In another series, TVUS was performed on 8,794 asymptomatic postmenopausal women as part of their routine gynecological check-up and 2.5% had a simple unilocular adnexal cyst. The risk of carcinoma was 0.6% among all patients and 2% of resected cysts. The most frequent histological diagnosis was a serous cystadenoma (84%) (Castillo et al. 2004). Incidental adnexal pathology was detected in 168 (5%) of 3,448 pre and post menopausal women undergoing CT. This study included patients with a known non-gynecological malignancy. Overall in this group of 168 women, 69% had benign disease, 1% had malignant adnexal masses and 30% had indeterminate lesions. In patients with a known malignancy the likelihood of an indeterminate lesion was higher than in patients with no known malignancy, 48% versus 30%. In addition, lesions were more likely to be benign in pre-menopausal women (81%) compared to post menopausal women (59%) (Slanetz et al. 1997). In a similar CT study looking at 2,869 women over 50 years of age, undergoing low dose CT colonography, 4% had incidental adnexal masses. After subsequent work-up including TVUS, MRI and surgical resection, no ovarian cancers were identified. However, in this study, four women subsequently developed ovarian cancer during a 15–44 month period in the group that revealed no adnexal mass on the index CT indicating that a normal CT does not exclude ovarian cancer (Pickhardt and Hanson 2010).

It becomes quite important therefore to evaluate an adnexal mass within the clinical context. Pre-menopausal, asymptomatic women are more likely to have benign lesions whilst post-menopausal, high risk patients have a higher risk of malignancy.

A. Sahdev (✉)
Department of Radiology, St Bartholomew's Hospital, Barts and The London NHS Trust and Queen Mary's School of Medicine and Dentistry, London, UK

Department of Diagnostic Imaging, King George V wing, St Bartholomew's Hospital, London, UK

B. Hamm, P. R. Ros (eds.), *Abdominal Imaging*, DOI 10.1007/978-3-642-13327-5_136,
© Springer-Verlag Berlin Heidelberg 2013

Table 130.1 Most frequent causes of adnexal masses

	Gynecological	Non-gynecological
Benign	Ovarian	Benign
	Physiological follicles and corpus luteum	Appendiceal, diverticular, Crohns, post surgical abscesses
	Tubo-ovarian/ovarian abscess	Urachal and congenital retroperitoneal cysts
	Ovarian torsion/infarction	Anterior meningocoele
	Endometrioma	Inclusion cysts
	Mature teratomas	Retroperitoneal pelvic haematomas
	Cystadenomas	
	Non-ovarian	
	Hydrosalphinx	
	Leiomyomas	
	Ectopic pregnancy	
	Pelvic endometriosis	
Malignant	Epithelial carcinomas of the ovary and fallopian tubes	Peritoneal metastases
	Germ cell tumors	Parametrial, pelvic nodal metastases
	Stromal and sex cord tumors	Carcinoma of the bowel and bladder
		Sacral, nerve sheath and retroperitoneal tumors

Causes of Adnexal Masses

As adnexal masses may be found in women of all ages, they have a wide variety of aetiologies. Table 130.1 summarize the most frequent causes of adnexal masses.

Evaluation

The diagnostic evaluation of an adnexal mass begins with a thorough history and physical examination. In most cases, however, history and physical examination alone are insufficient to make a diagnosis and imaging and laboratory studies, are necessary. The primary functions of imaging are to:

(a) Confirm the presence of an adnexal mass.
(b) Deduce the origin of the mass, in particular distinguish between ovarian and extra-ovarian disease.
(c) Determine whether the mass is benign or malignant.

The most serious concern arises when there is a possibility of malignancy in the discovered mass. There are several clinical and imaging methods of evaluation to determine the origin of an adnexal mass and the probability of a benign or malignant cause.

Important Indicators in Patient History

The likely etiology of an adnexal mass is strongly influenced by age of the patient. In infants, ovarian cysts are found in up to 5% of females and are caused by ovarian stimulation by persisting maternal oestrogens (Comparetto et al. 2005). These regress within the first few months of life as the maternal estrogen effects abate. Functional cysts are then extremely rare until menarche and the presence of an ovarian mass raises the likelihood of germ cell tumors, either benign or malignant. After menarche, in adolescence, the ovary becomes functional with cyclical cyst formation and the vast majority of adnexal masses are functional cysts. Neoplasms are rare, the commonest neoplasm at this age is a mature cystic teratoma. In adolescence and throughout childbearing age, in a sexually active woman, the combination of pelvic pain, vaginal bleeding or discharge and an adnexal mass should alert the examiner to the possibility of pelvic inflammatory masses including tubo-ovarian abscesses, ovarian torsion and ectopic pregnancy. Non gynecological causes, appendicitis and inflammatory bowel disease in particular, are an important differential in adolescence and young adults. In the 30–45 year range, endometriosis becomes an important cause for pelvic cystic masses due to ovarian or extra-ovarian endometriomas, haematosalpinges and pelvic scarring and fibrosis. Leiomyomas also become more common and pedunculated uterine, broad ligament and ovarian leiomyomas will present as solid or solid-cystic adnexal masses. Borderline malignant lesions increase in frequency and these are an important differential of complex cystic ovarian masses. As age increases, so does the risk of malignancy but ovarian cancer is rare below the age of 40 years. The most frequent primary epithelial ovarian carcinoma is the epithelial cystadenocarcinomas. In the perimenopausal and post menopausal period, estrogen sensitive lesions, leiomyomas and endometriosis regress. As the ovaries are no longer functioning, functional cysts do not occur. Most unilocular cysts are benign cystadenomas but there is now an increasing incidence of malignancy.

In pre-menopausal women, the cyclical history and the regularity of mensus is important when evaluating cystic ovarian lesions. A thin walled, simple cyst in the first half of the menstrual cycle is a dominant functional follicle whilst a thick walled cyst with rim perfusion in the second half of the menstrual cycle indicates a corpus luteal cyst. Women on the combined contraceptive pill may have suppressed follicular pattern whilst women on fertility enhancement have large ovaries and large bilateral ovarian cysts due to ovarian stimulation.

History of acute pain without fever associated with an adnexal mass lends to the diagnosis of hemorrhage or rupture of cysts, torsion or ectopic pregnancy. The association of fever favors appendicitis and pelvic inflammatory disease. Chronic cyclical pelvic pain is supportive of endometriosis or adenomyosis. Painless abdominal distension and complex adnexal masses are in keeping with malignancy.

Important Indicators in Patient Examination

On examination the presence of fixed irregular firm pelvic masses and ascites supports a malignant process whilst a smooth, mobile, cystic mass is more compatible with a benign process. Nodularity and tenderness in the Pouch of Douglas, thickened uterosacral ligaments and cyclical pain is in keeping with deep pelvic endometriosis. Unfortunately physical examination is rarely adequate to provide a firm diagnosis and may be limited by patient size and cooperation.

Biochemistry

The most frequently used and helpful biochemical tests in the evaluation of adnexal masses are urinary or serum pregnancy tests, white cell counts and tumors markers, CA125, alpha feto-protein (AFP) and human chorionic gonadotropin (HCG). CA125 is an antigen present on 80% of nonmucinous ovarian carcinomas. CA125 is often elevated in patients with ovarian cancer. The reported performance of CA125 as a marker for detection of ovarian cancer has varied greatly in the literature depending on threshold levels considered to represent malignancy, population group and study selection bias. CA125 may be raised by any cause for peritoneal irritation including inflammatory disease, endometriosis, cardiac or hepatic ascites and metastatic disease. However when only applied to post menopausal women, with no known malignancy, CA125 has a high sensitivity and specificity of 83% and 99% respectively for ovarian carcinoma (Tiss et al. 2010). AFP and HCG are markers for germ cell carcinomas of the testes and ovaries. Both are elevated in normal pregnancy as well as germ cell tumors of the ovaries usually occuring in adolescents and young women. Hence the type of marker elevation may help in characterizing a complex or solid adnexal mass seen on imaging.

Risk of Malignancy Index (RMI)

The risk of malignancy index is used to discriminate between malignant and benign pelvic masses. It is a scoring system which can be introduced easily into clinical practice to facilitate the selection of patients requiring further imaging or primary surgery at an oncological unit.

RMI score is based on menopausal status, ultrasound score and serum CA125.

RMI = CA125 level × menopausal status × US score

Menopausal status: 1 if premenopausal and 3 if postmenopausal.

Table 130.2 TVUS categorization of adnexal masses

Benign lesions	Malignant lesions	Indeterminate lesions
Simple cyst	1. Cyst with multiple thick irregular septae or walls	1. Complex mass which cannot be placed into either benign or malignant categories following thorough US evaluation including Doppler evaluation
1. Round, oval cysts	2. Nodule or nodules with Doppler flow	-Features suggestive but not characteristic of endometrioma or dermoid
2. Thin, smooth walls	3. Irregular cyst >5 cms	-Focal wall or septal calcification
3. Anechoic internal architecture		-Multiple septae
4. Size < 3 cm		-Nodule without Doppler flow
5. No solid component or septae		2. If origin of the mass cannot be determined
6. No Doppler flow		Lesions are commonly:
Haemorrhagic cyst		-Endometriomas
1. Low level internal echoes		-Mature teratomas
2. Debris in concave and dependent margins		-Adnexal fibroids
3. No internal flow		-Fibromas/fibrothecmas
Endometrioma		
1. Homogenous low level echoes		
2. No Doppler flow		
3. +/− echogenic foci in wall		
Dermoid		
1. Focal or diffuse dense hyperechoic component with dense acoustic shadowing		
2. Hyperechoic lines and dots in the cyst		
3. No internal Doppler flow		
Hydrosalpinx		
1. Tubular cystic mass		
2. Separate ovary		
3. Waist sign: "septae" not extending to the opposite side of the tubular lesion		
Peritoneal inclusion cyst		
1. Flaccid cyst following the contours of adjacent structures		
2. Ovary suspended within the mass or at the edge		
3. +/− septations		
4. No Doppler flow		

Ultrasound score: score of 0 (no features of malignancy), 1 (one feature of malignancy) or 3 (two or more features of malignancy)

The US features of malignancy are: bilaterality, solid areas, multilocular, ascites, evidence of metastases, 6–10 cm in size, complex solid/cystic mass with papillary or nodular projections, septa or walls > 3 mm in thickness, low impedance arterial flow on Doppler.

AN RMI score of less than 25 has less than 3% chance of malignancy and an RMI of greater than 250 has a 75% chance of malignancy. Using an RMI cut-off of 200, the sensitivity, specificity and PPV was 85%, 97% and 83% respectively. Patients with a RMI score of > 200 had, on average, 42 times the background risk of cancer (Jacobs et al. 1990; Tingulstad et al. 1996).

Imaging in Characterizing Adnexal Masses

Transvaginal ultrasound is the preferred modality for initial evaluation due to its ease of availability, low cost, good anatomical detail, high negative predictive

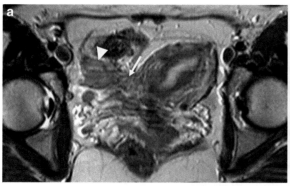
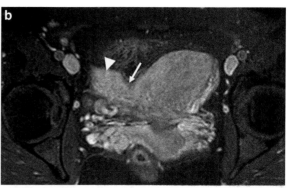

Fig. 130.1 MRI of a 34-year-old woman with an incidental solid adnexal mass on ultrasound. (**a**) Axial T2-weighted image showing a solid high T2 signal intensity mass in the right adnexa. The mass (*arrowhead*) has a pedicle (*arrow*) attaching the solid mass to the uterus. (**b**) Axial T1 fat-saturated image after gadolinium administration. The pedicle and solid mass enhance in time with the myometrium. The mass has the typical appearances of a pedunculated fibroid. The lesion was not resected but follow-up with ultrasound over 5 years showed stability

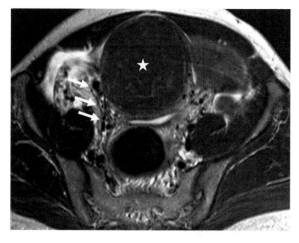

Fig. 130.2 Bridging vessel sign. Axial T2-weighted image showing an anterior subserosal fibroid (*asterisk*). Between the uterus and fibroid, there are serpinginous bridging veins (*arrows*) that confirm the uterine connection of the fibroid. These veins are the arcuate uterine vessels stretched by the subserosal fibroid

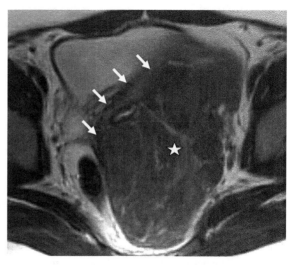

Fig. 130.3 Claw sign. Axial T2-weighted image from a 33-year-old woman investigated for menorrhagia and a solid adnexal mass on TVUS. The mass (asterisk) has low T2 signal intensity and normal cervical stroma (arrows) stretched around the mass with a "claw like" appearance. This sign implies the mass has a cervical origin as there is normal cervical stroma surrounding part of the mass

value and lack of ionizing radiation. A wide range of sensitivities and specificities, 85–100% and 52–100%, respectively, have been reported for detection of malignant ovarian masses using ultrasound (Brown et al. 1998; van Trappen et al. 2007). These variations are thought to be secondary to different operator expertise and patient body habitus.

The role of ultrasound is mainly in detection of adnexal masses and categorizing masses into:

(a) Benign.
(b) Malignant.
(c) Indeterminate categories.

The subsequent management of the mass will dependent on this US categorization. The European society of urological radiology (ESUR) and the American society of Radiologists in ultrasound have set out guidelines in the management, investigations and follow-up of US detected adnexal masses. Post menopausal women, or women with a high RMI, a mass demonstrating malignant US features and ancillary signs of malignancy such as ascites, omental cake, peritoneal deposits, and an

Fig. 130.4 (**a**) Sagittal T2-weighted image showing a large left hydrosalphinx with a "S" shape configuration. The *black arrow* shows the folds of the tubal wall. (**b**) Axial T2-weighed image of the same hydrosalphinx with a "C" shape configuration and a tubal fold appearing as a solid nodule along the right tubal wall (*white arrow*)

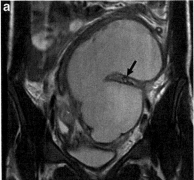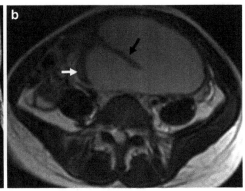

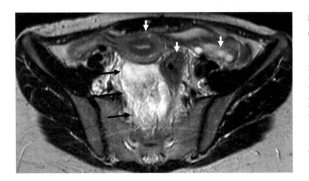

Fig. 130.5 Aggressive angiomyoma of the pelvis seen on TVUS as a solid adnexal mass. Axial T2-weighted imaging of a 42-year-old woman presenting with non-specific pelvic pain. There is a very high T2 signal intensity lesion (*black arrows*) filling the pelvis. It displaces the uterus, ovaries and recto-sigmoid junction anteriorly. The mass does not appear to originate from any pelvic organ. After surgical biopsy the lesion was confirmed as an aggressive angiomyoma

elevated CA125 undergo abdominal and pelvic CT for staging. Patients with a low RMI and entirely benign US features in a mass less than 4 cm in size require no further imaging. Masses above 4 cm are recommended to undergo US follow-up to ensure resolution. Patients with a low RMI, low or minimally elevated CA125 and an indeterminate mass on US have been shown to benefit from further MRI characterization avoiding unnecessary exploratory laparotomy (Sohaib et al. 2005; Spencer et al. 2010; Levine et al. 2010). In this group of patients less than 25% of adnexal masses prove to be malignant (Kinkel et al. 2005).

Table 130.2 summarizes US features used to categorize adnexal masses into the recommended three categories.

In women with a low or moderately raised RMI (between 0 and 100) and adnexal lesions considered indeterminate on US, contrast enhanced MRI has been

shown to be superior in characterizing adnexal masses (Sohaib et al. 2005; Yamashita et al. 1995; Komatsu et al. 1996). Both techniques are sensitive but MRI has greater specificity for blood, fat and fibrous tissue. This allows MRI to correctly identify endometriomas, dermoids, pedunculated fibroids, fibromas and fibrothecomas of the ovary which may appear malignant on TVUS.

MRI Evaluation of Adnexal Masses

The evaluation of adnexal masses on MRI requires a methodical approach describing its organ of origin, the signal characteristics of the mass and its anatomical relations in detail.

Organ of Origin

The relationship of the mass to the uterus and ovaries should be established using sagittal, axial and oblique T2 weighted images. If the mass lies lateral to the uterus, a coronal oblique plane is favored whilst the relations of a posterior or superior mass are best imaged in the axial oblique plane. Features that favor an ovarian origin include presence of surrounding follicles and the "beak" sign. The "beak" sign refers to an acute angle between the mass and ovarian stroma with a contiguous capsule surrounding both ovary and mass (Fig. 134.18). Another helpful feature is identification of ovarian veins extending into the lesion, thereby confirming an ovarian origin (Figs. 134.12, 134.14). The identification of ovaries separate and distant from the mass excludes an ovarian origin. Demonstration of a pedicle connecting the lesion to uterus confirms a pedunculated uterine mass usually a fibroid (Fig. 130.1).

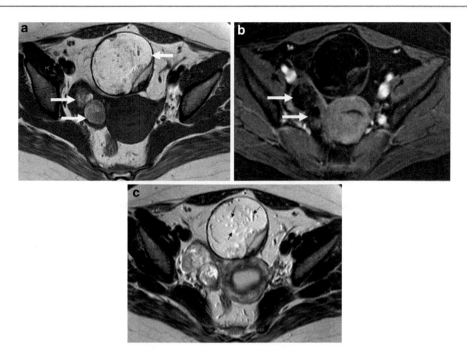

Fig. 130.6 Bilateral, multiple ovarian dermoid cysts. (**a**) Axial T1-weighted image showing a large left dermoid cyst and two smaller dermoids in the right ovary (*white arrows*). All contain extensive high T1 signal intensity tissue within the cysts along with areas of solid nodules. (**b**) Axial T1-weighted image with fat saturation. The areas of high T1 signal intensity seen in (**a**), lose signal intensity after fat saturation, typical of adipose tissue thereby confirming the lesions as dermoid cysts. (**c**) Axial T2-weighted image showing the fat droplet sign within the large left dermoid cyst. The *black arrows* show examples of the "droplets" which correspond to chemical shift artifact at the interface of suspended fat or sebum droplets within the dermoid cyst

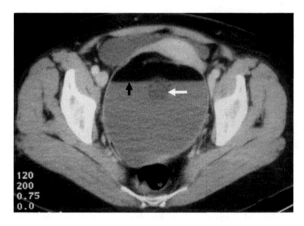

Fig. 130.7 Contrast-enhanced CT image of a large dermoid cyst with a striking fat-fluid level (*black arrow*) and a floating Rokitansky nodule (*white arrow*). In this instance there is no significant enhancement of the nodule but depending on its tissue constituents, the nodule can demonstrate significant enhancement

Subserosal fibroids also commonly demonstrate the "shared or bridging vessel sign." This describes the presence of tortuous prominent uterine vessels at the uterine-adnexal mass interface which supply

the mass thereby confirming its uterine origin (Fig. 130.2). Uterine masses may also demonstrate the "claw" sign that consists of normal myometrial tissue stretched around part or whole of the mass (Fig. 130.3). Fallopian tube masses have a tubular configuration which is appreciated usually on review of more than one plane of T2 weighted images. On MRI, hydrosalpinges appears as a C- or S-shaped cystic lesion. Characteristically, these have "incomplete septae" that arise from one wall but do not extend to another edge which are incomplete longitudinal folds representing the partially effaced mucosal plicae of the fallopian tube. These can sometimes be mistaken for mural nodules when the tube is markedly dilated (Fig. 130.4). Tubal masses are usually intimately adherent to the ovaries commonly forming "tubo-ovarian complexes" as the two structures may not be separable. This feature is frequently seen in pelvic inflammatory disease.

Adnexal masses may also arise from non-gynecological organs such as the rectum, appendix, retroperitoneal soft tissue and meninigocoeles. Retroperitoneal masses can usually be recognized as they

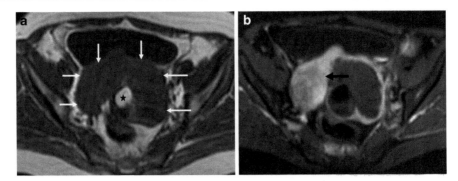

Fig. 130.8 Dermoid with squamous cell malignancy. (**a**) Axial T1-weighted image showing a large right ovarian dermoid cyst (*white arrows*) with a small pocket of high T1 signal intensity fat centrally (*asterisk*). (**b**) Post gadolinium enhanced T1-weighted image with fat saturation. The small pocket of high T1 signal intensity has lost signal in keeping with adipose tissue. There is a large solid enhancing lateral component (*black arrow*) which forms a large part of the dermoid but has extra-lesional extension. This capsular breech raises the possibility of malignancy and in this dermoid, a squamous cell carcinoma was confirmed

Fig. 130.9 Bilateral endometriomas. (**a**) TVUS image showing a cystic lesion containing diffuse, homogenous low level echoes throughout the cyst. No vascular flow is demonstrated within the lesion and the appearances are typical of an endometrioma. (**b**) Axial T1-weighted image demonstrating bilateral high T1 signal intensity ovarian lesions (*white arrows*). (**c**) Axial T2-weighted image demonstrating the lesions with intermediate to low T2 signal intensity. (**d**) Axial T1-weighted image with fat saturation. The bilateral lesions retain high signal in keeping with hemorrhage within endometriomas

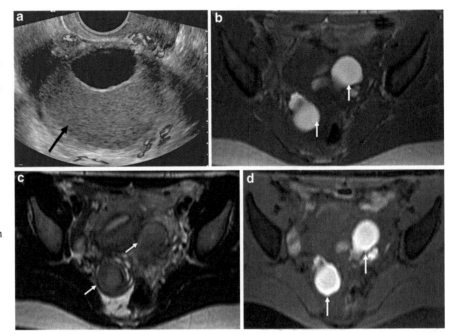

displace all pelvic organs extending into pre-sacral and ischio-rectal fat without appearing to arise from any pelvic organ (Fig. 130.5). The commonest tumors in this category are aggressive angiomyomas, haemangiopericytomas, smooth muscle tumors of unknown malignant potential and plexiform neurofibromas.

Signal Characteristics of the Mass

The signal characteristics of the adnexal mass on the different MR weightings, reflect the constituents of the lesion. These can be characterized by evaluating the T1, T2, T1 with fat saturation and post contrast images. Adnexal masses can be broadly categorized into lesions with:

(a) High T1 signal intensity.
(b) Low T2 signal intensity.
(c) Cystic-solid lesion.

High T1 Signal Intensity Masses

When the T1 signal intensity of the mass is similar to fat, the lesion is likely to be an ovarian teratoma or a haemorrhagic mass. When the T1 signal intensity is

Fig. 130.10 Endometriod carcinoma in an endometrioma. (**a**) Axial T1-weighted image with fat saturation demonstrating a right sided ovarian endometrioma with two papillary nodules in the wall (*arrows*). (**b**) Axial T1-weighted image with fat saturation and following gadolinium enhancement. The nodules have increased in signal intensity but due to the high background signal intensity of blood in the endometrioma, it can be difficult to be sure of enhancement. (**c**) Sagittal subtraction image. This is a post processed image generated by subtracting the pre from the post contrast enhanced images. Hence the high signal intensity in the endometrioma is nulled and only areas of enhancement are seen. The two mural nodules are seen as enhancing papillary lesions raising the likelihood of malignancy in the endometrioma. Surgical resection confirmed endometriod carcinoma in the nodules

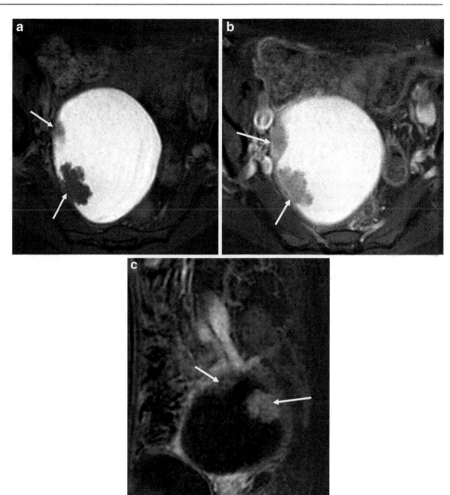

less than fat but higher than soft tissue, a mucin containing mass should be considered.

In ovarian teratomas, areas of high signal intensity represent mature adipose tissue and therefore on fat suppression sequences, these areas lose signal entirely. This confirms the presence of fat in the mass. Benign teratomas (dermoid cysts) account for 90% of ovarian teratomas. On T2 weighted images, dermoid cysts illustrate the "fat droplet sign" and the Rokitansky nodule (Figs. 130.6, 130.7). The fat droplet sign describes floating pockets of fat or sebum against the background fluid-cystic component of the dermoid. The low T1 and high T2 signal is a chemical shift artifact at the interface of the fat droplets and the fluid. Rokitansky nodule is a solid admixture of various tissues including hair, skin and teeth and

enhancement of the Rokitansky nodule is common. Dermoid cysts may also contain hemorrhage secondary to torsion. Malignant teratomas may also contain small pockets of fat. However these are generally large, >10 cm at presentation and unlike benign teratomas may consist almost entirely of solid tissue. The solid components can invade and extend beyond the capsule of the ovary. Malignant teratomas are more frequent in childhood and contain a wide range of malignant elements within the teratoma. In adults, the malignant component most commonly arises in skin elements causing squamous cell carcinomas (Fig. 130.8). Conversely, in fat poor dermoids, detection of fat may be very difficult and the adnexal mass mimics a malignant cystic-solid lesion (Outwater et al. 2001).

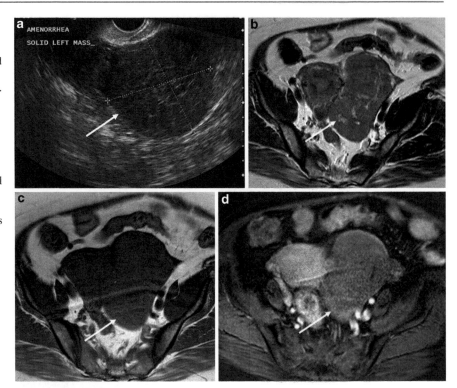

Fig. 130.11 Left ovarian fibrothecoma. (**a**) TVUS showing a solid left adnexal mass detected in a 35-year-old woman as part of investigations for amenorrhea. (**b**) Axial T2-weighted image showing the solid homogenous mass has intermediate to low signal intensity. (**c**) Axial T1-weighted image of the lesion with intermediate signal intensity. (**d**) Axial T1-weighted image with fat saturation shows the lesion has low level enhancement only. The T2 appearances and the low level enhancement are typical for a fibrothecoma

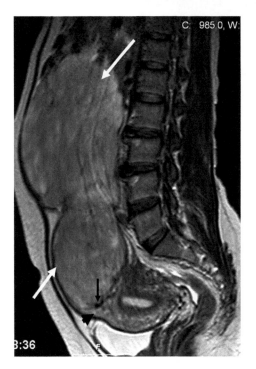

Fig. 130.12 Sagittal T2-weighted MR image demonstrating a large solid subserosal pedunculated fibroid with myxoid degeneration. The fibroid has a homogenous intermediate T2 signal intensity (*white arrows*). Its uterine origin is confirmed by the presence of the bridging veins (*black arrow*) and the claw sign (*arrowhead*)

Hemorrhage is seen as high T1 signal intensity but demonstrates variable T2 signal characteristics depending on the age of blood products present. Functional haemorrhagic cysts are unilateral, unilocular and have high T2 signal intensity (Fig. 134.20). Endometriomas are usually bilateral, complex and have low, intermediate or "shaded" T2 signal intensity (Fig. 130.9). The low T2 signal and shading is due to multiple episodes of bleeding and shortening of the T2 relaxation time not seen following a single episode of acute hemorrhage. Blood may also be a feature of acute hemorrhage in a malignant lesion. The diffuse high T1 signal of blood may mask enhancing solid nodules characteristic of malignant masses. In the author's experience, detection of these small nodules can be enhanced by use of subtraction images which null pre-contrast high T1 signal and demonstrate only enhancing tissue on subtracted images (Fig. 130.10). This technique also assists in the distinction between non-enhancing blood clot within an endometriomas and enhancing vegetations in a malignant lesion. No demonstration of enhancing tissue by this technique increases the certainty of a benign lesion.

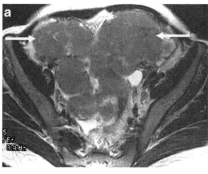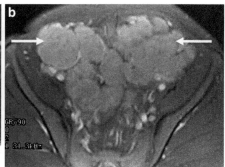

Fig. 130.13 Ovarian lymphoma. (**a**) Axial T2-weighted image showing large bilateral solid homogenous masses with a lobulated contour. (**b**) Axial T1-weighted image with fat saturation and gadolinium enhancement. The masses have uniform enhancement, both features are non-specific for malignancy and indistinguishable from metastatic disease or primary ovarian carcinomas particularly dysgerminomas in young women

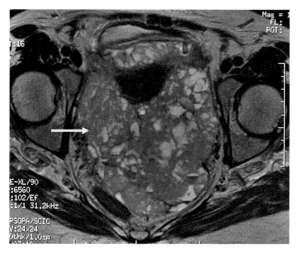

Fig. 130.14 Ovarian sarcoma. Axial T2-weighted image showing a large heterogenous intermediate T2 signal intensity mass filling the entire pelvis and displacing the uterus anteriorly. The appearances have no specific features of a sarcoma but the intermediate T2 signal and the solid mass with focal areas of high T2 signal intensity raise the suspicion of an aggressive malignancy

Low T2 Signal Intensity Lesions

Lesions with low T2 signal intensity may be either solid or cystic. Cystic lesions contain chronic hemorrhage and are most commonly endometriomas. These chronic endometriomas have high T1 signal and demonstrate no enhancement following contrast administration.

Solid low T2 signal intensity (signal lower than skeletal muscle) masses are fibrous tumors: fibromas or fibrothecomas of the ovary, Brenner tumors and pedunculated fibroids of the uterus. Fibromas and fibrothecomas demonstrate low or intermediate T1 signal intensity, minimal enhancement following administration of intravenous gadolinium and may have associated endometrial hyperplasia due to stromal estrogen secretion (Fig. 130.11). Pedunculated or subserosal fibroids have a uterine attachment. They demonstrate a wide range of T2W appearances varying according to the degree and type of degeneration within the fibroid. The T2 appearances range from homogenous T2 signal intensity, cystic areas of high T2 signal intensity and myxoid or hyaline degeneration seen as intermediate T2 signal. Hemorrhage or red degeneration is associated to pregnancy and areas of high T1 and high T2 signal intensity are seen within a background of a low T2 signal intensity mass (Figs. 130.16, 130.12) (Murase et al. 1999).

Solid Lesions with Intermediate T2 Signal Intensity

These masses have higher signal intensity than skeletal muscle. Primary ovarian epithelial carcinomas, dysgerminomas, lymphoma, metastases, atypical fibrothecomas and fibroids make up the majority of lesions in this category (Figs. 130.13, 130.14). There is too much overlap in the appearances on MRI and clinical and biochemical pointers should be sought. Dysgerminomas are malignant ovarian tumors in adolescent and young women and a clinical history of a rapidly growing pelvic mass usually leads to the correct diagnosis. In patients with a known carcinoma of the pancreas, stomach and colon, the possibility of metastases is supported by elevated CEA and CA19-9 tumor markers.

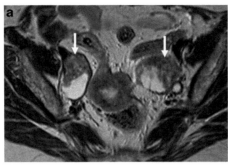
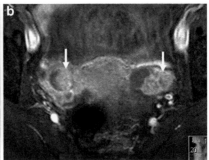

Fig. 130.15 Bilateral primary ovarian carcinomas. (**a**) Axial T2-weighted image with bilateral solid-cystic masses. The solid components (*arrows*) have irregular contours, intermediate signal intensity and on the left extend beyond the ovarian capsule. (**b**) Axial T1-weighted image with fat saturation and after gadolinium administration. There is avid enhancement of the solid components, typical of malignant masses

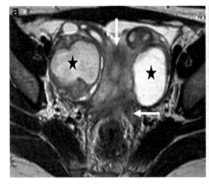
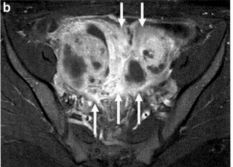

Fig. 130.16 Pelvic inflammatory disease. (**a**) Axial T2-weighted image with bilateral abnormal enlarged ovaries containing thick walled cystic lesions (*asterisks*) and no normal ovarian stroma. There is thickening of the fascial planes in the pelvis (*white arrows*). (**b**) Axial T1-weighted image with fat saturation and intravenous gadolinium. There is marked enhancement of the thick walls of the ovarian lesions, the ovarian capsule and all fascial planes of the pelvis. This thick sheet like enhancement of the fascial planes (*white arrows*) is typical of pelvic inflammatory disease. The ovarian lesions have typical appearances of ovarian abscesses

Complex Solid-Cystic Lesions with High T2 Signal Intensity

To characterize complex cystic-solid lesions, administration of intravenous gadolinium is contributory. Lesions demonstrating no enhancement are benign and include cystadenomas and hydrosalpinges. Irregular enhancement of septal nodules and soft tissue components are features of malignancy in primary epithelial carcinomas, metastases and borderline tumors (Fig. 130.15) (Sohaib et al. 2005).

Diffuse enhancement of pelvic fascial planes, diffuse enhancement of the peritoneum indicative of a reactive peritonitis and hyperaemia of pelvic vessels around thick walled cystic masses is indicative of inflammatory disease, pyosalpinges and ovarian abscesses (Fig. 130.16). The clinical presentation of the patients with fever and pelvic pain support inflammatory disease but on MRI and CT alone there is an overlap in the appearances of malignant and inflammatory diseases.

Summary

Most US indeterminate masses can be adequately characterized on MRI and its main strength is to confirm benign lesions in women with a low or intermediate probability of cancer. A summary of the diagnostic

Fig. 130.17 Summary of algorithm of MRI appearances

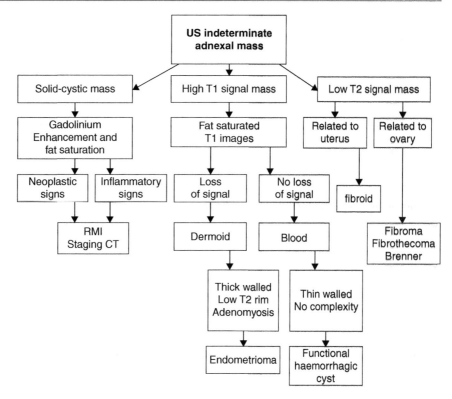

algorithm using MRI features is shown as Fig. 130.17. This allows optimal management decisions to be made for patient care. However, a small minority of masses will remain indeterminate on MRI due to overlap of appearances of malignant, inflammatory and rare benign tumor tumors. As malignancy cannot be confidently excluded in this small category, surgical resection is recommended.

References

Borgfeldt C, Andolf E. Transvaginal sonographic ovarian findings in a random sample of women 25–40 years old. Ultrasound Obstet Gynecol. 1999;13:345.

Brown DL, Doubilet PM, Miller FH, et al. Benign and malignant ovarian masses: selection of the most discriminating grayscale and Doppler sonographic features. Radiology. 1998;208:103–10.

Castillo G, Alcázar JL, Jurado M. Natural history of sonographically detected simple unilocular adnexal cysts in asymptomatic postmenopausal women. Gynecol Oncol. 2004;92:965.

Comparetto C, Giudici S, Coccia ME, Scarselli G, Borruto F. Fetal and neonatal ovarian cysts: what's their real meaning? Clin Exp Obstet Gynecol. 2005;32(2):123–5.

Jacobs I, Oram D, Fairbanks J, Turner J, Frost C, Grudzinskas JG. A risk of malignancy index incorporating CA 125, ultrasound and menopausal status for the accurate preoperative diagnosis of ovarian cancer. Br J Obstet Gynaecol. 1990;97(10):922–9.

Kinkel K, Lu Y, Mehdizade A, Pelte MF, Hricak H. Indeterminate ovarian mass at US: incremental value of second imaging test for characterization–meta-analysis and Bayesian analysis. Radiology. 2005;236(1):85–94.

Komatsu T, Konishi I, Mandai M, Togashi K, Kawakami S, Konishi J, Mori T. Adnexal masses: transvaginal US and gadolinium-enhanced MR imaging assessment of intratumoral structure. Radiology. 1996;198(1):109–15.

Levine D, Brown DL, Andreotti RF, Benacerraf B, Benson CB, Brewster WR, et al. Management of asymptomatic ovarian and other adnexal cysts imaged at US: Society of Radiologists in ultrasound consensus, conference statement. Radiology. 2010;256(3):943–54.

Murase E, Siegelman ES, Outwater EK, Perez-Jaffe LA, Tureck RW. Uterine leiomyomas: histopathologic features, MR imaging findings, differential diagnosis, and treatment. Radiographics. 1999;19:1179–97.

Outwater EK, Siegelman ES, Hunt JL. Ovarian teratomas: tumor types and imaging characteristics. Radiographics. 2001;21(2):475–90.

Pickhardt PJ, Hanson ME. Incidental adnexal masses detected at low-dose unenhanced CT in asymptomatic women age 50 and older: implications for clinical management and ovarian cancer screening. Radiology. 2010;257(1):144–50.

Slanetz PJ, Hahn PF, Hall DA, Mueller PR. The frequency and significance of adnexal lesions incidentally revealed by CT. Am J Roentgenol. 1997;168(3):647–50.

Sohaib SA, Mills TD, Sahdev A, Webb JA, Vantrappen PO, Jacobs IJ, Reznek RH. The role of magnetic resonance imaging and ultrasound in patients with adnexal masses. Clin Radiol. 2005;60(3):340–8.

Spencer JA, Forstner R, Cunha TM, Kinkel K, ESUR Female Imaging Sub-Committee. ESUR guidelines for MR imaging of the sonographically indeterminate adnexal mass: an algorithmic approach. Eur Radiol. 2010;20(1):25–35.

Tingulstad S, Hagen B, Skjeldestad FE, Onsrud M, Kiserud T, Halvorsen T, Nustad K. Evaluation of a risk of malignancy index based on serum CA125, ultrasound findings and menopausal status in the pre-operative diagnosis of pelvic masses. Br J Obstet Gynaecol. 1996;103(8): 826–31.

Tiss A, Timms JF, Smith C, Devetyarov D, Gentry-Maharaj A, Camuzeaux S, et al. Highly accurate detection of ovarian cancer using CA125 but limited improvement with serum matrix-assisted laser desorption/ionization time-of-flight mass spectrometry profiling. Int J Gynecol Cancer. 2010;20(9):1518–24.

van Trappen PO, Rufford BD, Mills TD, Sohaib SA, Webb JA, Sahdev A, Carroll MJ, Britton KE, Reznek RH, Jacobs IJ. Differential diagnosis of adnexal masses: risk of malignancy index, ultrasonography, magnetic resonance imaging, and radioimmunoscintigraphy. Int J Gynecol Cancer. 2007;17(1):61–7.

Yamashita Y, Torashima M, Hatanaka Y, Harada M, Higashida Y, Takahashi M, Mizutani H, Tashiro H, Iwamasa J, Miyazaki K, et al. Adnexal masses: accuracy of characterization with transvaginal US and precontrast and postcontrast MR imaging. Radiology. 1995;194(2):557–65.

131

Ovarian Cysts, Endometriosis

Anju Sahdev

Endometriosis is a benign entity that affects women of reproductive age. It is defined as the presence of endometrial tissue outside the uterus. The clinical manifestations of endometriosis are protean. The presence of endometrial tissue in the myometrium is termed adenomyosis. Superficial implants of endometrial tissue may occur throughout the peritoneal cavity, along serosal surfaces and in the abdominal wall. Deep infiltrating endometriosis occurs when implants infiltrate the peritoneum and serosa by at least 5 mm and involve visceral organs. Histologically, these lesions are characterized by fibromuscular hyperplasia around foci of endometriosis which sometimes contain small cavities (Koninckx et al. 1994). The majority of patients have superficial endometriosis, usually asymptomatic, with the commonest site of involvement being the ovaries, uterine ligaments, pouch of Douglas, serosal uterine surface, fallopian tubes, rectosigmoid junction, and bladder dome. Deep infiltrative endometriosis is symptomatic and causes significant morbidity including chronic pelvic pain, infertility, haematuria, and rectal pain and bleeding.

A variety of imaging techniques including TVUS, TRUS, CT, and MRI have been used to evaluate deep pelvic endometriosis. Ultrasound is best suited to the detection and follow-up of endometriomas and bladder lesions. Transrectal ultrasound can be used to detect infiltrative lesions of the serosa or wall of the bowel but this technique does not allow evaluation of the complete pelvis. The value of imaging in superficial endometriosis is limited as small scattered deposits are easily masked by bowel and hence laparoscopy remains the gold standard for diagnosis. The therapeutic options for patients depend on the location and extent of disease and the relative proportion of active and fibrous endometriosis. Active endometriotic deposits are receptive to medical hormone treatment whilst scarring fibrous endometriosis, when symptomatic requires surgical lysis.

Imaging Features

Increasingly in clinical practice, information on the distribution, pattern of disease, and ratio of active to fibrotic disease is provided by detailed TVUS and high resolution MR imaging of the pelvis.

Endometriomas

The ovary is the most commonly involved site, where endometriotic cysts may be termed "chocolate cysts" or "endometriomas." Extra-ovarian endometriomas have similar imaging characteristics but lie distant from the ovaries in the pelvis and occur anywhere in the abdomen and pelvis.

On high resolution TVUS, the sensitivity of detection of endometriomas is excellent, with reports of 83% sensitivity and 98% specificity.

A. Sahdev (✉)
Department of Radiology, St Bartholomew's Hospital, Barts and The London NHS Trust and Queen Mary's School of Medicine and Dentistry, London, UK

Department of Diagnostic Imaging, King George V wing, St Bartholomew's Hospital, London, UK

B. Hamm, P. R. Ros (eds.), *Abdominal Imaging*, DOI 10.1007/978-3-642-13327-5_138,
© Springer-Verlag Berlin Heidelberg 2013

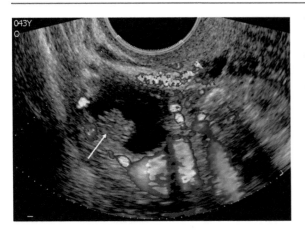

Fig. 131.1 TVUS showing a thick walled cyst in the right ovary with a mural non-enhancing nodule (*arrow*). In this patient, the diagnosis of endometriosis was known, the patient had a low RMI and the cyst was followed up with gradual resolution over 4 months

been achieved using standard T1 and T2 weighted sequences alone (Togashi et al. 1991). Endometriomas can appear complex, containing solid debris, clot, or calcification (Figs. 131.10, 131.2). The typically thin cyst wall shows contrast enhancement but, when fibrotic, can appear thick and irregular, mimicking malignancy. Malignant transformation is rare and only occurs in 0.6–0.8% of women with ovarian endometriosis (Takeuchi et al. 2006). The cause for the transformation is unclear but unopposed eostrogen effects are thought to contribute. Endometrioid and clear cell adenocarcinomas are the most common histological subtypes. On MRI, the most indicative finding for malignant transformation is the presence of enhancing mural nodules (Takeuchi et al. 2006). Unenhanced and contrast-enhanced subtraction images are valuable in detecting small enhancing nodules within the background of a T1-hyperintense endometriomas (Fig. 131.10).

Diagnostic accuracy may be enhanced by Doppler flow studies where blood flow in endometriomas is usually around the cyst with a resistive index above 0.45 (Bis et al. 1997).

There is a wide range of ultrasound appearances of endometriomas including multilocular cysts, cysts with diffuse, low level internal echoes (occur in 95% of endometriomas), and cysts with hyperechoeic foci within the wall (Patel et al. 1999) (Figs. 131.9, 131.1).

The role of CT, due to its poor specificity and high radiation dose, has been replaced by MRI. Endometriomas have nonspecific appearances appearing as solid, cystic, or mixed solid and cystic lesions, resulting in a broad overlap in appearances with abscesses, benign functional ovarian cysts or even malignant masses.

Cyclical bleeding within the cysts results in accumulation of blood products of different ages that contain very high concentrations of paramagnetic products from hemoglobin breakdown. Consequently, endometriomas have typically high T1 signal intensity and very high signal on fat-suppressed T1-weighted images. A wide range of T2 signal intensity has been observed, ranging from a fluid hyperintensity to complete signal void and low-signal-intensity shading (Woodward et al. 2001) which has been reported as characteristic of endometriomas. The detection and characterization on MRI is excellent and sensitivities and specificities of 90% and 98%, respectively, have

Deep Infiltrative Endometriosis

MRI performs well in detection of infiltrative endometriosis, with a sensitivity of 68% for lesions diffusely scattered in the pelvis, typically along the posterior uterine surface and in the rectovaginal septum (Bis et al. 1997). In deep pelvic endometriosis, fibrotic changes due to inactive tissue and scarring, results in distortion of the posterior vaginal fornix, uterus, and uterosacral ligaments. This distortion is clearly seen with a high sensitivity (94%) along with extra-ovarian endometriomas and haematosalpinges (Woodward et al. 2001). The positive predictive value of MRI for deep infiltrative endometriosis is 92% and the negative predictive value is 89% (Bazot et al. 2004). Although the main imaging sequences required are T1, multiplanar high resolution T2, and T1 with fat saturation, use of gadolinium contrast agents is useful to increase the sensitivity for detection of active endometrial deposits and secondly to distinguish between enhancing active endometrial tissue and non-enhancing fibrosis.

To best evaluate features of deep infiltrative endometriosis, the pelvis can be divided into posterior and anterior compartments relative to the uterus. The posterior compartment, which is most frequently involved in infiltrative endometriosis, comprises of the uterine surface, cervix, posterior vaginal wall, Pouch

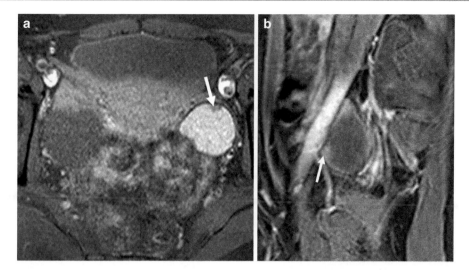

Fig. 131.2 Benign endometrioma. (**a**) Axial T2-weighted image of a left endometrioma with a small papillary nodule (*arrow*) in the anterior wall. (**b**) Axial T1-weighted image with fat saturation and intravenous gadolinium enhancement showing enhancement of the nodule (*arrow*). The endometrioma was resected but entirely benign with no malignancy despite the small enhancing nodule

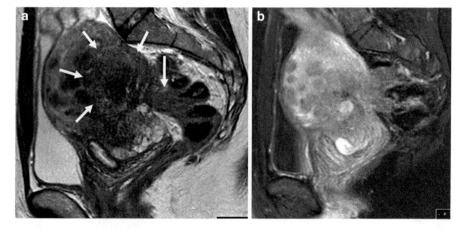

Fig. 131.3 Diffuse infiltrative endometriosis. (**a**) Sagittal T2-weighted image showing a large torus uterinus mass with an admixture of low and high T2 signal intensity. The mass involves the posterior surface of the cervix, uterus, and rectum. It causes retroversion of the uterus and extends posteriorly, involving the rectal serosa (*arrows*). (**b**) Sagittal T1-weighted image with fat saturation and intravenous gadolinium. There is pronounced enhancement of the torus uterinus and the dense sheet like mass around the rectal serosa and rectal wall suggesting active endometriosis

of Douglas, rectum, and the uterosacral ligaments. The anterior compartment consists of vesico-uterine pouch and bladder. In the posterior compartment, in order of frequency, the commonest sites of disease involvement are uterosacral ligaments, uterine and cervical surfaces, pouch of Douglas, bowel loops, and rectosigmoid junction. Bladder involvement is rarely solitary and occurs in association with deep posterior endometriosis (Bazot et al. 2004).

The diagnosis of infiltrative endometriosis is based on signal intensity abnormalities and morphological changes. Small endometriotic deposits are seen as scattered hyperintense foci on T1 and T1 fat saturated sequences. Small cavities of high T2 signal intensity

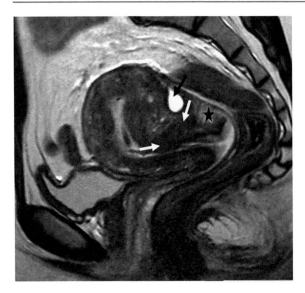

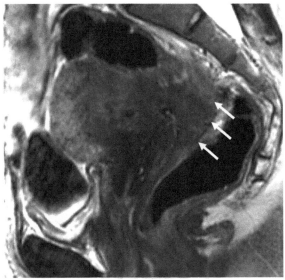

Fig. 131.4 Sagittal T2-weighted image showing a low T2 signal intensity torus uterinus mass (*white arrows*) with scarring causing upward displacement of the posterior fornix (*asterisk*) and retroversion of the uterus. A small loculated pocket of fluid is seen along the posterior uterine surface (*black arrow*)

Fig. 131.6 Sagittal T2-weighted image of a large torus uterinus endometriotic deposit along the posterior uterine surface extending to the rectovaginal fat, rectal serosa and the rectal wall. On imaging, the appearances can mimic a colorectal carcinoma; however the age of the patient, the typical location of the rectosigmoid junction, and clinical history would support endometriosis

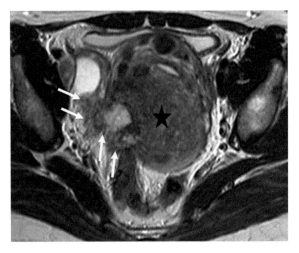

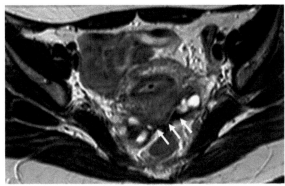

Fig. 131.5 Axial T2-weighted image showing a sheet of endometriotic tissue involving the posterior compartment, right ovary, and obliterating the right lateral uterosacral ligament. A large adenomyoma is also seen in the posterior myometrium (*asterisk*)

Fig. 131.7 Axial T2-weighted image with a dense fibrotic low T2 signal band posterior to the uterus (*arrows*). The fibrosis results in both ovaries being adherent to the posterior uterine surface and medially retracted. The medial retraction results in both ovaries lying in contact resulting in the kissing sign

are also indicative of endometriosis. Morphological changes in the posterior compartment include torus uterinus mass which is a mass or thickening along the upper posterior cervical surface which binds together the posterior uterine surface, the posterior vaginal fornix, and the medial portions of the uterosacral ligaments. This mass may either be mainly fibrotic with low T2 signal intensity causing extensive adhesions, active endometriotic tissue of high T2 signal intensity or an admixture of both. This causes shortening and thickening of uterosacral ligaments, retroverted uterus and raised posterior fornix sign

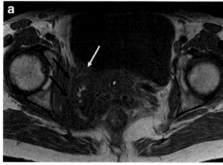 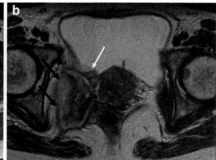

Fig. 131.8 Axial T1-weighted image with deep infiltrative endometriotic tissue along the right pelvic side wall with low T1 signal and small foci of high T1 signal intensity (*black arrows*). The endometriotic tissue extends into the posterior bladder wall (*white arrow*) including the bladder mucosa and the cervix

(Figs. 131.3, 131.4). Infiltration of the uterosacral ligaments includes the presence of irregular or regular nodules, fibrotic stellate bands, or thickening of the ligaments (Fig. 131.5). This thickening is palpable clinically within the adnexa. Associated inflammatory changes may occur causing enhancement on gadolinium administration. Obliteration of normal low T2 signal intensity of the cervix, vaginal wall and rectal wall, and loss of normal fat planes separating the vaginal and rectal walls are features of rectovaginal septal disease. Lesions at this site are almost always accompanied by endometriotic disease in other posterior compartment sites. Involvement of the rectal and bowel wall can be enhanced by use of intraluminal fluid installation, negative luminal contrast agents, and intravenous gadolinium.

The most frequent constellation of posterior compartment disease includes rectovaginal disease and torus uterinus mass. This results in upward displacement of the posterior vaginal fornix, anterior retraction and opposition of the rectum to the posterior vaginal wall, and obliteration of the pouch of Douglas with thickening of the uterosacral ligaments (Fig. 131.6).

Fibromuscular endometriosis in the broad ligaments causes retraction by fibrosis of the ovaries which come to lie along the posterior uterine surface. The ovaries may be so retracted, that they lie in the midline abutting each other resulting in the "kissing sign" (Fig. 131.7). Endometriosis may also result in a frozen pelvis where there is a block of endometriotic tissue which extends to multiple adjacent pelvic structures resulting in complete fusion of these structures. This block of endometriotic tissue is not amenable to surgical resection and a frozen pelvis has a high morbidity. These appearances have an overlap with pelvic inflammatory disease and disseminated pelvic peritoneal ovarian cancer.

Pelvic Visceral Endometriosis

The gastrointestinal tract may be involved in about 12% of cases and the urinary tract is affected in about 1% (Woodward et al. 2001). Gastrointestinal endometriosis usually involves the sigmoid colon and rectum. Endometrial implants first involve the bowel serosa followed by erosion into muscle causing bowel obstruction, pain, and rectal bleeding. Unlike neoplastic lesions, the mucosa is not affected. Typically, on barium enema studies, endometriotic lesions result in an irregular contour of the bowel wall, constricting or an eccentric intramural filling defect and loops of bowel may be tethered together. The commonest site of pelvic endometrial deposits is along the anterior wall of the mid rectum. Endometriosis less commonly involves the urinary tract with adhesions or endometriomas obstructing the ureters just below the pelvic brim. The bladder is affected in 84% of urinary tract endometriosis (Fig. 131.8). Endometrial implants on the posterior wall and dome of the bladder produce filling defects that are seen on intravenous urography and have multiple high signal foci on T1 and T2 weighted images. Bladder deposits cause cyclical haematuria or chronic cystitis.

References

Bazot M, Darai E, Hourani R, Thomassin I, Cortez A, Uzan S, Buy J. Deep pelvic endometriosis: MR imaging for diagnosis and prediction of extension of disease. Radiology. 2004;232:379–89.

Bis KG, Vrachliotis TG, Agrawal R, Shetty AN, Maximovich A, Hricak H. Pelvic endometriosis: MR imaging spectrum with laparoscopic correlation and diagnostic pitfalls. Radiographics. 1997;17:639–55.

Koninckx PR, Oosterlynck D, D'Hooghe T, Meuleman C. Deeply infiltrating endometriosis is a disease whereas mild endometriosis could be considered a non-disease. Ann NY Acad Sci. 1994;734:333–41.

Patel MD, Feldstein VA, Chen DC, Lipson SD, Filly RA. Endometriomas: diagnostic performance of US. Radiology. 1999;210:739–45.

Takeuchi M, Matsuzaki K, Uehara H, Nishitani H. Malignant transformation of pelvic endometriosis: MR imaging findings and pathologic correlation. Radiographics. 2006;26:407–17.

Togashi K, Nishimura K, Kimura I, Tsuda Y, Yamashita K, Shibata T, et al. Endometrial cysts: diagnosis with MR imaging. Radiology. 1991;180:73–8.

Woodward PJ, Sohaey R, Mezzetti Jr TP. Endometriosis: radiologic–pathologic correlation. Radiographics. 2001;21:193–216.

Ovary and Adnexa: Benign Neoplasms

132

Anju Sahdev

Like their malignant counterparts, benign neoplasms of the ovary are categorized according to their cell of origin. Figure 132.1 summarizes the benign ovarian tumors.

Benign Tumors of Epithelial Origin

Serous and Mucinous Cystadenomas

Although serous and mucinous cystadenomas may have characteristic imaging features, overlap exists and distinction between the two is not important, as their management is identical. They affect mainly women between 50 and 70 years and 30% are bilateral. The size can range from 5 to 35 cm. The larger lesions may cause symptoms related to size such as abdominal distension, pain, and ureteric obstruction. Serous cystadenomas are the commonest benign tumor accounting for about 15% of all epithelial neoplasms (Lowe 2007). On imaging, serous cystadenomas are mostly unilocular but may be multilocular with thin walls and smooth septae (Fig. 132.2). Small soft tissue papillary projections may also be present but these raise the possibility of a malignant mass on imaging. The cyst contents consist of clear serous fluid but may be bloody in torted

cystadenomas. Mucinous cystadenomas are usually multilocular, lined by mucin-producing epithelial cells or intestinal epithelium, and may be thick walled. They contain thick white mucus unless torsion has occurred. Mucinous cystadenomas have been known to occur in association with Brenner tumors and dermoids and hence may contain solid areas. On MRI imaging, due to the varying mucin and protein contents, mucinous cystadenomas usually demonstrate multiple locules of varying signal intensities on both T1-and T2-weighted images (Fig. 132.3) (Ghossain et al. 1991). Rupture of mucinous cystadenomas into the peritoneal cavity leads to spillage of mucin-secreting epithelium which results in pseudomyxoma peritonei. In this condition, there is unregulated production of mucin by the scattered mucin-producing cells within the whole peritoneum mimicking ascites on CT and MRI.

Brenner Tumors, Cystadenofibromas, and Adenofibromas

Brenner tumors consist of two components, transitional cell epithelium in small cystic spaces and dense fibrous stroma. It can therefore be considered as a mixed epithelial and mesodermal tumor. They occur in women between the ages of 30 and 60 years, 7% may be bilateral. Thirty percent of Brenner tumors may be found in association with mucinous cystadenomas or dermoids. The stromal component may secrete estrogens resulting in endometrial hyperplasia (Lowe 2007). These tumors are usually small (<2 cm) with low signal on T2-weighted images reflecting the dense fibrous component of the

A. Sahdev
Department of Radiology, St Bartholomew's Hospital, Barts and The London NHS Trust and Queen Mary's School of Medicine and Dentistry, London, UK

Department of Diagnostic Imaging, King George V wing, St Bartholomew's Hospital, London, UK

B. Hamm, P. R. Ros (eds.), *Abdominal Imaging*, DOI 10.1007/978-3-642-13327-5_139,
© Springer-Verlag Berlin Heidelberg 2013

Fig. 132.1 Benign ovarian
tumors

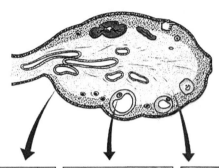

Epithelial origin	Germ cell	Stromal cell tumours
Cystadenomas -serous: 25% -mucinous: 20% Cystadenomas/adenofibromas Brenner tumours: 2–3%	Mature teratomas (dermoid cysts): 20–50% Monodermal teratomas: 3%	Fibromas and thecomas: 20% Sclerosing stromal tumours

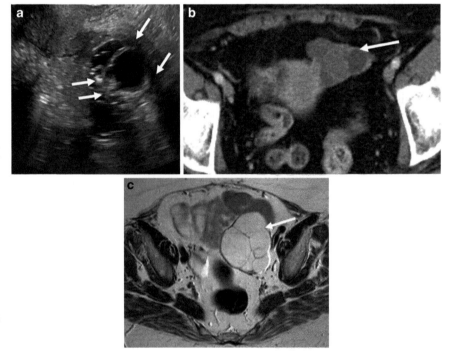

Fig. 132.2 Serous
cystadenoma.
(**a**) Transvaginal ultrasound
(TVUS) showing
a multilocular left ovarian
mass with several thin septa.
Small hyperechoic foci are
seen in the cyst septa. The
walls of the cyst are thickened
and irregular leading to further
investigations (*arrows*).
(**b**) Contrast enhanced CT
showing that the left adnexal
cyst contains several thin
smoothly enhancing septa and
no other ancillary features of
malignancy. (**c**) Axial
T2-weighted image showing
a predominantly cystic lesion
with thin, smooth, multiple
septa and no solid component
or thick wall. The appearances
on MRI are consistent with
a benign ovarian lesion

tumor (Fig. 132.4). The solid components show homogeneous enhancement on post contrast CT and MRI. Amorphous calcification may also be present and larger tumors may show cystic changes (Moon et al. 2000). These cystic changes lead on imaging, to an overlap with the appearances of cystadenofibromas. Cystadenofibromas and adenofibromas have an admixture of epithelial and fibrous tissue, with

Fig. 132.3 Bilateral mucinous cystadenomas. (**a**) Axial T2-weighted image. (**b**) Axial T1-weighted image. (**c**) Axial T1-weighted image with fat saturation. The images show bilateral cystic ovarian lesions with varying signal intensities on T1 and T2 images. The MRI shows a typical "stained glass" appearance with no solid components or irregularity of the septa or cyst wall

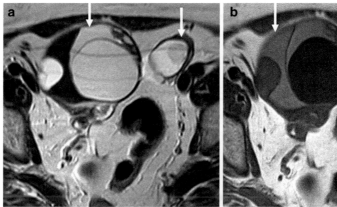

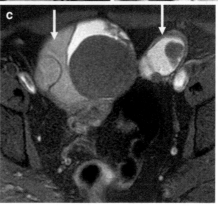

a dominant fibrous component. The imaging appearances are variable and dependent on the proportion of solid tissue which is of very low T2 signal intensity and cystic change. The tumors range from being entirely cystic to complex solid-cystic masses (Cho et al. 2004). The feature of very low T2 signal intensity of the solid components is useful to distinguish cystadenomas from malignant solid-cystic lesion (Fig. 132.5).

Sex Cord and Stromal Cells

Fibromas, Thecomas, Fibrothecomas

Fibromas, thecomas, and fibrothecomas are related solid tumors arising from stromal elements of the ovary. Fibromas are made up of bundles of benign fibroblasts and collagen arranged in whorls. Thecomas are composed of theca cells with abundant cytoplasmic lipid and varying fibrosis. The term "fibrothecoma" reflects the frequently observed histological overlap. Thecal cells produce estrogens and tumors with a dominant proportion of thecal cells having concomitant endometrial hyperplasia or endometrial carcinoma (Troiano et al. 1997). The MR imaging appearances of these tumors are similar with low signal intensity on T1- and T2-weighted images. Tumors with a dominant fibrous component show no or little enhancement after gadolinium administration while those with dominant thecal component have avid enhancement (Troiano et al. 1997; Outwater et al. 1997) (Figs. 132.11 and 132.6). Ovarian fibromas may be associated with ascites and pleural effusions that resolve after resection of the tumor, Meigs syndrome.

Germ Cell Tumors

Mature Teratomas of the Ovary (Dermoids)

These are tumors composed of mature, well-differentiated adult tissues, most commonly epidermis and adipose tissue. They occur at all ages but are

Fig. 132.4 (a) Axial T2-weighted image. (b) Axial T1-weighted image. (c) Axial T1-weighted image with fat saturation and intravenous gadolinium. A right adnexal solid-cystic complex mass is seen on T2-weighted images, the posterior component has solid areas of very low T2 signal intensity (white arrow). On T1 images, the anterior component has high T1 signal intensity which after fat saturation loses signal in keeping with fat in a dermoid cyst (black arrow). After gadolinium contrast, the solid component enhances avidly. The combination of findings is compatible with a fibrous tumor and dermoid cyst of the right ovary, confirmed at surgery

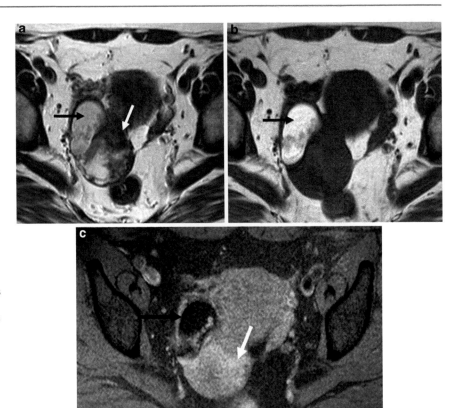

most frequent in young women with only 5% occurring in postmenopausal women (Vortmeyer et al. 1999). The gross pathologic appearance of dermoids is usually that of a unilocular cyst with a solid Rokitansky nodule that is composed of fat and hair (Fig. 136.7). Histologically, the cyst is lined with squamous epithelium and filled with sebaceous material. On occasion, mature teratomas may be entirely solid and contain epidermal components only, forming the rare epidermoid tumors. However, the majority contain tissues of epidermal and dermal origin and are called dermoids. Monodermal dermoids contain a single tissue type only, commonly, thyroid (strauma ovari), brain, or skin. Monodermal dermoids do not contain fat.

Mature dermoids show a variable appearance ranging from cystic to entirely solid lesions. The characteristic imaging feature is the presence of fat which is present in 95% of the tumors (Fig. 136.6). This has hyperechoic US appearances, low fatty attenuation on CT, and high T1 signal intensity on MR which is lost on fat saturated and out-of-phase chemical shift imaging sequences. Chemical shift imaging is particularly useful for fat poor dermoids (Imaoka et al. 1993). The imaging findings have been described in detail under "characterizing adnexal masses."

Summary

Benign tumors of the ovary are now commonly detected on modern imaging. Cystadenomas, dermoids, and fibrous tumors have characteristic appearances particularly on MRI and can be characterized with certainty. Adnexal masses with benign morphology can be periodically monitored as an alternative to surgery in selected patients.

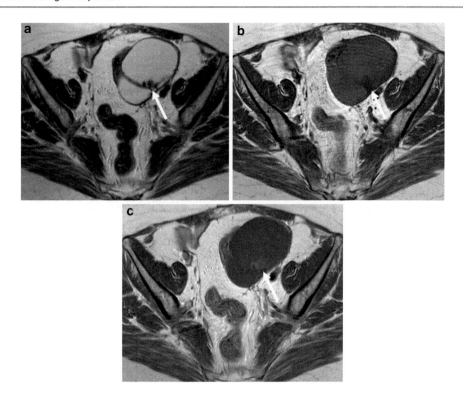

Fig. 132.5 (a) Axial T2-weighted image. (b) Axial T1-weighted image. (c) Axial T1-weighted image after administration of intravenous gadolinium. A left adnexal cystic lesion with septa and small low T2 signal intensity papillary nodules (arrow). The nodules also have very low T1 signal intensity and have moderate enhancement with gadolinium. The appearances are characteristic of a cystadenofibroma with the low T2 signal nodules characteristically fibrotic on MRI

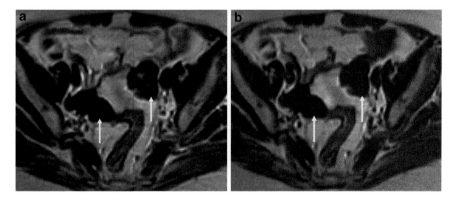

Fig. 132.6 (a) Axial T2-weighted image. (b) Axial T1-weighted image. Bilateral solid homogenous low T2 and low T1 signal intensity masses are incidentally detected in a postmenopausal woman investigated for unrelated abdominal pain. The masses have typical appearances of ovarian fibromas, confirmed on histological resection. The masses were resected at the patient's request but would normally undergo TVUS surveillance to ensure stability

References

Cho SM, Byun JY, Rha SE, Jung SE, Park GS, Kim BK, Kim B, Cho KS, Jung NY, Kim SH, Lee JM. CT and MRI findings of cystadenofibromas of the ovary. Eur Radiol. 2004; 14(5):798–804.

Ghossain MA, Buy JN, Lignères C, Bazot M, Hassen K, Malbec L, Hugol D, Truc JB, Decroix Y, Poitout P. Epithelial tumors of the ovary: comparison of MR and CT findings. Radiology. 1991;181:863–70.

Imaoka I, Sugimura K, Okizuka H, Iwanari O, Kitao M, Ishida T. Ovarian cystic teratomas: value of chemical fat saturation magnetic resonance imaging. Br J Radiol. 1993; 66(791):994–7.

Lowe D. The pathological features of ovarian neoplasms. In: Reznek RR, editor. Cancer of the ovary. Contemporary issues in cancer imaging. Cambridge: Cambridge University Press; 2007.

Moon WJ, Koh BH, Kim SK, Kim YS, Rhim HC, Cho OK, Hahm CK, Byun JY, Cho KS, Kim SH. Brenner tumor of the ovary: CT and MR findings. J Comput Assist Tomogr. 2000;24(1):72–6.

Outwater EK, Siegelman ES, Talerman A, Dunton C. Ovarian fibromas and cystadenofibromas: MRI features of the fibrous component. J Magn Reson Imaging. 1997;7(3):465–71.

Troiano RN, Lazzarini KM, Scoutt LM, Lange RC, Flynn SD, McCarthy S. Fibroma and fibrothecoma of the ovary: MR imaging findings. Radiology. 1997;204(3):795–8.

Vortmeyer AO, Devouassoux-Shisheboran M, Li G, Mohr V, Tavassoli F, Zhuang Z. Microdissection-based analysis of mature ovarian teratoma. Am J Pathol. 1999;154(4): 987–91.

Penelope Moyle and Evis Sala

Introduction

Ovarian cancer causes more deaths than any other cancer of the female reproductive system and accounts for 4% of all female cancers. In 2010, an estimated 1 in 71 women in the United States will develop ovarian cancer in their lifetime with an estimated 13,850 deaths (Cancer Facts and Figures 2010). However, death rates for ovarian cancer have been decreasing by 1.4% per year since 2002 which is partly due to accurate staging of ovarian carcinoma which is vital for the appropriate management and counseling of patients. Identifying the volume and locations of tumor is valuable in planning percutaneous tissue biopsy and triaging patients to either primary cytoreductive surgery, or primary platinum-based chemotherapy. This chapter will discuss the classification, risk factors, current imaging modalities, and staging of ovarian cancer to provide a comprehensive overview for the clinical radiologist.

Classification of Ovarian Tumors

The majority of ovarian cancers arise from the surface epithelial cells (85%), with the remaining 15% arising approximately equally from germ cells, sex cords or metastatic to the ovary (Krukenberg tumors) (Travassoli and Devilee 2003). The histological classification of invasive ovarian cancer is summarized in Table 133.1.

Each histological subtype is subdivided into benign, borderline, or malignant which reflects their clinical behavior and prognosis. Borderline ovarian tumors are a subset of epithelial ovarian tumors that usually occur in premenopausal women and have a favorable prognosis with almost 75% diagnosed at Stage I.

Risk Factors

While most cases of ovarian cancer are sporadic, the most important risk factor is a strong family history of breast or ovarian cancer. Women who have had breast cancer or who have tested positive for inherited mutations in BRCA1 or BRCA2 tumor suppressor genes are at increased risk. Studies suggest that preventive surgery to remove the ovaries and fallopian tubes in these women can decrease the risk of ovarian cancers. Other risk factors include increasing age, nulliparity, early menarche, late menopause, and long-term hormone replacement therapy. Rarer hereditary causes include Lynch II Syndrome, in which the carriers have multiple adenocarcinomas of the ovary, endometrium, and colon, and the Familial site-specific ovarian cancer syndrome, in which multiple family members are affected over several generations (Holschneider and Berek 2000).

P. Moyle (✉)
Department of Radiology, Hinchingbrooke Hospitals NHS Trust, Huntingdon, Cambridgeshire, UK

E. Sala
Memorial Sloan-Kettering Cancer Center, New York, NY, USA

B. Hamm, P. R. Ros (eds.), *Abdominal Imaging*, DOI 10.1007/978-3-642-13327-5_140,
© Springer-Verlag Berlin Heidelberg 2013

Table 133.1 Histological classification of invasive ovarian cancer

Epithelial tumors (85%)	*Serous*
	Mucinous
	Endometrioid
	Clear cell
	Brenner (transitional cell)
	Mixed epithelial
	Undifferentiated
	Carcinosarcoma
	Extraovarian peritoneal
Germ cell (5%)	
Sex cord (5%)	
Metastatic (5%)	*Colon, stomach, pancreas, breast*

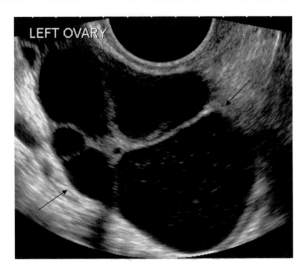

Fig. 133.1 A 48-year-old woman presented with left iliac fossa pain. TV US image demonstrates a well-defined cystic mass with multiple thick septa (*black arrows*). The left ovary could not be visualized separately from the lesion. US is important in the diagnosis of ovarian disease but is not suitable for accurate staging. Histology demonstrated a borderline serous cystadenoma

The Imaging Modalities Available in Staging Ovarian Malignancy

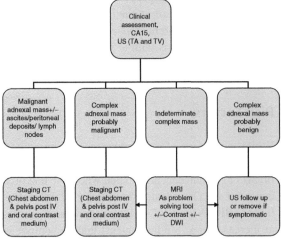

A summary of the appropriate imaging modalities to evaluate ovarian cancer

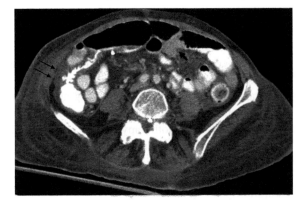

Fig. 133.2 A 56-year-old woman with Stage III ovarian serous cystadenocarcinoma. Contrast-enhanced CT demonstrates serosal soft tissue on the ascending colon (*double black arrows*) and on the transverse colon (*short black arrow*). Oral contrast medium significantly improves visualization of serosal deposits

Ultrasound

US is the primary imaging technique in the assessment of a suspected adnexal mass but not recommended as a staging modality for ovarian carcinoma (Forstner et al. 2010) (Fig. 133.1).

Computed Tomography

CT is the modality of choice for staging ovarian carcinoma as it is a quick, readily available whole body imaging technique and has a reported accuracy for all stages of 70–90%. Oral contrast medium is mandatory for the demonstration of serosal deposits on the bowel (Fig. 133.2). If Krukenberg tumors are suspected (bilateral metastatic adnexal masses), the thorax, abdomen, and pelvis can be examined to identify the primary tumor which can arise from the colon, stomach, pancreas, or breast (Fig. 133.3).

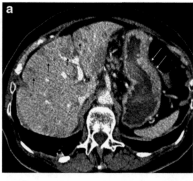
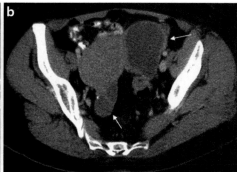

Fig. 133.3 A 66-year-old woman presented with abdominal pain and a change in bowel habit. Axial contrast-enhanced CT demonstrates (**a**) thickening at the greater curve of the stomach (*white arrows*) and multiple liver metastases (*black arrows*) and (**b**) bilateral predominantly cystic solid adnexal masses (*white arrows*). Histology confirmed a mucinous primary gastric tumor with Krukenberg tumors (metastatic disease to the ovaries)

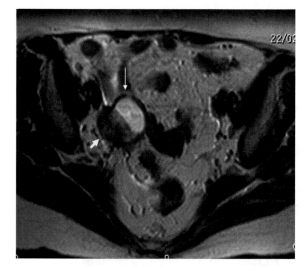

Fig. 133.4 A 66-year-old woman with right iliac fossa pain and a raised CA 125, but an initial pelvic ultrasound could not identify either ovary. (**a**) An axial T2W image demonstrates a right complex pelvic cyst containing a single fluid locule (*white arrow*) and a solid component not identified at US (*thick white arrow*). The MRI confirmed the high suspicion of malignancy indicated by the raised CA 125 and pain. Final histology identified a serous cystadenocarcinoma

Magnetic Resonance Imaging

MRI is a problem-solving tool and not the modality of choice for staging. MRI can characterize the origin of an adnexal mass and determine whether an indeterminate adnexal mass is benign or malignant. It reduces the number of unnecessary operations for benign lesions, reduces operating on inoperable cases, and can help triage patients to primary chemotherapy (Figs. 133.4, 133.5).

In staging of ovarian cancer, Diffusion Weighed Magnetic Resonance Imaging (DW-MRI) has a role to increase the reader's confidence, but also identifying metastatic lesions, peritoneal or serosal nodules that may be difficult to initially visualize on standard sequences; overall it can improve staging accuracy (Fig. 133.6) (Fujii et al. 2008) and is seen as complementary to contrast-enhanced MRI imaging.

[18]FDG Positron Emission Tomography–Computed Tomography (PET-CT)

PET/CT has a limited role in diagnosis and staging of ovarian malignancy as it is poor at detecting low grade and cystic tumors and has false positives in some benign disease. An increasing number of centers are using PET/CT in the preoperative evaluation of patients suspected to have ovarian cancer but its role is to reveal metastatic ovarian cancer and coexisting malignant tumors not aid diagnosis. However, PET/CT is highly sensitive and specific to evaluation of recurrent and residual disease and this is where it has a significant role (Gu et al. 2009) (Fig. 133.7).

Staging of Ovarian Cancer

There are two staging systems which can be used with ovarian malignancy: The International Federation of Gynecology and Obstetrics (FIGO), which is the most commonly and universally used (Benedet et al. 2000),

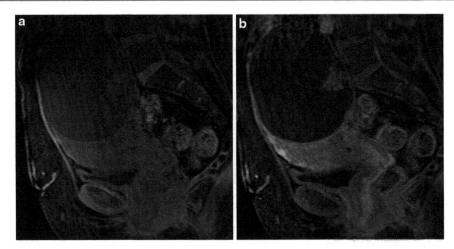

Fig. 133.5 A 42-year-old woman presented with a pelvic mass. (**a**) Unenhanced sagittal T1W fat saturated MR demonstrates a cystic solid mass arising from the pelvis. The solid areas are difficult to discern (*black arrow*). Dynamic contrast enhancement was performed to assess the complex mass in greater detail. (**b**) Post administration of intravenous gadolinium there was rapid enhancement of the solid tissue and septa within the mass. A selected immediately post contrast T1W fat saturated sagittal image illustrates the solid components are avidly enhancing (*black arrow*). Final histology confirmed a grade II mucinous cystadenocarcinoma

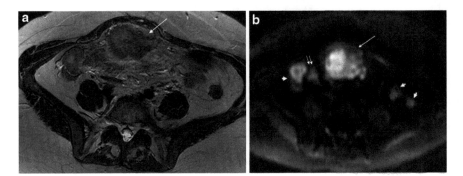

Fig. 133.6 A 47-year-old woman presented with abdominal pain. (**a**) Axial T2W MRI demonstrates a large omental deposit (*white arrow*). (**b**) Axial DWI at the same level demonstrates restricted diffusion not just at the obvious omental deposit seen on the T2W image (*white arrow*), but further areas of restricted diffusion indicating subtle peritoneal disease (*double white arrow*) and serosal disease (*white arrowheads*). DWI can increase readers' confidence and identify subtle peritoneal lesions difficult to discern on conventional MRI sequences

and the TNM classification based on clinical and/or pathological classification (Sobin et al. 2009) (Tables 133.2 and 133.3).

FIGO staging does not formally include radiology but the committee encourages the use of imaging techniques if available to assess the important prognostic factors such as resectable or residual disease and lymph node status. Understaging can occur with imaging; therefore, FIGO recommends a full final surgical staging with a hysterectomy, bilateral salpingo-oophorectomy, pelvic and paraaortic lymph node biopsies, omentectomy, peritoneal biopsies, and washings (Tables 133.2 and 133.3).

Stage I

The primary ovarian tumor can have a variable appearance but usually is a complex cystic solid mass with septae and/or papillary projections. It is an intraperitoneal structure and is always seen originating medial to the iliac vessels. In Stage IA, the tumor is limited to

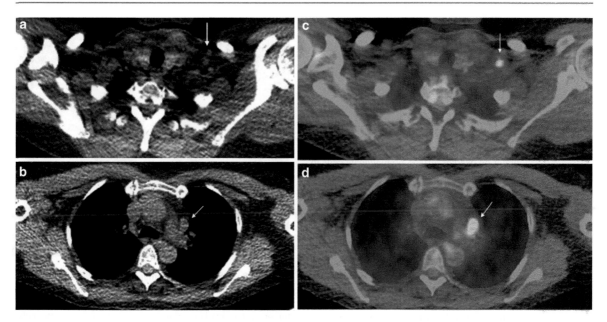

Fig. 133.7 A 43-year-old woman with known Stage IIIA serous cystadenocarcinoma of the ovary treated with chemotherapy and surgical debulking. Eight months after initial therapy CA 125 tumor markers were rising, yet there was no evidence on a standard CT of recurrence. A PET/CT was performed. (**a**) Initial attenuation correction CT identifies two 5 mm left supraclavicular lymph nodes (*white arrow*), and (**b**) a 7 mm pre-vascular lymph node (*white arrow*). (**c**) The fused PET/CT identifies increased uptake of FDG in one of the supraclavicular nodes (*white arrow*) and (**d**) the pre-vascular lymph node (*white arrow*) indicating metastatic tumor. Functional imaging with PET/CT is highly sensitive in detecting recurrent disease in morphologically normal tissue

one ovary with the capsule intact, no tumor is present on the ovarian surface, and no malignant cells in the ascites or peritoneal washings (Fig. 133.8). In Stage IB, the tumor is limited to both ovaries with the capsule intact, no tumor is present on the ovarian surface, and no malignant cells in the ascites or peritoneal washings. In Stage IC, the tumor is limited to one or both ovaries with either capsular rupture, tumor on ovarian surface and/or malignant cells in ascites or peritoneal washings. The 5-year survival statistics of Stage I tumor is 93% (Woodward et al. 2004).

Stage II

The tumor spreads locally with direct extension to the surrounding pelvic tissues but not into the upper abdomen. In Stage IIA disease, there is extension and/or tumor implants on the uterus or fallopian tube(s), but no malignant cells in the ascites or peritoneal washings. In Stage IIB disease, there is extension and/or implants on other pelvic tissues, but no malignant cells in the ascites or peritoneal washings (Fig. 133.9).

There must be careful evaluation of the fat planes surrounding the primary tumor, the uterus, and pelvic side-walls. If there is less than 3 mm between the tumor and the pelvic side-wall, this indicates pelvic side-wall invasion. Displacement or encasement of iliac vessels and invasion of the colon and/or bladder also changes surgical management. Due to the greater tissue contrast with MR imaging direct invasion of the tumor may be easier to identify with MR imaging than CT imaging. The 5-year survival of Stage II is 70%.

Stage III

Approximately 70% of patients have Stage III disease with peritoneal metastases at staging laparotomy (Buy et al. 1988). Intraperitoneal dissemination is the most common mode of tumor spread in ovarian carcinoma as tumor cells are shed from the primary tumor and follow the circulation of peritoneal fluid around the abdomen and pelvis. Peritoneal fluid flows from the Pouch of Douglas, along the paracolic gutters to the diaphragm and hence these are the key areas

Table 133.2 The FIGO and TNM staging of ovarian carcinoma

FIGO	TNM	Description
	Tx	Primary tumor cannot be assessed
	T0	No evidence of primary tumor
I	T1	Tumor limited to ovaries (one/both)
IA	T1a	Tumor limited to one ovary, capsule intact, no tumor on ovarian surface, no malignant cells in ascites or peritoneal washings[a]
IB	T1b	Tumor limited to both ovaries, capsule intact, no tumor on ovarian surface, no malignant cells in ascites or peritoneal washings[a]
IC	T1c	Tumor limited to one or both ovaries with any of the following: capsular rupture, tumor on ovarian surface, malignant cells in ascites or peritoneal washings[a]
II	T2	Tumor involves one or both ovaries with pelvic extensions or implants
IIa	T2A	Extension and/or implants on uterus/tube(s), no malignant cells in ascites or peritoneal washings
IIb	T2b	Extension and/or implants on other pelvic tissue, no malignant cells in ascites or peritoneal washings
[b]III	T3 and/ or N1	Tumor involves one or both ovaries with microscopically confirmed peritoneal metastasis outside the pelvis
IIIA	T3a	Microscopically confirmed peritoneal metastasis outside the pelvis (no macroscopic tumor)
IIIB	T3b	Macroscopically peritoneal metastasis outside the pelvis 2 cm or less in dimension
IIIC	T3c and/ or N1	Macroscopically peritoneal metastasis outside the pelvis greater than 2 cm and/or regional lymph nodes
[c]IV	M1	Distant metastasis beyond the peritoneal cavity

[a]The presence of ascites does not affect staging unless malignant cells are present.
[b]Liver capsule metastasis are T3/Stage III, liver parenchymal metastasis M1/
[c]Stage IV. Pleural effusion must have positive cytology.

Table 133.3 Regional lymph nodes (N) and distant metastasis (M)

FIGO	TNM	Description
	NX	Regional lymph nodes cannot be assessed
	N0	No regional lymph node metastasis
IIIC	N1	Regional lymph node metastasis
	MX	Distant metastasis cannot be assessed
	M0	No distant metastasis
IV	M1	Distant metastasis (not including peritoneal metastasis)

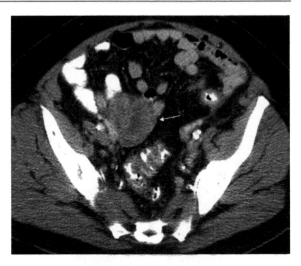

Fig. 133.8 A 50-year-old woman presented with an abdominal mass. Axial CECT demonstrates a well-defined solid right adnexal mass (*white arrow*). The capsule is intact with no tumor on the ovarian surface and no extension into the pelvic organs, peritoneal or lymph nodes. Laparotomy confirmed Stage IA endometrioid carcinoma of the right ovary

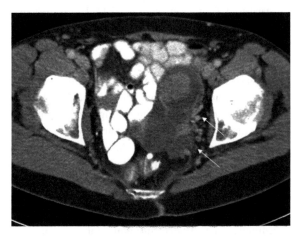

Fig. 133.9 A 62-year-old woman presented with left iliac fossa pain. Axial CECT demonstrates a complex cystic solid left adnexal mass abutting the left internal and external iliac vessels (*white arrows*) and less than 3 mm from the pelvic side-wall. The final pathology confirmed Stage IIB endometrioid adenocarcinoma

where peritoneal seeding and deposits occur. There is preferential flow along the right paracolic gutter and hence, the right side of the peritoneum and diaphragm should be especially scrutinized for metastatic disease. Understanding the locations that peritoneal disease

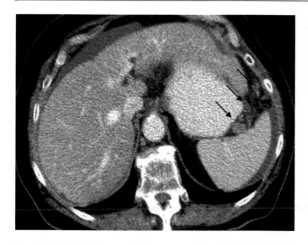

Fig. 133.10 A 65-year-old woman presented with abdominal fullness and a pelvic mass. Staging axial CECT identifies peritoneal disease in the gastrosplenic ligament, a very common site for peritoneal disease (*black arrows*). The final pathology confirmed Stage IIIa mucinous cystadenocarcinoma

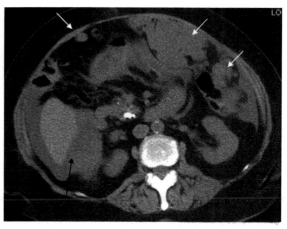

Fig. 133.12 A 74-year-old woman with a biopsy-proven serous cystadenocarcinoma of the ovary. Staging axial CECT demonstrates multiple >2 cm peritoneal deposits (*white arrows*) and ascites (*black arrow*), therefore, indicating Stage IIIB disease

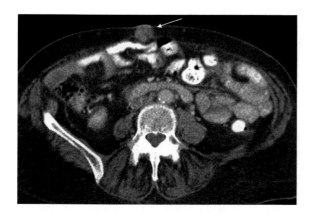

Fig. 133.11 A 79-year-old woman with Stage IIIB serous cystadenocarcinoma of the ovary. Staging axial CECT demonstrates a 15 mm "Sister Joseph's nodule." This is a metastasis in the umbilicus which occurs via peritoneal spread

occurs will help to accurately diagnose small deposits (Fig. 133.10).

Stage III disease reflects the presence of peritoneal dissemination with Stage IIIA demonstrating microscopic confirmed peritoneal metastasis outside the pelvis (no macroscopic tumor) and Stage IIIB demonstrating macroscopic peritoneal metastasis outside the pelvis which are 2 cm or less (Fig. 133.11). Stage IIIC demonstrates macroscopic peritoneal metastasis outside the pelvis which is greater than 2 cm and/or regional lymph nodes involved (Fig. 133.12).

Peritoneal deposits can be nodular to plaque-like and in some cases may appear cystic. Plaque-like serosal disease of the bowel can be a challenge to the radiologists; therefore, bowel thickening and irregularity should be considered as serosal disease, and oral contrast can greatly help identify serosal plaques.

The omentum is the commonest site for peritoneal tumor spread, and omental disease progresses from a fine reticular nodular pattern to focal nodular thickening, and then extensive thickening which is also called an "omental cake." Thickened omentum is one of the most accessible sites for the radiologist to perform a percutaneous tissue biopsy for histological diagnosis (Fig. 133.13). It has been shown to be safe, accurate, and a relatively quick technique using US or CT guidance (Griffin et al. 2009).

Subcapsular deposits of the liver and spleen typically cause scalloping. This may be difficult to differentiate from a parenchymal lesion if the deposit is large; therefore, reformatting to sagittal and coronal images is recommended. It is important to differentiate between the two lesions because a capsular deposit is Stage III/T3, but a liver parenchymal metastasis is Stage IV/M1 (Fig. 133.14).

Subcapsular scalloping can also occur in pseudomyxoma peritonei. This is a rare condition characterized by metastatic thick mucinous or gelatinous material on the surfaces of the peritoneal cavity causing mass effect (Fig. 133.15). Bowel loops are matted

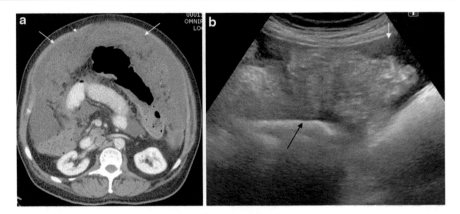

Fig. 133.13 A 46-year-old woman presented with abdominal bloating. (**a**) Staging axial CECT identifies extensive metastatic infiltration to the omentum – "omental cake" (*white arrows*) and ascites. (**b**) US demonstrates the infiltrated omentum (*black arrow*) and a small pool of ascites (*white arrow*) from which

an US-guided percutaneous biopsy was performed. If there is too much ascites, the thickened omentum can move within the fluid when trying to obtain a percutaneous biopsy. Ascites should be drained pre procedure to obtain the best results

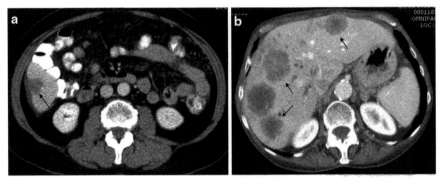

Fig. 133.14 (**a**) A 60-year-old woman with biopsy-proven mixed Mullerian tumor. Axial CECT identifies a subcapsular metastasis indenting into the liver parenchyma (*black arrow*) and unlike the parenchymal metastases does not have tissue surrounding it. This is in keeping with Stage III disease. (**b**) 51-year-old woman with biopsy-proven serous

cystadenocarcinoma. Axial CECT identifies multiple low attenuation lesions within the liver (*black arrows*) in keeping with parenchymal liver metastases, therefore Stage IV disease. Care must be taken to distinguish the exact location of liver metastases in ovarian malignancy

posteriorly rather than floating anterior and freely within fluid ascites, and fine septae may be visualized. Surgical resection of the insidious mucin is very difficult and repeated laparotomies may be needed (Levy et al. 2009). Peritoneal mucinous carcinomatosis can arise from mucinous carcinoma of the ovary, gastrointestinal tract or pancreas with peritoneal spread and is characterized by invasive, high-grade, poorly differentiated mucinous carcinoma with large extracellular pools of mucin. However, it is now widely accepted that the majority of cases of classic pseudomyxoma peritonei develop from low-grade mucinous carcinomas that arise

in the appendix, and that penetrate or rupture into the peritoneal cavity (Moran and Cecil 2003). If pseudomyxoma peritonei is suspected, MRI is the imaging of choice due to the greater tissue contrast for peritoneal nodules and the high T2-weighted signal intensity of the mucinous deposits.

Serous and mucinous cystadenocarcinomas produce unilocular/multilocular fluid-filled masses. Both the primary tumor and the metastatic peritoneal deposits can contain microcalcifications; in serous tumors, these are known as psammoma bodies, and in mucinous tumors as non-psammoma calcification.

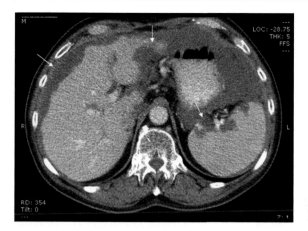

Fig. 133.15 A 66-year-old woman with a Stage IIIC mucinous cystadenocarcinoma of the ovary. Axial CECT demonstrates scalloping of the liver and spleen by thick gelatinous pseudomyxoma peritonei. The mass effect of the subcapsular gelatinous deposits gives the scalloped appearance (*white arrows*)

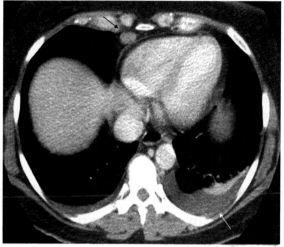

Fig. 133.16 A 52-year-old woman with biopsy-proven clear cell carcinoma of the ovary. Axial CECT demonstrates an enlarged 12-mm cardiophrenic lymph node (*black arrow*) which is one of the classical sites of nodal disease in ovarian malignancy. A left pleural effusion (*white arrow*) is also present which was drained and cytology contained malignant cells. Both these features indicate Stage IV disease

This tumor calcification can be seen on CT in up to 33% of cases (Mitchell 1986) and careful inspection of the peritoneal surfaces for calcification is needed.

Ovarian cancer also metastasizes through the lymphatic system. Peritoneal fluid drains through the large lymphatic capillary network of the diaphragm into the anterior mediastinal nodes which can become occluded by malignant cells. This then further blocks the absorption of peritoneal fluid and contributes to the accumulation of malignant ascites (Holschneider and Berek 2000). Large volumes of ascites usually indicate peritoneal metastasis even if cytology from the ascitic fluid is negative.

Lymph node involvement follows the ovarian veins to the paraaortic and paracaval nodes at the level of the renal hilum which is the most common site for metastatic adenopathy in ovarian cancer. Lymph vessels also pass through the broad ligament and involve the external iliac, hypogastric, and obturator chain and along the round ligament to involve the inguinal nodes.

There is increasing evidence that primary surgical evaluation of the lymph nodes by extensive systemic lymphadenectomy at the time of surgical staging is associated with an improved 5-year disease-specific survival, even when adjusted for age, stage, grade, and number of positive lymph nodes. This may be because occult micrometastatic disease that is resistant to chemotherapy is removed (Chan et al. 2007). Therefore, identifying enlarged lymph nodes preoperatively

will guide the surgeon in planning the retroperitoneal dissection. The 5-year survival rate of Stage III tumor is 37% (Woodward et al. 2004).

Stage IV

Stage IV disease is defined by distant metastasis beyond the peritoneal cavity and it occurs via hematogenous spread. It is the least common mode of tumor spread in ovarian carcinoma but typically occurs in the solid abdominal organs such as the liver, spleen, kidneys, adrenals, brain, and bone. Care must be taken when assessing the liver and spleen. Intraparenchymal Stage IV disease is usually less defined and surrounded by tissue while subcapsular Stage III disease is usually smooth and scalloped. Tumor extending into the falciform ligament (Stage III) can be mistaken for intraparenchymal disease and reformatted images are helpful in this assessment. Stage IV lung involvement includes either parenchymal disease or positive cytology in pleural effusions. Cardiophrenic lymph nodes larger than 5 mm should be regarded as suspicious for Stage IV (Fig. 133.16). Hematogenous metastases are uncommon at the time of diagnosis but can be the sites of recurrence and up to 50% of patients at autopsy

Table 133.4 The imaging criteria for predicting "non-optimally" resectable disease in ovarian cancer

Implants of size >2 cm: diaphragm, lesser sac, porta hepatis, falciform ligament, gall bladder fossa; gastrosplenic, gastrohepatic ligament and small bowel mesentery
Pelvic side-wall (<3 mm) or abdominal wall invasion
Retroperitoneal presacral disease
Parenchymal liver metastases and subcapsular liver metastases
Lymph node enlargement above the renal hilum

have hematogenous metastases (Holschneider and Berek 2000). The 5-year survival rate of Stage IV tumor is 25% (Woodward et al. 2004).

Non-resectable Disease

One of the most important aspects of imaging ovarian cancer is to help guide triaging the patients into primary surgery or primary chemotherapy. A multidisciplinary team approach is best to decide operable or non-optimally resectable disease, and this must be taken within the context of the patients pre disease health status. Table 133.4 describes the imaging criteria for predicting "non-optimally" resectable disease in ovarian cancer (Table 133.5).

Conclusion

The radiologist has an invaluable role in the care and management of patients with ovarian carcinoma. Accurate staging with identifying the volume and locations of tumor is needed in planning percutaneous tissue biopsy, triaging patients to either primary chemotherapy, or advising surgical planning for primary cytoreductive surgery.

Pearls to Remember

- US is the first-line imaging modality in women clinically suspected to have an adnexal mass/ovarian pathology.
- CT is the modality of choice for staging ovarian carcinoma. MRI is the modality of choice for problem solving.

Table 133.5 Mimics and differential diagnoses of ovarian cancer

Condition	Description
Hemorrhagic cyst	Unilateral adnexal cyst, "cob-web"/ septae or retracted clot. High SI on T1W imaging. Undergoes transformation and spontaneous resolution
Endometriosis/ Endometrioma[a]	Pelvic pain, cysts with homogenous low-level internal echoes. High SI T1W imaging. Shading and blood fluid levels
Dermoid/Teratoma	Cystic and solid masses containing fat
Ovarian metastases	Bilateral cystic solid masses usually in known malignancy
Tubo-ovarian abscess	Fever, raised inflammatory markers. Complex adnexal mass +/− sepiginous structures and free fluid
Actinomycosis	Often history of long-term IUCD. Infiltrative adnexal mass. Lack of ascites and nodes compared with volume of disease +/− fistula
TB	Tubo-ovarian abscess, ascites (90%) omental cake, mesenteric mass, calcified lymph nodes, tubes and ovaries can occur
Gastrointestinal stromal tumor (GIST)	Well-defined submucosal heterogenous mass, often large at presentation
Pedunculated or broad ligament leiomyoma (fibroid)	Well-defined mass which may be attached to the uterus by a pedicle or within the broad ligament
Leiomyomatosis disseminata	Multiple small nodules on the peritoneal surface mimicking a malignant process, but generally benign histological features. Many patients have uterine leiomyomas as well
Splenosis	Spontaneous transplantation of splenic tissue to unusual sites after splenic trauma. The splenic pulp implants appear as red-blue nodules on the peritoneum, omentum, and mesentery − similar to endometriosis
Meigs syndrome	Triad of ascites, pleural effusion, and ovarian fibroma which resolved once the fibroma has been removed

[a]It must be remembered that the tumor marker CA 125 is nonspecific and may be raised in a benign adnexal mass such as endometriosis.

- PET/CT has a limited role in diagnosis and staging of ovarian malignancy and is generally limited to evaluation of recurrent disease.
- FIGO is the most universally used staging system based on surgical staging, but imaging is complimentary to surgical staging.

- More than 70% of patients with ovarian cancer present with Stage III disease.
- Krukenberg tumors (bilateral metastatic cystic or solid adnexal masses) can arise from the colon, stomach, pancreas, or breast.
- Careful interrogation of the peritoneum for nodules especially in the gastrosplenic ligament, lesser sac and falciform ligament to diagnose Stage III disease.
- Cardiophrenic lymph nodes larger than 5 mm should be regarded as suspicious for Stage IV.

References

Benedet JL, Bender H, Jones III H, et al. FIGO staging and clinical practical guidelines in the management of gynaecological cancers. FIGO Committee on gynaecologic oncology. Int J Gynaecol Obstet. 2000;70:209–62.

Buy JN, Moss AA, Ghossain MA, et al. Peritoneal implants from ovarian tumors: CT findings. Radiology. 1988;169:691–4.

Cancer Facts and Figures. Atlanta: American Cancer Society; 2010. http://www.cancer.org/acs/groups/content/@nho/documents/document/acspc-024113.pdf

Chan JK, Urban R, Hu JM, Shin JY, Hussain A, Teng NN, et al. The potential therapeutic role of lymph node resection in epithelial ovarian cancer: a study of 13918 patients. BJ Cancer. 2007;96:1817–22.

Forstner R, Sala E, Kinkel K, Spencer JA. European Society of urogenital radiology. ESUR guidelines: ovarian cancer staging and follow-up. Eur Radiol. 2010;20:2773–80.

Fujii S, Matsusue E, Kanasaki Y, et al. Detection of peritoneal dissemination in gynecological malignancy: evaluation by diffusion-weighted MR imaging. Eur Radiol. 2008;18:18–23.

Griffin N, Grant L, Freeman SJ, et al. Image-guided biopsy in patients with suspected ovarian carcinoma: a safe and effective technique? Eur Radiol. 2009;19:230–5.

Gu P, Pan LL, Wu SQ, Sun L, Huang G. CA 125, PET alone, PET-CT, CT and MRI in diagnosing recurrent ovarian carcinoma: a systematic review and meta-analysis. Eur J Radiol. 2009;71:164–74.

Holschneider CH, Berek JS. Ovarian cancer: epidemiology, biology, and prognostic factors. Semin Surg Oncol. 2000;19:3–10.

Levy AD, Shaw JC, Sobin LH. Secondary tumors and tumor like lesions of the peritoneal cavity: imaging features with pathologic correlation. Radiographics. 2009;29:347–73.

Moran BJ, Cecil TD. The etiology, clinical presentation, and management of pseudomyxoma peritonei. Surg Oncol Clin N Am. 2003;12:585–603.

Sobin L, Gospodarowicz M, Wittekind C, editors. TNM classification of malignant tumours, Ovary (ICD-O C56). 7th ed. Chichester/Hoboken: Wiley-Blackwell; 2009.

Travassoli FA, Devilee T, editors. Pathology and genetics. Tumours of the breast and female genital organs. WHO classification of tumour. Geneva: WHO; 2003.

Woodward PJ, Hosseinzadeh K, Saenger JS. Radiologic staging of ovarian carcinoma with pathologic correlation. From the archives of the AFIP. Radiographics. 2004;24:225–46.

Adnexal Masses in Pregnancy

134

Matthias Meissnitzer and Rosemarie Forstner

Clinical Background

With prenatal screening, incidental finding of adnexal masses in pregnancy has become a well-recognized clinical problem. Adnexal masses are detected in 2–4% of pregnancies, and in 0.5% at cesarean section (Spencer and Robarts 2006; Kooninga et al. 1988).

The vast majority of these adnexal masses consist of benign functional cysts that will regress during pregnancy. Other common benign adnexal lesions in pregnancy include dermoid cysts, cystadenomas, endometriomas, and subserous uterine fibroids. Due to young age, the incidence of ovarian cancer ranges only from 0.004% to 0.04%. Tumor markers (e.g., CA125 or AFP) play a limited role, as they are physiologically elevated during pregnancy (Spencer and Robarts 2006).

The management of adnexal masses depends on size and morphology on US, clinical symptoms, and gestational age. In the clinical setting of an indeterminate adnexal mass under expectant sonographic follow-up, MRI has become an important adjunct in patient management (Fig. 134.1) (Woodfield et al. 2010). Unless malignancy is suspected, most experts recommend to postpone surgery to a point in time after 14 weeks of gestation in order to minimize the risk of fetal loss (Spencer and Robarts 2006).

Pain in a pregnant patient with an adnexal mass should alert to adnexal torsion. Adnexal masses larger than 5 cm in size, particularly dermoids and cystadenomas are prone to torsion (up to 5%), which is commonly found in the first trimester. Later, large adnexal lesions may cause obstructed labor.

Imaging Findings

The vast majority of benign adnexal lesions are sonographically *simple or hemorrhagic cysts* displaying typical imaging features and typically regressing during follow-up (Table 134.1) (Telischak et al. 2008).

Solid or complex cystic and solid tumors (Table 134.1) in pregnancy may represent *subserosal leiomyomas* with or without hemorrhage, and adnexal neoplasms including *fibrothecomas, luteuma in pregnancy, hyperreactio luteinalis, Brenner tumors, and ovarian malignancies.*

Luteomas in pregnancy are benign tumor-like lesions deriving from ovarian stroma or its derivatives which typically regress within 4 weeks postpartally. They are found bilaterally in one-third of cases and typically present as large tumors ranging between 6 and 10 cm in size. Hypersecretion of androgens may cause maternal acne. However, risk of virilization for a female fetus is low due to androgen protection by the placenta (Kao et al. 2005).

Approximately 1–3% of adnexal masses in pregnancy are malignant including *ovarian adenocancer, borderline tumors, sex-cord stromal tumors* (Fig. 134.2), *germ cell tumors, and Krukenberg tumors.* They present as solid or complex solid and

M. Meissnitzer (✉) • R. Forstner
Department of Radiology, Landeskrankenhaus Salzburg,
Paracelsus Medical University, Salzburg, Austria

B. Hamm, P. R. Ros (eds.), *Abdominal Imaging*, DOI 10.1007/978-3-642-13327-5_142,
© Springer-Verlag Berlin Heidelberg 2013

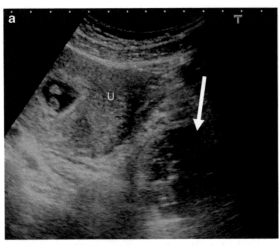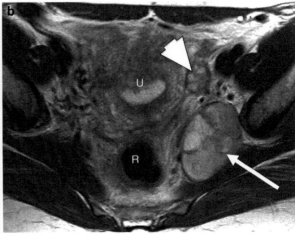

Fig. 134.1 Neurinoma of the left pelvic sidewall: Sonography (**a**) at 12 weeks of pregnancy demonstrates a left pelvic mass (*arrow*) of equivocal origin. Transaxial T2 MRI (**b**) identifies the mass (*arrow*) as clearly separated from the left ovary (*arrowhead*). Location and anterior displacement of vessels help to identify its extraperitoneal origin. Pregnant uterus (*U*), rectum (*R*)

Table 134.1 Morphologic appearance of adnexal masses

Predominant morphologic appearance	Differential diagnosis
Cystic	-Functional ovarian cysts -Cystadenoma
Cystic hemorrhagic	-Hemorrhagic cysts -Endometrioma
Fat	-Dermoids
Cystic and solid	-Hyperreactio luteinalis -Endometrioma -Cancer -Borderline tumors -Ovarian metastasis
Solid	-Leiomyoma -Fibrothecoma -Dysgerminoma -Luteoma -Ovarian metastasis

cystic lesions with typical imaging features of malignancy on MRI. Recently, Thomassin-Naggara et al. reported the added value of DWI in solid adnexal masses during pregnancy, with low SI on high b value images as a typical feature of a benign lesion (Thomassin-Naggara et al. 2009).

Solid components in an *endometrioma* may indicate rare malignant transformation, but when found during pregnancy it may also reflect decidualization due to progesterone effect (Telischak et al. 2008). Such endometrioma enlarges in size and may mimic ovarian cancer in Doppler US and in MRI. Reported imaging findings include smoothly lobulated mural nodules with prominent internal vascularity similar to decidualized endometrium. Such findings in an endometrioma may warrant expectant waiting and resection after surgery (Poder et al. 2008).

Appropriateness of Different Imaging Modalities

Sonography is the first-line modality to assess adnexal masses during pregnancy. In adnexal masses not regressing during follow-up and in sonographically indeterminate lesions MRI has become an important adjunct in further characterization (Spencer et al. 2010; Woodfield et al. 2010). In pregnancy routine use of Gadolinium should be avoided, as the risk to the fetus remains unknown (Kanal et al. 2007). However, DWI is emerging as a valuable alternative to further characterize complex adnexal masses (Thomassin-Naggara et al. 2009).

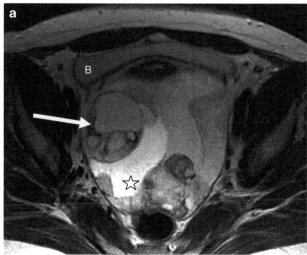 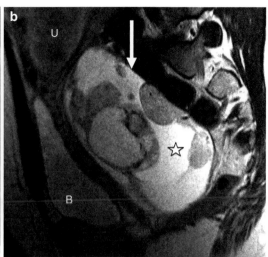

Fig. 134.2 Sertoli–Leydig cell tumor: A 30-year-old patient presenting with an extensive adnexal mass at 20 weeks of pregnancy. Transaxial T2 (**a**) and sagittal T2 MRI (**b**) show a well-delineated complex adnexal mass (*arrow*) with cystic and solid components and locules containing hemorrhagic fluid (*), but no evidence of fat. Imaging does not allow differentiation from other ovarian malignancies, such as ovarian cancer or Krukenberg tumor. Pregnant uterus (*U*), bladder (*B*)

References

Kanal E, Barkovich AJ, Bell C, et al. ACR Blue ribbon panel on MRI safety. ACR guidance document for safe MR practices. Am J Roentgenol. 2007;188:1447–74.

Kao HW, Wu CJ, Chung KT, et al. MR imaging of pregnancy luteoma: a case report and correlation with the clinical features. Korean J Radiol. 2005;6:44–6.

Kooninga PP, Platt LD, Wallace R. Incidental adnexal neoplasm at cesarean section. Obstet Gynecol. 1988;72:767–9.

Poder L, Coakley FV, Rabban JT, et al. Decidualized endometrioma during pregnancy: recognizing an imaging mimick of ovarian malignancy. J Comput Assist Tomogr. 2008;32:555–8.

Spencer CP, Robarts PJ. Management of adnexal masses in pregnancy. Obstet Gynecol. 2006;8:14–9.

Spencer JA, Forstner R, Cunha MT, Kinkel K. ESUR guidelines for MR imaging of the sonographically indeterminate mass. Eur Radiol. 2010;20:25–35.

Telischak NA, Yeh BM, Nj B, et al. MRI of adnexal masses in pregnancy. Am J Roentgenol. 2008;191:364–70.

Thomassin-Naggara I, Darai E, Cuenod CA, et al. Contribution of diffusion-weighted MR imaging for predicting benignity of complex adnexal masses. Eur Radiol. 2009;19:1544–52.

Woodfield CA, Lazarus E, Chen KC, et al. Abdominal pain in pregnancy: diagnosis and imaging unique to pregnancy-review. Am J Roentgenol. 2010;194:14–30.

Christian Bieg and Rahel A. Kubik-Huch

Septic Puerperal Ovarian Vein Thrombosis (SPOVT)

Clinical Background

Septic puerperal ovarian vein thrombosis (SPOVT) is an uncommon (1 of 2000 deliveries), but potentially lethal cause of postpartal fever and sepsis, most commonly reported in women after Cesarean section. The symptoms such as pelvic pain, fever, and elevated infection parameters are unspecific; therefore, imaging plays an important role to diagnose or exclude SPOVT. Common differential diagnoses include other infections, such as urinary tract infections, endomyometritis, infected hematomas after Cesarean section, or adnexal torsion (Kominiarek and Hibbard 2006; Akinbiyi et al. 2009).

Imaging Findings

Ultrasound is the imaging modality of first choice. Typical findings in patients with SPOVT are a dilated and tortuous course of the ovarian vein with evidence of an intraluminal blood clot and absent flow in color doppler ultrasound (CDUS).

In inconclusive cases, due to its availability, CT is often the next imaging modality, showing a dilatation of the ovarian vein itself with contrast-enhancement of the thickened vessel wall and perivascular stranding, the evidence of a hypodense intraluminal blood clot and associated secondary signs like an enlargement of the

uterus and an enhancing parauterin mass as correlate for the pelvic thrombophlebitis (Kubik-Huch et al. 1999; Virmani et al. 2010). If SPOVT is excluded, the adjacent organs can be evaluated. However, radiation dose is relatively high for this young group of female patients in childbearing age.

With the advantage of lack of ionizing radiation, MRI should therefore be the first additional imaging modality in cases of inconclusive ultrasound in patients with suspicion for SPOVT. MRI findings are equal to the other modalities with the additional possibility to differentiate between acute and subacute thrombus due to the signal intensity with a hyperintense signal both on the T1- and T2-weighted images in subacute clots (Virmani et al. 2010) and the assessment of the perivascular inflammatory changes that are best seen on contrast-enhanced T1-weighted fat-suppressed axial scans. With a sensitivity, specificity, and accuracy of 100% (Kubik-Huch et al. 1999), the MRI is the most reliable modality to prove or exclude SPOVT (Fig. 135.1).

Ovarian Torsion

Clinical Background

Ovarian torsion is an uncommon, but potentially life-threatening cause of pelvic pain in women, especially in those of childbearing age. Early diagnosis and treatment is essential to prevent ovarian infarction/necrosis and to allow for organ-preventing surgery. The symptoms, such as unilateral pelvic pain, nausea, vomiting, palpable abdominal mass, and peritoneal signs, are unspecific (Rha et al. 2002; Chang et al. 2008).

C. Bieg (✉) • R.A. Kubik-Huch
Institute of Radiology, Baden, Switzerland

B. Hamm, P. R. Ros (eds.), *Abdominal Imaging*, DOI 10.1007/978-3-642-13327-5_141,
© Springer-Verlag Berlin Heidelberg 2013

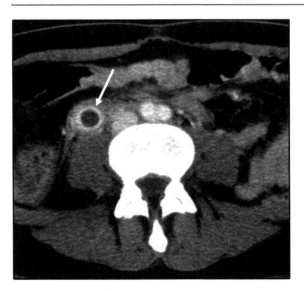

Fig. 135.1 *SPOVT of the right ovarian vein.* Contrast-enhanced CT shows an enlarged diameter of the right ovarian vein with absent flow (*arrow*), enhancement of the wall as well as inflammatory changes of the perivascular tissue

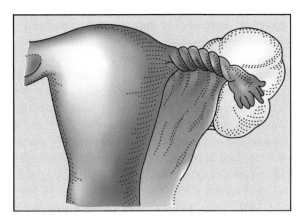

Fig. 135.2 *Ovarian torsion.* Illustration of left-sided ovarian torsion with a twisted vascular pedicle

Common differential diagnoses include appendicitis or follicle rupture.

The pathogenesis is an ovarian rotation around its vascular pedicle, causing a partial or complete obliteration of venous, lymphatic and, in later course or immediately, arterial flow.

In almost all cases, ovarian torsion is associated with an underlying, in some cases bilateral, benign ovarian tumor, for example, a mature cystic teratoma, but, especially in children and adolescents with hypermobility and laxity of ovary fixation. Torsion in

normal ovaries is also possible (Tschirch et al. 2004) and can cause recurrent, unspecific abdominal pain in cases of recurrent ovarian torsion and detorsion.

Imaging Findings

Typical sonographic findings are an enlarged ovary (>4 cm) with edematous stroma and an associated, in some cases bilateral solid, cystic, or mixed tumor. In CDUS, the blood flow may be absent, diminished, or normal (up to 67% of cases), dependent on the degree of vascular (arterial) compression. Associated findings include a dilatated and wall-thickened Fallopian tube (Diameter >10 mm), a deviation of the uterus toward the side of the twisted ovary as well as ascites. In some cases, twisted vascular pedicle can be seen as "whirlpool sign" (Chang et al. 2008) (Fig. 135.2). CT and MRI are indicated in cases with inconclusive ultrasound or as first-line imaging modality of choice in patients with recurrent and unspecific pelvic pain due to recurrent ovarian torsion and detorsion. Further examinations can be performed with contrast-enhanced CT or, due to lack of ionizing radiation preferably MRI. As additional information, CT and MRI may visualize hemorrhage and lack of ovarian enhancement after contrast-administration as suspicious signs of hemorrhagic infarction (Fig. 135.3).

Pelvic Congestion Syndrome

Clinical Background/Patient Management

Insufficiency of ovarian veins is seen in 10% of all women, of whom 60% suffer of dull pelvic pain (Belenky et al. 2002), aggravated after long-standing or postcoitus. The so-called pelvic congestion syndrome (PCS) is a frequent, but often missed diagnosis. Secondary manifestations can be vulval or thigh varicosities due to communications of ovarian vein to the pelvic and vulval venous plexus. Main causes for PCS are absent or incompetent vein valves, often in multiparous women. As an additional contributing factor, an elevated estrogen level is suggested, supported by the fact, that PCS is almost absent in postmenopausal women. Other, rare causes for a secondary ovarian vein insufficiency and PCS are a retroaortal left renal vein or their compression under the superior mesenteric artery, the

Fig. 135.3 *Sagittal T2-weighted MRI of the true pelvis. Left*: Enlarged right ovary with small cysts. Free fluid in the pouch of Douglas. *Right*: Thickened vascular pedicle between the right ovary and the bladder (From Tschirch et al. (2004) with permission)

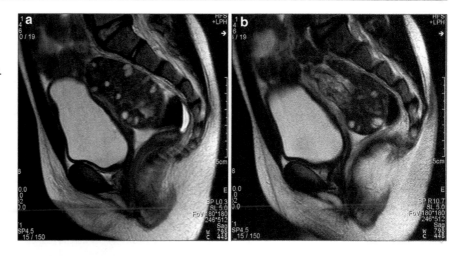

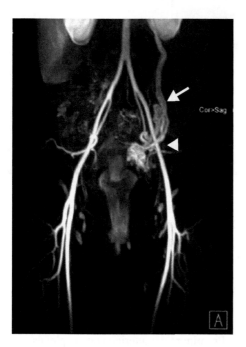

Fig. 135.4 Contrast-enhanced MR angiography, arterial phase: Early enhancement of the dilated and tortuous left ovarian vein (*arrow*) and dilated parauterine venous plexus (*arrowhead*)

so-called nutcracker phenomenon (D'Archambeau et al. 2004). The multidisciplinary diagnostic approach has to exclude other causes for pelvic pain and should encompass a gynecological (e.g., pelvic inflammation, endometriosis), gastrointestinal (e.g., bowel obstruction), and orthopedic (e.g., vertebral or hip-related pain) workup (Ignacio et al. 2008) (Fig. 135.4).

Therapy of choice is the vascular embolization that shows an improvement or complete relief of symptoms

in 68–83% of patients with pelvic pain and PCS (Maleux et al. 2000; Kim et al. 2006) (Fig. 135.5). Rarely (in < 3% of cases), complications like thrombophlebitis or pulmonary embolism of embolic agents (Freedman et al. 2010) were reported. Other treatment options include medical management using gonadotropin receptor agonists or surgical ovarian vein ligation with or without hysterectomy and ovarectomy; however, lower success rates in short- and long-term follow-up compared to embolization have been reported (Ignacio et al. 2008).

Imaging Findings

Imaging modality of first choice is the transabdominal or transvaginal ultrasound with CDUS. Typical findings in patients with PCS are dilatated ovarian veins (>6 mm, PPV 83.3%) with retrograde flow in CDUS and a slight predilection for the left side (Park et al. 2004). A thickened endometrium with dilatated arcuate veins in the myometrium and pelvic varicocele are other sonographic findings in PCS (Adams et al. 1990; Park et al. 2004). As additional information, the examination can be performed with Valsalva maneuvre or in standing position to avoid false negative findings (Freedman et al. 2010).

CT has only an additional role to exclude other causes of pelvic pain and PCS like the "Nutcracker" Syndrome or the retroaortal left renal vein. The insufficient veins can be seen as dilatated tubular vessels with contrast-enhancement. In MRI, especially in MR-venography, a dilatation of the ovarian vein with a diameter

Fig. 135.5 *Left*: Coronal view of a conventional venography with catheter inside the dilatated left ovarian vein and a dilatation of the parauterine venous plexus. *Right*: Coronal view after embolization: Multiple coils inside the left ovarian vein with complete embolization and lack of contrast inside the parauterine vein plexus

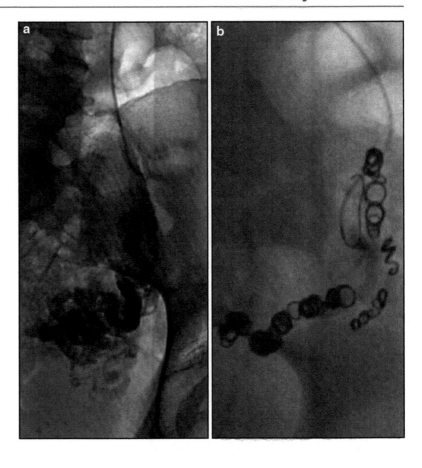

>7 mm, also seen as a normal variant in asymptomatic women, and a dilatation of the parauterin vein plexus, typically hyperintense or, due to the blood flow velocity, iso- or hypointense on T2-weighted images can be visualized (Freedman et al. 2010). Additional information can be obtained using a time-resolved MR-angiography (TR-MRA) to prove the reversed flow in the ovarian veins and to exclude or detect communicating vessels to the internal iliac veins (Kim et al. 2009).

Pearls to Remember

- SPOVT
  - Enlarged ovarian vein
  - Absent flow
  - Perivascular inflammation
- Ovarian torsion
  - Enlarged ovary
  - Twisted vascular pedicle
  - Reduced/absent flow
- Pelvic congestion syndrome
  - Enlarged ovarian vein
  - Retrograde flow
  - Prominent parauterine venous plexus

Appropriateness of Different Imaging Modalities

Due to its availability and the lack of radiation, sonography including CDUS is almost always the first-line imaging modality in evaluation of vascular disorders of the ovaries. In inconclusive cases or for further examinations, cross-sectional imaging, preferably using MRI, can be performed to establish the diagnosis and to exclude other, non-gynecological causes.

References

Adams J, Reginald PW, Franks S, Wadsworth J, Beard RW. Uterine size and endometrial thickness and the significance of cystic ovaries in women with pelvic pain due to congestion. Br J Obstet Gynaecol. 1990;97(7):583–7.

Akinbiyi A, Nguyen R, Katz M. Postpartum ovarian vein thrombosis – two cases and review of literature. Case Report Med. 2009;2009:101367.

Belenky A, Bartal G, Atar E, Cohen M, Bachar GN. Ovarian varices in healthy female kidney donors: incidence, morbidity, and clinical outcome. AJR. 2002;179:625–7.

Chang HC, Bhatt S, Dogra VS. Pearls and pitfalls in diagnosis of ovarian torsion. Radiographics. 2008;28:1355–68.

D'Archambeau O, Maes M, De Schepper AM. The pelvic congestion syndrome: role of the "Nutcracker Phenomenon" and results of endovascular treatment. JBR–BTR. 2004;87:1–8.

Freedman J, Ganeshan A, Crowe PM. Pelvic congestion syndrome: the role of Interventional radiology in the treatment of chronic pelvic pain. Postgrad Med J. 2010;86 (1022):704–10.

Ignacio EA, et al. Pelvic congestion syndrome: diagnosis and treatment. Semin Intervent Radiol. 2008;25(4):361–8.

Kim HS, Malhotra AD, Rowe PC, Lee JM, Venbrux AC. Embolotherapy for pelvic congestion syndrome: long-term results. J Vasc Interv Radiol. 2006;17(2 Pt 1):289–97.

Kim CY, Miller Jr MJ, Merkle EM. Time-resolved MR angiography as a useful sequence for assessment of ovarian vein reflux. AJR Am J Roentgenol. 2009;193(5):W458–63.

Kominiarek MA, Hibbard JU. Postpartum ovarian vein thrombosis: an update. Obstet Gynecol Surv. 2006;61(5):337–42.

Kubik-Huch RA, Hebisch G, Huch R, Hilfiker P, Debatin JF, Krestin GP. Role of duplex colour Doppler ultrasound, computed tomography and MR angiography in the diagnosis of septic puerperal ovarian vein thrombosis. Abdom Imaging. 1999;24(1):85–91.

Maleux G, Stockx L, Wilms G, Marchal G. Ovarian vein embolization for the treatment of pelvic congestion syndrome: long-term technical and clinical results. J Vasc Interv Radiol. 2000;11(7):859–64.

Park SJ, Lim JW, Ko YT, Lee DH, Yoon Y, Oh JH, Lee HK, Huh CY. Diagnosis of pelvic congestion syndrome using transabdominal and transvaginal sonography. AJR Am J Roentgenol. 2004;182(3):683–8.

Rha SE, et al. CT and MR imaging features of adnexal torsion. Radiographics. 2002;22:283–94.

Tschirch FTC, Kubik-Huch RA, Roth K, Wopmann M, Komminoth P, Otto R. Ovarian torsion in childhood. Praxis. 2004;93:1193–6.

Virmani V, Kaza R, Sadaf A, Fasih N, Fraser-Hill M (2010) Ultrasound, computed tomography, and magnetic resonance imaging of ovarian vein thrombosis in obstetrical and nonobstetrical patients. Can Assoc Radiol J.

Irene A. Burger, Susan J. Freeman, and Evis Sala

Multiple imaging techniques can be utilized to evaluate the uterus. Ultrasound is the initial examination of choice to diagnose benign and malignant uterine conditions. Magnetic resonance imaging (MRI) is the best technique for the evaluation of uterine anomalies, treatment planning of leiomyomas, and guiding treatment selection for uterine malignancies. Computerized tomography (CT) and positron emission tomography (PET)/CT have complementary roles with MRI in the staging of advanced cervical carcinoma and evaluating recurrent disease.

Ultrasound

Ultrasound (US) is the primary imaging modality in the initial assessment of the female pelvis and can be performed by a transabdominal or transvaginal approach. It is the initial investigation of choice in patients with acute pelvic pain, postmenopausal bleeding, suspected pelvic mass, and characterization of ovarian masses. It is also the primary imaging modality of choice in the investigation of amenorrhoea and suspected Mullerian tube anomalies.

Ultrasound has become invaluable in guiding a range of invasive procedures. For example,

US-guided biopsy and fluid aspiration (via transabdominal or transvaginal approach) are routinely used in the diagnosis of suspected gynecological malignancy. Following diagnosis, US has a role in guiding transvaginal drain placement and assessing appropriate positioning of brachytherapy devices in the treatment of cervical and endometrial malignancy. Intraoperative US can be utilized to assess completion of uterine evacuation and instrument placement, particularly when preoperative definition of anatomy has been suboptimal.

Saline infusion sonography (sonohysterography) can increase the detection of endometrial abnormalities and significantly increase the accuracy of endometrial sampling in women with peri- or postmenopausal bleeding, from a diagnostic rate of 52% (endometrial biopsy alone) to 89% (sampling following hysterosonography) (Moschos et al. 2009).

Transabdominal US requires a full bladder, as this provides a sonic window for optimal views of the uterus and ovaries. This examination utilizes 3.5 – 5 MHz curvilinear transducers. Transvaginal US is essential for more detailed views of the endometrium and adnexa. The patient must have an empty bladder for close apposition of the probe to the pelvic organs. As the transvaginal probes have higher frequencies of insonation (5–8 MHz), this provides improved image resolution but reduces the depth of field of view. Color, power, and spectral Doppler are used to assess abnormal vascularity.

US has many advantages in routine pelvic imaging:

- It is widely available
- Relatively inexpensive
- Quick
- Portable
- Requires no ionizing radiation or contrast medium

I.A. Burger (✉)
Divison of Nuclear Medicine, Department of Medical Radiology, University Hospital Zurich, Zurich, Switzerland

S.J. Freeman
University Department of Radiology, Addenbrooke's Hospital, Cambridge, UK

E. Sala
Memorial Sloan-Kettering Cancer Center, New York, NY, USA

B. Hamm, P. R. Ros (eds.), *Abdominal Imaging*, DOI 10.1007/978-3-642-13327-5_178,
© Springer-Verlag Berlin Heidelberg 2013

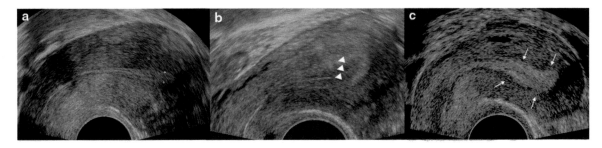

Fig. 136.1 Sagittal transvaginal US images of a normal premenopausal uterus: (**a**) early proliferative phase with well-defined endometrium (*cursors*); (**b**) trilaminar appearance of the endometrium in late proliferative phase, mid-cycle (*arrowheads*); and (**c**) hyperechoic thickening of endometrium in secretory phase (*arrows*)

However, the limitations of US include:

- Operator dependency
- Reduced image quality in obese patients
- Reduced image quality in the presence of overlying bowel gas

Although endovaginal, sonohystero- and endorectal US provide improved spatial resolution, CT or MRI of the pelvis and abdomen have higher sensitivity in the staging of pelvic malignancy, especially for evaluation of metastatic spread. However, US can be useful in assessing complications secondary to tumor, including hydronephrosis, distention of the uterine cavity, ascites and venous thrombosis.

Normal Ultrasound Anatomy

The normal uterus measures between 5 and 9 cm in length and is usually visualized in an anteverted position (in relation to the urinary bladder). The appearance of the endometrium changes throughout the menstrual cycle under the influence of different hormone levels (Fig. 136.1). In the proliferative phase of the cycle, the endometrium is sonographically well defined and may measure up to 8 mm in thickness. In midcycle, the endometrium assumes a trilaminar appearance and may measure up to 12–16 mm. During the secretory phase, the layers become hyperechoic due to the increasing complexity of glandular structure and secretions.

The postmenopausal uterus may decrease in size and an endometrial thickness of 5 mm serves as a threshold for endometrial biopsy (Arger 1992) (Fig. 136.2). An endometrial thickness of up to 8 mm is considered normal for those patients on hormonal therapy (Lin et al. 1991).

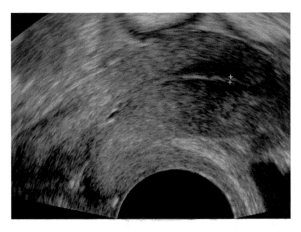

Fig. 136.2 Sagittal transvaginal US image of a postmenopausal uterus, with a normal endometrium thickness of 1 mm (*cursors*)

US is unable to adequately view the cervix and parametrial tissues even on transvaginal views. Clinical examination and Papanicolou smear test remain the gold standard in the detection of early cervical tumors. However, complications of cervical cancer can be readily detected, including parametrial spread causing hydronephrosis and tumor within the endocervical canal producing a distended uterine cavity.

In the normal cervix, anechoic nabothian cysts are commonly seen (Fig. 136.3). The Fallopian tubes are usually not identified unless distended with fluid.

Computed Tomography

Computed tomography (CT) has a limited role in the imaging of the female pelvis due to inherent poor soft tissue contrast. The advent of high-resolution multidetector CT in combination with multiplanar

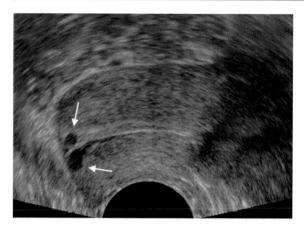

Fig. 136.3 Sagittal transvaginal US image of a normal premenopausal uterus demonstrating anechoic nabothian cysts within the cervix (*arrows*)

reformatting has provided some improvement in delineating pelvic pathology. However, magnetic resonance imaging remains the gold standard in pelvic cross-sectional imaging.

CT is utilized in the staging of advanced endometrial and cervical cancer when magnetic resonance imaging is contraindicated. It is also used to identify peritoneal nodules in serous papillary and clear cell carcinoma of the endometrium. In addition, CT has a role in the staging of uterine sarcomas and the detection of recurrent disease.

Most CT examinations of the abdomen and pelvis are performed following oral and intravenous (IV) contrast medium. Oral contrast medium (iodine-based solution) is consumed over a 48 h period, with the final dose 30 min prior to the CT. This regimen allows opacification of the entire gastrointestinal tract, enabling the radiologist to distinguish between bowel loops, lymphadenopathy, and the pelvic organs. IV contrast medium causes enhancement of blood vessels and viscera, permitting easier identification of lymphadenopathy and parenchymal lesions, particularly within the liver and spleen. Usually a dose of 90–120 mL nonionic, low osmolar iodine-based contrast medium is used at a concentration of 300–370 mg iodine/mL, ideally injected at 2–3 mL/s. Images are subsequently acquired in the portal venous phase, at 70 s postinjection.

Advantages of CT include:

- Fast data acquisition
- High spatial resolution
- Multiplanar reformatting capability

Disadvantages of CT include:

- Use of ionizing radiation
- Lack of tissue contrast within the pelvis
- Risk of renal impairment secondary to IV contrast medium

Before administration of IV contrast medium, the serum creatinine should therefore be determined to calculate the estimated glomerular filtration rate (eGFR). For patients at risk of renal impairment, (GFR < 60 mL/min/1.73 m^2) nephrotoxic drugs should be stopped (for example, nonsteroidal anti-inflammatory drugs, metformin, ACE inhibitors) and prophylactic medication (*N*-acetylcysteine) or pre-hydration should be considered. For patients with a very high risk of renal impairment (GFR < 30 mL/min/1.73 m^2), unenhanced CT or alternative imaging including MRI without contrast or FDG PET/CT could be performed (Goldfarb et al. 2009).

CT imaging utilizes ionizing radiation and therefore the possibility of pregnancy must be excluded prior to pelvic CT. The average dose received from an abdominopelvic CT is 10 mSv.

Recently, research has focused on techniques to reduce the dose received by patients undergoing CT examinations, while maintaining image quality. Automatic tube current modulation can decrease the average radiation dose for an abdominal/pelvic CT by up to 25%, without any reduction of the signal-to-noise ratio (Kalra et al. 2004). Furthermore, preliminary results of phantom studies suggest that iterative reconstruction of CT data could produce a dose reduction of 65%, without impairment of the signal-to-noise ratio (Silva et al. 2010).

Normal Computer Tomography Anatomy

CT examination displays the uterus as a triangular or ovoid soft-tissue structure behind the urinary bladder (Fig. 136.4). On unenhanced images, secretions within the endometrial canal can demonstrate a centrally located decreased attenuation. Following IV contrast medium administration, the myometrium enhances, which helps to delineate the endometrium which remains of lower attenuation.

The cervix has a rounded configuration and enhances less than the myometrium sometimes. This can produce a mass-like appearances which can be mistakenly taken for a cervical tumor. Sagittal

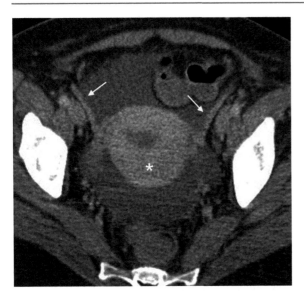

Fig. 136.4 Axial CT image of the pelvis. The presence of ascites helps to define the uterus (*asterisk*) and broad ligaments (*arrows*)

reformats can be helpful to avoid this pitfall if in doubt (Fig. 136.5). At the level of the fornix, the vagina is seen as a flat rectangle. The broad and round ligaments can be seen coursing laterally and anteriorly, respectively (Fig. 136.4). Occasionally, the uterosacral ligaments are depicted as arc-like structures extending from the cervix to the sacrum.

Positron Emission Tomography

Positron emission tomography (PET) and PET/CT has an increasing role in oncological imaging of a wide range of tumors. The most commonly used tracer is a glucose analogue: 2-[^{18}F]-fluoro-2-deoxy-D-glucose (FDG). FDG exploits the accelerated rate of glycolysis common to neoplastic cells to image tumors. For a variety of epithelial tumors, assessment with FDG

PET/CT is finding an increased usage in both staging and treatment response assessment (Cohade et al. 2003; Lardinois et al. 2003; von Schulthess et al. 2006). Although not yet accepted in official gynecological guidelines, there is emerging evidence that FDG PET/CT plays an important role in staging and restaging cervical carcinoma.

For pelvic malignancies, a partial body examination from the head to mid thigh is acquired. Patients need to fast at least 4 h prior to the PET/CT in order to keep insulin levels low. The blood glucose levels must be measured prior to FDG administration. If insulin levels are too high, FDG can be taken up by skeletal muscle, often leading to nondiagnostic examinations. A plasma glucose level of <7 mmol/L is recommended (Boellaard et al. 2010); however, if the study cannot be rescheduled or the patient is diabetic and normoglycemic control is not possible, higher glucose levels can be accepted. After IV injection of 300–700 MBq FDG, the patient needs to rest for 60 min in a warm room to prevent uptake of tracer in muscles and brown fat. As FDG is excreted via the urinary system, the patient is asked to empty their bladder immediately prior to imaging to reduce bladder activity possibly obscuring tracer uptake within the rest of the pelvis. With a PET/CT system, first a low-dose CT for attenuation correction is performed (40–120 mA and 80–140 kV). Afterward the PET acquisition starts, with frame times of 1.5–3 min and 7–8 frames the overall scan time is around 10–25 min. In single PET systems, the attenuation correction is performed with a transmission scan with Germanium (^{68}Ge). Such transmission scans are time-consuming (10 min) and the quality decreases with the decay of Germanium (half-life of 270 days).

The overall radiation burden varies with FDG dose and parameters for attenuation correction. With 350 MBq FDG and CT parameters of 80 mA/140 kV, the overall radiation dose is around 10 mSv (von Schulthess et al. 2006).

$$\text{Standardised Uptake Value (SUV)} = \frac{\text{activity in volume of interest (kBq/mL)} \times \text{body weight (kg)}}{\text{activity administered (MBq)}}$$

To report the activity, the FDG tissue uptake (kBq/mL) is usually divided by the injected dose (MBq) and multiplied with the body weight to obtain the standard uptake value (SUV). This value is supposed to represent metabolic activity of malignant lesions. A change in SUV after treatment therefore reflects metabolic

Fig. 136.5 CT images of the pelvis. (**a**) The cervix (*asterisk*) appears bulky on this axial CT image; (**b**) sagittal reformatted CT image is reassuring with no cervical mass identified

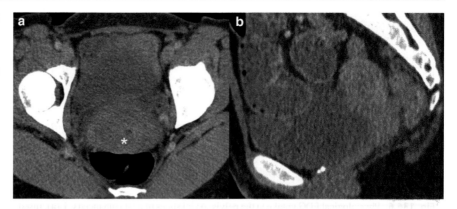

progression or remission. For therapy response assessment the PERCIST criteria suggest a cutoff at 30% decrease in SUV as evidence for partial metabolic response, whereas an increase of 30% is regarded as a progression (Wahl et al. 2009).

Advantages of PET/CT:
- Provides both functional and anatomical data
- Allows accurate detection and staging of tumors
- Permits tumor response assessment
  Disadvantages of PET/CT:
- Use of ionizing radiation (radio-isotope and attenuation correction CT)
- Long acquisition time
- Expensive
- Reduced availability of PET/CT imaging compared with CT or MRI

Normal PET/CT Physiology

FDG uptake and metabolism in both ovaries and uterus change throughout the menstrual cycle. Large studies in healthy volunteers showed increased FDG uptake in the endometrium during the late proliferative and early secretory phase of 56% of all women examined within this period, whereas during menses there was an increased FDG uptake in nearly all women. The mean FDG activity was higher during menses (SUV 4.6 ± 1.0, range 3.5–6.1) than during ovulation (SUV 3.3 ± 0.3, range 2.8–4.0) (Nishizawa et al. 2005) (Fig. 136.6). It is important to note that there is no physiological uptake of FDG in the postmenopausal uterus and ovaries.

Magnetic Resonance Imaging

The role of magnetic resonance imaging (MRI) in gynecology has evolved during the last three decades. MRI is now widely utilized to evaluate female pelvic pathology, due to its superb soft tissue contrast and spatial resolution as well as multiplanar capability. In addition, the lack of ionizing radiation and faster acquisition times (i.e., breathhold and breathing-independent) have increased patient acceptability and improved image quality.

Advantages of MRI imaging:
- Excellent soft tissue contrast and spatial resolution
- No ionizing radiation
- No IV iodinated contrast medium required – patient with renal failure and contrast medium allergy
  Disadvantages of MRI imaging:
- Not suitable for patients with pacemakers and certain metallic implants
- May cause claustrophobia
- Risk of nephrogenic systemic fibrosis secondary to gadolinium chelate administration in patients with renal impairment

Women undergoing pelvic MRI should always be asked a set of questions about hormonal status and previous therapy, as well as foreign bodies, to ensure adequate interpretation of the images. This can be done with a distributed questionnaire (Table 136.1).

Patient preparation and positioning are crucial in obtaining optimal results. Patients should fast for 4–6 h before the MRI examination in order to limit artifacts produced by small bowel peristalsis.

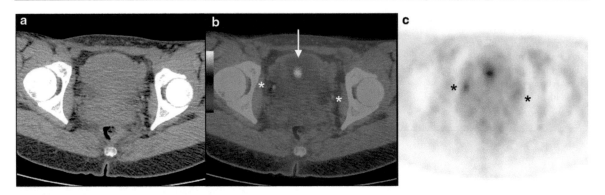

Fig. 136.6 Physiological FDG uptake in the pelvis. Axial slices of an unenhanced CT (**a**), fused PET/CT (**b**), and only PET (**c**) of the pelvis during early secretory phase. Mild FDG uptake in both ovaries (*) and in the uterine cavity (*arrow*) is detectable

Table 136.1 Questionnaire for women undergoing pelvic MRI

Menstrual status:	Premenopausal ☐	Postmenopausal ☐
Date of last period:		
Hormones: (OCP or estrogens)	Yes ☐	No ☐
Pregnancy:	Yes ☐	No ☐
Parity:	Null ☐ Multi ☐ Cesarean ☐	
Foreign bodies: (tampon, IUD, pessary)		
*Previous Surgery**	Yes ☐	No ☐
*Previous Radiotherapy**	Yes ☐	No ☐
*If * yes, Date:*		

Alternatively, an antiperistaltic agent (hyoscine butyl bromide or glucagon) may be administered intravenously before imaging. Ideally, the patient is asked to empty their bladder immediately prior to the MR examination, as a full bladder may degrade T2-weighted images due to ghosting and motion artifacts.

Selection of Coils

Patients are imaged in the supine position using a pelvic surface array multicoil. Use of a phase-array coil increases resolution and decreases imaging time. Endoluminal coils (endorectal and endovaginal) can provide high-resolution images of small tumors of the cervix or those with adjacent parametrial invasion. However, their field of view is limited for the detection of extrauterine extension to adjacent organs.

3.0 Versus 1.5 T MRI

3.0 Tesla (T) MR systems are increasingly implemented in clinical settings. The higher signal-to-noise (SNR) ratio allows either faster acquisition time or higher resolution. In the brain and musculoskeletal systems, this allows a clear benefit for image interpretation. In the abdomen and the pelvis 3.0 T is prone to artifacts, especially due to field heterogeneity which can deteriorate the image quality. This can be reduced with dielectric pads on the patient (water or sonography gel) (Kataoka et al. 2007). Despite the higher resolution in 3.0 T images, the overall accuracy is still considered equivocal compared to 1.5 T (Hori et al. 2009).

Examination Sequences and Imaging Planes

Standard imaging protocols for gynecological MR imaging include axial T1-weighted and T2-weighted images and sagittal T2-weighted images. T1-weighted images are useful in the detection of lymphadenopathy, as well as bone marrow metastases. Fat-saturation T1-weighted images are necessary to distinguish between blood products and fat, which both appear as high signal on T1-weighted images. For example, if T1-weighted imaging reveals an adnexal focus of high intensity, fat suppression will convert the focus to low intensity if fat containing or retain high signal with the presence of blood. Large field of view T1-weighted axial images of the entire pelvis and upper abdomen are essential to evaluate patients for lymphadenopathy in staging gynecological malignancies. T1-weighted gradient echo sequences can be employed as these are faster than spin-echo sequences but produce images of lower quality. The T2-weighted sequence is helpful in demonstrating pathology, as the presence of tumor causes distortion of the normal anatomy and signal characteristics on MR imaging. Coronal T2-weighted images are valuable in evaluating Mullerian duct anomalies and differentiating a pedunculated fibroid from an adnexal mass.

The MR sequences are individually adapted for the suspected/known pelvic pathology. Specific imaging protocols for endometrial and cervical carcinoma are described below.

Intravenous administration of gadolinium is used for staging endometrial carcinoma and distinguishing recurrent tumor from posttreatment fibrosis. Due to reported cases of nephrogenic systemic fibrosis after administration of gadolinium-based intravenous contrast agents, it is recommended to measure serum creatinine before administration and to use only if GFR is over 30 mL/min/1.73 m^2. For patients with impaired renal function, special restrictions and precautions should be considered such as immediate hemodialysis. If possible, alternative MR sequences should be utilized or if administration is deemed necessary, minimal dosing as well as written informed consent about risk and benefit is recommended (Kuo et al. 2007; Shellock and Spinazzi 2008).

Diffusion-weighted MRI (DW-MRI) is a functional method to evaluate the uterus and cervix. It has been shown to improve staging of myometrial invasion in endometrial cancer. In addition, DW-MRI has a role in identifying extrauterine disease and assessing response to chemo-radiotherapy in cervical carcinoma.

Endometrial Carcinoma

In addition to the basic imaging protocol described, high-resolution axial oblique T2-weighted fast spin-echo (FSE) images are acquired parallel to the short axis of the uterine corpus to evaluate the depth of myometrial invasion (Sala et al. 2007). Dynamic multiphase contrast-enhanced T1-weighted sequences through the uterus in the sagittal and axial oblique (parallel to the short axis of the uterine corpus) planes are routinely used to improve staging accuracy in endometrial cancer. The early enhancement phase (0 and 1 min postinjection of IV gadolinium) allows identification of early myometrial invasion, as the subendometrial zone enhances earlier than the bulk of

the myometrium, corresponding to the inner junctional zone (Kinkel et al. 2009). The equilibrium phase (2 min postinjection) allows better evaluation of deep myometrial invasion, while the delayed phase (4–5 min) enables better evaluation of cervical stroma invasion. The interface between tumor and myometrium should be assessed in at least two planes.

Functional imaging with diffusion-weighted magnetic resonance imaging (DW_MRI) has been demonstrated to be both sensitive and specific in the staging of endometrial carcinoma. Accurate assessment of the depth of myometrial invasion can be difficult by morphological criteria; this is seen particularly in polypoid tumors, where there is poor tumor to myometrium contrast, in adenomyosis or poor definition of the junctional zone (common in the postmenopausal uterus). It has been suggested that DW-MRI could replace dynamic contrast-enhanced imaging in staging of endometrial carcinoma (Rechichi et al. 2010; Sala et al. 2010).

Cervical Carcinoma

Cervical tumors are best seen on T2-weighted images, where they are demonstrated as exophytic or infiltrative soft tissue masses, of intermediate signal compared with the low signal of normal cervical stroma. The sagittal plane allows evaluation of tumor extension into the body of the uterus and vagina. The axial oblique T2-weighted FSE (parallel to the short axis of the cervix) enables accurate assessment of parametrial invasion (Balleyguier et al. 2010). The use of IV contrast medium is optional in staging of cervical carcinoma, as it does not improve staging accuracy compared with T2-weighted images (Balleyguier et al. 2010). However, the early phase of enhancement does significantly increase lesion conspicuity compared with T2-weighted images. Dynamic contrast-enhanced MRI (DCE-MRI) is a helpful noninvasive technique for assessing tumor response to treatment. Early increase in tumor perfusion has been shown to correlate with response to chemo-radiotherapy in carcinoma of the cervix (Mayr et al. 1996). Recently, intravenous ultrasmall particles of iron oxide (USPIO) have been shown to improve the detection of lymph node metastases independent of node size in patients with endometrial and cervical cancer (Keller et al. 2004).

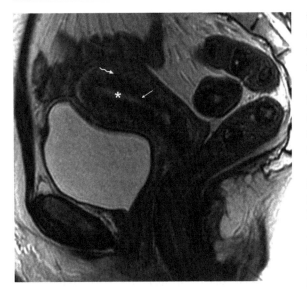

Fig. 136.7 T2-weighted sagittal MR image demonstrates the normal zonal architecture of a premenopausal uterus. The normal endometrium (*asterisk*), junctional zone (*straight arrow*) and myometrium (*curved arrow*) are clearly delineated

Normal MRI Anatomy

Pelvic anatomy is exquisitely demonstrated by MRI (Fig. 136.7). On T1-weighted sequences, the normal pelvic musculature and organs demonstrate homogeneous low to intermediate signal intensity. However, it is the contrast resolution of T2-weighted imaging that is the basis for the superb tissue characterization of MRI. On T2-weighted sequences the uterus, cervix, and vagina exhibit distinct layers of different signal intensity – the so-called zonal architecture.

Three distinct layers can be visualized on T2-weighted images. The endometrium yields high signal intensity. In comparison, the peripheral myometrium yields intermediate signal intensity, which is higher than that of striated muscle. Interposed between these two layers is a narrow band of lower signal intensity, the junctional zone, which corresponds to the innermost myometrium. The signal properties of the junctional zone reflect its lower water content compared with the remainder of the myometrium, which may be a function of its lower extracellular matrix/unit volume (Brown et al. 1991). There is no direct correlation between the three layers seen on MR images and the zonal architecture in sonography (Mitchell et al. 1990). The endometrial thickness varies with the menstrual cycle and measures up to 3 mm in the proliferative phase and up to 7 mm in

the secretory phase, in the sagittal plane. In postmenopausal women not receiving exogenous hormones, uterine zonal anatomy is often indistinct and the endometrium measures less than 5 mm.

Following the administration of intravenous gadolinium the zonal anatomy of the uterus is demonstrated on T1-weighted images. The endometrium and outer myometrium enhance to a greater extent than the junctional zone.

On T2-weighted imaging, the normal cervix demonstrates a central area of high signal intensity representing the endocervical glands and mucus. This is surrounded by low-signal-intensity stroma (elastic fibrous tissue). A rim of intermediate signal intensity similar to that of myometrium is seen around the periphery of the cervix due to the presence of smooth muscle. Occasionally, intermediate signal intensity cervical mucosal folds (plicae palmatae) can be seen interposed between the low-signal-intensity cervical stroma and the high-signal-intensity endocervical canal. In the cervical stroma hyperintense glandular cysts (nabothian cysts) can be visualized on T2-weighted images.

After the administration of IV gadolinium, the inner cervical mucosa and outer smooth muscle enhance more than the fibrocervical stroma. The parametrial tissues, vaginal walls, and submucosa also enhance with intravenous contrast medium.

References

Arger PH. Transvaginal ultrasonography in postmenopausal patients. Radiol Clin North Am. 1992;30(4):759–67.

Balleyguier C, Sala E, Da Cunha T, et al. Staging of uterine cervical cancer with MRI: guidelines of the European Society of Urogenital Radiology. Eur Radiol. 2010;21(5):1102–10.

Boellaard R, O'Doherty MJ, Weber WA, et al. FDG PET and PET/CT: EANM procedure guidelines for tumour PET imaging: version 1.0. Eur J Nucl Med Mol Imaging. 2010;37(1):181–200.

Brown HK, Stoll BS, Nicosia SV, et al. Uterine junctional zone: correlation between histologic findings and MR imaging. Radiology. 1991;179(2):409–13.

Cohade C, Osman M, Leal J, Wahl RL. Direct comparison of (18)F-FDG PET and PET/CT in patients with colorectal carcinoma. J Nucl Med. 2003;44(11):1797–803.

Goldfarb S, McCullough PA, McDermott J, Gay SB. Contrast-induced acute kidney injury: specialty-specific protocols for interventional radiology, diagnostic computed tomography radiology, and interventional cardiology. Mayo Clin Proc. 2009;84(2):170–9.

Hori M, Kim T, Murakami T, et al. MR imaging of endometrial carcinoma for preoperative staging at 3.0 T: comparison with imaging at 1.5 T. J Magn Reson Imaging. 2009;30(3):621–30.

Kalra MK, Maher MM, Toth TL, et al. Strategies for CT radiation dose optimization. Radiology. 2004;230(3):619–28.

Kataoka M, Isoda H, Maetani Y, et al. MR imaging of the female pelvis at 3 Tesla: evaluation of image homogeneity using different dielectric pads. J Magn Reson Imaging. 2007;26(6):1572–7.

Keller TM, Michel SC, Frohlich J, et al. USPIO-enhanced MRI for preoperative staging of gynecological pelvic tumors: preliminary results. Eur Radiol. 2004;14(6):937–44.

Kinkel K, Forstner R, Danza FM, et al. Staging of endometrial cancer with MRI: guidelines of the European Society of Urogenital Imaging. Eur Radiol. 2009;19(7):1565–74.

Kuo PH, Kanal E, Abu-Alfa AK, Cowper SE. Gadolinium-based MR contrast agents and nephrogenic systemic fibrosis. Radiology. 2007;242(3):647–9.

Lardinois D, Weder W, Hany TF, et al. Staging of non-small-cell lung cancer with integrated positron-emission tomography and computed tomography. N Engl J Med. 2003;348(25):2500–7.

Lin MC, Gosink BB, Wolf SI, et al. Endometrial thickness after menopause: effect of hormone replacement. Radiology. 1991;180(2):427–32.

Mayr NA, Yuh WT, Magnotta VA, et al. Tumor perfusion studies using fast magnetic resonance imaging technique in advanced cervical cancer: a new noninvasive predictive assay. Int J Radiat Oncol Biol Phys. 1996;36(3):623–33.

Mitchell DG, Schonholz L, Hilpert PL, Pennell RG, Blum L, Rifkin MD. Zones of the uterus: discrepancy between US and MR images. Radiology. 1990;174(3 Pt 1):827–31.

Moschos E, Ashfaq R, McIntire DD, Liriano B, Twickler DM. Saline-infusion sonography endometrial sampling compared with endometrial biopsy in diagnosing endometrial pathology. Obstet Gynecol. 2009;113(4):881–7.

Nishizawa S, Inubushi M, Okada H. Physiological 18 F-FDG uptake in the ovaries and uterus of healthy female volunteers. Eur J Nucl Med Mol Imaging. 2005;32(5):549–56.

Rechichi G, Galimberti S, Signorelli M, Perego P, Valsecchi MG, Sironi S. Myometrial invasion in endometrial cancer: diagnostic performance of diffusion-weighted MR imaging at 1.5-T. Eur Radiol. 2010;20(3):754–62.

Sala E, Wakely S, Senior E, Lomas D. MRI of malignant neoplasms of the uterine corpus and cervix. Am J Roentgenol. 2007;188(6):1577–87.

Sala E, Rockall A, Rangarajan D, Kubik-Huch RA. The role of dynamic contrast-enhanced and diffusion weighted magnetic resonance imaging in the female pelvis. Eur J Radiol 2010;76(3):367–85.

Shellock FG, Spinazzi A. MRI safety update 2008: part 1, MRI contrast agents and nephrogenic systemic fibrosis. Am J Roentgenol. 2008;191(4):1129–39.

Silva AC, Lawder HJ, Hara A, Kujak J, Pavlicek W. Innovations in CT dose reduction strategy: application of the adaptive statistical iterative reconstruction algorithm. Am J Roentgenol. 2010;194(1):191–9.

von Schulthess GK, Steinert HC, Hany TF. Integrated PET/CT: current applications and future directions. Radiology. 2006;238(2):405–22.

Wahl RL, Jacene H, Kasamon Y, Lodge MA. From RECIST to PERCIST: Evolving Considerations for PET response criteria in solid tumors. J Nucl Med. 2009;50(Suppl 1): 122S–50.

Congenital Uterine Anomalies

Penelope Moyle and Evis Sala

Introduction

Congenital uterine abnormalities (Müllerian duct anomalies) are a diverse and complex group of conditions which not only challenges the radiologist in obtaining optimal imaging but also in their interpretation. Many congenital uterine abnormalities will be detected incidentally and have no impact of the patient. They may present at menarche with an obstructed uterus or later in life if there are investigations for fertility or miscarriages. It must be remembered that these diagnosis can arouse painful emotions and or have life changing effects. Detailed anatomical imaging is paramount for patient management and for the planning of any surgical procedure aimed to reestablish normal anatomy and/or fertility.

This chapter will discuss the incidence, embryology, and classification and imaging modality available for the interpretation of congenital uterine abnormalities. Each individual condition will be discussed in detail to provide a comprehensive overview of congenital uterine abnormalities for the clinical Radiologist.

Epidemiology

The true incidence of uterine abnormalities is difficult to assess as studies have differences in data acquisition, and populations groups. A large meta-analysis of

P. Moyle (✉)
Department of Radiology, Hinchingbrooke Hospitals NHS Trust, Huntingdon, Cambridgeshire, UK

E. Sala
Memorial Sloan-Kettering Cancer Center, New York, NY, USA

573,138 women by Nahum (Nahum 1998) reported that uterine anomalies were identified in 0.17% of fertile women and 3.5% of infertile women (P < 0.00001). Overall the prevalence in the general population was 0.5%. The majority of women with congenital uterine abnormalities can naturally conceive but there is a significantly higher miscarriage rate, premature delivery, and abnormal fetal presentation at delivery.

The cause of congenital uterine abnormalities is considered to be sporadic or multifactorial, although environmental factors such as ionizing radiation, thalidomide, and diethylstilbestrol (DES) can also affect the developing genital tract.

Embryology

At 6 weeks of fetal life both male and female genital tracts have paired paramesonephric (Müllerian) ducts and mesonephric (Wolffian) ducts. In females the mesonephric ducts degenerate and by 12 weeks the paired paramesonephric ducts fuse from the vaginal plate, forming the primordial body of the uterus and the unfused lateral arms of the paramesonephric ducts form the Fallopian tubes (Moore and Persaud 1998). Initially separated by a septum the paramesonephric ducts fuse at their inferior margin to form a single lumen uterovaginal canal. The uterine septum regresses by apoptosis mediated by the lack of expression of the BCL-2 gene (Lee et al. 1998). If apoptosis does not occur there is a persistent septum. The upper 80% of the vagina is formed from the uterovaginal canal. The lower 20% is derived from the sinovaginal bulbs of the primitive urogenital

B. Hamm, P. R. Ros (eds.), *Abdominal Imaging*, DOI 10.1007/978-3-642-13327-5_179,
© Springer-Verlag Berlin Heidelberg 2013

sinus. The uterovaginal canal remains separate from the sinovaginal bulb by the horizontal vaginal plate. During third to fifth fetal months the vaginal plate lengths and contacts the urogenital sinus to form the hymen. The hymen usually ruptures in the perinatal period. The ovaries are derived from mesoderm, mesenchyme, and primordial germ cells (gonadal tissue) and their formation is separate process from the mesonephric or paramesonephric ducts. Therefore ovarian development is not usually associated with Mullerian duct abnormalities.

The urinary and genital system both arise from the dorsal mesodermal ridge. Abnormal differentiation of the mesonephric and paramesonephric ducts may also be associated with renal anomalies such as crossed ectopia, cystic renal dysplasia, duplex collecting systems, or renal agenesis. It is therefore important to image the urinary tract for presence of congenital uterine anomalies.

Imaging Techniques to Assess Congenital Uterine Abnormalities

Ultrasound

For the assessment of congenital uterine anomalies, imaging in the secretory phase (15–28 days typically) gives better delineation of the endometrium as the thickness and echogenicity is at its greatest to help delineate morphology (Caliskan et al. 2010).

Ultrasound examination should be performed both transabdominal and transvaginal.

Many studies have demonstrated 3D sonography with image reconstruction (Ghi et al. 2009) to be highly accurate in the assessment of uterine anomalies due to their surface and transparent reconstructions allowing accurate uterine contours and volumes to be produced. Bermejo (2010) compared 3D ultrasound with magnetic resonance imaging and found a very good concordance (kappa 0.88) with the relationship between cavity and fundus being visualized equally well with both techniques. Both 2D and 3D ultrasound should be complemented by careful gynecological exploration in order to identify any alterations in the cervix as this can be difficult to interpret.

Magnetic Resonance Imaging (MRI)

Magnetic resonance imaging (MRI) is the method of choice for evaluation of congenital uterine anomalies (Carrington et al. 1990). It can also be more acceptable to younger women or girls in which a transvaginal examination would not be appropriate. MRI is still more expensive and time consuming than CT or ultrasound but its spatial and contrast resolution with the lack of ionizing radiation make this technique suitable for the study of the female pelvis. MRI has the ability of volumetric and multiplanar acquisitions which are tools of unique utility in the characterization of the congenital anomalies of the female reproductive organs. The acquisition of oblique planes is very important in congenital uterine abnormalities: the axial oblique plane (parallel to the short axis of the uterus and perpendicular to the long axis of the uterus), and the coronal oblique plane (parallel to the long axis of the uterus and perpendicular to the short axis of the uterus). These will identify septa and the planes of the uterine horns. A coronal T2 of the abdomen is very helpful to exclude associated congenital renal anomalies.

Hysterosalpingography (HSG)

Hysterosalpingography (HSG) is the radiographic evaluation of the uterine cavity and fallopian tubes by fluoroscopic imaging of contrast medium. It is used predominantly in the evaluation of infertility and hence often diagnoses congenital uterine anomalies. The examination provides information on the endometrial canal and tubal patency. HSG has a number of limitations. It cannot evaluate non patent horns (rudimentary horns) or the external contour of the uterus. There can be difficulties in distinguishing a complete septate from a bicornuate uterus and if only one cervix is cannulated, differentiating a unicornuate from a didelphys uterus. There is also exposure to ionizing radiation which is also a consideration in young women (Simpson et al. 2006).

Table 137.1 The key features of uterovaginal congenital abnormalities as classified by the American Society of Reproductive Medicine

Congenital abnormality	Mullerian duct classification Buttram & Gibbons/American fertility Society AFS	Ovaries	Fallopian tubes	Uterus	Upper 2/3rds vagina	Lower 1/3rd vagina	Other features
Uterine agenesis/hypoplasia	Class I	Majority normal	Absent	Absent/hypoplastic	Absent	Present	
MRKH syndrome	Class I	Present	Present	Absent/hypoplastic	Absent	Present	Associated renal & skeletal abnormalities & deafness
Unicornuate uterus	Class IIa-d depending on presence of rudimentary horn	Present	Present	One uterine horn	Present	Present	Rudimentary horn present 65% cases
Uterus didelphys	Class III	Present	Present	Complete duplication of uterine horns and cervices	Present	Present	Longitudinal vaginal septum in 75%
Uterus bicornuate	Class IVa-b	Present	Present	Incomplete fusion fundal myometrium	Present	Present	Always a communication between the uterine horns
Septate uterus	Class V	Present	Present	Fibrous septum between the two uterine horns	Present	Present	No uterine fundal cleft
Arcuate uterus	Class VI	Present	Present	Smooth indentation of fundal endometrial canal			No division of uterine horns, normal fundal contour
In utero DES exposure	Class VII	Present	Shortened, sacculations, stenosis	Hypoplastic narrow, irregular, constriction bands	Present	Present	Uterine length not exceeding 6 cm
Vaginal septae		Present	Present	Present	Fibrous septum	Fibrous septum	Possible associated hematometrocolpos

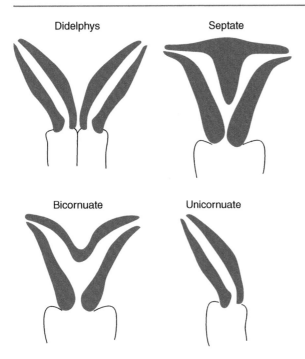

Fig. 137.1 A schematic illustration of the fundamental uterine anomalies

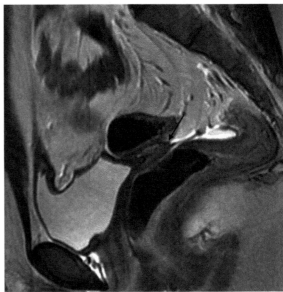

Fig. 137.2 Uterine hypoplasia: sagittal T2-weighted image demonstrates a small fibrous remnant (*black arrow*) where the uterus would be expected

Classification of Uterine Anomalies

Uterovaginal congenital anomalies can be described upon the different degrees of non-fusion or non-resorption of the Mullerian ducts and vaginal plate development. This classification was first described by Buttram and Gibbons in 1979 and modified by the American Fertility Society in 1988 (now called the American Society of Reproductive Medicine). This is the most widely accepted classification and the key features of each condition are summarized in Table 137.1. A schematic illustration of the fundamental uterine anomalies is demonstrated in Fig. 137.1.

Uterine Agenesis or Hypoplasia (Class I)

The nondevelopment or rudimentary development of the Mullerian ducts results in uterine agenesis or hypoplasia in a 46XX karyotype females. It comprises 5–10% of Mullerian duct anomalies. The uterus can either be hypoplastic or absent (agenesis), with only a fibrous remnant and veins present where the uterus was expected (Fig. 137.2). Rarely a contracted endometrial cavity is present resulting in hematometra at puberty. The upper 2/3 of the vagina is absent or atretic in both uterine hypoplasia and agenesis.

An important key feature is that the ovaries are normal in the majority of these patients, although they may be situated more cranially in the lower quadrants of the abdomen. This distinguishes the condition from gonadal dysgenesis, androgen insensitvity syndrome, and pseudohermaphrodites (male).

Mayer–Rokitansky–Kuster–Hauser (MRKH) syndrome encompasses vaginal and uterine agenesis or hypoplasia with intact ovaries and Fallopian tubes. There are associated anomalies of the urinary tract (40–50%), skeletal system (10–12%), and deafness (10–25%) (Pittock et al. 2005). Inguinal hernias are frequently seen in these patients.

Two subsets of MRKH syndrome exist: Type I (90%) encompasses vaginal agenesis and uterine agenesis but the fallopian tubes and ovaries are normal. Type II (10%) encompasses vaginal agenesis and uterine hypoplasia with two separate uterine horns which may be symmetric or asymmetric and rarely associated with functioning endometrium. There is hypoplasia of one or both fallopian tubes but the ovaries are normal. MRKH is the second most common cause of primary amenorrhea.

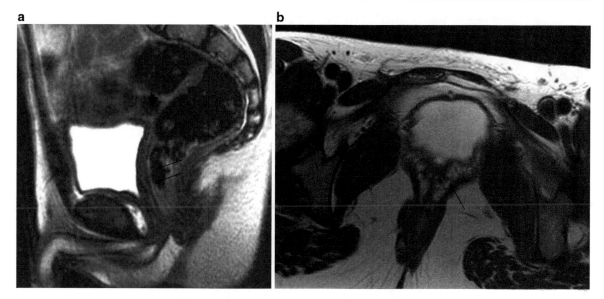

Fig. 137.3 Mayer–Rokitansky–Kuster–Hauser (MRKH) syndrome. (**a**) Sagittal T2-W image demonstrating agenesis of the uterus (*black arrowhead*). The lower vagina is present (*black arrows*). (**b**) Axial T2-W image demonstrates a bulge at the posterior aspect of the bladder (*black arrow*) due to the absent vaginal tissues. The rectum is now posterior to the bladder

HSG has no role in the evaluation of uterine agenesis or hypoplasia.

On ultrasound a normal uterus cannot be identified at the vagina apex. A hypoplasic uterus without an echogenic endometrium may be seen. Vaginal hypoplasia or agenesis will be evident from the prior clinical examination.

MRI is the best imaging modality to assess the extent of the aplasia/hypoplasia and the degree of development of the lower vagina (Fig. 137.3). It is important not to mistake connective tissue or veins around a fibrous remnant for a uterus or likewise a vagina. The uterus is defined as hypoplastic when it is small in size, with an atrophic endometrium and the myometrium has a lower than expected signal intensity on T2-weighted images. Rarely the T1-weighted image will identify high signal intensity hematometra in a contracted endometrial cavity. A fast acquisition through the upper abdomen is useful to assess the presence of both kidneys. The role of MRI is to describe the anatomy for the reconstructive surgical planning and to differentiate MRKHS from vaginal aplasia, which is the result of failure of the vaginal plate to form or cavitate; in this case the uterus has a normal anatomy. Women with uterine agenesis or hypoplasia cannot carry a pregnancy, but in vitro fertilization and surrogacy is still possible for these women, and for this reason is useful to localize normal ovaries.

Unicornuate Uterus (Class II)

The unicornuate uterus occurs when one Mullerian duct fails to elongate or develop causing an asymmetric uterus with or without a small rudimentary horn. It comprises of approximately 20% of Mullerian duct anomalies with an associated rudimentary horn in 65% of cases. The rudimentary horn may have an endometrial cavity (32%) which can be communicating (10%), or non-communicating (22%) with the dominant cavity. A small atretic fallopian tube is usually seen if a rudimentary horn is present (Troiano and McCarthy 2004). Both ovaries are present with a normal cervix and vagina.

Overall the above subdivides the classification into Class IIa – unicornuate with cavity and communicating rudimentary horn. Class IIb – unicornuate with cavity, and non-communicating rudimentary horn. Class IIc – unicornuate with no cavity. Class IId – unicornuate with no communicating horn.

Patients with unicornuate uterus may be asymptomatic and an incidental finding.

They may present at puberty with cyclical pain if there is an obstructed endometrial cavity. There is an increased risk of endometriosis in patients with an obstructed horn possibly due to retrograde expulsion of menstrual products. Normal pregnancy can occur

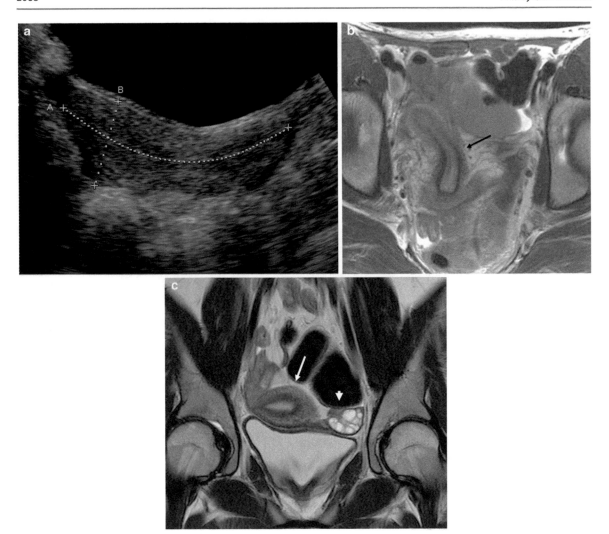

Fig. 137.4 Unicornuate uterus. (**a**) Transabdominal US (longitudinal section) showing a unicornuate uterus. The "banana" or fusiform appearance can be difficult to appreciate on ultrasound. (**b**) Axial T2-W image in the same patient demonstrating a unicornuate uterus (*black arrow*) which has a "banana" shaped single uterine horn. (**c**) A coronal T2-W image demonstrates only the right uterine horn which deviates from the midline (*white arrow*). The left ovary is normal (*white arrowhead*)

but there is an increased rate of spontaneous abortions, premature birth, and abnormal fetal lie. Many functional non-communicating horns present during or after the third decade of life with acute obstetric uterine rupture (Jayasinghe et al. 2005) and, therefore, surgical removal before pregnancy is recommended.

Renal anomalies are more commonly associated with unicornuate uterus than any other Müllerian duct anomaly and can be seen in approximately 40% of cases. Ipsilateral renal aplasia is the commonest (67%) but horseshoe kidney, cystic dysplasia, duplex systems are also described (Fedele et al. 1996).

HSG imaging may demonstrate a small cervix and contrast medium fills a fusiform or "banana" shaped endometrial cavity shifted off the midline. One fallopian tube will fill. A rudimentary horn may fill with contrast medium only if communicating and, therefore, HSG cannot assess non-communicating horns.

On ultrasound a unicornuate uterus can be difficult to detect as the elliptical shape can be difficult to appreciate. The midline shift of the uterus can be helpful but careful inspection is needed to identify both cornu. A rudimentary horn can be mistaken for a leiomyoma (Fig. 137.4).

Fig. 137.5 Uterus didelphys. Coronal T2-W image demonstrates two divergent uterine horns and cavities (*black arrows*) with two cervices seen in the same plane. There is no communication between the two uterine cavities. The normal right ovary can be identified on this image (*thick black arrowhead*)

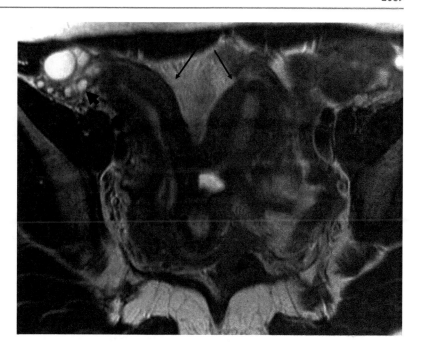

MRI is the imaging of choice if a unicornuate uterus is suspected. It can assess if there is a rudimentary horn containing endometrium, a communication to the main endometrium or complications of the rudimentary horn such as a hematocolpos. MRI is also the best anatomical map prior to surgery if the remnant is to be removed. A unicornuate uterus is curved and elongated with tapering of the fundal segment off the midline ("banana" shaped), with a normal uterine zonal anatomy (endometrium, junctional zone, and peripheral zone) (Fig. 137.4). The rudimentary horn, if present, has low signal intensity on T2-weighted images. The optimal sequence to demonstrate a unicornate uterus is the FSE T2WI axial oblique (long axis) view. The optimal sequence to demonstrate a rudimentary horn is the FSE T2WI coronal oblique (short axis) view. T1WI with fat saturation post intravenous Gadolinium administration may help demonstrate a rudimentary horn if the T2WI is indeterminate.

Uterus Didelphys (Class III)

Uterus didelphys occurs when two Müllerian ducts develop normally but they fail to fuse giving complete duplication of uterine horns and cervices with no communication between the duplicated endometrial or endocervical cavities (8). It comprises of approximately 5% of Müllerian duct anomalies and a longitudinal vaginal septum is associated in 75% of these anomalies. Occasionally there may be associated complications of a transverse vaginal septum which causes obstruction and hematocolpos. Patients with this condition may be completely asymptomatic but again there is an increased spontaneous abortion and premature births. There is an increased risk of endometriosis if there is an obstruction due to retrograde menstrual flow.

Care must be taken when performing an HSG because if only one cervix is cannulated the appearances would be of a unicornuate uterus with one fallopian tube. Both cervices must be cannulated to demonstrate two fusiform separate endometrial and endocervical canals.

Ultrasound demonstrated widely divergent uterine horns with two distinct cervices and no connecting endometrium.

A uterus didelphys is best appreciated on MRI, with coronal oblique T2-weighted images. In this plane it is possible to image the two uterine horns and the two cervices with normal appearance of the endometrial and myometrium layers (Fig. 137.5).

The longitudinal vaginal septum is optimally imaged with a short axis view of the vagina. A transverse septum can be present occasionally which is best demonstrated on axial oblique T2-weighted images. If the transverse

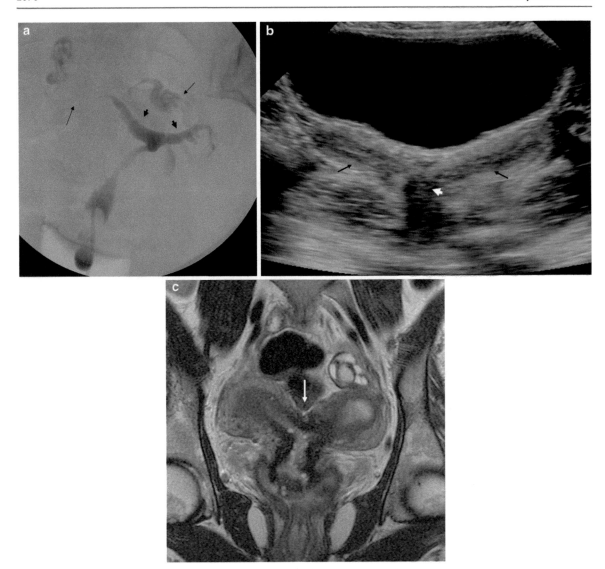

Fig. 137.6 Bicornuate uterus. (**a**) HSG examination demonstrates widely divergent horns (*black arrowheads*) with an intercornual angle >105° and an intercornual distance >4 cm. There is a communication between the uterine horns and only one cervix is identified (bicornuate unicollis). Each fusiform horn has a single fallopian tube (*thin black arrows*). (**b**) Transvaginal ultrasound of a bicornuate uterus (different patient). There is a large fundal cleft >1 cm with widely divergent symmetric horns (*black arrows*) and normal bilateral symmetrical endometrial complexes which communicate (*white arrow*). (**c**) Coronal T2-W image (different patient) demonstrates a concave uterine fundal contour >1 cm (*white arrow*) between divergent uterine horns with an intercornual distance >4 cm. The endometrial cavities are normal. One cervix is identified and the appearances are of a bicornuate unicollis uterus

septum causes obstruction with hematocolpos and/or hematometrocolpos, the T1W images before and after fat saturation demonstrates the high SI blood products. A single shot fast spin echo (SSFSE) coronal T2WI of the abdomen is recommended to assess the kidneys for any associated congenital anomalies.

Uterus Bicornuate (Class IV)

Partial fusion of normally developed Mullerian ducts result in the presence of bicornuate uterus. It comprises of approximately 10% of Mullerian duct anomalies.

There is incomplete fusion of the fundal myometrium with a fundal cleft >1 cm separating divergent but symmetrical uterine horns. There are two subdivisions of this class:.Class IVa demonstrates a fundal cleft extending to the internal os. Class IVb demonstrates a fundal cleft variable in length ending proximal to the internal os. There must be a communication between the uterine horns to make the diagnosis. A bicornuate uterus may be associated with only one cervix (bicornuate unicollis) or with two cervices (bicornuate bicollis).

Patients with a bicornuate uterus have higher risk for pregnancy loss, preterm delivery, and malpresentation with a spontaneous abortion rate of approximately 30% (Rackow and Arici 2007).

HSG demonstrates widely divergent horns with an intercornual angle >105° and an intercornual distance >4 cm suggestive of a bicornuate uterus. Each fusiform horn has a single fallopian tube (Fig. 137.6). As only the endometrial cavities are assessed and not the external uterine contour there can be a similar appearance to a septate uterus on a HSG. The septate uterus usually has an acute angle between the uterine horns (<75%) (Braun et al. 2005) but as these different entities have different treatments and prognoses further imaging should be sought to clarify the appearances.

Ultrasound images demonstrate a large fundal cleft >1 cm with widely divergent symmetric horns and normal bilateral symmetrical endometrial complexes (Fig. 137.6). Care must be sought if there is extreme anteversion, retroflexion, or leiomyomas as this can make the fundus appearance convex.

The T2WI coronal oblique plane is very useful to demonstrate the fundal cleft, wide divergence, and normal zonal anatomy with the two endometrial cavities communicating which is essential for the diagnosis (Fig. 137.6).

Septate Uterus (Class V)

The septate uterus is the most common Müllerian duct abnormality comprising of approximately 55% of Mullerian duct anomalies. It results from the normal development of the Müllerian ducts but with incomplete resorption of the final fibrous septum between the two uterine horns. The extension of the fibrous septum is variable and may reach the external cervical os. Unlike the bicornuate uterus the septate uterus does not have a fundal cleft, its uterine fundal contour being flat, convex, or mildly <1 cm concave (Mueller et al. 2007). This key point helps to differentiate between the septate and bicornuate uterus which have different surgical procedures. This differentiation is also clinically relevant as the septate uterus has the worst obstetric outcome of all Müllerian duct anomalies with a high abortion rate and pregnancy complication rate compared to bicornuate uterus (Rackow and Arici 2007). These complications are related to the lack of blood supply to the fibrous septum and the length of septum does not correlate with the obstetric outcome. The septum can be removed at hysteroscopy which significantly increases the chance of at term pregnancy.

As described above there is a significant degree of overlap between the findings on HSG of a septate uterus and bicornuate uterus. A septate uterus on HSG demonstrates an acute angle between the contrast filled endometrial cavities, and the cavities are smaller and narrow than a bicornuate uterus (Fig. 137.7). There is only 55% accuracy for differentiating a septate from a bicornuate uterus on HSG (Reuter and Daly 1989).

Transvaginal ultrasound demonstrates echogenic endometrial cavities separated at the fundus by the intermediate echogenicity fundal myometrium without a cleft. The septum is a fibrous hypoechoic structure (Fig. 137.7). If a coronal oblique image (true orthogonal view along the long axis of the uterus) can be obtained and a line drawn between the apices of the endometrial cavities at the ostia of the fallopian tubes, the fundus will be > 5 mm over this line. A bicornuate uterus would have its prominent fundal cleft below or at or <5 mm above this interostial line. It is the relationship of the fundal cleft that helps distinguish the two entities.

MRI best demonstrates the presence of the fibrous septum on the coronal oblique T2-weighted images. This allows the fundal contour to be assessed as described above. The superior segment of septum is isotense with the myometrium while the lower septum demonstrates low SI fibrous tissue. The septum can be complete (Fig. 137.7) or partial (Fig. 137.7). A SSFSE coronal T2WI image to assess the kidneys for associated anomalies is recommended.

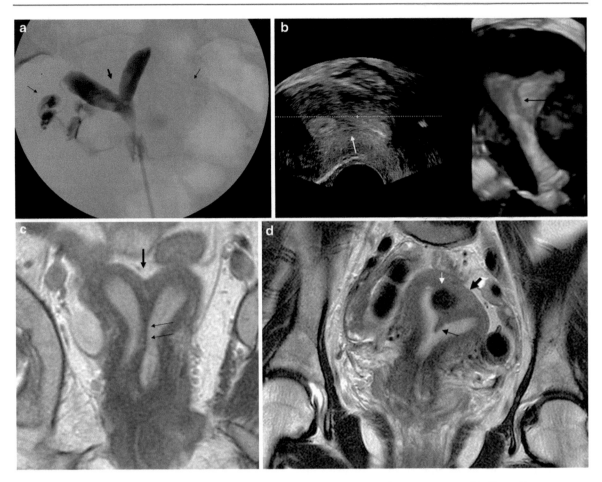

Fig. 137.7 Septate uterus. (**a**) HSG examination demonstrates an acute angle between the contrast-filled endometrial cavities (*thick black arrow*). Both fallopian tubes are present (*thin black arrows*). Since HSG examination does not outline the fundal myometrium to evaluate a cleft, care must be taken interpreting the images as differentiation between a bicornuate uterus and septate uterus can be challenging. (**b**) 2D transvaginal ultrasound (*left hand-side image*) demonstrates echogenic endometrial cavities separated at the fundus by the intermediate echogenicity fundal myometrium without a cleft (*white arrow*). 4D reconstructed ultrasound (*right hand-side image*) of the same uterus demonstrating a septum as a thin linear fibrous structure (*black arrow*). (**c**) Coronal oblique T2-weighted image (different patient) demonstrates a low SI complete fibrous septum (*thin black arrows*). Only a small fundal indentation (*thick black arrow*) is noted and the uterine horns are not divergent. (**d**) Coronal oblique T2-weighted image (different patient) demonstrates a small low SI incomplete fibrous septum (*thin black arrow*). There is no fundal indentation (*thick black arrow*). An incidental leiomyoma is noted in the fundal myometrium (*white arrow*)

Arcuate Uterus (Class VI)

An arcuate uterus is caused by mild focal thickening of the uterine fundal myometrium with a minor indentation of the endometrial cavity.

HSG demonstrates a single cavity with broad saddle shaped indentation of endometrium at the fundus. If the ratio of fundal height to length between the cornu is less than 10% an adverse reproductive outcome is not expected (Wolfman and Ascher 2006).

Ultrasound demonstrates a normal uterine contour but a broad fundal indentation of normal myometrium.

Coronal oblique imaging best demonstrates the MRI mild focal thickening of the uterine fundal myometrium as described (Fig. 137.8).

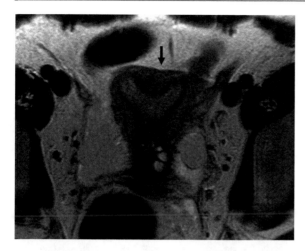

Fig. 137.8 Arcuate uterus. A Coronal oblique T2-weighted image demonstrates mild focal thickening of the uterine fundal myometrium (saddle shaped fundus) with a minor indentation of the endometrial cavity (*black arrow*)

Anomaly Associated with In Utero Exposure of Diethylstilbestrol (DES) (Class VII)

Diethylstilboestrol is a synthetic estrogen given to women experiencing spontaneous abortion, premature deliveries, and other pregnancy complications between 1948 and 1971. Clear cell carcinoma of the cervix was found to be associated with its use and hence it was discontinued, but DES was also found to affect the embryologic development of the female genital tract. Not all the daughters of women will have problems as it is dependent on the dose and when it was administered (second trimester most damaging). However, DES exposed women are less likely than unexposed women to have full-term live births and more likely to have had premature births, spontaneous pregnancy losses, or ectopic pregnancies (Kaufman et al. 2000).

HSG demonstrates a small "T" shaped endometrial cavity and constriction bands (thickening of the junctional zone). The fallopian tubes may be short, irregular with sacculations and the endocervical canal may be stenosed and cannulation difficult. HSG is the best imaging tool to demonstrate these findings if clinically suspected.

At ultrasound it can be difficult to appreciate the classic "T" shaped endometrium and constriction bands but the length of the uterus does not exceed 6 cm.

T2-weigted MRI best appreciates the "T" shaped endometrial cavity and focal thickened junctional zone to give indentations of constriction bands (Kaufman et al. 1980).

Vaginal Septae

Abnormal fusion of the Mullerian ducts with the vaginal bulb gives rise to a transverse vaginal septum. If there is obstruction, the vaginal bulb becomes dilated and may contain fluid, debris or blood (hematocolpos) or with distention of the endometrium (hematometrocolpos). The septum most commonly is identified at the junction of the middle and upper third of the vagina and can be obstructive or nonobstructive in nature. Obstructive vaginal septae may present at menarche with severe abdominal or pelvic pain and there is an increased risk of endometriosis due to the retrograde flow of menstrual products.

HSG does not have a role to evaluate transverse vaginal septae.

Ultrasound can identify a hematometrocolpos (distended vagina and endometrium) as a cystic mass with low level internal echoes of blood products surrounded by the myometrial wall. The actual septum may be difficult to appreciate as a low echogenic fibrous transverse line.

MRI is the imaging modality of choice. The septum is best characterized on the sagittal T2-weighted image by low signal intensity fibrous tissue septa with loss of normal vaginal zonal anatomy. T1-weighted images with fat suppression are useful to assess the presence of blood products within a hematometrocolpos (Miller and Breech 2008) (Fig. 137.9).

Complete Androgen Insensitivity Syndrome

Complete androgen insensitivity syndrome (CAIS) or testicular feminization syndrome is not a congenital uterine anomaly but patients have often been raised as female until investigation for primary amenorrhea discovers the true diagnosis.

It is caused by complete end organ resistance to androgens and the patients have a 46XY karyotype

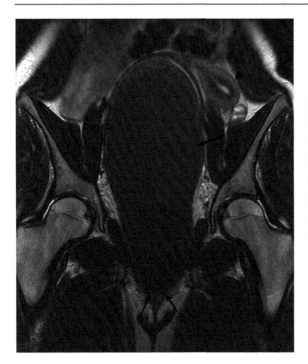

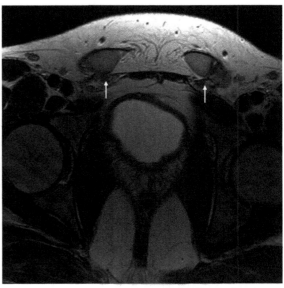

Fig. 137.9 A Coronal T2-weighted image demonstrates a low SI vaginal septum (*double black arrows*) causing obstruction to the vagina. The normal uterus (*black arrowhead*) is displaced superiorly and to the left by the much distended vagina (*single black arrow*). The obstructing low signal intensity vaginal septum is causing a hematocolpos (*double black arrow*)

Fig. 137.10 T2-W axial image demonstrates bilateral oval intermediate signal masses within the inguinal canals (*white arrows*). They are hyperintense to muscle and hypointense relative to fat with a low SI rim on T2-weighted imaging. These are undescended testes within the inguinal canals. No male external genitalia was identified and the patient had a diagnosis of complete androgen insensitivity

with functioning testes but a female phenotype. With the absence of Mullerian duct derivatives there is agenesis of the uterus, fallopian tubes, and upper 2/3 of the vagina. The testes are present, although usually undescended with 70% along the common or external iliac chains, 25% in the inguinal canal, and 5% in the retroperitoneum. It is important to search for testes as there is an increased risk of germ cell tumors developing in the undescended testes (risk of tumor increases to 10% at puberty and peaks 30% by 50 years).

MRI is the imaging modality of choice is the diagnosis is suspected to confirm the absent uterus, fallopian tubes, and ovaries. The testes have a signal intensity typically hyperintense to muscle, hypointense relative to fat but lower than normal gonads. A low SI rim on T2-weighted imaging is helpful to distinguish the gonads from lymph nodes (Oakes et al. 2008) (Fig. 137.10).

Pearls to Remember

– Renal anomalies are commonly associated with congenital uterine anomalies.
– Unicornuate uterus can have a rudimentary horn which is communicating or non-communicating.
– Unicornuate uterus has a "banana" shaped endometrial cavity shifted off the midline with one ipsilateral fallopian tube.
– Uterus didelphys has widely divergent uterine horns with two distinct cervices and non-communicating endometrium-associated vaginal septum 75% of cases.
– Bicornuate uterus has widely divergent horns, large fundal cleft, intercornual angle >105°, and intercornual distance >4 cm. There is a communication between the uterine horns.
– Septate uterus does not have a fundal cleft, its uterine fundal contour being flat, convex, or mildly <1 cm concave. It usually has an acute angle between the uterine horns (<75%).

- There is only 55% accuracy for differentiating a septate from a bicornuate uterus on HSG.
- Transverse vaginal septum can cause hematocolpos or hematometrocolpos.

References

Bermejo C, Martínez Ten P, Cantarero R, Diaz D, Pérez Pedregosa J, Barrón E, Labrador E, Ruiz López L. Three-dimensional ultrasound in the diagnosis of Müllerian duct anomalies and concordance with magnetic resonance imaging. Ultrasound Obstet Gynecol. 2010;35(5):593–601.

Braun P, Grau FV, Pons RM. Enguix DP Is hysterosalpingography able to diagnose all uterine malformations correctly? A retrospective study. Eur J Radiol. 2005;53(2):274–9.

Buttram Jr VC, Gibbons WE. Müllerian anomalies: a proposed classification. (An analysis of 144 cases). Fertil Steril. 1979;32(1):40–6.

Caliskan E, Ozkan S, Cakiroglu Y, Sarisoy HT, Corakci A, Ozeren S. Diagnostic accuracy of real-time 3D sonography in the diagnosis of congenital Mullerian anomalies in high-risk patients with respect to the phase of the menstrual cycle. J Clin Ultrasound. 2010;38(3):123–7.

Carrington BM, Hricak H, Nuruddin RN, et al. Mullerian duct anomalies: MR imaging evaluation. Radiology. 1990;176:715–20.

Fedele L, Bianchi S, Agnoli B, Tozzi L. Vignali M Urinary tract anomalies associated with unicornuate uterus. J Urol. 1996;155(3):847–8.

Ghi T, Casadio P, Kuleva M, Perrone AM, Savelli L, Giunchi S, Meriggiola MC, Gubbini G, Pilu G, Pelusi C. Pelusi G Accuracy of three-dimensional ultrasound in diagnosis and classification of congenital uterine anomalies. Fertil Steril. 2009;92(2):808–13.

Jayasinghe Y, Rane A, Stalewski H, Grover S. The presentation and early diagnosis of the rudimentary uterine horn. Obstet Gynecol. 2005;105(6):1456–67.

Kaufman RH, Adam E, Binder GL, Gerthoffer E. Upper genital tract changes and pregnancy outcome in offspring exposed in utero to diethylstilbestrol. Am J Obstet Gynecol. 1980;137(3):299–308.

Kaufman RH, Adam E, Hatch EE, Noller K, Herbst AL, Palmer JR, Hoover RN. Continued follow-up of pregnancy outcomes in diethylstilbestrol-exposed offspring. Obstet Gynecol. 2000;96(4):483–9.

Lee DM, Osathanondh R, Yeh J. Localization of Bcl-2 in the human fetal müllerian tract. Fertil Steril. 1998;70(1):135–40.

Miller RJ, Breech LL. Surgical corrections of vaginal anomalies. Clin Obstet Gynecol. 2008;51:223–36.

Moore KL, Persaud TV (1998) The urogenital system: the development of the genital system. The Developing Human. Clinically orientated embryology 6th ed. Philadelphia: Saunders, 1998.303

Mueller GC, Hussain HK, Smith YR, et al. Müllerian duct anomalies: comparison of MRI diagnosis and clinical diagnosis. AJR Am J Roentgenol. 2007;189:1294–302.

Nahum GG. Uuterine anomalies. How common are they, and what is their distribution among subtypes? J Reprod Med. 1998;43(10):877–87.

Oakes MB, Eyvazzadeh AD, Quint E, Smith YR. Complete androgen insensitivity syndrome-a review. J Pediatr Adolesc Gynecol. 2008;21:305–10.

Pittock ST, Babovic-Vuksanovic D, Lteif A. Mayer-Rokitansky-Küster-Hauser anomaly and its associated malformations. Am J Med Genet A. 2005;135(3):314–6.

Rackow BW, Arici A. Reproductive performance of women with müllerian anomalies. Curr Opin Obstet Gynecol. 2007;19(3):229–37.

Reuter KL, Daly DC. Cohen SM Septate versus bicornuate uteri: errors in imaging diagnosis. Radiology. 1989; 172(3):749–52.

Simpson Jr WL, Beitia LG, Mester J. Hysterosalpingography: a reemerging study. Radiographics. 2006;26(2):419–31.

The American Fertility Society classifications of adnexal adhesions, distal tubal occlusion, tubal occlusion secondary to tubal ligation, tubal pregnancies, müllerian anomalies and intrauterine adhesions. Fertil Steril. 1988; 49(6):944–55.

Troiano RN, McCarthy SM. Mullerian duct anomalies: imaging and clinical issues. Radiology. 2004;233(1):19–34.

Wolfman DJ, Ascher SM. Magnetic resonance imaging of benign uterine pathology. Top Magn Reson Imaging. 2006;17:399–407.

Patricia Noël and Caroline Reinhold

Introduction

Benign uterine conditions of myometrial or endometrial origin are frequent and an accurate diagnosis is mandatory in order to provide the patient the best treatment alternatives. Although transvaginal ultrasound (TVS) remains the primary imaging modality in their assessment, magnetic resonance imaging (MRI) has an added value, acting as a problem-solving tool in several conditions, as well as being a reproducible imaging modality for follow-up when conservative therapy is chosen. The following conditions will be discussed specifically: adenomyosis, leiomyomas, endometrial hyperplasia, and polyps.

Adenomyosis

Adenomyosis is the presence of ectopic endometrial glands and stroma embedded within the myometrium. This induces a hypertrophic reaction to surrounding smooth muscle cells which is another important element of the diagnosis. Its actual prevalence remains unknown. Detection rate in past surgical series varies from 5% to 70% (Azziz 1989). The most commonly used criteria at pathology for depth of penetration of endometrial glands is 2 mm. The prevalence increases as the number of sections increases. Studies that have sectioned the uterus systematically every 1 cm have found the prevalence to be as high as 70%. A clinical and pathological distinction is made between superficial and deep adenomyosis (Azziz 1989). In the superficial form of adenomyosis, the ectopic endometrial glands and stroma reside within the inner myometrium, and are unlikely to cause symptoms. In the deep form, the ectopic glands and stroma invade the myometrium deeply and there is a correlation with uterine enlargement and symptoms. The adenomyotic endometrial glands do not typically undergo cyclical bleeding, reflecting the predominance of endometrial zona basalis which is relatively refractory to hormonal stimuli. The exact etiology of adenomyosis is unknown. The hypothesis of a basement membrane defect at the endometrial-myometrial interface has been suggested, as well as endometrial glands migration through lymphatic or vascular channels (Griffin et al. 2010). Risk factors have been described inconsistently, and include hereditary factors, uterine trauma from childbirth or abortion, chronic endometritis, and hyperestrogenemia. Women are affected during their reproductive and perimenopausal years, most commonly during the fifth and sixth decades (Ascher et al. 2003). Although adenomyosis may be asymptomatic, pelvic pain, hypermenorrhea, and uterine enlargement have been described as clinical symptoms and signs. Symptoms have been shown to correlate with the extent of the disease.

Clinical diagnosis of adenomyosis cannot be made reliably, as it may mimic several other conditions such as uterine leiomyomas, endometriosis, and dysfunctional uterine bleeding. While historically the treatment of severe adenomyosis has been

P. Noël (✉)
Department of Radiology, Universite Laval, Quebec, Canada

C. Reinhold
Department of Radiology, McGill University Health Center, Montreal General Hospital, Montreal, Quebec, Canada

B. Hamm, P. R. Ros (eds.), *Abdominal Imaging*, DOI 10.1007/978-3-642-13327-5_180,
© Springer-Verlag Berlin Heidelberg 2013

hysterectomy, conservative treatment and emerging uterine sparing surgical techniques have been described, making an accurate diagnosis of the condition even more important. Hormonal treatment such as levonorgestrel intrauterine device has been demonstrated equivalent to hysterectomy in controlling hemoglobin level and health-related quality of life, but with superior effect on psychological and social life (Ozdegirmenci et al. 2011). Uterine artery embolization (UAE), initially thought to be ineffective for adenomyosis, has shown to cause significant clinical and symptomatic improvements on a short- and long-term basis in more than 75% of patients (Popovic et al. 2011). Ultrasound-guided high-intensity focused ultrasound ablation is under investigation with promising results (Zhou et al. 2011).

Several studies have addressed the capabilities of transvaginal ultrasound (TVUS) versus MRI in the diagnosis of adenomyosis. Reinhold et al. have demonstrated endovaginal ultrasound to be as accurate as MRI at diagnosing diffuse adenomyosis with sensitivities and specificities of 89% for both modalities (Reinhold et al. 1996). Another study, although involving a smaller group of patients, concluded that MRI was better ($p < 0.02$) at diagnosing adenomyosis than TVUS. The study did not use real-time US, which can account for the lower sensitivity of US in their series (Ascher et al. 1994). Bazot et al. showed similar accuracy of TVUS and MRI for the diagnosis of adenomyosis, except when other conditions such as leiomyomas were associated, in which cases MRI was superior than TVUS (Bazot et al. 2001). In a recent systematic review assessing test accuracy for detection of adenomyosis, pooled sensitivity and specificity of TVUS were 72% and 81% and of MRI 77% and 89%, respectively (Champaneria et al. 2010).

Transvaginal ultrasound characteristics of adenomyosis include: (1) ill-defined areas of heterogeneous myometrial echotexture, caused by echogenic islands of heterotopic endometrial tissue surrounded by hypoechoic smooth muscle, (2) asymmetric thickening of anterior or posterior myometrial wall, (3) subendometrial cysts, (4) subendometrial echogenic linear striations and (5) poor definition of the endometrial-myometrial junction (Reinhold et al. 1996, 1999) (Fig. 138.1a). The presence of myometrial cysts in a poorly defined area with abnormal echotexture is highly specific of the diagnosis, although its sensitivity does not exceed 40–60%.

At color Doppler, blood vessels follow their vertical course in myometrial areas of involvement, in comparison to fibroids, where they are located at the periphery of the lesions. The limitations of US remain body habitus and lack of reproducibility due to operator experience. Recently, the performances of 2D-TVUS and 3D-TVUS have been compared for the diagnosis of adenomyosis, resulting in similar accuracy, specificity, and likelihood ratio, but in significantly greater sensitivity and negative predictive value for 3D-TVUS (Exacoustos et al. 2011). At sonohysterography, the same signs as for TVUS are present, in addition to myometrial cracks, which are seen as elongated tracks of fluid extending from the endometrial cavity in the myometrium.

MRI criteria for the diagnosis of adenomyosis rely on T2-weighted (T2W) sequences, where lesions mostly consist of low SI areas, frequently giving an appearance of diffuse or focal thickening of the junctional zone. This reflects the smooth muscle hyperplasia accompanying the heterotopic endometrial tissue. The junctional zone, which corresponds to the inner myometrium, is normally of low signal intensity. Junctional zone thickness ≥ 12 mm has been demonstrated to be the optimal cut-off value for diagnosing adenomyosis in both premenopausal and postmenopausal patients (Reinhold et al. 1996). A junctional zone < 8 mm typically excludes the disease. When the junctional zone thickness is between 8 and 12 mm, ancillary findings such as relative thickening of the junctional zone in a localized area, poorly defined borders, and high signal intensity foci on T1-weighted (T1W) and T2W sequences suggest the presence of adenomyosis (Reinhold et al. 1999). Bright T2W foci in areas of low signal intensity in the myometrium are seen in 50% of patients. They represent islands of heterotopic endometrial tissue, cystic dilatation of herniated glands, or hemorrhagic foci. Linear striations of high signal intensity radiating out from the endometrium into the myometrium may be seen as well, representing direct invasion of the endometrium into the myometrium. These striations may become coalescent resulting in an appearance of pseudo-widening of the endometrium. Areas of hemorrhage within glands represented by high signal intensity spots on T1W imaging are less frequently observed. Their occurrence is not well understood, since in adenomyosis, the basal layer of the endometrium is involved, and not the functional layer, and the

Fig. 138.1 (a) Sagittal transvaginal ultrasound (TVUS) shows heterogeneous myometrium in an enlarged uterus. There are linear hypoechoic strands (*arrow*) in a patient with adenomyosis. (b) Axial T2WI in the same patient shows thickening of the junctional zone in the dorsal myometrium with high SI foci (*arrow*) representing heterotopic endometrium in keeping with focal adenomyosis. (c) Axial T1WI with fat suppression at the same level shows heterogeneous aspect of the involved myometrium with tiny high SI foci (*arrow*) representing hemorrhage within the endometrial glands. Also noted are bilateral ovarian endometriomas (*asterisks*). (d) Sagittal T1W FS with intravenous gadolinium shows heterogeneous enhancement of the involved myometrium with hypoenhancement of the heterotopic endometrial glands (*arrows*) giving the characteristic "swiss-cheese" appearance

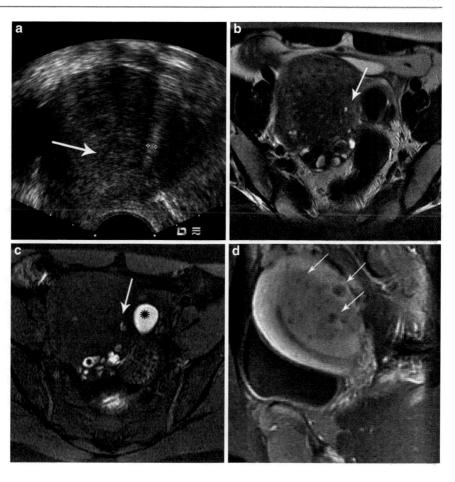

herniated glands are relatively refractive to hormonal stimuli. After extracellular gadolinium contrast agent administration, the wall of the endometrial glands may enhance, but the cystically dilated glands lumen do not, and this may give a swiss-cheese appearance to the myometrium (Ascher et al. 2003) (Figs. 138.1b, c, d and 138.2a, b).

Adenomyosis may be focal (Fig. 138.2b) or diffuse, but other subtypes, such as adenomyomas and cystic adenomyosis, may occur. Cystic adenomyosis is a subtype of adenomyosis resulting from hemorrhage in a focus of adenomyosis. It manifests as a well-circumscribed, cystic myometrial mass, which exhibits signs of hemorrhage at different stages on MR imaging. It is typically surrounded by a low T2W SI rim (Fig. 138.3b, c, d). Adenomyoma is a nodular form of adenomyosis, which on MRI appears as a well-circumscribed mass with foci of high signal intensity on T2W sequences (Fig. 138.3a). Small foci of hemorrhage may appear as areas of increased signal

on the T1W sequences. Adenomyomas can be submucosal, intramural, or subserosal.

Adenomyosis must be differentiated from leiomyomas, since treatment options vary. There can be imaging overlap between focal adenomyosis or adenomyomas and leiomyomas, but MRI helps in making this distinction. The appearance favors focal adenomyosis when the lesion has poorly defined margins, when it is elliptical and extends along the endometrial line, and when it has little mass effect on the endometrium relative to its size (Togashi et al. 1989). Pitfalls to avoid are the presence of myometrial contractions, which can be differentiated from adenomyosis by their transient nature as well as changing appearance over time. Myometrial contractions tend to focally distort the endometrial line (Fig. 138.2d), which is not the case with focal adenomyosis. The junctional zone thickness and appearance varies during the menstrual cycle, and decreased signal of the myometrium during the

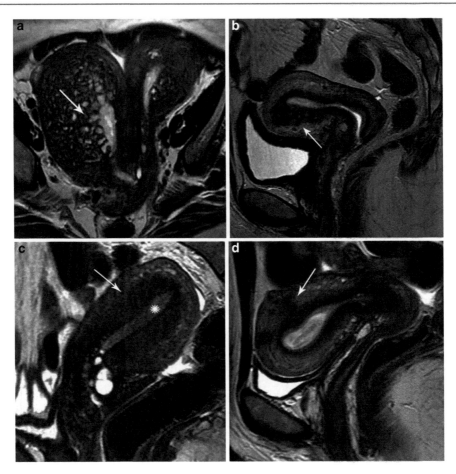

Fig. 138.2 (a) Axial T2WI shows asymmetric thickening of the junctional zone in a patient with didelphic uterus. There are hyperintense linear striations (*arrow*) extending from the endometrium into the myometrium representing endometrial glands. The findings are consistent with diffuse adenomyosis. (b) Sagittal T2WI in a different patient shows focal thickening (arrow) of the junctional zone at the ventral aspect of the myometrium containing bright foci, corresponding to focal adenomyosis. (c) Sagittal T2WI in a patient during her menstrual phase shows low signal intensity of the endometrium (*asterisk*) in keeping with blood. Junctional zone (*arrow*) appears ill defined and thickened which is due to uterine peristalsis. (d) Sagittal T2WI shows an ill-defined low signal intensity focus in the myometrium (*arrow*) which exerts mass effect on the endometrium but not on the outer myometrial contour. This was not observed on other acquisitions on the same patient and was consistent with a transient myometrial contraction

menstrual-early proliferative phase may cause apparent widening of the junctional zone (Fig. 138.2c). As such, MR imaging for adenomyosis is optimally performed in the late proliferative phase (Takeuchi et al. 2010).

Leiomyomas

Leiomyomas or fibroids are the commonest female genital tract neoplasm. They occur in 20–30% of reproductive aged females. They are benign and histologically consist of smooth muscle cells arranged in a whorl-like pattern with a variable amount of collagen, extracellular matrix, and fibrous tissue. They are well demarcated by a pseudocapsule of areolar tissue. They are estrogen-receptive tumors; thus, they can increase in size during pregnancy or with the use of oral contraceptive pills and shrink after menopause. Most of them occur in the uterine corpus and are classified according to their location. They can be intramural (the most common, within the substance of the myometrium), subserosal (beneath the serosa, when more than 50% of the volume extends outside the uterine contour), or submucosal (projecting within the endometrial canal, the most symptomatic,

Fig. 138.3 (a) Sagittal T2WI in another patient shows a diffusely enlarged uterus. There is an ill-defined posterior and fundal hypointense myometrial mass (*arrow*) that is distinct from the junctional zone and contains foci of high signal intensity. It mildly distorts the uterine contour. This is consistent with adenomyoma. Partly seen is a hematosalpinx (*asterisk*) on the superior aspect of the uterus. (b) Axial T2WI in another patient shows a myometrial mass (*arrow*) consisting of a low intensity rim with hyperintense center. (c) On the corresponding axial T1WI with fat suppression the center is high signal (*arrow*). This is consistent with cystic adenomyosis. (d) Sagittal TVUS in a different patient shows a subserosal myometrial cyst (*arrow*) with a thick wall that proved to be cystic adenomyosis

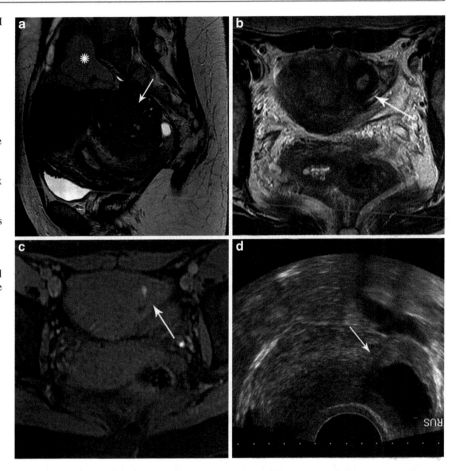

associated with dysmenorrhea, menorrhagia, and infertility) (Ascher et al. 2003). Less frequently, they can occur in the uterine cervix (5%), the broad ligament, or even completely detached from the genital tract where they parasitize the abdominal vasculature. As they enlarge, they may outgrow their blood supply, resulting in ischemia and degeneration that can be hyaline, cystic, myxoid, fatty, hemorrhagic (red or carneous), and sarcomatous (Ueda et al. 1999). Most women with uterine leiomyomas are asymptomatic. When symptomatic, they can present with abnormal uterine bleeding, but pressure symptoms, pain, infertility, miscarriage, and palpable mass may occur, as well as acute torsion.

According to a study by Duelhom et al. (2002), MRI and US are equally accurate in ascertaining the presence of leiomyomas, but MRI is superior for the mapping of individual leiomyomas, especially when they are numerous (more than 4) and of increased volume (more than 375 ml). MRI was also superior in this series in defining uterine embedment and position of leiomyomas, irrespective of the number or size of lesions. TVUS may be limited by acoustic shadow generated by leiomyomas that limit visualization of subjacent lesions, as well as by a very large uterus that extends outside the field of view (Dueholm et al. 2002). In a recent paper comparing US and MR before uterine artery embolization, MR was more accurate than US in characterizing uterine leiomyomas (Rajan et al. 2011). MRI also has capabilities in differentiating pedunculated leiomyomas from adnexal masses, as well as focal adenomyosis and transient myometrial contractions from leiomyomas. Moreover, MRI may also allow assessment of the ovaries in patients with enlarged uterus where clinical assessment is unsatisfactory.

The initial imaging modality of choice for assessment of uterine leiomyomas is ultrasound. TVUS allows better evaluation of the endometrium and submucosal fibroids than transabdominal US, especially in obese patients and when there is overlying bowel gas. US shows an enlarged uterus, with contour abnormalities as well as focal masses that are of variable echogenicity (usually hypoechoic, but can also be iso- to hyperechoic as well). There may be shadowing from calcification. The echogenicity of leiomyomas may vary when there is internal degeneration such as anechoic areas in cystic degeneration or echogenic areas due to calcification or hemorrhage. The sensitivity of ultrasound is operator dependent and has been reported to range from 63% to 99% (Dueholm et al. 2002). Limitations of TVUS include mapping of leiomyomas in very large uteri as well as detection of subserosal leiomyomas. A combined transabdominal and transvaginal US approach is sometimes warranted in patients with large myomatous uteri. US sometimes fails at differentiating leiomyomas from adenomyosis.

Because of its limited tissue contrast, CT is not useful in the evaluation of uterine leiomyomas unless they are calcified.

MRI has excellent soft tissue contrast resolution, and is therefore the imaging modality of choice for pretreatment planning (Dueholm et al. 2002), as well as for follow-up after conservative therapy. Typical leiomyomas will manifest on MRI as sharply marginated masses of lower signal intensity than the myometrium on T2W sequences, with a variable degree of enhancement, typically slightly less than the myometrium. Their signal will vary according to the presence or absence of associated degeneration. Sixty percent of leiomyomas will show very low T2W signal intensity, with little enhancement representing various degree of hyaline degeneration (Fig. 138.4a, b) (Ueda et al. 1999). Edema, although not a proper type of degeneration, is often present and will manifest as high signal intensity on T2W imaging in a leiomyoma, that will enhance after contrast administration. This also characterizes the hypercellular subtype of leiomyoma (Fig. 138.4c), which consists of compact smooth muscle cells without intervening collagen. Cystic degeneration will manifest as round areas of low T1W signal intensity and high T2W signal intensity without enhancement (Fig. 138.5). Myxoid degeneration (gelatinous material) will result in areas of bright T2W signal intensity with mild delayed enhancement. Red degeneration appears as a bright signal intensity mass on T1W with low signal intensity on T2W, and absence of enhancement (Fig. 138.6). Leiomyosarcomas are rare occurrences. In a large series of hysterectomies performed for presumed benign leiomyomas, their frequency was reported as

0.11% and 0.49% (Takamizawa et al. 1999). Although most leiomyosarcomas are thought to arise de novo, case reports have shown histological transition from benign to malignant leiomyomas. Imaging criteria for differentiating one from the other are poorly validated. From a small retrospective study, several MR features are associated with an increased likelihood of malignancy, including greater than 50% high T2W signal intensity, tiny bright T1W foci, well-demarcated nonenhancing lesions within a mass, indistinct borders, and invasion of adjacent structures (Tanaka et al. 2004) (Fig. 138.7). Rapid enlargement of an apparent leiomyoma is also a poor predictor of malignancy, and in the absence of organ invasion or nodal disease, an indeterminate uterine mass is more likely an atypical leiomyoma than a leiomyosarcoma (Ueda et al. 1999). There may also be a role of diffusion-weighted imaging and ADC measurement in differentiating benign cellular and degenerated leiomyomas from leiomyosarcomas (Tamai et al. 2008).

Presence of calcifications may be manifested by signal voids on MR, although these voids are nonspecific and may as well represent fast flowing blood.

MR may differentiate a subserosal leiomyoma from an adnexal mass. It is the most accurate imaging modality in differentiating a leiomyoma from adenomyosis (Weinreb et al. 1990).

Hysterectomy has for a long time been the treatment modality of choice for uterine fibroids, but medical conservative therapies and minimally invasive therapies have developed in recent years. The use of GnRH antagonists to induce a medical menopause is widespread, and can be considered either as a treatment or as a mean of size reduction before definitive therapy. Decrease in size by 30–60% as well as reduction in blood flow has been reported under this therapy (Weeks et al. 1999). Laparoscopic and hysteroscopic myomectomy are conservative alternative therapies. A precise delineation with MRI of the thickness of the myometrium surrounding the leiomyoma allows adequate surgical planning. Uterine artery embolization (UAE) has been extensively used since 1995. The procedure involves femoral artery catheterization, cannulation of the uterine arteries and injection of particles, leading to ischemia of fibroids and subsequently reducing their size. All large series comparing UAE to hysterectomy have favored embolization over hysterectomy in terms of efficacy (80–90% symptoms

Fig. 138.4 (a) On this sagittal T2WI, there is diffuse thickening of the junctional zone (*arrow*) consistent with diffuse adenomyosis. There is a concomitant subserosal leiomyoma (*asterisk*) manifested by a well-defined hypointense mass distorting the uterine contour. (**b**) On this sagittal T1WI FS after gadolinium, there is no enhancement in the central portion of the leiomyoma (*asterisk*) in keeping with hyaline degeneration. The thickened junctional zone enhances slightly less (*arrow*) than the myometrium. (**c**) Sagittal T2WI shows a myometrial mass (*arrow*) that is of intermediate signal intensity with a peripheral area of low signal intensity. This mass is consistent with an intramural leiomyoma that proved to be cellular (it did enhance intensely after gadolinium [not shown]). (**d**) Sagittal T2WI shows a high SI subserosal mass (*white arrow*) as well as a pedunculated endocavitary hypointense mass (*black arrow*). These are consistent with a subserosal pedunculated leiomyoma as well as pedunculated submucosal leiomyoma. (**e**) Sagittal T2WI in the same patient after hysteroscopic resection of the endocavitary leiomyoma and uterine artery embolization. There is no residual endocavitary lesion. The subserosal leiomyoma (*arrow*) has reduced in size, but still shows an intermediate signal intensity and appeared to regrow after the procedure

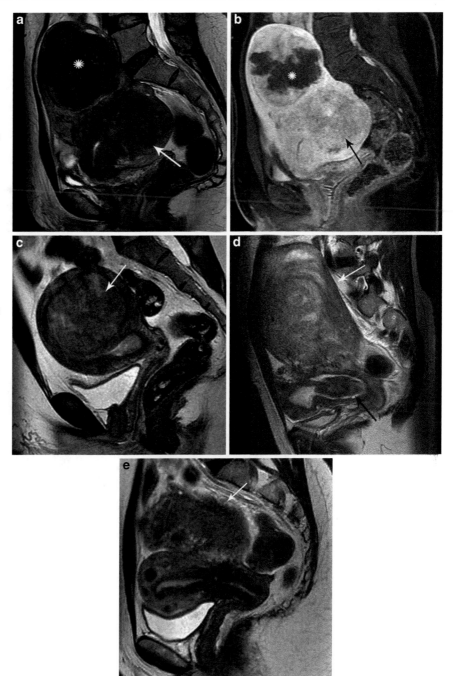

reduction for menorrhagia, pain, and bulk-related symptoms) and rate of complications (1–4%) (Spies et al. 2004).

MR-guided focused ultrasound therapy is increasingly used with good results so far, 75% reduction of symptoms (Shen et al. 2009).

MRI may help in the selection of the type of invasive treatment (i.e., myomectomy versus hysterectomy

versus UAE) (Fig. 138.4d, e). Hemorrhagic or necrotic leiomyomas do not respond to UAE and are best treated by myomectomy or hysterectomy. The presence of ovarian-uterine artery anastomosis on contrast-enhanced MRI may be associated with lower UAE success rates and amenorrhea. MRI is valuable in the follow-up of patients who have undergone myomectomy as recurrence occurs in up

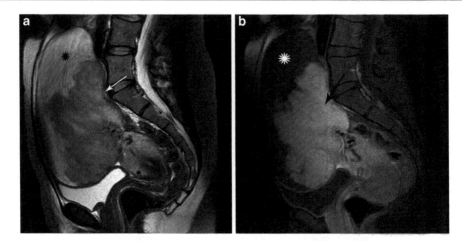

Fig. 138.5 (a) Sagittal T2WI shows a pedunculated subserosal uterine mass that is mostly of intermediate signal intensity (*arrow*) with an anterior portion showing very high signal intensity (*asterisk*). (b) Sagittal T1WI FS after gadolinium in the same patient shows avid enhancement (*arrow*) of the portion that is intermediate signal intensity on T2WI and no enhancement of the portion (*asterisk*) that is bright on T2WI. At surgery this proved to be a cellular leiomyoma with portions of cystic degeneration

Fig. 138.6 (a) TVUS of a patient with acute pelvic pain shows a well-defined hypoechoic mass (*arrow*) that is not vascularized at color Doppler. (b) Sag T2WI in the same patient shows a well-delineated intramural myometrial mass (*arrow*) with a peripheral low signal intensity halo and a heterogeneous high signal intensity center. (c) Ax T1WI FS in the same patient shows that the mass exhibits high signal intensity in keeping with hemorrhagic content. (d) Subtraction imaging after iv gadolinium in the same patient shows no enhancement of the mass (*arrow*). The findings are consistent with hemorrhagic degeneration of a leiomyoma

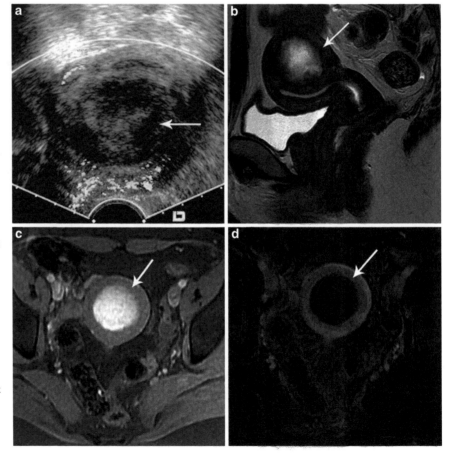

Fig. 138.7
(**a**) Transabdominal ultrasound of a woman with enlarging abdomen shows a heterogeneous uterine mass (*arrow*). (**b**) Sagittal T2WI shows the mass has heterogeneous signal intensity with areas of very high signal intensity (*asterisk*) and areas of intermediate signal intensity (*black arrow*). The inferior aspect of the mass is lobulated (*white arrow*). (**c**) Axial T1WI with fat suppression shows corresponding areas of high signal intensity within the mass (*arrow*), in keeping with hemorrhagic degeneration. (**d**) Sagittal T1WI fat suppressed after iv gadolinium shows heterogeneous enhancement with areas of absence of enhancement (*arrow*). Patient had surgery because of growing of the mass and pressure symptoms. The histopathological diagnosis was leiomyosarcoma

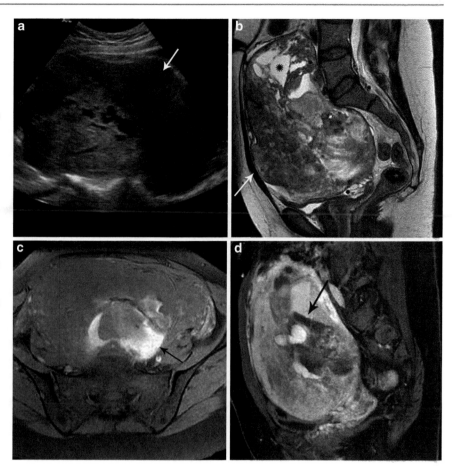

to 15% of patients. On follow-up MRI after embolization, fibroids typically show absence of enhancement with areas of T1W high signal intensity and variable signal intensity on T2WI. Between 3 months and a year after embolization, progressive liquefaction of the fibroid with increase in signal intensity on T2W imaging will occur and with successful infarction, some decrease in size will follow.

Endometrial Hyperplasia

Endometrial hyperplasia represents a diffuse abnormal proliferative response of the endometrium to estrogen stimulation. It is subdivided into hyperplasia without and with cytologic atypia. The risk of evolution toward malignancy is different among the two groups, being less than 2% with the former and 23% in the latter (Kurman and Norris 1994). It is a common sequela of unopposed estrogens or sequential estrogen-progesterone hormone replacement therapy in postmenopausal women. In premenopausal women, it is associated with hyperestrogenic conditions such as polycystic ovary syndrome, obesity, anovulatory cycles, as well as some estrogen producing tumors such as granulosa cell tumors and thecomas. Tamoxifen therapy is also a risk factor for the development of endometrial hyperplasia. Patients typically present with abnormal genital bleeding. Histologically there is excessive proliferation of endometrial glands with an increase in the glands-to-stroma ratio. Treatment depends on histologic findings, atypical hyperplasia being usually treated by hysterectomy given the risk of malignant degeneration, while simple and complex hyperplasia usually undergo a trial of progesterone therapy with follow-up imaging or endometrial sampling.

Endometrial hyperplasia cannot be prospectively diagnosed on imaging. Patients will commonly be referred to TVUS for postmenopausal bleeding. On TVUS, endometrial hyperplasia usually presents as diffuse echogenic homogeneous thickening of the

Fig. 138.8 (**a**) Sagittal TVUS shows nonspecific diffuse echogenic endometrial thickening (*arrow*) in a woman with postmenopausal bleeding. (**b**) Sagittal T2WI in the same patient shows that the endometrial complex is thickened (*arrow*) and slightly hypointense to the normal expected endometrial signal. (**c**) Sagittal T1 FS early after gadolinium shows that the lesion enhances more than the underlying endometrium and does not disrupt the subendometrial line (*arrow*). The appearance is nonspecific and mimics stage 1A endometrial carcinoma. (**d**) Sagittal T1 FS delayed after gadolinium shows that there is progressive enhancement of the lesion (*arrow*). This turned out to be atypical endometrial hyperplasia

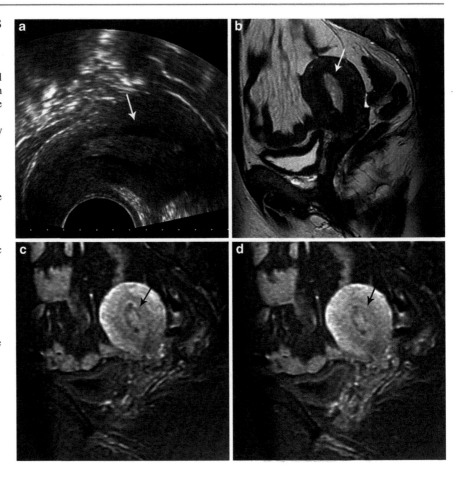

endometrium (Fig. 138.8a), although it may be focal. Small cystic anechoic foci may be encountered (Reinhold and Khalili 2002). Atypical hyperplasia may be more heterogeneous. On color Doppler US, several feeding vessels are visualized. Sonohysterographic appearance is similar. The appearance on US is not specific and may mimic other endometrial conditions including endometrial carcinoma. In postmenopausal patients presenting with vaginal bleeding and an endometrial thickness greater than 5 mm, endometrial sampling is necessary (Smith-Bindman et al. 1998), unless the patient is under hormonal replacement therapy, where endometrial thickness up to 8 mm may be accepted.

MRI has no role in endometrial hyperplasia evaluation. It can however be used as a problem-solving tool in cases where endometrial sampling is not possible to confirm endometrial thickness measured at US and avoid pseudothickening due to position of the uterus or concomitant adenomyosis. MR can also characterize an endometrial thickening as an endometrial polyp. However, the imaging characteristics of endometrial hyperplasia are nonspecific, and may mimic stage 1A endometrial carcinoma, cystic atrophy, and endometrial polyps (Reinhold and Khalili 2002). Endometrial hyperplasia will manifest as diffuse or less commonly focal thickening of the endometrial complex. The endometrial-myometrial border remains well defined. On T2W sequences, the signal of the lesion will be iso- or slightly hypointense to the normal endometrium (Fig. 138.8). After gadolinium, it may follow the signal of the normal endometrium, with an early hypoenhancement relative to the myometrium and later iso- or hyperenhancement. It may also remain hypoenhancing relative to the myometrium even on delayed imaging. Small hypointense foci representing cystic glandular dilatations may also be seen on delayed imaging (Reinhold and Khalili 2002).

There is an emerging role of diffusion-weighted imaging in differentiating endometrial carcinoma from normal endometrium or benign endometrial conditions. Recent studies have shown a significantly

Fig. 138.9 (**a**) Sagittal TVUS shows an endocavitary hyperechoic lesion (*long arrow*) that causes deviation of the endometrial hyperechoic interface(*short arrow*). (**b**) Sagittal TVUS with color Doppler in the same patient shows that the lesion is vascularized and exhibits a feeding vessel (*arrow*). The findings are consistent with an endometrial polyp

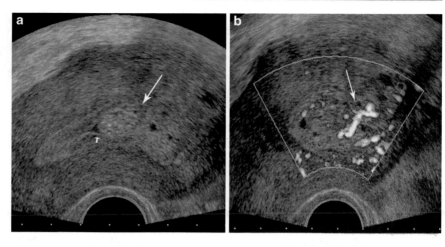

lower ADC measurement in stage 1A endometrial carcinoma than in normal endometrium or endometrial polyps or hyperplasia, without overlap between the ADC values of endometrial carcinoma and benign uterine pathology (Takeuchi et al. 2009). More work is needed to validate this data.

Endometrial Polyps

Endometrial polyps are common, occurring in 10% of women and being multiple in 20%. They consist in a localized outgrowth of endometrium covered by epithelium and may contain a mixture of three elements in varying degrees: stroma of dense fibrous tissue, thick-walled vascular channels, and endometrial glands. The incidence of endometrial polyps is higher in patients treated with tamoxifen (8–36%) than in the general population (0–10%) (Ascher et al. 2000). They are most commonly seen in perimenopausal and postmenopausal women. They are usually asymptomatic, but may result in postmenopausal bleeding when ulceration and necrosis occurs. They can be isolated or associated with endometrial hyperplasia and carcinoma. They are associated with a 0.5% risk of malignancy. They can be sessile or pedunculated, and typically occur in the uterine fundus or cornua (Reinhold and Khalili 2002). Polyps developing in the setting of tamoxifen therapy tend to be larger (mean diameter, 5 cm) than polyps not related to tamoxifen, and show more cystic glandular dilatation (Ascher et al. 2000).

TVUS is the imaging modality of choice. Endometrial polyps present as ovoid echogenic masses projecting in the endometrial lumen. A localized deviation of the central hyperechoic line representing the endometrial interface may be a clue to the presence of an endometrial polyp. At Doppler US, a feeding vessel may be identified (Fig. 138.9). Sonohysterography has been proven more accurate than TVUS in detection, localization, and characterization of endometrial pathology. It can make a precise diagnosis in cases where TVUS only shows endometrial complex thickening. An endometrial polyp will appear as a homogeneous echogenic smoothly marginated mass that does not disrupt the endometrial lining. It is isoechogenic to the endometrium. It projects in the endometrial cavity on a stalk or forms an acute angle with the underlying endometrium. Endometrial polyps can be readily differentiated from submucosal leiomyomas using sonohysterography. Submucosal leiomyomas demonstrate a myometrial origin, and are usually hypoechoic, heterogeneous, round, and attenuating. On color Doppler, they show diffuse vascularity or a rim of peripheral flow instead of a single feeding vessel (Reinhold and Khalili 2002).

MRI can be used in patients with indeterminate findings or if sampling is not possible. The appearance on MRI is variable (Figs. 138.10 and 138.11). Endometrial polyps can be slightly lower in signal intensity than the endometrium on T2W imaging, although they can also be isointense and present as focal or diffuse endometrial thickening. They can also be heterogeneous with cystic areas, especially when large. A low T2W signal intensity fibrous core has also been described. The presence of a fibrous core and intralesional cysts favors a benign polyp (Grasel et al. 2000). On T1W imaging, they appear isointense to the endometrium. On MR the differential diagnosis includes submucosal

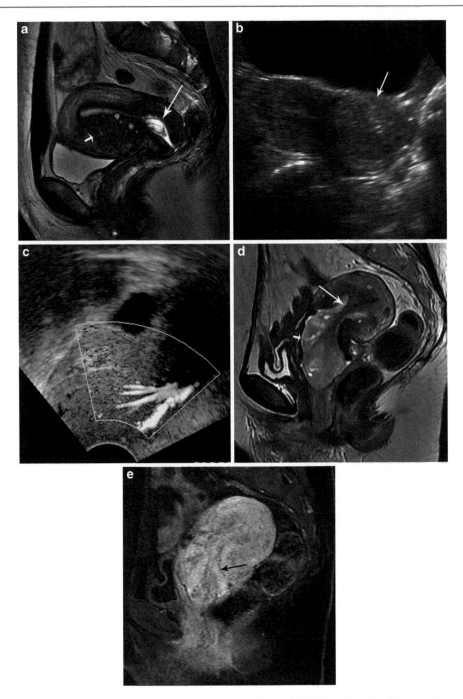

Fig. 138.10 (a) Sagittal T2WI shows an endocervical high SI lesion (*long arrow*) that contains a linear low SI core. The lesion is consistent with an endometrial polyp arising from the isthmus and extending into the endocervical canal. Also noted in this patient are characteristic findings of focal adenomyosis with focal thickening of the junctional zone (*short arrow*) containing bright foci. (b) Sagittal TAS shows in another patient with menorrhagia, a hyperechoic endocervical mass (*arrow*). (c) Sagittal TVUS with color Doppler shows the mass is connected to the endometrium by a vascularized pedicle. (d) Sagittal T2WI shows the mass has high SI (*short arrow*) and connects to the myometrial fundus through a low SI pedicle (long arrow). (e) Sagittal T1WI with fat suppression after intravenous gadolinium shows intense enhancement of the mass and of its pedicle (*arrow*). At resection, the histologic diagnosis was an adenomyomatous polyp

Fig. 138.11 (a) Sagittal T2WI shows focal endometrial thickening (*arrow*), that is isointense to the remainder of the endometrium. (**b**) Axial T2WI in the same patient shows that the endometrial thickening is centered on the right cornua (*arrow*), sparing the left cornua. (**c**) Axial T1WI fat suppressed early after intravenous gadolinium shows the lesion (*long arrow*) enhances more than the underlying endometrium (*short arrow*). (**d**) Sagittal T1W fat-suppressed delayed image after intravenous gadolinium shows persistence of the hyperenhancement of the lesion (*arrow*). The findings are consistent with an endometrial polyp. There is also a left ovarian dermoid (*asterisk*) seen on this image

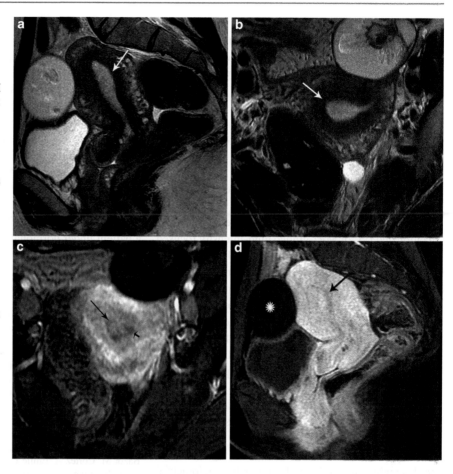

fibroid, endometrial hyperplasia, and endometrial carcinoma. Submucosal fibroids are usually hypointense on T2W imaging and myometrial in origin, thereby allowing differentiation to be made. After gadolinium administration, the enhancement of endometrial polyps is variable. Small polyps typically show early enhancement, appearing bright against the hypoenhancing endometrial background. A vascular stalk may also be identified during the arterial phase. On delayed imaging, polyps tend to be slightly hypointense relative to the endometrial complex, but remain hyperintense or isointense relative to the myometrium. A heterogeneous pattern of enhancement is associated with large polyps. The addition of gadolinium sequences improves the detection of endometrial polyps.

Although the diagnosis of endometrial polyps can accurately be performed by imaging, women with postmenopausal bleeding usually undergo endometrial sampling and removal of the polyp because of the symptomatology, the possibility of foci of atypical hyperplasia and/or carcinoma in a benign appearing polyp, as well as the possible coexistence of endometrial polyp and endometrial carcinoma in the same patient.

In conclusion, imaging has a great value in the assessment of benign uterine pathology and helps orient the patient toward the best possible therapy.

Choice of Imaging Modality

Ultrasound (US) and, especially, transvaginal ultrasound (TVUS) are the primary imaging modality in the evaluation of abnormal uterine bleeding. They can accurately diagnose benign uterine conditions such as adenomyosis and leiomyomas, and detect endometrial thickening. Sonohysterography has an added value in the evaluation of endocavitary lesions, allowing differentiation of submucosal leiomyomas from endometrial lesions such as polyps and nonspecific endometrial thickening.

Magnetic resonance imaging (MRI) is the most accurate imaging modality in the evaluation of adenomyosis and uterine leiomyomas. It acts as a problem-solving tool, helps in therapy planning, and is a reproducible imaging modality for follow-up under conservative treatment. MRI as TVUS can assess the endometrial thickness, but cannot differentiate benign from malignant endometrial thickening.

Clinical Impact of Imaging on Patient Management

With the advent of uterine sparing surgical techniques for adenomyosis and leiomyomas, as well as minimally invasive techniques such as uterine artery embolization and US- or MRI-guided high-intensity focused ultrasound therapy, imaging, especially with MRI, allows proper selection of patients for these procedures, as well as adequate surgical planning.

In the particular setting of leiomyomas, imaging can precisely assess the location of a leiomyoma, as well as its content and degeneration, allowing one to make the right choice of therapy, and if surgery is chosen, deciding on a hysteroscopic, laparoscopic, or open approach.

In front of abnormal uterine bleeding in a postmenopausal patient, imaging has a high sensitivity for detection of endometrial thickening, but cannot differentiate benign from malignant thickening. Endometrial sampling should be performed when endometrial thickness is more than 5 mm on TVUS, unless the patient is under hormonal replacement therapy, where endometrial thickness up to 8 mm may be accepted.

Endometrial polyps detected on imaging should also be resected, because they can coexist with endometrial carcinoma, and may contain foci of atypical hyperplasia or carcinoma.

Pearls to Remember

Benign uterine lesions such as adenomyosis and leiomyomas cannot be clinically differentiated, both manifesting with abnormal uterine bleeding and uterine enlargement. Both TVUS and MRI are highly accurate in their diagnosis, but MRI has an added value in precise anatomical delineation of lesions for treatment planning, identification of types of degeneration in leiomyomas, and provides a reproducible imaging modality for follow-up after treatment.

TVUS is the imaging modality of choice for the assessment of endocavitary lesions. Sonohysterography and MRI may help in differentiating submucosal leiomyomas from endometrial polyps and nonspecific endometrial thickening, by demonstrating the fibrous stalk of a polyp and the myometrial origin of a submucosal leiomyoma.

Endometrial thickening can be secondary to endometrial hyperplasia or endometrial carcinoma, and imaging cannot differentiate one from another. Endometrial sampling is necessary in a postmenopausal patient when the measured endometrial thickness is more than 5 mm or more than 8 mm in a patient under hormonal replacement therapy.

References

Ascher SM, Arnold LL, Patt RH, Schruefer JJ, Bagley AS, Semelka RC, Zeman RK, Simon JA. Adenomyosis: prospective comparison of MR imaging and transvaginal sonography. Radiology. 1994;190(3):803–6.

Ascher SM, Imaoka I, Lage JM. Tamoxifen-induced uterine abnormalities: the role of imaging. Radiology. 2000;214:29–38.

Ascher SM, Jha RC, Reinhold C. Benign myometrial conditions: leiomyomas and adenomyosis. Top Magn Reson Imaging. 2003;14(4):281–304.

Azziz R. Adenomyosis: current perspectives. Obstet Gynecol Clin North Am. 1989;16:221–35.

Bazot M, Cortez A, Emile D, et al. Ultrasonography compared with magnetic resonance imaging for the diagnosis of adenomyosis: correlation with histopathology. Hum Reprod. 2001;16:2427–33.

Champaneria R, Abedin P, Daniels J, Balogun M, Khan KS. Ultrasound scan and magnetic resonance imaging for the diagnosis of adenomyosis: systematic review comparing test accuracy. Acta Obstet Gynecol Scand. 2010;89(11):1374–84.

Dueholm M, Lundorf E, Hansen ES, Ledertoug S, Olesen F. Accuracy of magnetic resonance imaging and transvaginal ultrasonography in the diagnosis, mapping, and measurement of uterine myomas. Am J Obstet Gynecol. 2002;186(3):409–15.

Exacoustos C, Brienza L, Di Giovanni A, Szabolcs B, Romanini ME, Zupi E, Arduini D. Adenomyosis: three-dimensional sonographic findings of the junctional zone and correlation with histology. Ultrasound Obstet Gynecol. 2011;37(4):471–9.

Grasel RP, Outwater EK, Siegelman ES, Capuzzi D, Parker L, Hussain SM. Endometrial polyps: MR imaging features and distinction from endometrial carcinoma. Radiology. 2000;214(1):47–52.

Griffin Y, Sudigali V, Jacques A. Radiology of benign disorders of menstruation. Semin Ultrasound CT MR. 2010;31(5):414–32.

Kurman RJ, Norris HJ. Endometrial hyperplasia and related cellular changes. In: Kurman RJ, editor. Blaustein's pathology of the female genital tract. 4th ed. Berlin/Heidelberg/New York: Springer; 1994. p. 411–37.

Ozdegirmenci O, Kayikcioglu F, Akgul MA, Kaplan M, Karcaaltincaba M, Haberal A, Akyol M. Comparison of levonorgestrel intrauterine system versus hysterectomy on efficacy and quality of life in patients with adenomyosis. Fertil Steril. 2011;95(2):497–502.

Popovic M, Puchner S, Berzaczy D, Lammer J, Bucek RA. Uterine artery embolization for the treatment of adenomyosis: a review. J Vasc Interv Radiol. 2011;22(7):901–9.

Rajan DK, Margau R, Kroll RR, Simons ME, Tan KT, Jaskolka JD, Kachura JR, Sniderman KW, Beecroft JR, Haider M. Clinical utility of ultrasound versus magnetic resonance imaging for deciding to proceed with uterine artery magnetic resonance imaging for deciding to proceed with uterine artery embolization for presumed symptomatic fibroids. Clin Radiol. 2011;66(1):57–62.

Reinhold C, Khalili I. Postmenopausal bleeding: value of imaging. Radiol Clin North Am. 2002;40(3):527–62.

Reinhold C, McCarthy S, Bret PM, et al. Diffuse adenomyosis: comparison of endovaginal US and MR imaging with histopathologic correlation. Radiology. 1996;199:151–8.

Reinhold C, Tafazoli F, Mehio A, et al. Uterine adenomyosis: endovaginal US and MR imaging features with histopathologic correlation. Radiographics. 1999;19:S147–60.

Shen SH, Fennessy F, McDannold N, Jolesz F, Tempany C. Image-guided thermal therapy of uterine fibroids. Semin Ultrasound CT MR. 2009;30(2):91–104.

Smith-Bindman R, Kerlikowske K, Feldstein VA, Subak L, Scheidler J, Segal M, Brand R, Grady D. Endovaginal ultrasound to exclude endometrial cancer and other endometrial abnormalities. JAMA. 1998;280(17):1510–17.

Spies JB, Cooper JM, Worthington-Kirsch R, et al. Outcome of uterine embolization and hysterectomy for leiomyomas: results of a multicenter study. Am J Obstet Gynecol. 2004;191:22–31.

Takamizawa S, Minakami H, Usui R, et al. Risk of complications and uterine malignancies in women undergoing hysterectomy for presumed benign leiomyomas. Gynecol Obstet Invest. 1999;48:193–6.

Takeuchi M, Matsuzaki K, Nishitani H. Diffusion-weighted magnetic resonance imaging of endometrial cancer: differentiation from benign endometrial lesions and preoperative assessment of myometrial invasion. Acta Radiol. 2009;50(8):947–53.

Takeuchi M, Matsuzaki K, Nishitani H. Manifestations of the female reproductive organs on MR images: changes induced by various physiologic states. Radiographics. 2010;30 (4):1147.

Tamai K, Koyama T, Saga T, et al. The utility of diffusion-weighted MR imaging for differentiating uterine sarcomas from benign leiomyomas. Eur Radiol. 2008;18:723–30.

Tanaka YO, Nishida M, Tsunoda H, et al. Smooth muscle tumors of uncertain malignant potential and leiomyosarcomas of the uterus: MR findings. J Magn Reson Imaging. 2004;20:998–1007.

Togashi K, Ozasa H, Konishi I, et al. Enlarged uterus: differentiation between adenomyosis and leiomyoma with MR imaging. Radiology. 1989;171:531–4.

Ueda H, Togashi K, Konishi I, Kataoka ML, Koyama T, Fujiwara T, Kobayashi H, Fujii S, Konishi J. Unusual appearances of uterine leiomyomas: MR imaging findings and their histopathologic backgrounds. Radiographics. 1999;19: S131–45.

Weeks AD, Wilkinson N, Arora DS, et al. Menopausal changes in the myometrium: an investigation using a GnRH agonist model. Int J Gynecol Pathol. 1999;18:226–32.

Weinreb JC, Barkoff ND, Megibow A, Demopoulos R. The value of MR imaging in distinguishing leiomyomas from other solid pelvic masses when sonography is indeterminate. Am J Roentgenol. 1990;154:295–9.

Zhou M, Chen JY, Tang LD, Chen WZ, Wang ZB. Ultrasound-guided high-intensity focused ultrasound ablation for adenomyosis: the clinical experience of a single center. Fertil Steril. 2011;95(3):900–5.

Shilpa Liyanage, Nishat Bharwani, and Andrea G. Rockall

Imaging plays an important role in the multidisciplinary management of uterine corpus malignancies. The diagnosis of these tumors is made on histology and staging is surgico-pathological using the Federation of Gynecology and Obstetrics (FIGO) system (Pecorelli 2009). Magnetic resonance imaging (MRI) has emerged as the most widely used imaging technique and is useful in characterization, staging, treatment planning, and subsequent follow-up. MR imaging elegantly demonstrates disease extent and can suggest more aggressive histological subtypes which would necessitate a more radical surgical approach.

Endometrial Carcinoma

Incidence

Carcinoma of the endometrium is the most prevalent cancer of the female genital tract in North America and Western Europe and is the fourth most frequent site of cancer in women (Cancer Research UK; National Cancer Institute). The incidence is greatest in the postmenopausal population and, as a result, its incidence is climbing due to increased life expectancy as well as rises in obesity (Amant et al. 2005a; Kitchener and Trimble 2009). In the United Kingdom, the incidence of new cases in 2007 was 7,536 (24/100,000), with 1,500 deaths in 2008 (Cancer Research UK). In the United States in 2010, there were 43,470 new cases (23.9/100,000) of endometrial cancer and 7,950 deaths (National Cancer Institute). Therefore, despite being a relatively common malignancy, it is not a leading cause of death, with a 10-year survival rate of 75%, partly because 75–80% of women present at an early stage with postmenopausal or intermenstrual bleeding (Cancer Research UK).

Etiology

Endometrial cancer is associated with several recognized risk factors. Any condition which results in prolonged unopposed estrogen stimulation of the endometrial lining can predispose to endometrial hyperplasia, which then increases the risk of developing atypical hyperplasia and subsequent endometrial cancer. Estrogen excess can be exogenous (unopposed estrogen therapy) or endogenous, for example in obese patients, those with ovarian malfunction or in patients with estrogen-secreting tumors, such as theca-cell tumors of the ovary (Rose 1996). Nulliparity is also associated with an increased risk (Epplein et al. 2008). Long-term use of tamoxifen, is another recognized risk factor (Polin and Ascher 2008; Swerdlow and Jones 2005). This risk is dependent on the duration of treatment, but increases if there has been previous use of estrogen replacement during the

S. Liyanage
Imaging, Bart's Cancer Centre, King George V Wing
St Bartholomew's Hospital, West Smithfield, London, UK

N. Bharwani
Imaging, Bart's Cancer Centre, King George V Wing
St Bartholomew's Hospital, West Smithfield, London, UK

Department of Radiology, St Mary's Hospital, Imperial College Healthcare NHS Trust, London, UK

A.G. Rockall (✉)
Imperial College Healthcare NHS Trust, London, UK

B. Hamm, P. R. Ros (eds.), *Abdominal Imaging*, DOI 10.1007/978-3-642-13327-5_181,
© Springer-Verlag Berlin Heidelberg 2013

Table 139.1 Risk groups for pelvic and para-aortic nodal disease in endometrial cancer (Cragun et al. 2005)

Risk group	Features
High	Any age and all three features listed below:
	1. Grade 3 adenocarcinoma
	2. >50% deep myometrial invasion
	3. Lymphovascular space invasion
Intermediate	>50 years and any two of the above features
	>70 years and any one of the above features
Low	Grade 1 and 2 adenocarcinoma and no or superficial myometrial invasion

menopause or if the patient is also obese (Swerdlow and Jones 2005; Bernstein et al. 1999). Endometrial cancer may also occur as part of hereditary non-polyposis colorectal cancer (HNPCC) and screening for endometrial cancer in such cases may be effective (Kwon et al. 2008).

Clinical Features and Initial Diagnosis

Endometrial cancer primarily presents in postmenopausal women in the sixth to seventh decades, with only very few women diagnosed under the age of 35 (Cancer Research UK). Patients most commonly present with postmenopausal bleeding which usually occurs early in the course of the disease. Premenopausal patients may present with abnormal menstrual or intermenstrual bleeding, or occasionally as part of the investigation of infertility.

The diagnosis of endometrial cancer is made at histology. Imaging techniques cannot reliably distinguish between benign and malignant endometrial abnormalities. Many patients presenting with postmenopausal bleeding have a benign cause such as endometrial atrophy or polyps but endometrial cancer accounts for 7–14% of cases (Gull et al. 2003). Evaluation of the pelvis with transvaginal ultrasound is the first-line imaging test, with particular attention to the endometrial thickness (see Ultrasound section below). If the endometrium is thickened or abnormal bleeding continues, endometrial sampling is performed. Histopathological diagnosis and tumor grade can be either obtained as an outpatient, using a pipelle biopsy sampling technique, or by hysteroscopic assessment with dilatation and curettage under anesthesia.

Prognostic Factors

When the tumor is discovered in the early stages, the overall prognosis of endometrial carcinoma is good; more than 80% present with stage 1 disease and the 5-year survival rate is 85% (National Cancer Institute).

The prognosis of endometrial carcinoma depends on the age of the patient, histological tumor grade, cell type, tumor stage, and lymph node status (Kosary 1994; Creasman et al. 1987). A recent study by Todo et al. in 2010 supports these findings where the presence of para-aortic nodal metastases had the most impact on prognosis (hazard ratio of 3.07 compared with a hazard ratio of 1.81 for age over 56 years and a hazard ratio of 1.87 for Grade 3 or non-endometriod histology) (Todo et al. 2010).

The risk factors for pelvic and para-aortic lymph node metastases are summarized in Table 139.1 and include the depth of myometrial and cervical invasion, tumor grade and tumor occupying more than one-third of the uterine cavity. One large study demonstrated in Grade 3 tumors there was a 9% incidence of nodal metastases if only superficial myometrial invasion was present (involving the inner third), but this figure increased to 34% when deep myometrial invasion was present (involving the outer third) (Creasman et al. 1987). The depth of myometrial invasion is also an independent prognostic factor; in patients with no myometrial invasion and low-grade histology, the 5-year survival rate is 95%, compared with 42% in patients with tumor invasion into the outer half of the myometrium and high-grade histology (Amant et al. 2005a).

Staging and Treatment

Clinical staging of endometrial carcinoma is inaccurate and often underestimates the extent of disease (Creasman et al. 1999). As a result, the International Federation of Gynecology and Obstetrics (FIGO) reclassified the staging of endometrial carcinoma in 1988 as a surgico-pathological staging system (Shepherd 1989) and this was again revised in 2009 (Table 139.2) (Pecorelli 2009; Creasman 2009). Full FIGO staging entails a total abdominal hysterectomy (TAH), bilateral salpingo-ophrectomy (BSO), peritoneal washings, and evaluation and sampling of pelvic and para-aortic lymph nodes. FIGO classification is independent of radiological assessment.

Table 139.2 2009 revised FIGO staging of endometrial carcinoma with corresponding MR findings (Pecorelli 2009; Creasman 2009)

Stage	FIGO staging	MRI findings
Stage I[a]	Tumor confined to the corpus uteri	
1A	Tumor extending to <50% of myometrial depth	Signal intensity of tumor extends into the <50% of myometrium. Partial or full thickness disruption of the junctional zone
1B	Tumor extending to >50% of myometrial depth	Signal intensity of tumor extends into >50% of myometrium Full thickness disruption of the junctional zone
Stage II[a]	Tumor invades cervical stroma, but does not extend beyond the uterus	Internal os and endocervical canal are widened. Disruption of low signal intensity cervical stroma
Stage III[a]	Local and/or regional spread of the tumor	
IIIA	Tumor invades the serosa of the corpus uteri and/or adnexa	Disruption of continuity of outer myometrium. Irregular uterine configuration; peritoneal or adnexal deposit
IIIB	Vaginal and/or parametrial involvement	Segmental loss of hypointense vaginal wall; parametrial invasion
IIIC	Metastases to pelvic and/or para-aortic lymph nodes	Regional or para-aortic nodes >1 cm in short-axis diameter
IIIC1	Positive pelvic nodes	
IIIC2	Positive para-aortic lymph nodes +/− positive pelvic lymph nodes	
Stage IV[a]	Tumor invades bladder and/or bowel mucosa, and/or distant metastases	
IVA	Tumor invasion of bladder and/or bowel mucosa	Tumor signal intensity disrupts normal bladder or rectal wall
IVB	Distant metastases, including intra-abdominal metastases and/or inguinal lymph nodes	Tumor in distant sites or organs

Malignant mixed Müllerian tumors (MMMTs) are included in this classification
[a]Positive cytology obtained at peritoneal washings should be recorded but does not alter any stage

Although lymphadenectomy is a component of formal FIGO staging of endometrial carcinoma, the overall rate of lymph node involvement in endometrial cancer is low (5–8%) and lymphadenectomy carries a reported complication risk of up to 17–19%, requires increased anesthetic and operating times and needs the expertise of a specialized oncological surgeon (McMeekin et al. 2001; Morrow et al. 1991; Tozzi et al. 2005). As a result, only around 30% of endometrial cancer patients undergo lymphadenectomy in the United States as a whole, increasing to 48.3% in specialized cancer centers (Partridge et al. 1996). The role of lymphadenectomy in the management of endometrial cancer is currently an area of controversy in gynecological oncology with some conflicting evidence regarding the survival benefits associated with the procedure (Dowdy and Mariani 2010; Benedetti et al. 2008; Kitchener et al. 2009; Todo et al. 2010). However, in patients who are at high risk of nodal metastases, most centers continue to perform lymphadenectomy.

In most centers, surgical planning is dependent upon preoperative assessment of prognostic risk factors. Patients at low risk of extrauterine spread (Grade 1 or 2 histology, FIGO Stage <1B) may be treated with simple TAH and BSO, thus reducing the number of unnecessary lymph node dissections (Hardesty et al. 2000). However, any suspicious appearing nodes identified on preoperative imaging or at the time of surgery will be resected. In patients with high-risk disease (Grade >2, FIGO Stage >1A), full surgical staging including lymphadenectomy is recommended.

Controversy still surrounds the use of adjuvant therapy in endometrial carcinoma and as yet there is no consensus (Kong et al. 2008). In patients with low- or intermediate-risk disease, external beam radiotherapy (EBRT) can reduce the risk of pelvic relapse, but has no impact on overall survival (Creutzberg et al. 2000). However, in patients with high-risk disease, EBRT is associated with a 10% survival advantage (Johnson and Cornes 2007). Vaginal brachytherapy (VBT) is associated with reduced toxic effects and a recently published study has demonstrated that VBT is as effective as EBRT for the prevention of vaginal recurrence following surgery in intermediate to high-risk patients and therefore should become the standard of care (Nout et al. 2010). Chemotherapy can be used in the context of aggressive histological subtypes, either as part of a clinical trial or as a palliative measure (Kong et al. 2008).

Imaging

Preoperative imaging techniques for the assessment of uterine and extrauterine disease in endometrial carcinoma include ultrasound, CT, FDG-PET/CT, and MRI.

Ultrasound

Transvaginal ultrasound (TVUS) is the initial imaging modality of choice for evaluation of the endometrium in patients with abnormal uterine bleeding. Careful assessment of the endometrial thickness is required and using a threshold of 5 mm or greater in postmenopausal women provides a sensitivity of higher than 95% for malignancy (Minagawa et al. 2005). Imaging is unable to confidently differentiate benign entities from malignancy and, therefore, if the endometrium is thickened, sampling must be undertaken to obtain a histological diagnosis (Davidson and Dubinsky 2003). If a patient remains symptomatic despite negative imaging then a biopsy is obligatory.

Ultrasound signs of endometrial carcinoma include heterogeneity and irregular endometrial thickening (Fig. 139.1). Myometrial invasion is suggested if there is loss of the subendometrial halo or if there is a heterogenous myometrium with areas of increased echogenicity. The sensitivity for detecting deep myometrial invasion on ultrasound has been reported between 88% and 93% with diagnostic accuracies of 68–81% (DelMaschio et al. 1993; Fishman et al. 2000). However, direct comparison of TVUS with gadolinium-enhanced MRI confirms that MRI is superior in the assessment of myometrial invasion (Yamashita et al. 1993; Kim et al. 1995).

Computed Tomography (CT)

On contrast-enhanced CT, endometrial cancer is usually of slightly lower attenuation than the myometrium, but delineation of the tumor is difficult as there is relatively little contrast difference between tumor and the myometrium (Ascher and Reinhold 2002). CT is not sensitive or specific enough to assess the depth of myometrial invasion or cervical involvement (Hardesty et al. 2001). For detection of deep myometrial invasion, the sensitivity and specificity are 83% and 42%, respectively (Hardesty et al. 2001), with an overall staging accuracy of between 58% and 76% (Connor et al. 2000). CT is most commonly used in the assessment of advanced disease and performs as well as MRI in identifying extrauterine spread and identifying nodal

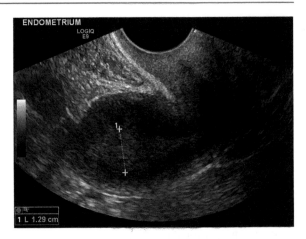

Fig. 139.1 Endometrial carcinoma on transvaginal ultrasound. The endometrial stripe (measured) is thickened to 13 mm by a hyperechoic soft tissue mass in a woman with postmenopausal bleeding

metastases (Kinkel et al. 1999). It is also used in patients where disease recurrence is suspected.

FDG-PET/CT

For initial staging, FDG-PET/CT has a limited role in assessing primary tumor extension within the pelvis (Kitajima et al. 2011). The primary role for FDG-PET/CT in endometrial carcinoma is for the detection of extrauterine and recurrent disease. Direct comparison of MRI with FDG-PET/CT has demonstrated no statistically significant difference in the detection of lymph node metastases in patients with endometrial cancer (Park et al. 2008). There was a high negative predictive value for nodal involvement (94–96%) on both imaging modalities. However, FDG-PET/CT was able to detect distant metastatic deposits with a sensitivity of 100% and a specificity of 94% (Park et al. 2008).

For nodal metastases, a sensitivity of 50% and a specificity of 86% have been reported, on a per patient basis. A study demonstrated the sensitivity of FDG-PET/CT in detecting involved nodes of 4 mm or less was 16.7%; for nodes measuring between 5 and 9 mm was 66.7%; and for nodes 10 mm or greater was 93.3% (Kitajima et al. 2008). However, most experts conclude that FDG-PET/CT is not generally considered sensitive enough to replace lymph node dissection.

Magnetic Resonance Imaging (MRI)

MRI is considered the most accurate imaging modality for preoperative assessment of endometrial carcinoma due to its excellent soft tissue contrast resolution.

Fig. 139.2 (a) Sagittal T2-weighted and (b) sagittal post-contrast images in a patient with a high-grade tumor. The margin of the tumor is difficult to delineate on the T2-weighted image. (b) Following contrast, the tumor (*) enhances to the same extent as the myometrium, which may be seen in high-grade tumors

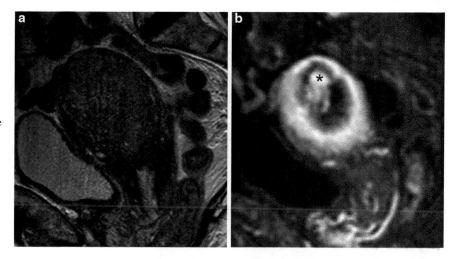

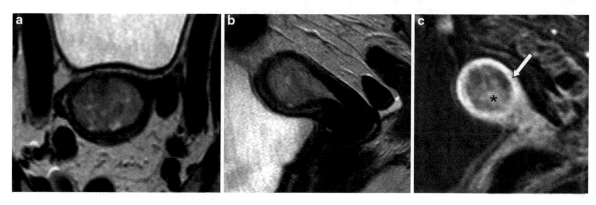

Fig. 139.3 Endometrial carcinoma in a postmenopausal woman with marked thinning of the myometrium. (a) Axial and (b) sagittal T2-weighted images demonstrate a large volume of tumor within the endometrial cavity compressing and stretching the myometrium. The depth of myometrial invasion is difficult to assess as a result. The postoperative histopathology revealed invasion of less than 50% of the myometrium, FIGO 1A. (c) The sagittal post-contrast image depicts the typical bright enhancement of the myometrium (*arrow*) with intermediate enhancement of the tumor (*)

Overall accuracies have been reported at 83–92% (Kim et al. 1995; Hricak et al. 1991). The greatest value of MRI is probably in evaluating tumors that may be at risk of extrauterine spread, where a tumor mass is seen at ultrasound and histology is Grade 2 or 3. The MRI findings corresponding to the FIGO stage of endometrial cancer are summarized in Table 139.2.

Tumor Appearance and Pitfalls

The normal zonal uterine anatomy is clearly delineated on T2-weighted imaging, where the normal endometrium is of high signal intensity, with a lower signal intensity junctional zone and intermediate signal intensity of the myometrium. Carcinoma of the endometrium is usually isointense to the myometrium on T1-weighted sequences and of lower signal intensity than the endometrial lining on the T2-weighted sequences. On T1-weighted post-contrast images, the tumor typically enhances less avidly than the normal myometrium and on dynamic contrast enhancement, enhances more slowly than myometrium. Occasionally, high-grade tumors may be very vascular and enhance to the same extent as the myometrium (Fig. 139.2).

Pitfalls in staging of endometrial cancer on MRI include blood in the uterine cavity due to tumor hemorrhage or recent dilatation and curettage, extreme thinning of the myometrium (Fig. 139.3), poor natural contrast between the tumor and myometrium, leiomyomata, and adenomyosis (Fig. 139.4) (Rockall et al. 2007; Scoutt et al. 1995).

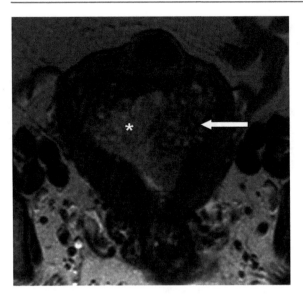

Fig. 139.4 Axial T2-weighted image shows endometrial cancer (*) in a patient with extensive adenomyosis (*arrow*). The depth of myometrial invasion is difficult to determine. The postoperative histopathology revealed deep myometrial invasion, FIGO IB

Preoperative MRI Staging

The criteria used in the FIGO staging system may be applied to preoperative MRI.

Stage I

Stage I tumors are confined to the uterine corpus and comprise over 80% of cases. In Stage IA disease, there is usually focal or diffuse thickening of the endometrium by tissue that is of lower signal intensity than normal endometrium. Post-contrast T1-weighted images help to differentiate viable tumor from debris in the endometrial cavity (Sironi et al. 1992).

Myometrial invasion (of less than 50% for Stage IA) may be diagnosed when the intermediate signal of the tumor is seen breeching the junctional zone and extending into the myometrium on T2-weighted and post-contrast images (Fig. 139.5). Subtle irregularity may be seen between the margin of the tumor and the junctional zone in cases of early invasion. In cases where the junctional zone is not visible or indistinct, a smooth interface between the endometrium and myometrium is considered to represent an intact myometrium.

Tumor that extends through more than 50% of the myometrium represents Stage IB disease (Fig. 139.6). However, an outer stripe of normal myometrial tissue remains intact. The degree of invasion should be assessed on both the T2-weighted images in the sagittal and oblique axial views as well as post-contrast images. Contrast-enhanced imaging may improve the delineation of myometrial invasion where the poorly enhancing tumor is seen within the avidly enhancing myometrium (Fig. 139.6) (Frei et al. 2000; Barwick et al. 2006). The reported sensitivities for the depth of myometrial invasion are between 70% and 95% and specificities between 80% and 95% (Barwick et al. 2006; Sala et al. 2007).

Stage II

Stage II disease is direct invasion of the cervical stroma (Fig. 139.7). Identification is important as 50–67% of patients with Stage II disease have lymph node involvement or other sites of extrauterine disease (Rockall et al. 2007; Mariani et al. 2001). Normal cervical stroma is usually hypointense on T2-weighted imaging and endometrial carcinoma is intermediate to high signal intensity. The assessment of cervical involvement may be improved on late dynamic post-contrast T1-weighted imaging, which can help distinguish between true invasion and a polypoid tumor protruding into the endocervical canal (Ascher and Reinhold 2002).

On T2-weighted sequences, tumor extends into and widens the endocervix and internal os with disruption of the hypointense fibrocervical stroma by hyperintense tumor. The overall accuracy of MRI in predicting cervical involvement is reported as 90–92%, with sensitivities of 75–80% and specificities of 94–96% (Seki et al. 1997; Manfredi et al. 2004; Toki et al. 1998; Rockall et al. 2007).

Stage III

Stage III disease is classified as disease outside the uterus but not outside the true pelvis. In Stage IIIA disease, there is invasion of the uterine serosa or adnexa. On the T2-weighted images, tumor may be seen to extend beyond the outer margin of the uterus and, on the contrast-enhanced T1-weighted imaging, there is loss of the normal rim of brightly

Fig. 139.5 Endometrial carcinoma FIGO IA. (**a**) Sagittal T2-weighted and (**b**) axial oblique T2-weighted MRI. There is intermediate T2 signal intensity soft tissue within the endometrium (*). Focal breach of the junctional zone is evident, and there is subtle irregularity between the margin of the tumor and the junctional zone (*arrow*)

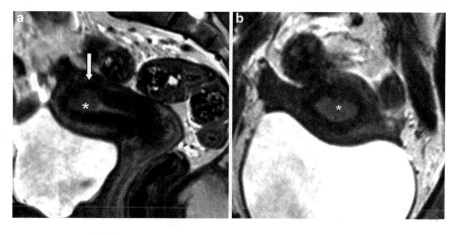

Fig. 139.6 Endometrial cancer FIGO 1B. (**a**) The tumor (*) is poorly defined on the T2-weighted axial image in this case and depth of myometrial invasion is difficult to assess. (**b**) Axial and (**c**) sagittal dynamic post-contrast images show the poorly enhancing tumor invading greater than 50% of the myometrial depth (*arrow*)

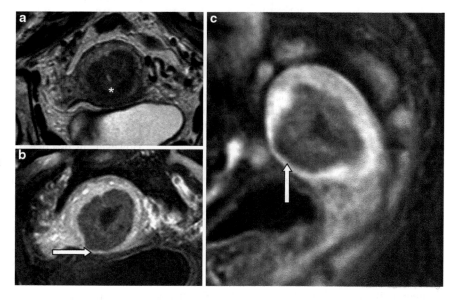

enhancing myometrium. Tumor deposits may be identified in the adnexa, even in the absence of serosal invasion, especially with high-grade or serous papillary tumors. In the 2009 revision of FIGO staging, positive peritoneal cytology from peritoneal washings alone does not constitute Stage IIIA disease. Cytological findings should be reported but no longer influence staging.

In Stage IIIB disease (Fig. 139.8), there is tumor involvement of the vagina or parametria, either by direct extension or as metastatic disease. On T2-weighted imaging, intermediate signal intensity tumor is seen to invade through the low intensity cervix or vaginal wall.

Regional nodal involvement indicates Stage IIIC disease; IIIC1 indicates involvement of pelvic nodes (Fig. 139.9), whereas Stage IIIC2 indicates positive para-aortic nodes with or without pelvic nodal involvement. Lymph nodes are hypointense on T1-weighted images and of intermediate intensity on T2-weighted images (Rockall et al. 2005). Nodal metastases correspond to drainage sites of involved portions of the uterus (Mariani et al. 2001). The diagnosis of nodal involvement on CT and MRI uses size criteria with a threshold of 1 cm short axis diameter. This results in a low sensitivity for the detection of lymph node metastases and diagnosis on MRI remains unsatisfactory (Rockall et al. 2005; Manfredi et al. 2004). Recent studies using ultrasmall particles of iron oxide, a lymph-node-specific MRI contrast agent, have shown a significant increase in the sensitivity of MRI for the diagnosis of nodal metastases (Rockall et al.

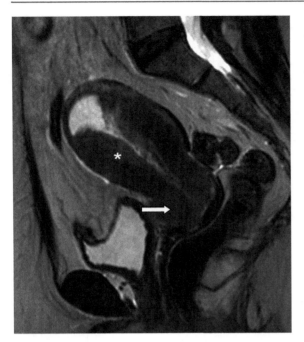

Fig. 139.7 Endometrial carcinoma FIGO stage II. Sagittal T2-weighted image demonstrates tumor in the endometrial cavity (*) which extends into the endocervical canal and invades the cervical stroma (*arrow*)

2005). However, these agents have not received FDA approval and research is underway to see if newer agents and techniques can improve specificity.

Stage IV

Direct infiltration of the bladder or bowel mucosa indicates Stage IVA disease (Fig. 139.10). This is seen as loss of the low signal intensity wall of the bladder or rectum on the T2-weighted images and tumor nodules in the wall of the invaded organ (Ascher and Reinhold 2002). MRI can often suggest invasion earlier than it is detected clinically, as formal FIGO staging requires visualization of tumor within the lumen of the involved organ.

In Stage IVB disease, there are distant metastatic deposits or intra-abdominal peritoneal deposits with or without inguinal lymph node involvement. Peritoneal deposits may be outlined by ascites and are best seen on delayed contrast-enhanced images, but deposits of less than 1 cm may be difficult to identify on any imaging modality (Ascher and Reinhold 2002). Distant spread to lung, liver, and bone is rare at presentation

and usually occurs hematogenously, the lung being the most common site involved.

Uterine Sarcomas

Uterine sarcomas are rare aggressive tumors of mesenchymal origin which account for 2–3% of all uterine malignancies. On MRI, cases that arise in the endometrium may be indistinguishable from endometrial carcinoma. Cases that arise in the myometrium, usually leiomyosarcoma, may be indistinguishable from atypical or degenerating fibroids. Uterine sarcomas differ from endometrial carcinomas with regard to their clinical behavior, pattern of spread, and management. Where possible, suggesting the diagnosis preoperatively is important as it can alter management by changing the extent of primary surgery and/or lymphadenectomy or by indicating surgical management, rather than embolization or focal treatment, of a suspicious fibroid. If there is a suspicion of a sarcoma on pipelle sampling or on imaging, the patient should be treated in a specialist gynecology-oncology unit. However, in practice, the sarcomatous nature of the tumor may only be established after hysterectomy, either within what was thought to be a fibroid preoperatively or within an endometrial lesion that was not thought to be sarcomatous on initial pipelle sampling.

Sarcomas are classified according to their tissue components. A pure sarcoma consists of a single sarcomatous element, whereas a mixed sarcoma consists of multiple different elements. A homologous sarcoma arises from tissues normally found within the uterus, whereas a heterologous sarcoma arises from elements not normally found within the uterus.

Traditionally, uterine sarcomas have been divided into three main subtypes: (1) malignant mixed Müllerian tumor (MMMT), also known as uterine carcinosarcoma; (2) endometrial stromal sarcoma (ESS); and (3) leiomyosarcoma (LMS). Other rarer subtypes include smooth muscle tumors of uncertain malignant potential (SMTUMP), undifferentiated high-grade sarcoma, and uterine rhabdomyosarcoma. However, recent immunohistochemical and molecular studies suggest that MMMT are metaplastic carcinomas in which the mesenchymal components retain epithelial features. Therefore, some researchers argue that MMMTs are better classified as an aggressive form of endometrial carcinoma (Rosai 2004). Indeed, the most recent FIGO

Fig. 139.8 Endometrial carcinoma FIGO IIIB. (**a**) Sagittal and (**b**) axial T2-weighted images demonstrate tumor within the endometrial cavity extending into the myometrium (*), cervix, and parametrium (*arrow*)

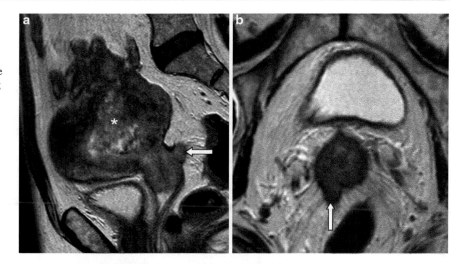

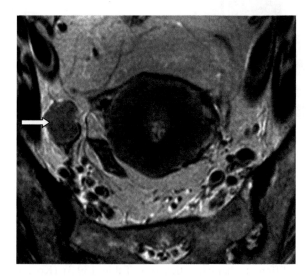

Fig. 139.9 Endometrial carcinoma FIGO IIIC1. Oblique axial T2-weighted image demonstrates an enlarged right external iliac lymph node (*arrow*) in a patient who also has extensive cervical stromal involvement

classification system (Pecorelli 2009) includes MMMT under the same staging system as endometrial carcinoma, whereas other uterine sarcomas come under a separate classification (Table 139.2).

Malignant Mixed Müllerian Tumor (MMMT)/Uterine Carcinosarcoma

MMMTs account for approximately 50% of all uterine sarcomas (Harlow et al. 1986) and can arise anywhere along the Müllerian axis.

These tumors have a high incidence of lymphatic spread and peritoneal seeding and higher rates of pulmonary metastases than other uterine malignancies (Amant et al. 2005b; Vaidya et al. 2006). Associations with prior radiotherapy for an unrelated pelvic malignancy and long-term tamoxifen have been made (Huang et al. 2006; Bergman et al. 2000; Curtis et al. 2004). Patients have a poorer prognosis than those with endometrial carcinoma with 5-year survival rates between 33% and 39% (Nielsen et al. 1989; Callister et al. 2004).

MMMTs do not have a pathognomic appearance on MRI and are most commonly indistinguishable from endometrial carcinomas (Fig. 139.11) (Sahdev et al. 2001; Bharwani et al. 2010). However, radiological suspicion should increase in the presence of large heterogeneous, infiltrative tumors or when tumoral enhancement equals or exceeds that of normal myometrium (Fig. 139.12) (Bharwani et al. 2010). The radiological literature also describes large heterogeneous pelvic masses with prominent pockets of high T2-weighted signal intensity, indicating necrosis and hemorrhage (Worthington et al. 1986). At presentation, MMMTs more often demonstrate deep myometrial invasion, cervical stromal invasion, and metastatic nodal disease than would be expected with an endometrial carcinoma of a similar size (Shapeero and Hricak 1989; Teo et al. 2008; Bharwani et al. 2010).

MR imaging features of recurrent disease are similar to those of the primary tumor.

Fig. 139.10 Endometrial carcinoma FIGO IVA. (**a**) Sagittal and (**b**) oblique axial T2-weighted images demonstrate a large tumor replacing and distorting the corpus. There is breach of the uterine serosa and invasion of the adjacent sigmoid colon (*arrow*). The tumor (*) exhibits restricted diffusion on the DWI (**c**) and the ADC map (**d**)

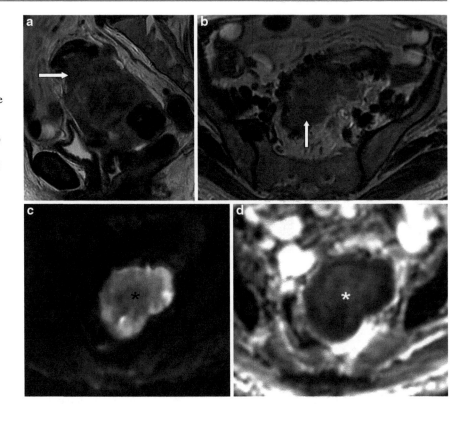

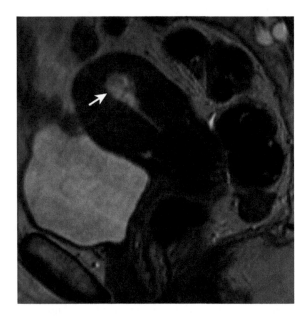

Fig. 139.11 Sagittal T2-weighted image demonstrating a small malignant mixed Müllerian tumor at the uterine fundus (*arrow*) with only superficial myometrial invasion. The imaging appearance is indistinguishable from an endometrial carcinoma

Endometrial Stromal Sarcoma (ESS)

ESSs account for 10% of primary uterine sarcomas (Harlow et al. 1986). They can be subdivided into low- and high-grade categories, which have distinctly different characteristics (see Table 139.3) (Koyama et al. 1999). These two categories are not thought to be part of a disease spectrum (Evans 1982).

ESSs commonly appear as either endometrial thickening or as a polypoid mass of homogeneous high T2 signal intensity (Fig. 139.13). Necrosis or hemorrhage may also be seen (Koyama et al. 1999; Sahdev et al. 2001).

The radiological literature describes several imaging findings which may suggest the diagnosis of ESS. These distinguishing features are more likely to be seen with high-grade ESS than with low-grade tumors (Koyama et al. 1999; Ueda et al. 2001; Sahdev et al. 2001). These include:

- Extensive myometrial involvement (which is often poorly marginated) with multiple intratumoral flow voids due to neovascularity.

Fig. 139.12 Sagittal T2-weighted image (**a**) showing a large, heterogeneous malignant mixed Müllerian tumor expanding the endometrial cavity and extending into the endocervical canal. There was no evidence of cervical stromal invasion on MRI or histology. Axial T1-weighted fat suppressed images (**b**) show peripheral soft tissue components and regions of high T1-weighted signal intensity in keeping with hemorrhage (*). Following gadolinium administration (**c**), some of the peripheral soft tissue nodules are seen to enhance less than the adjacent myometrium (*black arrowheads*) while other areas enhance avidly (*black arrow*). (**d**) The conspicuity of the enhancing soft tissue components (*black arrowheads*) is increased by using subtraction techniques on the dynamic contrast-enhanced MRI sequence

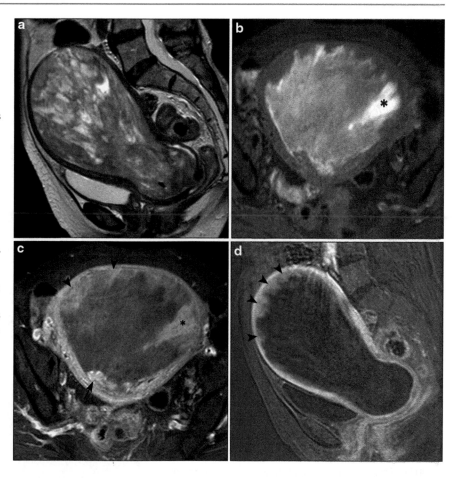

Table 139.3 Differentiation between high- and low-grade endometrial stromal sarcoma (Koyama et al. 1999)

	Low-grade ESS	High-grade ESS
Patient age	Younger (mean 39 years)	Older (mean 61 years)
Preoperative histology	Difficult to distinguish from benign endometrial stromal cells on pipelle	Diagnosis readily established on pipelle specimen
Clinical features	Indolent	Aggressive
	Distant metastases rare	Rapidly metastasizing

- Multiple marginal tumor nodules and intramyometrial worm-like extension.
- Bands of low T2-weighted signal intensity within areas of myometrial involvement which represent preserved normal myometrium.
- Continuous tumor extension along vessels or ligaments due to marked vascular and lymphatic invasion, with separate myometrial tumor nodules seen within invaded vessels.
- Tumor enhancement is commonly heterogeneous and the same as or greater than normal myometrium (in contrast with endometrial carcinoma, which enhances less than normal myometrium).

Leiomyosarcoma (LMS)

LMSs account for approximately one-third of primary uterine sarcomas (Harlow et al. 1986). It is thought that most arise de novo, but they may rarely result from sarcomatous transformation within a benign leiomyoma. The distinction between LMS and benign leiomyoma is increasingly important now that uterus-preserving procedures, such as uterine artery embolization and high-intensity focused ultrasound, are more commonplace.

Fig. 139.13 (a) Sagittal T2-weighted, (b) axial T2-weighted, and (c) axial T1 fat-suppressed images demonstrating a heterogeneous mass (*) with a large exophytic component arising at the fundus and replacing the majority of the uterus. Pockets of high T1 and T2 signal intensity (*) represent areas of hemorrhage. This tumor was histologically proven to represent a low-grade endometrial stromal sarcoma

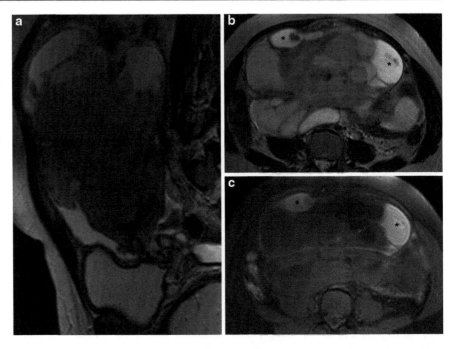

On MRI, LMSs cause massive uterine enlargement with either multiple sarcomatous nodules or confluent invasion. The tumor is typically heterogeneous with extensive (>50%) areas of high T2 signal intensity (Fig. 139.14) (Sahdev et al. 2001; Tanaka et al. 2004). These areas are isointense to water in areas of degeneration and slightly hyperintense to the outer myometrium in areas of increased cellularity and vascularity. There are irregular central regions of low T1 signal intensity, suggesting extensive necrosis, which may contain hyperintense T1 signal areas, indicating intratumoral hemorrhage (Sahdev et al. 2001). However, signal intensity is not a reliable indicator of malignancy. In contrast to benign leiomyomas, which have a sharply defined margin, LMS margins are usually irregular and ill defined. Foci of calcification may also be present, but are not well seen on MRI and are best visualized on CT (Rha et al. 2003).

Sarcomatous transformation is reported in approximately 0.2% of benign leiomyomas. MRI cannot reliably differentiate LMS from a benign degenerating leiomyoma. However, features suggestive of sarcomatous transformation within a benign leiomyoma include irregular margins and rapid growth. Recent studies suggest that diffusion-weighted MRI may be a potential tool in making this distinction (Tamai et al. 2008).

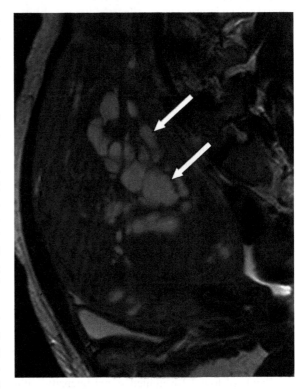

Fig. 139.14 Sagittal T2-weighted image showing a large heterogeneous tumor entirely replacing the uterine body and containing multiple regions of high T2 signal intensity. This tumor was histologically proven to be a leiomyosarcoma

Fig. 139.15 (a) Sagittal and (b) axial T2-weighted images demonstrating a primary colorectal tumor (*). The intermediate signal intensity endometrial mass lesion seen to invade the anterior myometrium (*white arrow*) was histologically proven to represent an endometrial metastasis

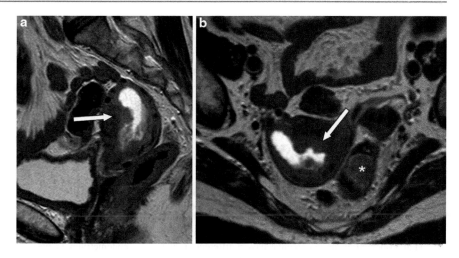

Lymphoma

Malignant lymphoma involving the uterus is rare. Primary uterine lymphoma is extranodal non-Hodgkin lymphoma confined to the uterus without evidence of other sites of involvement at the time of initial diagnosis. Secondary uterine lymphoma occurs when uterine involvement is part of a more generalized systemic process. Secondary lymphoma more commonly affects the uterine corpus than the cervix and the commonest histological subtype is diffuse large B-cell lymphoma followed by follicular lymphoma (Kosari et al. 2005; Harris and Scully 1984).

Patients most commonly present with vaginal bleeding or discharge and pelvic pain as with other uterine malignancies. Systemic B symptoms such as fever and weight loss are only rarely seen. Uterine lymphoma is treated with chemotherapy and radiotherapy rather than surgically and therefore differentiation is crucial. It has a good prognosis if correctly diagnosed, but the diagnosis may be overlooked due to nonspecific clinical and imaging features (Harris and Scully 1984; Kawakami et al. 1995).

Uterine lymphoma can present as a small mass or diffuse infiltration involving both the endometrium and myometrium. The tumor is typically of homogeneous intermediate T2-weighted signal intensity, low T1-weighted signal intensity, and demonstrates moderate enhancement following intravenous contrast medium (Kawakami et al. 1995; Kimura et al. 1991;

Kim et al. 1997; Goto et al. 2007; Suzuki et al. 2000). One group has described the finding of apparent septations following contrast medium, resulting in a nodular appearance, (Goto et al. 2007) although this has not been described elsewhere. With secondary lymphoma, lymphadenopathy is also demonstrated elsewhere in the body.

Metastases

The uterus is a rare site for metastatic disease from extrapelvic organs. The most common primary sites of malignancy are the breast (43%) or gastrointestinal tract (29%) (Fig. 139.15) (Kumar and Hart 1982). Less common sites include pancreas, lung, melanoma, and kidney. Prognosis is generally poor, as patients tend to have widespread metastatic disease. The uterine corpus is more commonly involved in direct extension from an adjacent pelvic tumor (Metser et al. 2003).

Imaging findings of the uterine lesion are generally nonspecific with the presence of an intermediate T2-weighted signal intensity mass causing partial or complete loss of the junctional zone. Generally, imaging will show clear evidence of a primary lesion elsewhere.

Summary

Imaging has assumed increasing importance in the diagnosis and management of malignancies of the uterine corpus, in particular endometrial carcinoma.

This trend reflects the need to obtain accurate staging and early disease detection to provide optimal treatment and minimize morbidity and mortality. Although not officially incorporated in the FIGO staging system, MRI is widely accepted as the most reliable imaging modality for staging and follow-up.

References

Amant F, Moerman P, Neven P, Timmerman D, Van Limbergen E, Vergote I. Endometrial cancer. Lancet. 2005a;366(9484): 491–505.

Amant F, Cadron I, Fuso L, Berteloot P, de Jonge E, Jacomen G, et al. Endometrial carcinosarcomas have a different prognosis and pattern of spread compared to high-risk epithelial endometrial cancer. Gynecol Oncol. 2005b;98(2):274–80.

Ascher SM, Reinhold C. Imaging of cancer of the endometrium. Radiol Clin North Am. 2002;40(3):563–76.

Barwick TD, Rockall AG, Barton DP, Sohaib SA. Imaging of endometrial adenocarcinoma. Clin Radiol. 2006;61 (7):545–55.

Benedetti PP, Basile S, Maneschi F, Alberto LA, Signorelli M, Scambia G, et al. Systematic pelvic lymphadenectomy vs. no lymphadenectomy in early-stage endometrial carcinoma: randomized clinical trial. J Natl Cancer Inst. 2008;100(23):1707–16.

Bergman L, Beelen ML, Gallee MP, Hollema H, Benraadt J, van Leeuwen FE. Risk and prognosis of endometrial cancer after tamoxifen for breast cancer. Comprehensive Cancer Centres' ALERT Group. Assessment of Liver and Endometrial cancer Risk following Tamoxifen. Lancet. 2000; 356(9233):881–7.

Bernstein L, Deapen D, Cerhan JR, Schwartz SM, Liff J, McGann-Maloney E, et al. Tamoxifen therapy for breast cancer and endometrial cancer risk. J Natl Cancer Inst. 1999;91(19):1654–62.

Bharwani N, Newland A, Tunariu N, Babar S, Sahdev A, Rockall AG, et al. MRI appearances of uterine malignant mixed Mullerian tumors. AJR Am J Roentgenol. 2010;195 (5):1268–75.

Callister M, Ramondetta LM, Jhingran A, Burke TW, Eifel PJ. Malignant mixed Mullerian tumors of the uterus: analysis of patterns of failure, prognostic factors, and treatment outcome. Int J Radiat Oncol Biol Phys. 2004;58(3):786–96.

Cancer Research UK. Cancer stats 2011. http://info.cancerresearchuk.org/cancerstats

Connor JP, Andrews JI, Anderson B, Buller RE. Computed tomography in endometrial carcinoma. Obstet Gynecol. 2000;95(5):692–6.

Cragun JM, Havrilesky LJ, Calingaert B, Synan I, Secord AA, Soper JT, et al. Retrospective analysis of selective lymphadenectomy in apparent early-stage endometrial cancer. J Clin Oncol. 2005;23(16):3668–75.

Creasman W. Revised FIGO staging for carcinoma of the endometrium. Int J Gynaecol Obstet. 2009;105(2):109.

Creasman WT, Morrow CP, Bundy BN, Homesley HD, Graham JE, Heller PB. Surgical pathologic spread patterns of endometrial cancer. A Gynecologic Oncology Group Study. Cancer. 1987;60(8 Suppl):2035–41.

Creasman WT, DeGeest K, Disaia PJ, Zaino RJ. Significance of true surgical pathologic staging; a Gynecologic Oncology Group Study. Am J Obstet Gynecol. 1999;181(1):31–4.

Creutzberg CL, van Putten WL, Koper PC, Lybeert ML, Jobsen JJ, Warlam-Rodenhuis CC, et al. Surgery and postoperative radiotherapy versus surgery alone for patients with stage-1 endometrial carcinoma: multicentre randomised trial. PORTEC Study Group. Post Operative Radiation Therapy in endometrial carcinoma. Lancet. 2000;355(9213):1404–11.

Curtis RE, Freedman DM, Sherman ME, Fraumeni Jr JF. Risk of malignant mixed mullerian tumors after tamoxifen therapy for breast cancer. J Natl Cancer Inst. 2004;96(1): 70–4.

Davidson KG, Dubinsky TJ. Ultrasonographic evaluation of the endometrium in postmenopausal vaginal bleeding. Radiol Clin North Am. 2003;41(4):769–80.

DelMaschio A, Vanzulli A, Sironi S, Spagnolo D, Belloni C, Garancini P, et al. Estimating the depth of myometrial involvement by endometrial carcinoma: efficacy of transvaginal sonography vs MR imaging. AJR Am J Roentgenol. 1993;160(3):533–8.

Dowdy SC, Mariani A. Lymphadenectomy in endometrial cancer: when, not if. Lancet. 2010;375(9721):1138–40.

Epplein M, Reed SD, Voigt LF, Newton KM, Holt VL, Weiss NS. Risk of complex and atypical endometrial hyperplasia in relation to anthropometric measures and reproductive history. Am J Epidemiol. 2008;168(6): 563–70.

Evans HL. Endometrial stromal sarcoma and poorly differentiated endometrial sarcoma. Cancer. 1982;50(10):2170–82.

Fishman A, Altaras M, Bernheim J, Cohen I, Beyth Y, Tepper R. The value of transvaginal sonography in the preoperative assessment of myometrial invasion in high and low grade endometrial cancer and in comparison to frozen section in grade 1 disease. Eur J Gynaecol Oncol. 2000;21(2):128–30.

Frei KA, Kinkel K, Bonel HM, Lu Y, Zaloudek C, Hricak H. Prediction of deep myometrial invasion in patients with endometrial cancer: clinical utility of contrast-enhanced MR imaging-a meta-analysis and Bayesian analysis. Radiology. 2000;216(2):444–9.

Goto N, Oishi-Tanaka Y, Tsunoda H, Yoshikawa H, Minami M. Magnetic resonance findings of primary uterine malignant lymphoma. Magn Reson Med Sci. 2007;6(1):7–13.

Gull B, Karlsson B, Milsom I, Granberg S. Can ultrasound replace dilation and curettage? A longitudinal evaluation of postmenopausal bleeding and transvaginal sonographic measurement of the endometrium as predictors of endometrial cancer. Am J Obstet Gynecol. 2003;188(2): 401–8.

Hardesty LA, Sumkin JH, Nath ME, Edwards RP, Price FV, Chang TS, et al. Use of preoperative MR imaging in the management of endometrial carcinoma: cost analysis. Radiology. 2000;215(1):45–9.

Hardesty LA, Sumkin JH, Hakim C, Johns C, Nath M. The ability of helical CT to preoperatively stage endometrial carcinoma. AJR Am J Roentgenol. 2001;176(3):603–6.

Harlow BL, Weiss NS, Lofton S. The epidemiology of sarcomas of the uterus. J Natl Cancer Inst. 1986;76(3):399–402.

Harris NL, Scully RE. Malignant lymphoma and granulocytic sarcoma of the uterus and vagina. A clinicopathologic analysis of 27 cases. Cancer. 1984;53(11):2530–45.

Hricak H, Rubinstein LV, Gherman GM, Karstaedt N. MR imaging evaluation of endometrial carcinoma: results of an NCI cooperative study. Radiology. 1991;179(3):829–32.

Huang YT, Huang KG, Ueng SH, Shaw SW. Irradiation-induced uterine malignant mixed mullerian tumor. Taiwan J Obstet Gynecol. 2006;45(4):353–5.

Johnson N, Cornes P. Survival and recurrent disease after postoperative radiotherapy for early endometrial cancer: systematic review and meta-analysis. BJOG. 2007;114(11): 1313–20.

Kawakami S, Togashi K, Kojima N, Morikawa K, Mori T, Konishi J. MR appearance of malignant lymphoma of the uterus. J Comput Assist Tomogr. 1995;19(2):238–42.

Kim SH, Kim HD, Song YS, Kang SB, Lee HP. Detection of deep myometrial invasion in endometrial carcinoma: comparison of transvaginal ultrasound, CT, and MRI. J Comput Assist Tomogr. 1995;19(5):766–72.

Kim YS, Koh BH, Cho OK, Rhim HC. MR imaging of primary uterine lymphoma. Abdom Imaging. 1997;22(4):441–4.

Kimura I, Togashi K, Tsutsui K, Nakano Y, Konishi J, Taii S, et al. MR imaging of gynecologic lymphoma. J Comput Assist Tomogr. 1991;15(3):500–1.

Kinkel K, Kaji Y, Yu KK, Segal MR, Lu Y, Powell CB, et al. Radiologic staging in patients with endometrial cancer: a meta-analysis. Radiology. 1999;212(3):711–8.

Kitajima K, Murakami K, Yamasaki E, Fukasawa I, Inaba N, Kaji Y, et al. Accuracy of 18F-FDG PET/CT in detecting pelvic and paraaortic lymph node metastasis in patients with endometrial cancer. AJR Am J Roentgenol. 2008;190(6):1652–8.

Kitajima K, Murakami K, Kaji Y, Sakamoto S, Sugimura K. Established, emerging and future applications of FDG-PET/CT in the uterine cancer. Clin Radiol. 2011;66(4):297–307.

Kitchener HC, Trimble EL. Endometrial cancer state of the science meeting. Int J Gynecol Cancer. 2009;19(1):134–40.

Kitchener H, Swart AM, Qian Q, Amos C, Parmar MK. Efficacy of systematic pelvic lymphadenectomy in endometrial cancer (MRC ASTEC trial): a randomised study. Lancet. 2009;373(9658):125–36.

Kong A, Powell M, Blake P. The role of postoperative radiotherapy in carcinoma of the endometrium. Clin Oncol (R Coll Radiol). 2008;20(6):457–62.

Kosari F, Daneshbod Y, Parwaresch R, Krams M, Wacker HH. Lymphomas of the female genital tract: a study of 186 cases and review of the literature. Am J Surg Pathol. 2005;29(11):1512–20.

Kosary CL. FIGO stage, histology, histologic grade, age and race as prognostic factors in determining survival for cancers of the female gynecological system: an analysis of 1973-87 SEER cases of cancers of the endometrium, cervix, ovary, vulva, and vagina. Semin Surg Oncol. 1994;10(1):31–46.

Koyama T, Togashi K, Konishi I, Kobayashi H, Ueda H, Kataoka ML, et al. MR imaging of endometrial stromal sarcoma: correlation with pathologic findings. AJR Am J Roentgenol. 1999;173(3):767–72.

Kumar NB, Hart WR. Metastases to the uterine corpus from extragenital cancers. A clinicopathologic study of 63 cases. Cancer. 1982;50(10):2163–9.

Kwon JS, Sun CC, Peterson SK, White KG, Daniels MS, Boyd-Rogers SG, et al. Cost-effectiveness analysis of prevention strategies for gynecologic cancers in Lynch syndrome. Cancer. 2008;113(2):326–35.

Manfredi R, Mirk P, Maresca G, Margariti PA, Testa A, Zannoni GF, et al. Local-regional staging of endometrial carcinoma: role of MR imaging in surgical planning. Radiology. 2004;231(2):372–8.

Mariani A, Webb MJ, Keeney GL, Podratz KC. Routes of lymphatic spread: a study of 112 consecutive patients with endometrial cancer. Gynecol Oncol. 2001;81(1):100–4.

McMeekin DS, Lashbrook D, Gold M, Scribner DR, Kamelle S, Tillmanns TD, et al. Nodal distribution and its significance in FIGO stage IIIc endometrial cancer. Gynecol Oncol. 2001;82(2):375–9.

Metser U, Haider MA, Khalili K, Boerner S. MR imaging findings and patterns of spread in secondary tumor involvement of the uterine body and cervix. AJR Am J Roentgenol. 2003;180(3):765–9.

Minagawa Y, Sato S, Ito M, Onohara Y, Nakamoto S, Kigawa J. Transvaginal ultrasonography and endometrial cytology as a diagnostic schema for endometrial cancer. Gynecol Obstet Invest. 2005;59(3):149–54.

Morrow CP, Bundy BN, Kurman RJ, Creasman WT, Heller P, Homesley HD, et al. Relationship between surgical-pathological risk factors and outcome in clinical stage I and II carcinoma of the endometrium: a Gynecologic Oncology Group study. Gynecol Oncol. 1991;40(1):55–65.

National Cancer Institute. Surveillance Epidemiology and End Results. Cancer Statistics. US National Institutes of Health, 2011. http://seer.cancer.gov/statistics

Nielsen SN, Podratz KC, Scheithauer BW, O'Brien PC. Clinicopathologic analysis of uterine malignant mixed Mullerian tumors. Gynecol Oncol. 1989;34(3):372–8.

Nout RA, Smit VT, Putter H, Jurgenliemk-Schulz IM, Jobsen JJ, Lutgens LC, et al. Vaginal brachytherapy versus pelvic external beam radiotherapy for patients with endometrial cancer of high-intermediate risk (PORTEC-2): an open-label, non-inferiority, randomised trial. Lancet. 2010;375(9717):816–23.

Park JY, Kim EN, Kim DY, Suh DS, Kim JH, Kim YM, et al. Comparison of the validity of magnetic resonance imaging and positron emission tomography/computed tomography in the preoperative evaluation of patients with uterine corpus cancer. Gynecol Oncol. 2008;108(3): 486–92.

Partridge EE, Shingleton HM, Menck HR. The National Cancer Data Base report on endometrial cancer. J Surg Oncol. 1996;61(2):111–23.

Pecorelli S. Revised FIGO staging for carcinoma of the vulva, cervix, and endometrium. Int J Gynaecol Obstet. 2009;105(2):103–4.

Polin SA, Ascher SM. The effect of tamoxifen on the genital tract. Cancer Imaging. 2008;8:135–45.

Rha SE, Byun JY, Jung SE, Lee SL, Cho SM, Hwang SS, et al. CT and MRI of uterine sarcomas and their mimickers. AJR Am J Roentgenol. 2003;181(5):1369–74.

Rockall AG, Sohaib SA, Harisinghani MG, Babar SA, Singh N, Jeyarajah AR, et al. Diagnostic performance of nanoparticle-enhanced magnetic resonance imaging in the diagnosis of lymph node metastases in patients with endometrial and cervical cancer. J Clin Oncol. 2005;23(12):2813–21.

Rockall AG, Meroni R, Sohaib SA, Reynolds K, Alexander-Sefre F, Shepherd JH, et al. Evaluation of endometrial carcinoma on magnetic resonance imaging. Int J Gynecol Cancer. 2007;17(1):188–96.

Rosai J. Female reproductive system. In: Rosai J, editor. Rosai and Ackerman's surgical pathology. Edinburgh: Mosby; 2004. p. 1483–1761. 2011.

Rose PG. Endometrial carcinoma. N Engl J Med. 1996;335(9):640–9.

Sahdev A, Sohaib SA, Jacobs I, Shepherd JH, Oram DH, Reznek RH. MR imaging of uterine sarcomas. AJR Am J Roentgenol. 2001;177(6):1307–11.

Sala E, Wakely S, Senior E, Lomas D. MRI of malignant neoplasms of the uterine corpus and cervix. AJR Am J Roentgenol. 2007;188(6):1577–87.

Scoutt LM, McCarthy SM, Flynn SD, Lange RC, Long F, Smith RC, et al. Clinical stage I endometrial carcinoma: pitfalls in preoperative assessment with MR imaging. Work in progress. Radiology. 1995;194(2):567–72.

Seki H, Azumi R, Kimura M, Sakai K. Stromal invasion by carcinoma of the cervix: assessment with dynamic MR imaging. AJR Am J Roentgenol. 1997;168(6):1579–85.

Shapeero LG, Hricak H. Mixed Mullerian sarcoma of the uterus: MR imaging findings. AJR Am J Roentgenol. 1989;153(2):317–9.

Shepherd JH. Revised FIGO staging for gynaecological cancer. Br J Obstet Gynaecol. 1989;96(8):889–92.

Sironi S, Colombo E, Villa G, Taccagni G, Belloni C, Garancini P, et al. Myometrial invasion by endometrial carcinoma: assessment with plain and gadolinium-enhanced MR imaging. Radiology. 1992;185(1):207–12.

Suzuki Y, Tamaki Y, Hasegawa M, Maebayashi K, Mitsuhashi N. Magnetic resonance images of primary malignant lymphoma of the uterine body: a case report. Jpn J Clin Oncol. 2000;30(11):519–21.

Swerdlow AJ, Jones ME. Tamoxifen treatment for breast cancer and risk of endometrial cancer: a case-control study. J Natl Cancer Inst. 2005;97(5):375–84.

Tamai K, Koyama T, Saga T, Morisawa N, Fujimoto K, Mikami Y, et al. The utility of diffusion-weighted MR imaging for differentiating uterine sarcomas from benign leiomyomas. Eur Radiol. 2008;18(4):723–30.

Tanaka YO, Nishida M, Tsunoda H, Okamoto Y, Yoshikawa H. Smooth muscle tumors of uncertain malignant potential and leiomyosarcomas of the uterus: MR findings. J Magn Reson Imaging. 2004;20(6):998–1007.

Teo SY, Babagbemi KT, Peters HE, Mortele KJ. Primary malignant mixed mullerian tumor of the uterus: findings on sonography, CT, and gadolinium-enhanced MRI. AJR Am J Roentgenol. 2008;191(1):278–83.

Todo Y, Kato H, Kaneuchi M, Watari H, Takeda M, Sakuragi N. Survival effect of para-aortic lymphadenectomy in endometrial cancer (SEPAL study): a retrospective cohort analysis. Lancet. 2010;375(9721):1165–72.

Toki T, Oka K, Nakayama K, Oguchi O, Fujii S. A comparative study of pre-operative procedures to assess cervical invasion by endometrial carcinoma. Br J Obstet Gynaecol. 1998;105(5):512–6.

Tozzi R, Malur S, Koehler C, Schneider A. Analysis of morbidity in patients with endometrial cancer: is there a commitment to offer laparoscopy? Gynecol Oncol. 2005; 97(1):4–9.

Ueda M, Otsuka M, Hatakenaka M, Sakai S, Ono M, Yoshimitsu K, et al. MR imaging findings of uterine endometrial stromal sarcoma: differentiation from endometrial carcinoma. Eur Radiol. 2001;11(1):28–33.

Vaidya AP, Horowitz NS, Oliva E, Halpern EF, Duska LR. Uterine malignant mixed mullerian tumors should not be included in studies of endometrial carcinoma. Gynecol Oncol. 2006;103(2):684–7.

Worthington JL, Balfe DM, Lee JK, Gersell DJ, Heiken JP, Ling D, et al. Uterine neoplasms: MR imaging. Radiology. 1986;159(3):725–30.

Yamashita Y, Mizutani H, Torashima M, Takahashi M, Miyazaki K, Okamura H, et al. Assessment of myometrial invasion by endometrial carcinoma: transvaginal sonography vs contrast-enhanced MR imaging. AJR Am J Roentgenol. 1993;161(3):595–9.

Malignant Conditions of the Cervix

140

K. Downey and N. M. DeSouza

Introduction

Worldwide, cervical cancer is the second most common cancer among women with an estimated 530,000 new cases and 275,000 deaths in 2008 (World Health Organization statistics). Most cervical cancer cases occur in developing countries, where they account for 15% of all female cancers. In developed countries, cervical cancer cases represent about 3.6% of new female cancers with the risk of diagnosis of 0.64%.

In developed countries, screening programs with papanicolau (pap) smear cytology performed every 3 years on women up to the age of 45 years have contributed greatly to early detection of cancer and led to a dramatic reduction in mortality. Screening is often not available in developing countries with resultant high rates of late-stage cervical cancer. The success of screening is largely dependent on the recognition of a well-defined preinvasive cancerous change defined as cervical intraepithelial neoplasia (CIN) and cervical glandular intraepithelial neoplasia (CGIN). Following the detection of abnormal cells, colposcopy is carried out and a cone or loop biopsy specimen obtained for histopathology to determine the grade of CIN or CGIN. Left untreated, 70% of CIN 3 and CGIN 3 (severe dyskaryosis) lesions will progress to invasive cervical cancer. Tumors are usually squamous (~70%) or adenocarcinomas (~30%) arising from the cervical epithelium in a background of intraepithelial neoplasia. Rarer histological variants include minimal deviation adenocarcinoma, cervical lymphoma, neuroendocrine variants, and metastases to the cervix.

The most widely used staging system for cervical cancer is the Federation Internationale de Gynécoligic et Obstétrique (FIGO) classification (Table 140.1). In early stages of carcinoma, the most important observation is the definition of the tumor and whether or not it has extended to the parametrium as this separates a surgical from a nonsurgical management approach. Currently, the FIGO staging is entirely clinical, relying on colposcopy and examination under anesthesia (EUA) which involves palpation together with cytoscopy and sigmoidoscopy. However, this assessment is often inaccurate because although the findings may give a reasonable indication of the size and extent of disease in exophytic tumors, in tumors with an endophytic component and in lesions located within the endocervical canal, the clinical assessment of disease is unreliable resulting in substantial underestimation. Also, while an experienced clinician can usually detect gross invasion of the parametria, early invasion invariably goes undetected. Furthermore, EUA does not detect lymph node metastases or distant metastatic disease. Imaging technologies are invaluable in providing accurate information for calculating tumor volume and for investigating the spread of disease to the parametrium and lymph nodes. Precise staging of the disease with imaging also

K. Downey
Cancer Research UK and EPSRC Cancer Imaging Centre, Institute of Cancer Research and Royal Marsden NHS Foundation Trust, Sutton, UK

N.M. DeSouza (✉)
Cancer Research UK and EPSRC Cancer Imaging Centre, Institute of Cancer Research and Royal Marsden NHS Foundation Trust, Sutton, UK

MRI Unit, Royal Marsden Hospital, Sutton, Surrey, UK

B. Hamm, P. R. Ros (eds.), *Abdominal Imaging*, DOI 10.1007/978-3-642-13327-5_182,
© Springer-Verlag Berlin Heidelberg 2013

Table 140.1 FIGO staging for carcinoma of the cervix

FIGO stage	Tumor extent
1A	Carcinoma cervix confined
1: $\leq$3 mm deep x $\leq$7 mm wide	Preclinical invasive
2: 3–5 mm deep x $\leq$7 mm wide	
1B	Carcinoma cervix confined
1: $\leq$4 cm	>5 mm deep and 8 mm wide
2: >4 cm	
2A	Beyond uterus but not pelvic sidewall or
1: $\leq$4 cm	lower one third Vagina
2: >4 cm	No parametrial invasion
2B	Beyond uterus but not pelvic sidewall or lower one third vagina Parametrial invasion
3A	Invasion of the lower one third vagina No pelvic sidewall invasion
3B	Invasion of the lower one third vagina Pelvic sidewall invasion/hydronephrosis/ nonfunctioning kidney
4A	Extension beyond the true pelvis or bladder/rectal involvement Spread of growth to adjacent organs
4B	Extension beyond the true pelvis or bladder/rectal involvement Spread to distant organs

Source: Pecorelli (2009)

provides a prognosis, allows the institution of correct treatment, and permits comparison of different treatment protocols.

Choice of Imaging Modality

Imaging with transabdominal ultrasound does not improve the accuracy of clinical staging because of poor image quality and difficulty in interpretation. Transrectal ultrasound produces clearer views of the cervix but definition of tumor from normal cervix is still poor. Cross-sectional imaging modalities such as computed tomography (CT), magnetic resonance imaging (MRI), and positron emission tomography (PET) are preferred diagnostic techniques for staging tumor and planning treatment of patients with cervical cancer. These imaging technologies have a significant impact in determining the management pathway for these patients and thus for improving their overall survival rates.

CT can be used to measure the size of the cervix and to detect any enlarged lymph nodes, obstruction of the ureter, and lung or liver metastases. As with ultrasound, however, the value of CT is limited because the normal cervix and cervical carcinomas have similar attenuation values, so that the tumor can only be recognized if it alters the contour or size of the cervix. Over the past several years, it has been clearly demonstrated that MRI is superior to any other imaging modality for evaluating disease extent. MRI is now an integral part of preoperative assessment of cervical cancer, in monitoring response to treatment and in detection of recurrence. PET with 2-[fluorine-1] fluroro-2-deoxy-D-glucose (FDG) may also be used in cervical cancer staging and follow-up and is useful in evaluating lymph node involvement and for detecting distant metastases.

Optimizing Spatial Resolution in Cervical Imaging

To maximize signal and thus improve spatial resolution, high field strength scanners are increasingly being advocated in oncology. Three Tesla (T) scanners offer increased SNR, but suffer from increased field inhomogeneity and, hence, artifacts, although data acquisition over small fields of view (e.g., over the cervix), are less prone to these effects. Cervix images at 3 T have been shown to be equivalent diagnostically to those at 1.5 T, although qualitative analysis of image homogeneity in the same dataset was felt to be inferior at 3 T (Hori et al. 2009). The benefits of imaging patients with cancer of the cervix at 3 T over 1.5 T therefore remain to be established.

To examine the pelvis effectively, a receiver in the form of a multichannel pelvic-phased array coil is the preferred option. However in extremely large patients where the fill factor of the patient in the body receive coil of the scanner is maximal, the body coil may provide equally good pelvic images. The use of a multichannel array also allows parallel imaging which reduces scan time without a significant reduction in signal-to-noise ratio. A four channel array is the norm, but increasingly manufacturers are producing eight or larger numbers of coil arrays. Positioning the patient in the coil is also important, as coverage from the pelvic floor to the lower para-aortic nodal chains is essential.

The resolution of the primary tumor on MR imaging may be further improved by using endocavitary receiver coils. Although coils may be sited in the rectum for this purpose, they are less comfortable than a vaginally sited coil. Endorectal coils give high-resolution images of the posterior cervix, but the anterior margin of the tumor and its relation to the bladder base is often difficult to define because of drop-off of signal. Endovaginal coils give very high-resolution images of the cervix and adjacent parametrium (deSouza et al. 1996). Balloon design–shaped coils are available that are of single loop geometry. A solenoid design endovaginal coil that envelops the cervix provides a signal-to-noise ratio advantage. The ring is 37 mm in diameter and is useful for delineating smaller tumors and early parametrial invasion (deSouza et al. 1996). When an endocavitary coil is used, immobilization of the coil is key to obtaining high-quality images. Balloon coils use the balloon itself as an immobilization device, but it is important to place a sandbag over the coil handle to further reduce motion. With the ring design coil, an external clamp is used to grasp the handle. Endovaginal coils are surprisingly well tolerated even in patients with larger tumors and are a particular advantage in assessing patients prior to fertility-sparing surgery. The endovaginal coil also may be combined with an external pelvic array in a multi-coil arrangement. This technique may be used to image more advanced stages of cervical carcinoma. The clinical value of this precise imaging technique is substantial. Armed with accurate information about the volume and extent of cervical disease, the clinician can take rational decisions about therapy. The outcome of different treatments can be interpreted more easily if the initial tumor has been defined accurately.

Clinical Impact of Imaging on Patient Management

Early studies confirmed superiority of MRI in staging cervical cancer compared to surgical staging (Togashi et al. 1989) and reported accuracies with MRI between 76% and 85%. Other studies showed that detection of the primary tumor on T2-weighted MRI was superior to CT (sensitivity 75 vs. 51%, $p < 0.005$) with substantial improvements in staging (accuracy 75–77 vs. 32–69%, $p < 0.025$) (Ho et al. 1992). Where available, therefore, MRI has become the modality of choice for detecting and staging the disease; in women with bulky stage Ib disease it is preferable to identify those who have a high risk of requiring postoperative radiotherapy because of

microscopic nodal disease as chemotherapy at the outset may be a better treatment option than having to undergo both radical surgery and radiotherapy.

There is increasing evidence that young women with small volume invasive disease which does not extend deep into the cervix might be treated successfully by radical removal of the cervix, so conserving their fertility. This conservative treatment was initially limited to ectocervical tumors because hitherto it had been impossible to accurately determine the extent of small endocervical lesions. Improved spatial resolution of MRI with use of an endovaginal technique allows a precise definition of the size and location of the tumor and lends greater confidence to the selection of women for whom such conservative surgical treatment might be appropriate. Fast spin-echo T2-weighted sequences provide best image contrast for delineating extent of disease within the cervix and hence the patient's suitability for trachelectomy (Peppercorn et al. 1999). Volume (3-D) imaging also provides the information necessary to calculate tumor volumes, which is of prognostic significance. Recently, diffusion-weighted MRI has shown higher accuracy than T2-weighted imaging alone for tumor detection (Charles-Edwards et al. 2008).

A common dilemma is the management of women following incomplete excision by loop diathermy or cone biopsy of stage Ia1 microinvasive tumors, adenocarcinoma in situ, or high-grade squamous intraepithelial disease. In some of these women, the lesion removed is just the tip of the iceberg. An invasive cancer remains lurking in the cervix. The conventional options are observation with a repeat smear in 4–6 months, a repeat cone biopsy, or a simple hysterectomy. Each of these has obvious disadvantages. Endovaginal MR imaging can exclude a gross lesion so that either a simple hysterectomy or a repeat smear may be performed without prejudicing the patient's prognosis. If necessary, the scan can be repeated at intervals to monitor progression.

Disease Staging

Imaging the Primary Tumor

Cervical cancer is recognized as a high signal intensity mass within the normally low signal intensity cervix on T2-weighted MRI (Fig. 140.1). Distortion of the low

Fig. 140.1 Organ-confined
cervical cancer: T2-weighted
sagittal (**a**), (FSE 2,370/90 ms
[repetition time/time to echo,
TR/TE]) and coronal (**b**),
(2,000/90 ms [TR/TE]) images
using an endovaginal coil
demonstrate an intermediate
signal intensity mass arising
from the anterior right lip of
the cervix (*arrows*). There is
a clear demarcation of normal
cervix seen around this lesion
(*arrowhead* in **b**) indicating no
evidence of parametrial
extension

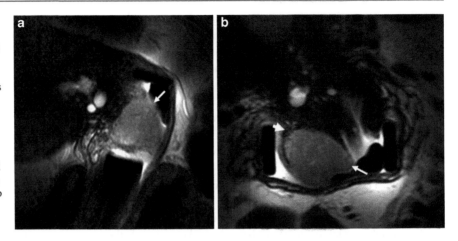

signal ring of inner cervical stroma may be apparent and any breaks in the ring representing tumor extension into the parametrium may be identified. MRI is also accurate in showing the relationship of the tumor to the internal os if trachelectomy is being considered (Peppercorn et al. 1999). Tumor volumes are estimated by drawing regions of interest around the tumor margins on successive T2-weighted scans and then computing the tumor volume per slice from the product of the area and the slice thickness. Volumes obtained with MR imaging correlate well with those obtained by histomorphometric methods but only weakly with clinical stage (Burghardt et al. 1989).

Although dynamic enhancement has been reported as valuable in accurate assessment of cervical invasion by tumor (Yamashita et al. 2000), there is general agreement that these images do not add to the information available on post-enhancement scans.

With an endovaginal MRI technique, the acquired in-plane resolution of ~0.4 mm means that very small cervical lesions with volumes as low as 0.2 cm³ and early spread or lack of spread to the parametrium can be demonstrated (Fig. 140.1). The precise definition of the size and location of small tumors with this technique lends greater confidence to the selection of women for fertility-sparing surgery. The sensitivity of endovaginal MR imaging compared to histology as the gold standard for detecting the presence of stage I tumors is 97.2%, specificity 80%, positive predictive value 97.2%, and negative predictive value 80% (deSouza et al. 2000). This compares well with quoted figures of 75% sensitivity and 70% specificity of conventional MR techniques (Hori et al. 2009). However, as patients are often referred following

positive cone biopsies when distortion of the cervix local hematoma or granulation tissue makes image interpretation difficult, false-positives may occur. In such cases, additional contrast mechanisms such as diffusion-weighted imaging in conjunction with the T2-weighted images are proving invaluable for differentiating granulation tissue from residual tumor (Charles-Edwards et al. 2011).

Imaging Local Spread

In initial studies comparing MRI, CT, and EUA with histological findings after radical hysterectomy, an accuracy rate for parametrial involvement of 87–90% for MR imaging, 55–80% for CT, and 82.5% for examination under anesthesia was seen (Ho et al. 1992). On MRI, extracervical extension is best defined using T2-weighted fast spin-echo sequences; fat suppression techniques do not provide additional benefits (Lam et al. 2000). Contrast enhancement has not proved beneficial: In a series of 73 patients, FSE T2-weighted images had an accuracy of 83% for determining parametrial extension (compared to 65% for T1-weighted gadolinium-enhanced images and 72% for T1-weighted gadolinium-enhanced fat-suppressed images). The high negative predictive value (95%) for the exclusion of parametrial tumor invasion is the principal contributor to the staging accuracy obtained with FSE T2-weighted imaging.

On T2-weighted MRI, an intact low signal intensity stripe of residual, normal stroma of the cervix seen peripheral to the tumor mass indicates that no extracervical spread is present, a break indicates

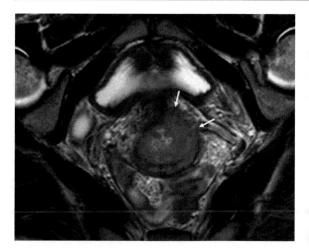

Fig. 140.2 Extracervical extension of cervical tumor: T2-weighted axial image (FSE 5,540/90 ms [repetition time to echo/time to echo, TR/TE]) through the pelvis using an external phased array receiver coil demonstrates a large tumor arising from the cervix. On the *left*, anteriorly there is disruption of the normal cervical stroma lateral to the mass, which extends out into the parametrial tissue (*arrows*)

extension of tumor into the adjacent parametrium. Where there is extensive involvement with tumor, no residual normal stroma may be demonstrated. The intermediate signal intensity of the tumor is seen extending into and blending with the high signalintensity of parametrial fat (Fig. 140.2). The use of three plane T2-weighted MRI to assess extracervical invasion is optimal: The oblique plane (perpendicular to the tumor) is used for determining parametrial invasion; the sagittal plane for extension into the uterine body, bladder, and rectum (Fig. 140.3); and the axial plane for determining extension into the bladder and rectum.

An intravenous urogram (IVU) is now obsolete as part of the staging process as it is superseded by MR imaging.

Nodal Involvement

Lymph node involvement in cervical cancer is often assessed with CT. The major drawback for this is that nodes must be enlarged to be detectable. Thus, metastases less than 1 cm in diameter will not be identified. In vivo tissue characterization based on relaxation times or signal intensities does not support differentiation of metastatic from hyperplastic nodes. MRI

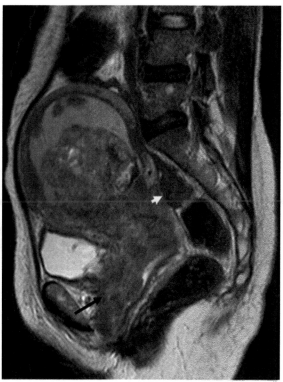

Fig. 140.3 Large cervical tumor involving bladder and bowel: T2-weighted sagittal image (FSE 3,357/125 ms [repetition time/ time to echo TR/TE]) through the pelvis demonstrates a large mass involving the cervix and uterine body, invading bladder wall and urethra anteriorly (*arrow*) and adherent to rectal wall posteriorly (arrowhead), indicating stage 4 disease

therefore, like CT, relies on changes in the size of the lymph nodes, since the tumor deposits themselves are not highlighted (Fig. 140.4). T1-weighted and STIR sequences in the coronal plane and T2-weighted sequences in the transverse plane (Fig. 140.3) provide optimal size information and allow measurements of the long and short axes of any visualized lymph nodes.

A lymph node–specific MR contrast agent has been developed that allows the identification of malignant nodal infiltration independent of the lymph node size. This novel MR contrast agent is classified as a nanoparticle (mean diameter, 30 nm), and is composed of an iron oxide core, coated with low molecular weight dextran (ultrasmall particles of iron oxide, USPIO). A significant increase in sensitivity, with no loss of specificity has been demonstrated for the detection of malignant lymph nodes with USPIOs in patients with cervical and endometrial cancer

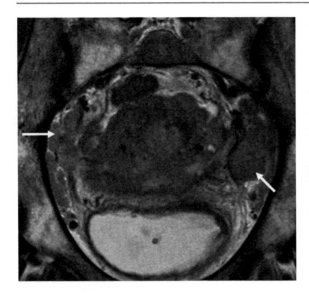

Fig. 140.4 Cervical tumor metastatic to pelvic lymph nodes. T2-weighted coronal oblique image (FSE 4,000/100 ms [repetition time/time to echo, TR/TE]) through the pelvis demonstrates bilateral iliac lymphadenopathy (*arrows*) metastatic from a large cervical tumor

(Rockall et al. 2005). On a node-by-node basis, the sensitivity increased from 29% using standard size criteria to 93% using USPIO criteria. On a patient-by-patient basis, sensitivity increased from 27% using standard size criteria to 100% using USPIO criteria.

The role of positron emission tomography (PET) for detecting metastatic pelvic lymph nodes is still being debated. Small single-center studies claim a 91–96% sensitivity and 96–100% specificity for detecting nodes involved with tumor (Loft et al. 2007) (Fig. 140.5), while results from other studies are much poorer. Urinary residues of [18]FDG in the ureters remain a source of false-positive results. Quantitation suggests that a $SUV_{max} \geq 3.3$ for lymph nodes is a significant adverse factor in those patients with nodal enlargement (Yen et al. 2008).

Unusual Histological Subtypes

Minimal Deviation Adenocarcinoma

Minimal deviation adenocarcinoma (MDA) of the cervix or adenoma malignum is a relatively rare variant of mucinous adenocarcinoma. It was first described in 1975 by Silverburg and Hurst and accounts for less than 3% of all cervical adenocarcinomas. It is typically

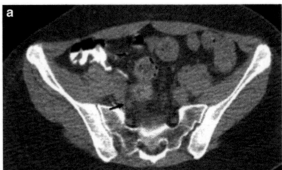

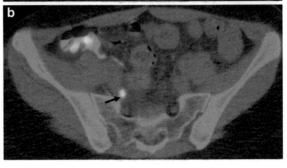

Fig. 140.5 Cervical tumor metastatic to pelvic lymph nodes. Axial CT scan (**a**), with corresponding [18]FDG-PET/CT slice (**b**), demonstrates a small right external iliac lymph node in a that is metabolically active in b (*arrows*). The node is difficult to appreciate on the CT scan alone

a low-grade epithelial tumor with prominent mature glandular tissue similar to that of normal benign glands but with nuclear anaplasia or stromal invasion and commonly presents with a watery vaginal discharge or dysfunctional uterine bleeding.

Accurate diagnosis of minimal deviation adenocarcinoma is challenging but important as delayed diagnosis often results in late presentation. Pap smear can be diagnostically unreliable because histological features resemble normal cervical glands (Li et al. 2010). Confirmation of MDA requires deep cervical biopsies such as a cervical conization specimen and relies on immunohistochemical antigen detection such as HIK1083.

MRI is the imaging modality of choice. On T2-weighted images, MDA can appear as pure enlargement of the cervix or as a fine villous lesion (Fig. 140.6) but is more commonly seen as a multicystic mass extending from the endocervical glands to the deep cervical stroma with a variable volume of thin, interdigitating solid elements. The cystic lesions are relatively isointense or slightly hypointense to the cervix on T1-weighted images and hyperintense on T2-weighted images. Both solid

Fig. 140.6 Minimal deviation adenocarcinoma confined to the cervix. T2-W sagittal (**a**) (FSE 2,500/80 ms [TR/TE]) and axial (**b**) (FSE 2,500/80 ms [TR/TE]) images through the cervix using an endovaginal coil show diffuse, ill-defined intermediate cervix signal intensity within the cervical stroma (*arrows*). Dilated endocervical glands typical of this entity are seen (*arrowheads*)

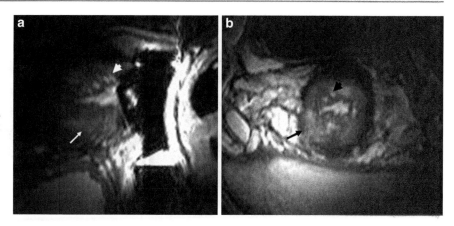

and cystic components enhance after contrast administration (Itoh et al. 2000).

Common incidental dilated endocervical glands (Nabothian cysts) are usually situated superficially within the cervix and can be confused with MDA if they extend into the deep stromal tissue of the cervix. Another mimic of minimal deviation adenocarcinoma is a "Tunnel cluster": A particular type of Nabothian cyst in which the endocervical glands display multicystic dilatation (Sugiyama 2007). Infection such as *Neisseria gonorrhoeae* and *Chlamydia trachomatis* can infect the glandular epithelium and cause endocervicitis and vaginal discharge and result in MR appearances similar to MDA. The clinical picture is critical in differentiating these cases.

As with squamous and adenocarcinomas of the cervix, MDA is staged using the FIGO system. The mean survival is approximately 5 years for patients with stage I, 38.1 months with stage II, 22.8 months with stage III, and 5.4 months for patients with stage IV disease (Li et al. 2010). It is relatively insensitive to chemotherapy and radiotherapy and usually treated with surgery if diagnosed early.

MDA has been associated with Peutz–Jeghers syndrome (pigmentation of the buccal mucosa and multiple intestinal harmatomas) and mucinous tumors of the ovary.

Cervical Lymphoma

Secondary infiltration of the cervix is common with advanced stage lymphoma but primary cervical lymphoma is rare. Only 1% of primary non-Hodgkin's lymphoma occurs within the genitourinary system and primary cervical lymphoma accounts for less than 1% of all cervical malignancies. Age range at diagnosis is wide (20–80 years) with the median age in reported studies varying from 40 to 52 years.

Most patients present with dysfunctional uterine bleeding; it is less common to present with an abdominal mass, urinary symptoms, or systemic symptoms (Marin et al. 2002). Clinical features are nonspecific and are shared with other cervical malignancies. Pap smear is often normal in the presence of primary lymphoma of the cervix; one large case series found that only 50% of cervical lymphomas had an abnormal Pap smear (Chan et al. 2005). Biopsy is therefore needed to make a definitive histological diagnosis.

Both the FIGO and the Ann Arbor systems for extra-nodal lymphoma are used for staging primary cervical lymphoma (Table 2).

It is important to distinguish lymphoma from cervical carcinoma, as the management and prognosis of these two groups differ. As with other cervical tumors, MRI is the modality of choice for delineating local extent and staging the disease using T2-weighted images. The imaging features of cervical lymphoma can be nonspecific but lymphoma should be suspected if there is a bulky, diffuse infiltrating mass. The majority of lesions are in excess of 4 cm in diameter at diagnosis. Lymphomas are hypointense on T1-weighted imaging relative to the myometrium and hyperintense on T2-weighted images (Marin et al. 2002). They often spare the cervical mucosa with preservation of stromal features and if they extend into the uterus, the low signal junctional zone is also often spared. Avid and diffuse contrast enhancement is another feature of primary

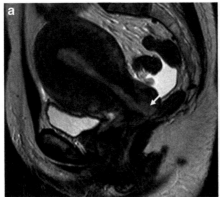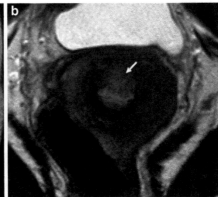

Fig. 140.7 Cervical metastasis from breast cancer: T2-weighted sagittal (**a**) (FSE 3,876/126 ms [TR/TE]) and axial (**b**) (FSE 4,401/100 ms [TR/TE]) images through the pelvis showing an intermediate signal intensity mass within the cervix (*arrows*) in a patient with metastatic breast cancer. Although this lesion is radiologically indistinguishable from a primary cervical tumor, it was histologically confirmed as metastatic breast cancer. The uterine body shows junctional zone hyperplasia and there is free fluid in the rectouterine pouch

cervical lymphoma (Marin et al. 2002). These features help differentiate cervical lymphomas from carcinomas (Marin et al. 2002). CT and [18]FDG-PET are useful for completion of staging and the latter has also been found to be useful in posttreatment follow-up (Bural et al. 2007).

Primary cervical lymphomas are predominantly of B-cell NHL origin (and diffuse B-cell subtype) and generally have a favorable prognosis. However, due to the relative rarity of these tumors in comparison to cervical carcinomas, there is no established treatment protocol and no current treatment meta-analysis exists. These nonepithelial tumors are often treated less radically than their epithelial counterparts with either chemotherapy alone, especially if fertility preservation is desired, or in combination with radiotherapy and or surgery (Okamoto et al. 2003).

Neuroendocrine Tumors

Neuroendocrine tumors of the cervix are rare, accounting for <5% of all cervical cancers. They usually present with abnormal vaginal bleeding. These tumors are characterized by a high incidence of early nodal and distant metastases, resulting in poorer prognosis than other subtypes of cervical cancers (Chan et al. 2003). Imaging protocols are identical to those for squamous and adenocarcinomas of the cervix. However, lesions can be hypo- or hyperintense compared to normal cervical stroma. In the former case, the use of gadolinium enhancement can be helpful in delineating the tumor and defining its extent.

Neuroendocrine tumors have an aggressive clinical course and those of the cervix histologically and clinically share similarities with small-cell lung cancer. Prognosis therefore is poor, with median survival durations in patients with localized, regional, and distant disease of 34, 14, and 5 months, respectively. Management is by primary chemotherapy and is based on the established role of cisplatin and etoposide in metastatic small-cell lung cancer.

Cervical Metastases

Metastases to the cervix are exceedingly rare and when they occur are often from a primary tumor in the breast. The literature primarily consists of isolated case reports. They can present with abnormal vaginal bleeding, but they often are asymptomatic. They may be discovered incidentally during routine pelvic surveillance of patients with malignancy; only surveillance can detect these secondary lesions early.

On imaging, it is not possible to differentiate a primary cervical carcinoma from a metastasis (Fig. 140.7). MRI is the diagnostic modality of choice; however, it should be emphasized that, in most cases, only accurate immunohistochemical investigation, particularly if performed on the primary lesion as well, can solve differential diagnostic problems and allow the clinician to establish appropriate treatment.

Depending on the presence of other metastatic sites, aggressive treatment of isolated cervical metastasis should be performed when feasible with surgery; otherwise, systemic chemotherapy with taxane could be sufficient in increasing survival.

Imaging as a Prognostic Biomarker

In cervical cancer, there has been considerable interest in using tumor size or volume as a prognostic biomarker: A retrospective study of 275 surgically treated women with stage Ib–IIb cervical cancer with negative lymph nodes showed a strong correlation between tumor diameter and prognosis (Comerci et al. 1998). Measuring tumor volume on MRI is of paramount importance: It has been shown that it is the size of tumor burden that determines the outcome rather than invasion beyond the anatomical margins of the uterus (Soutter et al. 2004).

The presence of involved lymph nodes upstages the disease and carries a poor prognosis. The risk of nodal disease may also be predicted from the tumor to cervix quotient and independently from the presence of parametrial spread (Biewenga et al. 2011).

Imaging in Treatment Planning

Following MRI, if disease is confined to the cervix, a surgical option is preferred. If MRI indicates disease outside the cervix, radiation therapy is required. [18]FDG PET also has a role in this regard because of improved detection of para-aortic lymph nodes (PALN), and results in reduced PALN relapses, but it has not been shown to improve survival because numbers of patients with treatment modification were small (n = 7) (Tsai et al. 2010).

Increasingly, [18]FDG-PET/CT is being advocated to aid delivery of intensity-modulated radiation therapy (IMRT): In 452 patients treated with curative intent (135 with IMRT) based on [18]FDG-PET/CT, the IMRT group showed better overall survival, although recurrence-free survival did not reach statistical significance (Kidd et al. 2010).

In smaller tumors, MRI is being investigated for brachytherapy planning, but requires MRI-compatible applicators to minimize artifacts and distortions. Shapes of the clinical target volumes and organs at risk also differ with CT and MRI planning which could lead to altered target dosing so that more work is needed in this area.

Monitoring Treatment Response

Serial MR imaging may be used before and after primary radiation therapy to assess tumor response. In addition, T2-weighted or diffusion-weighted techniques provide additional contrast (compared to CT and ultrasound) to distinguish fibrosis from residual tumor. Techniques such as DCE-MRI can be useful to monitor the effects of targeted cytostatic agents where there is an early switch-off of vascular response before a reduction in tumor size.

Despite the efficacy of chemoradiotherapy, $\sim$20% of patients will relapse within 5 years. Identification of these patients at early time points after treatment would be helpful to deliver an individualized therapeutic approach at the outset. DCE-MRI quantitative parameters of the exchange rate constants K^{trans} and K_{ep} (and semiquantitative parameters of peak time, slope, maximum slope, and contrast enhancement ratio) after 2 and 5 weeks of treatment in one small study have been shown to provide early prediction of primary tumor control and disease-free survival (Donaldson et al. 2010). Tumor volumes and regression ratios as early as 2 weeks into radiotherapy have been shown to correlate strongly with local recurrence: A volume of $<$40 cm^3 and a ratio of $<$20% from baseline at 1 month had an 89% sensitivity and an 87% specificity for predicting local recurrence (Wang et al. 2010).

An increase in ADC derived from DW-MRI seen after 15 days of therapy has also been shown to indicate response (Liu et al. 2009). Pretreatment ADCs for complete responders were significantly lower than those of partial responders with a negative correlation between pretreatment ADCs and percentage size reduction after 2 months of chemoradiation. There is also a role for [18]FDG-PET in response assessment wherein residual metabolically active disease 3 months after completion of treatment may be used to guide additional therapy (Schwartz et al. 2009).

Summary

In cervical cancer, MRI is the mainstay of disease detection and staging. Use of high spatial resolution imaging is particularly important if fertility-sparing procedures are being considered. At the opposite extreme, MRI identifies those at higher risk who may need radiation or chemoradiation therapy. In these cases, a preoperative [18]FDG-PET/CT scan may be useful for stratifying patients for adjuvant therapies. In more advanced disease where chemoradiotherapy is the primary treatment modality, MRI may be used for radiation therapy planning and is gaining an increasing role if dose redistribution with techniques such as intensity-modulated radiotherapy are being considered. [18]FDG-PET/CT is useful to guide decisions on irradiating para-aortic nodal chains; it is also a key modality in detecting recurrent disease, although in future it may be superseded by newer MRI techniques such as diffusion-weighted imaging for identifying pelvic recurrence.

Newer techniques in both MRI and PET are being implemented for use as prognostic biomarkers. In particular, DW-MRI has become an invaluable tool in the diagnostic armamentarium of this disease. Radiotracers that report on hypoxia and tumor receptor status will also gain increasing importance as we move to an era of personalized medicine.

Acknowledgments We acknowledge the support received from the CRUK and EPSRC Cancer Imaging Centre in association with the MRC and Department of Health (England) grant C1060/A10334, and NHS funding to the NIHR Biomedical Research Centre.

References

Biewenga P, van der Velden J, Mol BW, Stalpers LJ, Schilthuis MS, van der Steeg JW, et al. Prognostic model for survival in patients with early stage cervical cancer. Cancer. 2011;117:768–76.

Bural GG, Shriaknthan S, Houseni M, Alavi A. FDG-PET is useful in staging and follow-up of primary uterine cervical lymphoma. Clin Nucl Med. 2007;32:748–50.

Burghardt E, Hofmann HM, Ebner F, Haas J, Tamussino K, Justich E. Magnetic resonance imaging in cervical cancer: a basis for objective classification. Gynecol Oncol. 1989;33:61–7.

Chan JK, Loizzi V, Burger RA, Rutgers J, Monk BJ. Prognostic factors in neuroendocrine small cell cervical carcinoma: a multivariate analysis. Cancer. 2003;97:568–74.

Chan JK, Loizzi V, Magistris A, Hunter MI, Rutgers J, DiSaia PJ, et al. Clinicopathologic features of six cases of primary cervical lymphoma. Am J Obstet Gynecol. 2005;193:866–72.

Charles-Edwards EM, Messiou C, Morgan VA, De Silva SS, McWhinney NA, Katesmark M, et al. Diffusion-weighted imaging in cervical cancer with an endovaginal technique: potential value for improving tumor detection in stage Ia and Ib1 disease. Radiology. 2008;249:541–50.

Charles-Edwards E, Morgan V, Attygalle AD, Giles SL, Ind TE, Davis M, et al. Endovaginal magnetic resonance imaging of stage 1A/1B cervical cancer with A T2- and diffusion-weighted magnetic resonance technique: effect of lesion size and previous cone biopsy on tumor detectability. Gynecol Oncol. 2011;120:368–73.

Comerci G, Bolger BS, Flannelly G, Maini M, de Barros LA, Monaghan JM. Prognostic factors in surgically treated stage IB-IIB carcinoma of the cervix with negative lymph nodes. Int J Gynecol Cancer. 1998;8:23–6.

deSouza NM, Scoones D, Krausz T, Gilderdale DJ, Soutter WP. High-resolution MR imaging of stage I cervical neoplasia with a dedicated transvaginal coil: MR features and correlation of imaging and pathologic findings. AJR Am J Roentgenol. 1996;166:553–9.

deSouza NM, Whittle M, Williams AD, Sohail M, Krausz T, Gilderdale DJ, et al. Magnetic resonance imaging of the primary site in stage I cervical carcinoma: A comparison of endovaginal coil with external phased array coil techniques at 0.5 T. J Magn Reson Imaging. 2000;12:1020–6.

Donaldson SB, Buckley DL, O'Connor JP, Davidson SE, Carrington BM, Jones AP, et al. Enhancing fraction measured using dynamic contrast-enhanced MRI predicts disease-free survival in patients with carcinoma of the cervix. Br J Cancer. 2010;102:23–6.

Ho CM, Chien TY, Jeng CM, Tsang YM, Shih BY, Chang SC. Staging of cervical cancer: comparison between magnetic resonance imaging, computed tomography and pelvic examination under anesthesia. J Formos Med Assoc. 1992;91:982–90.

Hori M, Kim T, Murakami T, Imaoka I, Onishi H, Tomoda K, et al. Uterine cervical carcinoma: preoperative staging with 3.0-T MR imaging – comparison with 1.5-T MR imaging. Radiology. 2009;251:96–104.

Itoh K, Toki T, Shiohara S, Oguchi O, Konishi I, Fujii S. A comparative analysis of cross sectional imaging techniques in minimal deviation adenocarcinoma of the uterine cervix. BJOG. 2000;107:1158–63.

Kidd EA, Siegel BA, Dehdashti F, Rader JS, Mutic S, Mutch DG, et al. Clinical outcomes of definitive intensity-modulated radiation therapy with fluorodeoxyglucose-positron emission tomography simulation in patients with locally advanced cervical cancer. Int J Radiat Oncol Biol Phys. 2010;77:1085–91.

Lam WW, So NM, Yang WT, Metreweli C. Detection of parametrial invasion in cervical carcinoma: role of short tau inversion recovery sequence. Clin Radiol. 2000;55:702–7.

Li G, Jiang W, Gui S, Xu C. Minimal deviation adenocarcinoma of the uterine cervix. Int J Gynaecol Obstet. 2010;110:89–92.

Liu Y, Bai R, Sun H, Liu H, Zhao X, Li Y. Diffusion-weighted imaging in predicting and monitoring the response of uterine cervical cancer to combined chemoradiation. Clin Radiol. 2009;64:1067–74.

Loft A, Berthelsen AK, Roed H, Ottosen C, Lundvall L, Knudsen J, et al. The diagnostic value of PET/CT scanning in patients with cervical cancer: a prospective study. Gynecol Oncol. 2007;106:29–34.

Marin C, Seoane JM, Sanchez M, Ruiz Y, Garcia JA. Magnetic resonance imaging of primary lymphoma of the cervix. Eur Radiol. 2002;12:1541–5.

Okamoto Y, Tanaka YO, Nishida M, Tsunoda H, Yoshikawa H, Itai Y. MR imaging of the uterine cervix: imaging-pathologic correlation. Radiographics. 2003;23:425–45.

Pecorelli S. Revised FIGO staging for carcinoma of the vulva, cervix and endometrium. Int J Gynaecol Obstet. 2009;105(2):103–4.

Peppercorn PD, Jeyarajah AR, Woolas R, Shepherd JH, Oram DH, Jacobs IJ, et al. Role of MR imaging in the selection of patients with early cervical carcinoma for fertility-preserving surgery: initial experience. Radiology. 1999;212:395–9.

Rockall AG, Sohaib SA, Harisinghani MG, Babar SA, Singh N, Jeyarajah AR, et al. Diagnostic performance of nanoparticle-enhanced magnetic resonance imaging in the diagnosis of lymph node metastases in patients with endometrial and cervical cancer. J Clin Oncol. 2005;23:2813–21.

Schwartz JK, Grigsby PW, Dehdashti F, Delbeke D. The role of 18 F-FDG PET in assessing therapy response in cancer of the cervix. J Nucl Med. 2009;50:6S–73.

Soutter WP, Hanoch J, D'Arcy T, Dina R, McIndoe GA, deSouza NM. Pretreatment tumour volume measurement on high-resolution magnetic resonance imaging as a predictor of survival in cervical cancer. BJOG. 2004;111:741–7.

Sugiyama K, Takehara Y. MR findings of pseudoneoplastic lesions in the uterine cervix mimicking adenoma malignum. Br J Radiol. 2007;80:878–83.

Togashi K, Nishimura K, Sagoh T, Minami S, Noma S, Fujisawa I, et al. Carcinoma of the cervix: staging with MR imaging. Radiology. 1989;171:245–51.

Tsai CS, Lai CH, Chang TC, Yen TC, Ng KK, Hsueh S, et al. A prospective randomized trial to study the impact of pretreatment FDG-PET for cervical cancer patients with MRI-detected positive pelvic but negative para-aortic lymph-adenopathy. Int J Radiat Oncol Biol Phys. 2010;76:477–84.

Wang JZ, Mayr NA, Zhang D, Li K, Grecula JC, Montebello JF, et al. Sequential magnetic resonance imaging of cervical cancer: the predictive value of absolute tumor volume and regression ratio measured before, during, and after radiation therapy. Cancer. 2010;116:5093–101.

Yamashita Y, Baba T, Baba Y, Nishimura R, Ikeda S, Takahashi M, et al. Dynamic contrast-enhanced MR imaging of uterine cervical cancer: pharmacokinetic analysis with histopathologic correlation and its importance in predicting the outcome of radiation therapy. Radiology. 2000;216:803–9.

Yen TC, See LC, Lai CH, Tsai CS, Chao A, Hsueh S, et al. Standardized uptake value in para-aortic lymph nodes is a significant prognostic factor in patients with primary advanced squamous cervical cancer. Eur J Nucl Med Mol Imaging. 2008;35:493–501.

141

Uterus: Follow-up and Detection of Recurrent Disease

Tristan Barrett, Hebert A. Vargas, and Evis Sala

Introduction

Recurrent uterine or cervical cancer can be defined as the presence of a new, recurrent disease following definitive treatment with a curative intent. For cervical cancer, as with ovarian cancer, a cutoff of >6 months post-therapy is used to distinguish recurrent from residual disease (Liyanage et al. 2010). However, this time-scale is somewhat arbitrary and the distinction does not impact on management, making it less clinically relevant. The imaging of recurrent disease in endometrial carcinoma and uterine sarcoma is essentially identical, thus we employ the term "uterine cancer" herein.

Regardless of the treatment employed, recurrence typically occurs at early time points: >75% of cervical cancer recurrences and up to 87% of uterine cancer recurrences occur within 3 years of treatment (Sohaib et al. 2007; Lai 2004). Recurrence can be divided into four general categories which progressively involve disease more distal from the primary site and bring a worse overall prognosis (Choi et al. 2000). The four broad categories being local recurrence at the primary site or involving the pelvic organs or lymph nodes, extension to the pelvic sidewall, metastases to lymph nodes outside the pelvis, and distant metastases.

T. Barrett (✉)
Department of Radiology, School of Clinical Medicine,
Addenbrooke's Hospital and University of Cambridge,
Cambridge, UK

H.A. Vargas
Radiology Department, Memorial Sloan-Kettering Cancer
Center, New York, NY, USA

E. Sala
Memorial Sloan-Kettering Cancer Center, New York, NY, USA

Follow-up is necessary to identify such patients and in particular to recognize recurrence at the earliest possible stage. Cure rates of up to 80% can be achieved in patients with locally recurrent uterine cancer (Creutzberg et al. 2003) and the outcome of patients presenting with locally recurrent cervical cancer is significantly improved in comparison to those with distal disease (Poolkerd et al. 2006; Baalbergen et al. 2001).

Patient Management

There are several guidelines pertaining to the postoperative follow-up of patients with cervical or uterine cancer. The consensus is that follow-up should be clinical and involve a combination of history taking, physical examination, and vaginal examination (NCCN 2011; Emons et al. (2009); Elit et al. 2009). Serum CA-125 levels are sometimes elevated in cases of primary cervical or uterine cancer; in such patients monitoring of serum levels can be a useful means of detecting recurrence (Gadducci et al. 2004). Patients should also be educated on symptoms which may indicate recurrence and to seek early advice if these develop. Symptoms include vaginal bleeding or discharge, pelvic/abdominal pain, cough and shortness of breath, edema, loss of appetite, and weight loss. Although some authors have suggested selecting out uterine cancer patients that are at higher risk for closer follow-up (Tjalma et al. 2004), there is no consensus agreement on this and the guidelines recommend broadly the same follow-up for all types of uterine and cervical cancer. Surveillance is performed every 3–4 months during the first 2 years where the risk of recurrence is highest, every 6 months for

B. Hamm, P. R. Ros (eds.), *Abdominal Imaging*, DOI 10.1007/978-3-642-13327-5_183,
© Springer-Verlag Berlin Heidelberg 2013

the next 3 years, and annually thereafter. During follow-up appointments, the increased risk of breast, ovarian, and colon cancer in patients with uterine cancer should be considered (Baekelandt et al. 2009). The National Comprehensive Cancer Network recommends cervicovaginal cytology assessment with a Papanicolaou smear test at every follow-up appointment for cervical cancer and at alternate appointments for uterine neoplasms. However, some authors disagree on the use of "Pap" smears on the basis of their poor detection of recurrence in asymptomatic patients following treatment for cervical cancer (Bodurka-Bevers et al. 2000; Elit et al. 2009).

Imaging

Imaging plays a key role in confirming recurrence but is only recommended if there is a clinical suspicion during follow-up assessment. Ultrasound plays a role in image-guided biopsy for confirmation of recurrence; however, it is not used for primary detection of recurrent disease. Chest radiographs previously formed part of the routine follow-up but have a low sensitivity and by definition cannot detect locoregional recurrence, thus are no longer recommended. MRI, CT, and more recently PET-CT are established methods of detecting recurrent uterine or cervical cancer and the choice will be dictated by the clinical context along with other considerations (Son et al. 2010). MRI is more optimal for assessing suspected local recurrence and is also better for evaluation following radiotherapy. Postoperative complications are better assessed by CT. When distant metastases are suspected either CT or PET-CT are preferable to MRI. In the context of suspected lymph node involvement, PET-CT has a greater sensitivity and specificity than either MRI or CT.

An appreciation of the expected posttreatment appearances in patients with uterine and cervical cancer is essential for each of the imaging modalities; this is covered in subsequent chapters.

Appropriateness of Different Imaging Modalities

MRI is considered optimal for depicting local or pelvic recurrence due to its excellent soft tissue resolution as compared to CT. MRI is additionally the preferred modality for patients post radiotherapy where posttherapy fibrosis and recurrence can be better distinguished; PET-CT interpretation may be compromised by physiological uptake within the adjacent urinary bladder.

MRI: Technique

There are subtle differences in the protocols and sequences acquired when assessing for recurrent disease as opposed to the primary staging of disease. Patient preparation remains the same, with advice to fast for approximately 4 h beforehand and to empty the bladder immediately prior to scanning. The use of antispasmodic agents is strongly recommended in order to further reduce artifact from bowel peristalsis. A pelvic- or cardiac-phased array coil is preferred over a body coil to decrease scan time and improve image resolution (Yu et al. 1998). Standard MR protocols for assessment of recurrent uterine or cervical cancer include axial T1- and T2-weighted images, coronal and sagittal T2-weighted images, and post-contrast images in the axial plane. In addition to the standard anatomical sequences, the use of diffusion-weighted (DW) imaging is becoming commonplace (Sala et al. 2010).

MRI: Features of Recurrence

Locoregional recurrence of cervical and uterine cancer and involvement of the pelvic muscles is better depicted by MRI than CT (Jeong et al. 2003). Local recurrence is typically demonstrated as an irregular vaginal vault mass with a low signal intensity on T1 and a heterogeneous high-signal intensity on T2-weighted imaging, and displays heterogeneous enhancement following contrast administration (Choi et al. 2000; Jeong et al. 2003) (Fig. 141.1). Lesions may be cystic or contain a necrotic center which will appear of low signal intensity on T1 and high signal on T2-weighted imaging (Fig. 141.2). Local recurrence with invasion of adjacent organs such as the bladder or rectum is characterized by the loss of the intervening fat plane and direct extension of the mass into these structures. MRI has been shown to predict bladder invasion with an accuracy of 99% (Kim and Han 1997); findings include nodularity or

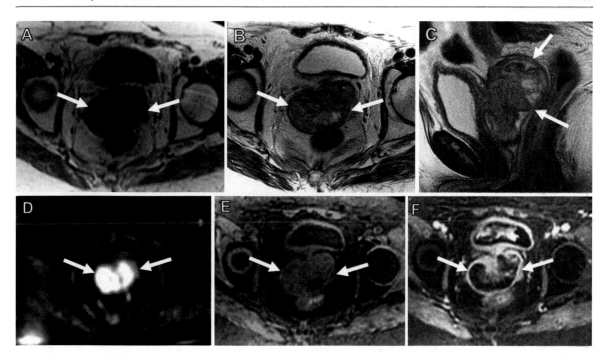

Fig. 141.1 *MRI demonstrating local recurrence of uterine cancer following total abdominal hysterectomy.* Axial T1-weighted (**a**), axial (**b**) and sagittal (**c**) T2-weighted images. The recurrent tumor appears as an irregular mass with a relatively homogeneous low T1 signal (*arrows* in **a**) and a heterogeneous, predominantly high signal intensity on T2-weighted imaging (*arrows* in **b** and **c**). Axial DWI *b*-400 s/mm^2 (**d**), and axial fat-suppressed T1 images before (**e**) and after (**f**) gadolinium administration. The mass demonstrates a high signal on DWI consistent with restricted diffusion (*arrows* in **d**) and displays heterogeneous, predominantly peripheral enhancement following contrast administration (*arrows* in **f**)

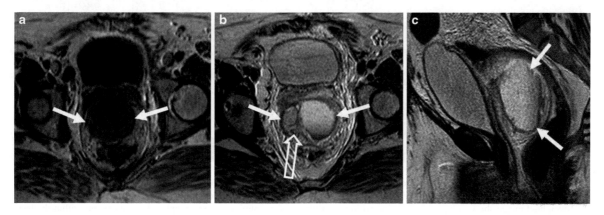

Fig. 141.2 *MRI of uterine cancer local (cystic) recurrence.* (**a**) Axial T1-weighted image shows local tumor recurrence, which is of homogeneous low signal intensity (*arrows*). Axial (**b**) and sagittal (**c**) T2-weighted images confirm the cystic nature of the mass which is predominantly of high T2 signal intensity (*arrows*) and contains internal septations (*open arrow* in **b**)

irregularity of the bladder base (Fig. 141.3), fistula formation with the tract appearing as high signal on T2-weighted imaging, and/or locules of air within the bladder. Pelvic sidewall invasion is diagnosed when the tumor extends to ≤3 mm from the sidewall and/or there is encasement or distortion of the vessels. More advanced signs of pelvic wall extension include infiltration of the muscles by tumor, with asymmetrical enlargement and contrast enhancement (Hricak and Yu 1996) (Fig. 141.4). Local lymph node

Fig. 141.3 *MRI demonstrating locoregional recurrence of cervical cancer with bladder invasion following radiotherapy.* Axial (**a**) and sagittal (**b**) T2-weighted images show subtle, irregular nodularity at the bladder base which is of intermediate T2 signal (*arrows*), as well as loss of the fat plane between the cervix and bladder. High *b*-value (b = 700 s/mm^2) axial (**c**) and sagittal (**d**) DW-MR images more easily identify the tumor infiltration as high signal at the bladder base (*arrows*)

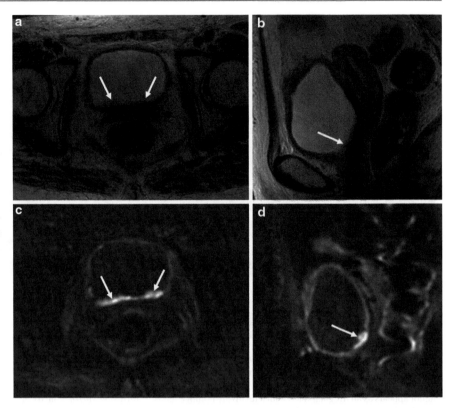

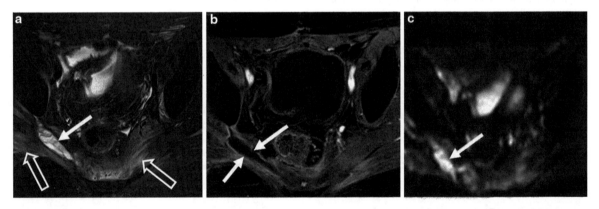

Fig. 141.4 *MRI of recurrent cervical cancer with pelvic side-wall invasion, following radiotherapy.* (**a**) Fat-saturated axial T2-weighted image shows a high-signal lesion within the right piriformis muscle (*arrow*), additional areas of high signal are noted within the gluteus maximus muscles bilaterally (*open arrows*) due to post-radiotherapy change. (**b**) Fat-saturated axial T1-weighted image 2 min after intravenous administration of gadolinium shows peripheral enhancement within the lesion (*arrows*). (**c**) Axial DW-MRI *b*-700 s/mm^2 demonstrates restricted diffusion within the lesion (*arrow*)

involvement includes the obturator, internal iliac, and external iliac groups; extra-pelvic nodal groups include the common iliac, sacral, and more distal nodal stations (Choi et al. 2000; Jeong et al. 2003). MRI relies mainly on size criteria (≥1 cm in short axis diameter) and basic morphological features to determine metastatic involvement; however, these criteria lack specificity and do not match the sensitivity of PET-CT. Bone metastases and abdominal spread can be well demonstrated by MRI but time constraints and patient comfort mean that dedicated imaging outside the pelvis is not performed,

Table 141.1 Pitfalls and potential false positive and negative results with PET imaging and diffusion-weighted MR imaging

	PET	DW-MRI
False negative	Physiological uptake along the renal tract limits adjacent nodal assessment	Tumors with low cellularity
	Physiological uptake in the bladder limits assessment of the surgical bed	Small mucosal deposits due to the high DW-MRI signal of bowel mucosa
	Small volume disease or lymph nodes (< 7 mm)	
	Cystic or necrotic lymph nodes	
	Small tumors	
	Non-FDG-avid tumors	
	CT component may be unenhanced and is not equivalent to diagnostic CT	
False positive	Inflammatory tissue uptake	"T2-shine through" effect
	Granulation tissue up to 6 months post surgery or radiotherapy	
	Reactive lymph nodes	
	Brown fat uptake	
	Muscle uptake	

FDG [18] F-Fluorodeoxyglucose; *DW-MRI* diffusion-weighted imaging

thus CT or PET-CT are better in this regard and for the detection of lung metastases.

Multiphase dynamic contrast-enhanced MRI (DCE-MRI) has been shown to improve accuracy in the differentiation of recurrence from postsurgical or radiotherapy change in gynecological malignancies, with early enhancement demonstrated within tumor tissue (Kinkel et al. 1997). However, it is at the early time points that differentiation of such changes is most difficult and this study only assessed a small percentage of cases within 6 months of treatment. DCE-MRI also plays an important role in the evaluation of response to chemoradiotherapy (Sala et al. 2010).

Diffusion-weighted MRI is increasingly being used for assessment of gynecological malignancies and is now routinely employed in most centers. DW-MRI provides information on the random motion of water molecules at a cellular level and is typically restricted in tumors due to their high cellularity. Sequences are acquired at multiple "*b*-values" in order to generate an apparent diffusion coefficient (ADC) map. DW-MRI benefits from a short acquisition time, furthermore it can provide functional information, and highlight abnormal areas due to its good lesion-to-background ratio (Liyanage et al. 2010). Although studies have not directly assessed the value of DW-MRI for detection of recurrent cervical or uterine cancer, the addition of DWI to conventional anatomical images may increase reader confidence (Sala et al. 2010) (Fig. 141.3). However, DW-MRI has a number of potential

pitfalls (Table 141.1). False positive results may occur due to high-signal "T2-shine through" effect on b-value images. This can be avoided by reading the ADC map, which will be of high signal in "T2 shine through" but low in tumors with restricted diffusion. False negative results may occur in tumors of low cellularity.

CT

CT is the preferred modality for assessment of suspected distal metastases or postoperative complications. A single-phase examination is sufficient, which should ideally be performed following oral contrast preparation and in the portal venous phase of intravenous enhancement.

Local recurrence typically mimics the imaging features of the primary tumor, appearing as a heterogeneous soft tissue mass, which is iso- or hypo-enhancing relative to the surrounding stroma (Fig. 141.5). Alternatively, pelvic recurrences may have a low attenuation cystic/necrotic appearance with minimal soft tissue (Pannu et al. 2001). However, CT is inferior to MRI in the assessment of local recurrence and in differentiating recurrence from posttherapy changes. Postoperative complications such as lymphoceles, seromas, infection, and hemorrhage are well demonstrated by CT (Jeong et al. 2003; Pannu et al. 2001). These can be confidently diagnosed and

Fig. 141.5 *CT demonstrating local recurrence of uterine carcinoma after surgery.* Axial (**a**) and sagittal reformatted (**b**) portal venous phase CT images demonstrate a heterogeneous soft tissue mass within the surgical bed (*arrows*), which is hypo-enhancing relative to the surrounding stroma

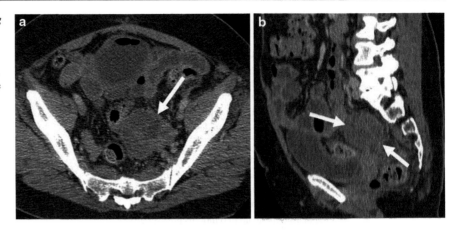

Fig. 141.6 *Follow-up CT showing distal recurrence in four different patients following treatment for primary uterine carcinoma.* Axial CT image of the mid abdomen (**a**) reveals a multi-lobulated mesenteric mass (*arrows*); axial image of the upper abdomen (**b**) shows bilobar liver metastases (*open arrows*), with subcapsular solid (*white arrow*) and cystic implants (*black arrow*) posterior to the right liver lobe. Axial CT of the lungs (**c**) shows multiple pulmonary metastases (*arrows*). Axial CT image of the upper abdomen (**d**) demonstrating an enlarged, irregular pericardiophrenic lymph node (*arrow*)

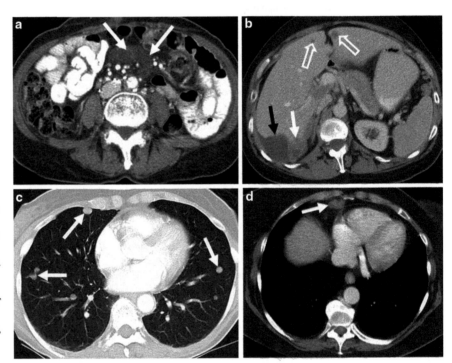

differentiated from recurrent disease in the appropriate clinical context and based on the relatively short post-procedural time frame in which they typically present. Post-radiotherapy complications such as fistulae, strictures, and osteonecrosis can also be well demonstrated by CT (Jeong et al. 2003).

CT is preferred to MRI for assessment of distant metastatic disease, benefiting from its faster acquisition time which limits artifact from respiratory motion and bowel peristalsis, and also has fewer contraindications compared to MR imaging. Abdominal metastatic disease may manifest as ascites, peritoneal thickening or nodularity, or soft tissue masses within the mesentery or solid organs, particularly the liver (Jeong et al. 2003) (Fig. 141.6). Thoracic metastases typically present as pleural effusions or multiple lung nodules; in the case of squamous cell carcinoma of the cervix these are occasionally cavitatory. Bone metastases usually occur due to direct extension from adjacent nodes, are more common in the lumbar spine, and are typically lytic in nature (Jeong et al. 2003). Lymph node metastases are diagnosed by size criteria and basic morphological features, but as with MRI assessment suffers from a reduced sensitivity and specificity.

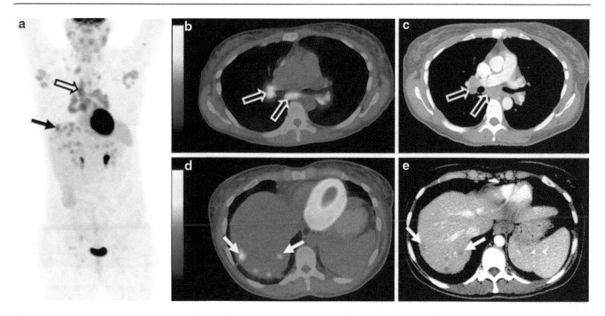

Fig. 141.7 *PET-CT whole-body field of view depicting distal metastatic disease in recurrent cervical cancer.* (**a**) Single maximum-intensity projection (MIP) PET image indicates multiple liver metastases (e.g., *black arrow* in **a**) and extensive hilar (e.g., *open arrow* in **a**), mediastinal, axillary, and cervical lymphadenopathy. Axial fused PET-CT image (**b**) and axial contrast-enhanced CT (**c**) confirm bilateral hilar and sub-carinal lymphadenopathy (*open arrows* in **b**, **c**). Axial fused PET-CT image (**d**) and axial contrast-enhanced CT (**e**) confirm multiple liver metastases (*white arrows* in **d**, **e**)

PET-CT

^{18}F-Fluorodeoxyglucose (FDG) positron emission tomography (PET) can be combined with CT to provide both functional and anatomical information. PET benefits from its whole-body field of view, which is particularly useful for identifying extra-pelvic disease in gynecological malignancies (Fig. 141.7). With its increased availability, PET-CT is rapidly becoming established as the technique of choice for assessing nodal involvement and the presence of distal recurrence in cervical and uterine cancer.

PET-CT is being increasingly utilized for the initial staging workup of cervical cancer, evaluating response to therapy, and for long-term follow-up (Grigsby 2009). PET is known to be more accurate than CT or MRI at assessing nodal involvement (Son et al. 2010) (Fig. 141.8). There is good evidence for the efficacy of PET in the assessment of recurrent cervical cancer, with Yen et al. showing an added benefit of PET alone over CT or MRI in 73.8% (93/126) of cases of recurrent cervical cancer (Yen et al. 2006). PET was particularly useful in the evaluation of extra-pelvic disease, and in the correction of false negative CT/MRI results. PET additionally shows promise for accurate monitoring of response to chemoradiotherapy

in the metastatic and neoadjuvant settings (Schwarz et al. 2009). It has been suggested that due to its high sensitivity and positive predictive value, PET/CT should be the modality of choice for evaluating extra-pelvic disease prior to considering pelvic exenteration in cases of confirmed cervical cancer recurrence (Son et al. 2010). The role of PET in uterine cancer is less well defined, due to the current lack of clinical data. Small studies have shown PET/CT to be accurate in the detection of recurrent uterine cancer with a sensitivity of 93% and a specificity of 93% (Kitajima et al. 2008). In another study, PET/CT helped modify the diagnosis or treatment plan in 7 out of 31 (22.6%) patients (Chung et al. 2008).

Despite the great potential of PET-CT and its increasing use in cervical and uterine cancer, PET has a number of limitations and potential pitfalls, some of which cannot always be overcome by combining PET with CT (Table 141.1). Furthermore, CT interpretation may be limited by a lack of intravenous contrast and is not of equivalent quality to a diagnostic CT. Reactive lymph nodes are often FDG-avid, while metastatic necrotic or cystic nodes/deposits or small volume nodes (5–7 mm) may be falsely negative (Sironi et al. 2004). Physiological uptake may be difficult to differentiate from disease avidity: renal tract

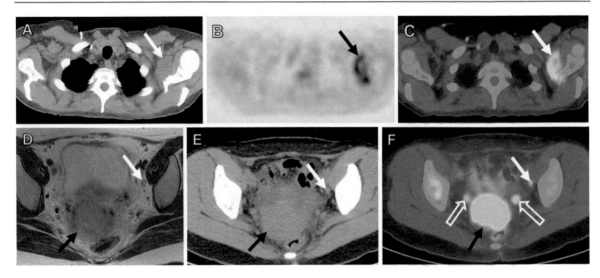

Fig. 141.8 *Advantage of PET-CT over CT and MRI.* Axial CT (**a**), axial PET (**b**), and axial fused PET-CT (**c**) images demonstrate a left axillary soft tissue mass (*arrows*) in a patient with recurrent uterine cancer. The lesion is harder to appreciate on the non-contrast-enhanced CT, with increased lesion conspicuity on the PET and fused images. Axial T2-weighted MRI (**d**), axial CT (**e**), and axial fused PET-CT image (**f**) at the same level in a patient with recurrent cervical cancer. A recurrent mass is seen within the surgical bed (*black arrows* in **d, e, f**). A left internal iliac lymph node (*white arrows* in **d, e, f**) was considered normal on the basis of size (5 mm) and morphology at MRI and CT, but avid tracer uptake on PET-CT indicates metastatic involvement. Tracer uptake is noted in both distal ureters (*open arrows* in **f**)

uptake may mask adjacent nodal activity, and the close proximity of the bladder to the surgical bed may compromise assessment of disease recurrence in this location (Blake et al. 2006). Uptake within brown fat or muscle tissue can also lead to false positive results; however, co-localization by CT should make this less of an issue (Truong et al. 2004). Additionally, granulation tissue may be FDG-avid within the first 3 months and up to 6 months following surgery or radiotherapy (Belhocine and Grigsby 2005).

- DW-MRI has not been evaluated for recurrent disease but improves reader confidence.
- CT is optimal for evaluation of postoperative complications and is superior to MRI for assessing distant metastatic disease.
- PET-CT is the best modality for assessing nodal involvement and is preferable for assessing distance metastatic disease.
- PET-CT should be used to evaluate distal disease prior to consideration of pelvic exenteration for recurrent disease.

Pearls to Remember

- Follow-up is primarily clinical. The role of imaging is to detect and localize recurrence when this is clinically suspected.
- Recurrence is most common in the first 3 years.
- An appreciation of the normal postoperative appearances is essential for image interpretation.
- MRI is the modality of choice for evaluating local recurrence and in assessment post-radiotherapy.
- DCE-MRI can evaluate response to chemoradiotherapy and may help differentiate recurrent disease from postoperative or radiotherapy changes.

Conclusion

Follow-up of cervical or uterine cancer is essential in order to detect recurrence at an early stage, when localized disease is potentially curable. Imaging does not play a role in routine surveillance of such patients, but is necessary to confirm recurrence when clinically suspected. MRI, CT, and PET-CT all have advantages and potential interpretation pitfalls, and each has a niche role to play in the workup of suspected recurrence. MRI is primarily used for the detection of local recurrence and the assessment of patients post radiotherapy. DW-MRI and DCE-MRI are useful adjuncts that improve diagnostic accuracy and reader confidence and help in the monitoring of response post chemoradiotherapy. CT plays a key role in diagnosing complications in the immediate postsurgical stage and still has a role to play in the assessment of distal disease. The recent development and increased availability of PET-CT has changed the workup of patients with suspected recurrence, its increased sensitivity and specificity particularly for nodal involvement and distal disease has made it the first-line modality for assessment of suspected recurrent disease with distal metastases.

References

Baalbergen A, Helmerhorst TJM, Burger CW. Prognostic factors that predict survival after relapse of cervical cancer. CME J Gynecol Oncol. 2001;6:391–7.

Baekelandt MM, Castiglione M. On behalf of the ESMO Guidelines Working Group. Endometrial carcinoma: ESMO clinical recommendations for diagnosis, treatment and follow-up. Ann Oncol. 2009; 20(Suppl 4): iv29–iv31

Belhocine TZ, Grigsby PW. FDG PET and PET-CT in uterine cancers. Cancer Ther. 2005;3:201–18.

Blake MA, Singh A, Setty BN, Slattery J, Kalra M, Maher MM, Sahani DV, Fischman AJ, Mueller PR. Pearls and Pitfalls in interpretation of abdominal and pelvic PET-CT. Radiographics. 2006;26(5):1335–53.

Bodurka-Bevers D, Morris M, Eifel PJ, Levenback C, Bevers MW, Lucas KR, Wharton JT. Posttherapy surveillance of women with cervical cancer: an outcomes analysis. Gynecol Oncol. 2000;78(2):187–93.

Choi JI, Kim SH, Seong CK, Sim JS, Lee HJ, Do KH. Recurrent uterine cervical carcinoma: spectrum of imaging findings. Korean J Radiol. 2000;1(4):198–207.

Chung HH, Kang WJ, Kim JW, Park NH, Song YS, Chung JK, Kang SB. The clinical impact of [(18)F]FDG PET/CT for the management of recurrent endometrial cancer: correlation with clinical and histological Wndings. Eur J Nucl Med Mol Imaging. 2008;35:1081–8.

Creutzberg CL, Van Putten WLJ, Koper PC, Jobsen JJ, Wárlám-Rodenhuis CC, De Winter KA, Lutgens LC, van den Bergh AC, van der Steen-Banasik E, Beerman H, van Lent M; PORTEC Study Group. Survival after relapse in patients with endometrial cancer: results from a randomized trial. Gynecologic Oncology. 2003; 89(2):201–09.

Elit L, Fyles AW, Devries MC, Oliver TK, Fung-Kee-Fung M, Gynecology Cancer Disease Site Group. Follow-up for women after treatment for cervical cancer: a systematic review. Gynecol Oncol. 2009; 114(3):528

Emons G, Kimmig R. Uterus Commission of the Gynecological Oncology Working Group (AGO). Interdisciplinary S2k guidelines on the diagnosis and treatment of endometrial carcinoma. J Cancer Res Clin Oncol. 2009; 135:1387–91.

Gadducci A, Cosio S, Carpi A, Nicolini A, Genazzani AR. Serum tumor markers in the management of ovarian,

endometrial and cervical cancer. Biomed Pharmacother. 2004;58(1):24–38.

Grigsby PW. Role of PET in gynecologic malignancy. Curr Opin Oncol. 2009;21(5):420–4.

Hricak H, Yu KK. Radiology in invasive cervical cancer. AJR Am J Roentgenol. 1996;167:1101–8.

Jeong YY, Kang HK, Chung TW, Seo JJ, Park JG. Uterine cervical carcinoma after therapy: CT and MR imaging findings. Radiographics. 2003;23:969–81.

Kim SH, Han MC. Invasion of the urinary bladder by uterine cervical carcinoma: evaluation with MR imaging. AJR Am J Roentgenol. 1997;168:393–7.

Kinkel K, Ariche M, Tardivon AA, Spatz A, Castaigne D, Lhomme C, Vanel D. Differentiation between recurrent tumor and benign conditions after treatment of gynecologic pelvic carcinoma: value of dynamic contrast-enhanced subtractionMRimaging. Radiology. 1997;204:55–63.

Kitajima K, Murakami K, Yamasaki E, Hagiwara S, Fukasawa I, Inaba N, Kaji Y, Sugimura K. Performance of FDG-PET/CT in the diagnosis of recurrent endometrial cancer. Ann Nucl Med. 2008;22(2):103–9.

Lai CH. Management of recurrent cervical cancer. Chang Gung Med J. 2004;27(10):711–7.

Liyanage SH, Roberts CA, Rockall AG. MRI and PET scans for primary staging and detection of cervical cancer recurrence. Womens Health (Lond Engl). 2010;6(2):251–67.

NCCN. National Comprehensive Cancer Network (NCCN) guidelines. 2011. www.nccn.org. Accessed 11 May 2011.

Pannu HK, Corl FM, Fishman EK. CT evaluation of cervical cancer: spectrum of disease. Radiographics. 2001;21(5):1155–68.

Poolkerd S, Leelahakorn S, Manusirivithaya S, Tangjitgamol S, Thavaramara T, Sukwattana P, Pataradule K. Survival rate of recurrent cervical cancer patients. J Med Assoc Thai. 2006;89(3):275–82.

Sala E, Rockall A, Rangarajan D, Kubik-Huch RA. The role of dynamic contrast-enhanced and diffusion weighted magnetic resonance imaging in the female pelvis. Eur J Radiol. 2010;76(3):367–85.

Schwarz JK, Grigsby PW, Dehdashti F, Delbeke D. The role of 18 F-FDG PET in assessing therapy response in cancer of the cervix and ovaries. J Nucl Med. 2009;50(Suppl 1):64S–73.

Sironi S, Messa C, Mangili G, Zangheri B, Aletti G, Garavaglia E, Vigano R, Picchio M, Taccagni G, Maschio AD, Fazio F. Integrated FDG PET/CT in patients with persistent ovarian cancer: correlation with histologic findings. Radiology. 2004;233(2):433–40.

Sohaib SA, Houghton SL, Meroni R, Rockall AG, Blake P, Reznek RH. Recurrent endometrial cancer: patterns of recurrent disease and assessment of prognosis. Clin Radiol. 2007;62(1):28–34.

Son H, Kositwattanarerk A, Hayes MP, Chuang L, Rahaman J, Heiba S, Machac J, Zakashansky K, Kostakoglu L. PET/CT evaluation of cervical cancer: spectrum of disease. Radiographics. 2010;30(5):1251–68.

Tjalma WA, van Dam PA, Makar AP, Cruickshank DJ. The clinical value and the cost-effectiveness of follow-up in endometrial cancer patients. Int J Gynecol Cancer. 2004;14(5):931–7.

Truong MT, Erasmus JJ, Munden RF, Marom EM, Sabloff BS, Gladish GW, Podoloff DA, Macapinlac HA. Focal FDG uptake in mediastinal brown fat mimicking malignancy: a potential pitfall resolved on PET/CT. AJR Am J Roentgenol. 2004;183(4):1127–32.

Yen TC, Lai CH, Ma SY, Huang KG, Huang HJ, Hong JH, Hsueh S, Lin WJ, Nq KK, Chang TC. Comparative benefits and limitations of (18)F-FDG PET and CT-MRI in documented or suspected recurrent cervical cancer. Eur J Nucl Med Mol Imaging. 2006;33:1399–407.

Yu KK, Hricak H, Subak LL, Zaloudek CJ, Powell CB. Preoperative staging of cervical carcinoma: phased array coil fast spin-echo versus body coil spin-echo T2-weighted MRimaging. AJR Am J Roentgenol. 1998;171(3):707–11.

Helen Clare Addley and Caroline Reinhold

Patient Management

Gynecological malignancies are common accounting for 10–15% of all female malignancies with ovarian and endometrial carcinoma accounting for 80% of these (Kehoe 2006). Gynecological cancers are usually treated by surgery, chemotherapy, and/or radiotherapy. The management of patients with malignant gynecological disease depends upon the grade and stage of the malignancy and organ of origin. The assessment for the most appropriate treatment strategy involves a multidisciplinary approach with input from radiology, histopathology, gynecology, and oncology.

In endometrial cancer, early stage disease (stage 1A, grade 1–2) is usually treated by surgery alone without chemoradiotherapy whereas more advanced stages or grades are treated with a combination of surgery and radiotherapy. In cervical cancer, chemoradiotherapy is used when tumors are greater than 4 cm or the stage is 2B or more. In ovarian cancer, chemotherapy has an important role in neoadjuvant treatment prior to surgery in nonresectable cases and also in patients where optimal surgical resection has not been achieved.

Following treatment, imaging plays a crucial role in assessing tumor response and detecting tumor recurrence. In disease recurrence, there are further treatment options available to such patients, most often chemoradiotherapy, but also further surgery such as exenteration can also be an option in a select group of patients.

H.C. Addley (✉) • C. Reinhold
Department of Radiology, McGill University Health Center,
Montreal General Hospital, Montreal, Quebec, Canada

Role of Chemoradiotherapy

Chemoradiotherapy has a primary role in the treatment of endometrial, cervical, and ovarian cancers as well as in combination with surgery and in the treatment of disease recurrence.

The role of chemoradiotherapy depends upon the treatment stratification of an individual patient. Chemotherapy is used as neoadjuvant treatment in advanced ovarian cancer and in some cases in advanced cervical cancer. Adjuvant chemotherapy is used following surgery in ovarian cancer and in advanced endometrial cancer. Primary chemoradiotherapy is used for the management of advanced cervical cancer (stages 2B or greater) or when the size of the tumor is 4 cm or greater (Delaney et al. 2004).

Adjuvant radiotherapy is used for node-positive cervical cancer treated surgically or in cases with close surgical margins. Adjuvant radiotherapy for cervical cancer following surgery can be either brachytherapy alone or used in combination with external beam radiotherapy. Radiotherapy in endometrial carcinoma is used following surgery in patients with advanced stage disease (stage 1B or greater or grade 3 disease) extending into the outer myometrium or outside the uterus. In ovarian cancer radiotherapy is recommended only in stage 4 disease as a palliative treatment (Delaney et al. 2004).

Radiotherapy Planning

Planning the area of intended radiation therapy is important to ensure that the target and any other local disease such as nodal areas are covered in such a way

B. Hamm, P. R. Ros (eds.), *Abdominal Imaging*, DOI 10.1007/978-3-642-13327-5_184,
© Springer-Verlag Berlin Heidelberg 2013

that there is as minimal irradiation of adjacent structures as possible. Pelvic irradiation affects other adjacent structures included in the radiation field, which are not intentionally targeted and can therefore result in gastrointestinal and genitourinary complications in particular.

Intrauterine and intracavitary brachytherapy is used following external beam radiotherapy to produce a focused high dose of radiation to a local area of the uterus or cervix. Perforation of the uterus occurs in approximately 8% of cases, and usually occurs at the time of placement of the brachytherapy device (Barnes et al. 2007). Three-dimensional imaging used to guide applicator placement avoids this complication, and helps to reduce radiation dose in brachytherapy for treatment of cervical cancer by accurate tandem placement (Viswanathan 2008).

In the future, decreased radiation of adjacent structures may be possible with the advent of intensity-modulated radiation therapy (IMRT) which has been implemented with the aim to achieve as high a dose as possible to the target without surrounding radiation of other organs (Georg et al. 2006). This technique has been reported to decrease the amount of radiation dose to the bladder and rectum by 23%, and to the small bowel by 50% (Portelance et al. 2001).

In addition to the affect on adjacent structures, dose limitation during radiotherapy planning is also important to reduce the risk of future malignancy. The absolute risk of occurrence of sarcomas following radiotherapy for gynecologic malignancies has been estimated to be as high as 0.8% (Mark et al. 1996).

Expected Appearances Post Chemoradiotherapy

Imaging of the post-chemoradiotherapy female pelvis is particularly challenging due to the alteration of the normal anatomy and loss of the tissue planes (Addley et al. 2010). It can be difficult to interpret if the appearances are due to expected changes following chemoradiotherapy or if there is a complication or disease recurrence. Awareness of the expected imaging findings following chemoradiotherapy, as well as the imaging findings of the common complications, is important to guide future management of these patients successfully.

Primary Tumor

Cervical tumors treated with radiotherapy will undergo follow-up MR examinations following radiotherapy treatment to assess treatment response and guide future treatment decisions. The treatment response to radiotherapy is assessed by a measurable decrease in tumor size and therefore volume of disease (Vincens et al. 2008). Treatment response and decrease in tumor volume can be seen as early as 2 months following treatment and predicts a good prognosis (Flueckiger et al. 1992). It is important not to perform follow-up imaging too early (less than 8 weeks) following radiotherapy treatment as the appearances can be misleading.

Following treatment with radiotherapy, the signal characteristics of the primary tumor changes and the soft tissue and fat planes within the pelvis become more indistinct. Fibrosis and contraction of the primary tumor occurs resulting in lower signal intensity and volume of disease (Fig. 142.1). The adjacent soft tissues are also likely to undergo a similar process of fibrotic change, therefore, appearing to be of low signal intensity and causing difficulty in distinguishing the pelvic anatomical planes from the primary tumor.

Because of the difficulty in distinguishing between the fat planes and the tumor post radiotherapy, and the fact that many of these patients will have parametrial invasion at presentation, it is a common pitfall on post-radiotherapy MRI that fibrosis mimics tumor recurrence in the parametrium. In these cases, therefore, where there was initial parametrial invasion, intravenous contrast medium can be helpful in distinguishing between radiotherapy induced parametrial fibrosis and residual or recurrent disease (Hricak et al. 1993). Tumor tends to enhance earlier than fibrosis and should be compared to the pretreatment imaging appearances as recurrent tumor typically has the same dynamic contrast enhancement characteristics as the original tumor.

The signal intensity of the tumor is also important as the very low signal intensity of fibrotic changes is reassuring and should be compared to the initial pre-radiotherapy MR appearances where the tumor is typically of intermediate signal intensity (Fig. 142.2). The signal intensity can also be compared to adjacent pelvic sidewall muscle on T2-weighted images and is suspicious for recurrence if it is of increased signal intensity compared to muscle (Weber et al. 1995). The reconstitution of the

Fig. 142.1 Sagittal T2-weighted images before (**a**) and following (**b**) radiotherapy in a patient with stage 4 cervical carcinoma with the cervical mass (*white arrow*, **a**) invading the rectosigmoid colon (*white arrowhead*, **a**). Following radiotherapy the mass has resolved and the cervix is seen as low signal intensity (*white arrow*, **b**) with a low signal intensity linear plaque extending from the cervix to the rectum at the site of the previous disease

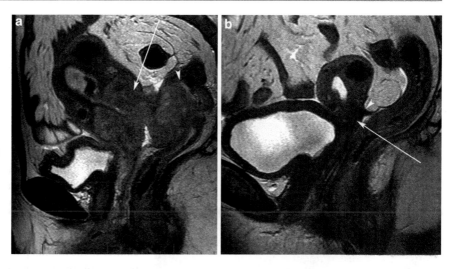

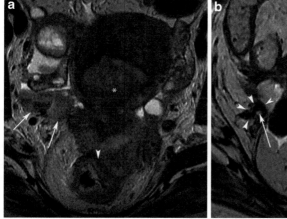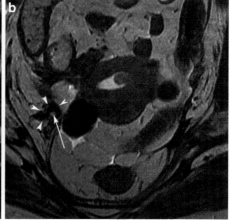

Fig. 142.2 Axial T2-weighted images before (**a**) and following (**b**) radiotherapy for stage 4 cervical carcinoma. Before radiotherapy the cervical cancer is seen as intermediate signal intensity mass (*asterisk*, **a**) with large mass extending posteriorly invading the rectum (*white arrowhead*, **a**) and parametrial disease on the right (*white arrows*, **a**). Following radiotherapy the intermediate signal mass has resolved but remaining low signal intensity can be seen in the right parametrium (*white arrowheads*, **b**) encircling the ureter (*white arrow*, **b**) consistent with post-radiotherapy fibrosis

normal low-signal intensity cervical stroma is the most reliable indicator of a tumor-free post-radiation cervix (Hricak et al. 1993).

Uterus and Cervix

Radiotherapy treatment in the postmenopausal patient does not produce any visible significant changes on the posttreatment MRI examination of the postmenopausal uterus. In premenopausal patients, however, changes in the signal intensity of the uterus are readily identified. The distinction between the junctional zone and outer myometrium is lost and after 6 months the endometrium becomes thin and of low signal intensity (Arrive et al. 1989).

Visible changes in the appearance of the cervix on MR can be seen as early as 3 months following radiotherapy in both pre- and postmenopausal patients. Before radiotherapy, the tumor distorts the normal

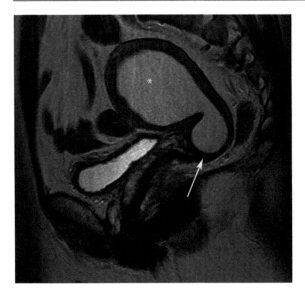

Fig. 142.3 Sagittal T2-weighted image in a patient following radiotherapy for cervical carcinoma demonstrates distension of the endometrial cavity (*asterisk*) secondary to cervical stenosis following radiotherapy with no mass lesion seen at the level of the obstruction at the os (*white arrow*)

imaging in such symptomatic patients by ultrasound examination can readily identify the distended fluid-filled endometrial cavity although further imaging with MR examination to detect the cause of the obstruction is usually necessary.

Ovaries

Following radiation treatment the ovaries gradually decrease in size and signal intensity with loss of physiological follicles, which is seen as a late appearance after at least 6 months (Hricak et al. 2006). The changes seen on MR examination of the ovaries are similar to the normal physiological changes seen in the ovaries of postmenopausal patients and reflect the decline in ovarian function following radiotherapy.

Therefore, in premenopausal patients who will be undergoing pelvic radiotherapy the function of the ovaries may be maintained by surgically placing them out of the radiation field. This procedure is called ovarian transposition and the common locations to place the ovaries are laterally within the pelvis, or in the lower abdomen in the paracolic gutters and anterior to the psoas muscles (Fig. 142.4) (Sella et al. 2005). The procedure of placing the ovaries out of their normal anatomical location does not increase their risk for primary or secondary malignancy (Feeney et al. 1995). The transposed ovaries can easily be mistaken for peritoneal disease because of their abnormal anatomical location, which is in sites typical for peritoneal malignant soft tissue deposits. Therefore, careful interrogation for the presence of follicles in the soft tissue mass is helpful to avoid this pitfall as well knowledge of the surgical history and age of the patient.

zonal anatomy of the cervix with stromal disruption and replacement with the intermediate signal tumor. Following radiotherapy and in patients with a successful disease response the zonal anatomy of the cervix once again becomes distinctly defined and the cervical stroma is of homogeneous low signal intensity. A widened endocervical canal and high signal in the cervical stroma at this stage can occur and in isolation are not necessarily signs of disease recurrence (De Graef et al. 2003). Progressive decrease in the signal intensity of the cervical stoma over time will exclude residual or recurrent tumor.

Cervical os stenosis may occur as a complication of radiotherapy fibrosis at the os and typically takes a few months to develop, becoming visible at the earliest between 3 and 6 months following treatment (Hricak et al. 2006) (Fig. 142.3). Tumor at the os can also cause stenosis and resultant distension of the endometrial cavity. Careful assessment of the appearances at the os for intermediate signal intensity or mass consistent with malignancy is therefore crucial. Obstruction of the uterus can lead to accumulation of fluid in the uterus causing hematometrium or resulting in infection and pyometrium. Although most patients are asymptomatic, in the case of pyometrium and infection, acute

Bowel

Both the large and small bowels are susceptible to radiation damage and can demonstrate a change in their appearances. The complications of such radiation damage are discussed in the later section of gastrointestinal complications. The expected changes that occur in asymptomatic patients and are readily seen on follow-up MR imaging are changes in the large bowel which is relatively static and close in anatomical location to the targeted gynecological

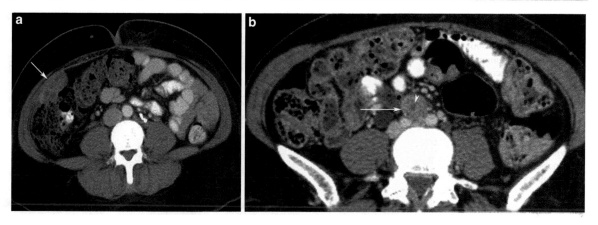

Fig. 142.4 Axial CT images of two patients who had undergone ovarian transposition demonstrating the variable positions that the ovaries can be transposed to. The ovaries can be positioned adjacent to the anterior abdominal wall in the abdomen (*white arrow*, **a***) as well as an incision made in the retroperitoneum on either side so that the ovaries lie adjacent to the psoas muscles or adjacent to the retroperionteal vessels (*white arrow*, **b**). In either position they may be mistaken for either peritoneal deposits or lymphadenopathy and close observation for the low attenuation follicles (*white arrowhead*, **b**) in the ovary will be helpful in their distinction. * Reproduced with permission from radiographics.rsna.org: Pelvic imaging following chemotherapy and radiation therapy for gynecologic malignancies (Addley et al. 2010)

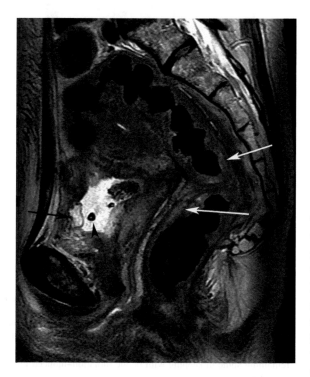

Fig. 142.5 Sagittal T2-weighted image in a patient following radiotherapy for cervical carcinoma. The submucosa of the rectum is of high T2-weighted signal and thickened (*white arrows*) in keeping with post-radiation appearances. In addition there is mucosal edema of the urinary bladder wall (*black arrow*) which has double J ureteric stents in situ (*black arrowhead*)

disease. The radiation treatment results in an increased signal intensity of the rectal and sigmoid submucosa on T2-weighted imaging (Fig. 142.5). This is most often a finding seen on early follow-up imaging and resolves gradually. In long-term follow-up an increase of the perirectal space due to fatty deposition is a normal finding post radiotherapy (Capps et al. 1997).

Urinary Bladder

The bladder is the most radiosensitive organ of the urinary system and is often included in the radiation field for treatment of gynecological malignancy and therefore often shows changes on follow-up imaging. Initially, the bladder wall becomes edematous and then symmetrically thickened. MRI shows the earliest changes of the bullous mucosal edema as high signal intensity on T2-weighted images while the bladder wall is of normal thickness (<5 mm). Following administration of intravenous contrast medium the mucosa enhances avidly and can be mistaken for malignancy if not correlated with the T2-weighted appearances, which are typical for demonstrating the undulating mucosal wall (Fig. 142.6). These changes are typically asymptomatic but can progress to more

Fig. 142.6 Axial
T2-weighted image (**a**) and
T1-weighted image following
intravenous gadolinium (**b**)
demonstrating mucosal edema
of the urinary bladder
occurring post-radiation
treatment. The mucosal edema
is seen as an inner low signal
intensity undulating line
(*white arrow*, **a**) which
enhances avidly following
gadolinium (*white arrow*, **b**)

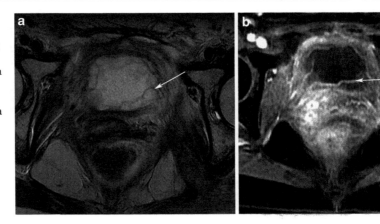

severe changes seen in radiation cystitis, which is discussed under the later heading of urological complications.

Bones

Radiation causes fatty conversion of the bone marrow, which can be seen as increased signal intensity of the bones on both T1- and T2-weighted images. These changes are the earliest readily detectable change following radiotherapy and can occur as early as 2 weeks following radiotherapy and persist for years (Yankelevitz et al. 1991). The well-demarcated signal intensity changes that occur are often very striking and are due to the boundary of the radiation field therefore only affecting the bone marrow subject to the radiotherapy (Fig. 142.7).

Although typically the fatty changes produce high signal intensity of those bones included in the radiation field, initially while the conversion from hemopoetic to fatty marrow occurs, there may be patchy differences in signal intensity characteristics. These patchy changes in signal intensity may be misinterpreted as metastatic bone disease unless the radiologist is aware of the process of the fatty bone marrow conversion and the timing of the patient's radiotherapy treatment. Later changes of radiation treatment cause osteopenia resulting from the diffuse decrease in bone density. This may progress to areas of insufficiency fractures, which will be discussed in the musculoskeletal complications section. As demineralization occurs, focal areas of demineralization may occur first and are difficult to distinguish from lytic metastases and should be correlated with other imaging investigations such as bone scintigraphy

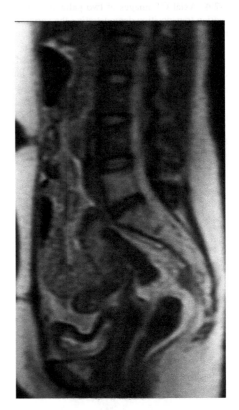

Fig. 142.7 Sagittal localizer image of a larger field of view than the focused sequences of the MR pelvis examination allows distinction of the fatty change affecting the bones of the pelvis in the radiation field compared to those outside of the field. The sacrum and L5 vertebra are of much higher signal than the remaining spine in keeping with pelvic radiation–induced fatty conversion

(Iyer et al. 2001). In contrast to age-related osteopenia, which is typically diffuse, osteopenia following radiotherapy can be patchy and radiation-induced osteitis and remodeling can occur resulting in areas of sclerosis and mottling as well as lysis (Fig. 142.8).

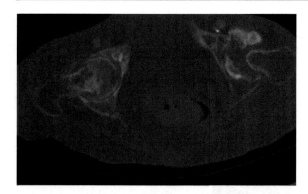

Fig. 142.8 Axial CT image of patient following radiotherapy demonstrating osteitis with both lytic and sclerotic areas of the affected bones

Complications Post Chemoradiotherapy

Complications following chemoradiotherapy are important to recognize as patients may be asymptomatic at the time of their follow-up MR examination and prompt diagnosis ultimately improves patient management. In addition, it is important to have knowledge of the more common complications following chemoradiotherapy to avoid the interpretation pitfall of reporting benign complications as malignant disease. The following section aims to address the most common complications that arise following chemoradiotherapy by categorizing them according to the physiological system affected. As with the expected changes, the complications can also be thought of in terms of the anatomy of the organ of origin that is subjected to the pelvic radiation field for the radiotherapy complications. The complications following chemotherapy are systemic and therefore are better categorized under the physiological systems. Awareness of the imaging findings of the common complications is important to guide future management of these patients successfully.

Gastrointestinal

The gastrointestinal tract is sensitive to the effects of radiation, which is dose dependent, and therefore gastrointestinal complications occur commonly following radiation treatment with 75% of patients complaining of diarrhea and gastrointestinal symptoms acutely. 1–5% of patients treated with 45–55 Gy external

beam radiation treatment suffer from chronic radiation injury to the colon and rectum (Donner 1998). The actively proliferating mucosa of the rectum and sigmoid colon undergo acute damage that results in proctitis of the rectum and colitis of the colon.

The changes in the rectum and colon can be seen on different imaging modalities but are most often assessed using CT and MR imaging. On CT imaging, the appearances are typically of uniform thickening and enhancement of the bowel wall. Over time this can undergo fibrotic changes, which can progress to areas of stricturing and bowel obstruction proximal to the strictures. On MR imaging the findings are similar to CT imaging, although the layers of the bowel are more readily distinguished than on CT imaging. Following intravenous contrast medium there is increased submucosal bowel wall enhancement on contrast-enhanced T1-weighted images. Furthermore, there is loss of definition between the muscle layers on T1-weighted images.

As the small bowel has more motility than the large bowel and is not fixed in position, the small bowel is usually subjected to lower doses of pelvic radiation. The small bowel is, however, more radiosensitive than the large bowel. Therefore, when the small bowel is affected by radiation changes, the results can be more problematic than in the large bowel. Enteritis of the small bowel typically involves the relatively more fixed terminal ileum. As with the large bowel, the changes can be seen on both CT and MR examinations appearing as bowel wall thickening and submucosal edema (Fig. 142.9). Chronic changes such as fibrosis can lead to stenotic segments. Fibrotic strictures may in turn lead to small bowel obstruction. In such cases, surgery may be required, but the segments are typically fibrosed to each other and the adjacent soft tissues resulting in challenging surgery and the possibility that many segments may have to be resected (Fig. 142.10).

Neutropenic colitis otherwise called typhlitis may occur infrequently following chemotherapy, which causes subsequent neutropenia and immunosuppression. The pattern of bowel involvement is characteristic as typhlitis typically affects the cecum and ascending colon resulting in segmental gross circumferential bowel wall thickening with surrounding fat stranding and free fluid (Fig. 142.11). Patients with typhlitis are typically very unwell with lower abdominal pain, guarding, and fever in comparison to the

Fig. 142.9 Axial CT image (a) and sagittal T2-weighted MR image (b) and T1-weighted image following intravenous gadolinium (c) of small bowel enteritis following radiotherapy. On the CT the increased mucosal enhancement of the involved small bowel (*black arrow*, a) and thickening of its wall are demonstrated as well as a similar process occurring in the sigmoid colon (*white arrow*, a). Note the moderate amount of associated free fluid. On MR imaging there is increased T2-weighted signal of the mucosa (*white arrow*, b) with avid enhancement of the affected bowel wall following gadolinium

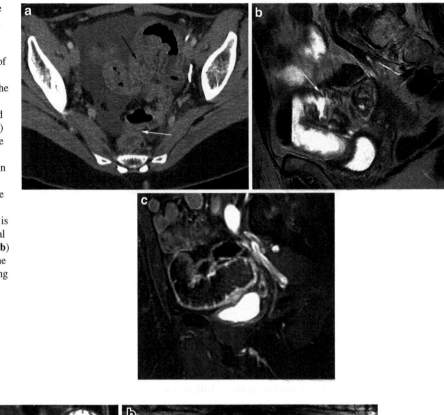

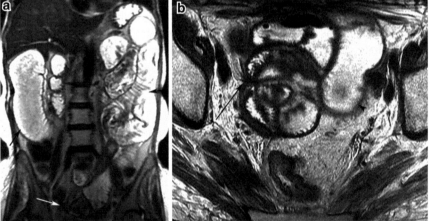

Fig. 142.10 Coronal (a) and axial (b) T2-weighted images following radiotherapy for cervical carcinoma. The patient had been complaining of intermittent colicky abdominal pain. MR images demonstrated multiple distended small bowel loops filled with fluid (*black arrows*, a) with collapsed loops of distal ileum in the right lower quadrant (*white arrow*, a). The transition point was seen at the site of a low signal intensity linear area in the right lower quadrant (*black arrow*, b). The appearances are in keeping with radiation-induced fibrosis and subsequent small bowel tethering and obstruction. This was confirmed at surgery where a small bowel resection and primary anastomosis was performed

patients with radiotherapy changes only who may often be asymptomatic despite their imaging appearances. In typhlitis, CT is the examination of choice rather than MR imaging as CT can clearly demonstrate the extent of the typhlitis and the complication of transmural necrosis and impending perforation which may ultimately lead to frank perforation and uncontrolled sepsis (Hoeffel et al. 2006).

Fig. 142.11 Axial (**a**) and sagittal reformatted image (**b**) of a patient following chemotherapy for ovarian carcinoma. There is gross bowel wall thickening (*black arrow*, **b**) and mucosal enhancement (*black arrow*, **a**) of the cecum and to a much lesser extent the ascending colon (*white arrow*, **b**) with associated ascites (*white arrowhead*, **b**). The distribution of the findings and the severity are in keeping with typhlitis

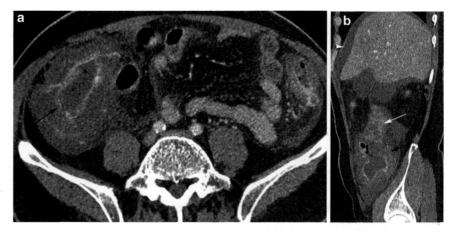

Following chemotherapy treatment, a small amount of ascites alone is a common finding. The presence of a large amount of ascites, however, is not an expected finding and therefore should prompt careful detection of the cause. In particular, images should be carefully assessed to detect any peritoneal deposits in addition to the ascites, which is consistent with recurrence of disease. If there is clinical doubt as to whether the ascites is malignant, an ultrasound guided tap for a sample of the fluid can be obtained and sent for cytology.

Urological

As with the bowel, radiation damage to the urinary bladder is dose dependent with lower doses of radiation (up to 30 Gy) having the potential to cause mild cystitis and higher doses (70 Gy) causing more severe changes with longer term effects. Radiation cystitis is not uncommon and is quoted to occur in up to 12% of cases (Iyer et al. 2001). The findings are often detected on routine follow-up imaging as the patients may be asymptomatic and the appearances of the bladder wall thickening on imaging are often worse than the clinical symptoms.

Radiation cystitis can be seen on both CT and MR imaging as thickening and increased enhancement of the bladder wall. MR imaging, however, is better at distinguishing the muscular layers of the bladder and is often the imaging modality of choice in routine follow-up for local disease assessment. The severe radiation changes result in bladder wall thickening and high signal intensity of the outer bladder wall on T2-weighted images. This is in contradistinction to mucosal edema,

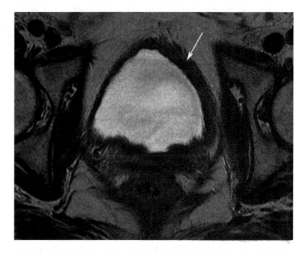

Fig. 142.12 Axial T2-weighted image following radiotherapy demonstrating a small volume, thick-walled urinary bladder which has a low signal intensity thickened wall (*white arrow*) in keeping with chronic changes of radiation-induced fibrosis

which is seen on the inner bladder wall. Following the administration of intravenous contrast medium there is increased enhancement of the mucosal layer on contrast-enhanced T1-weighted images.

If severe radiation damage to the urinary bladder occurs, the inflammation of the bladder wall can cause hemorrhage and even necrosis of the mucosa. At this severity the patient is symptomatic with hematuria and even passage of clots.

A long-term complication of radiotherapy treatment of the urinary bladder is a chronically small-volume urinary bladder, which is unable to fully distend because of the bands of fibrosis in its wall (Fig. 142.12). These fibrotic bands appear as thin bands of low signal intensity on the inner aspect

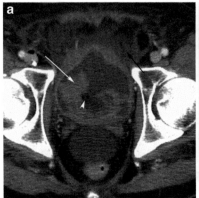
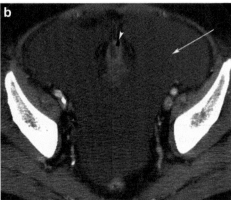

Fig. 142.13 Axial CT images of a patient following radiotherapy with sudden onset of severe suprapubic pelvic pain and inability to urinate. Axial CT image at the level of the urinary bladder demonstrates a catheter in situ (*white arrowhead*, **a**) with intermediate attenuation contents in a dependent position within the bladder (*white arrow*, **a**) in keeping with hemorrhage. The urinary bladder wall is thickened and there is adjacent low attenuation free fluid (*black arrow*, **a**). At the level of the bladder dome more cranially in the pelvis there is a large amount of fluid (*white arrow*, **b**) and a bubble of gas can be seen adjacent to the bladder dome but outside of the bladder lumen in the bladder wall (*white arrowhead*, **b**). The appearances are consistent with acute bladder rupture

of the bladder (Sugimura and Okizuka 2002). In addition, another recognized late complication following radiotherapy treatment is perforation of the urinary bladder. This is a very rare occurrence but is a life-threatening event when it occurs and necessitates prompt diagnosis (Fig. 142.13) (Addar et al. 1996).

In comparison to the urinary bladder, the distal ureters are less commonly affected by pelvic radiation. Soft tissue fibrosis of the tissues adjacent to the ureters in the parametria and pelvic sidewalls may, however, cause tethering of the ureters resulting in stricture formation and proximal dilatation (Fig. 142.14). The resulting dilatation and hydroureter ultimately leads to hydronephrosis in the long term. Careful interpretation of the site of ureteric stricture is therefore necessary in reporting of follow-up MRI studies as residual or recurrent parametrial disease may also cause stricture of the ureter and subsequent hydroureter. In comparison to the stricture of malignant disease, fibrotic strictures will appear as areas of low signal intensity linear tethering rather than an intermediate signal intensity mass. In addition, the ureteric stricture from radiation treatment is smoothly tapered rather than with an abrupt change in caliber as in malignancy. Delayed CT examination following intravenous contrast medium when the ureters are opacified is helpful in outlining the ureteric contour and provides information of how abrupt and irregular the stricture is. The timing

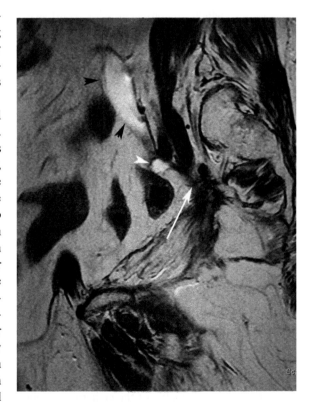

Fig. 142.14 Sagittal T2-weighted image of a patient following radiotherapy demonstrates hydroureter (*black arrowheads*) with obliteration of the ureteric lumen (*white arrowhead*) at the site of low signal intensity linear areas (*white arrow*) in keeping with radiation-induced fibrosis

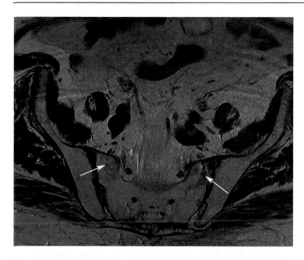

Fig. 142.15 Axial T2-weighted MR image demonstrating increased signal intensity of the pelvic bones in keeping with post-radiotherapy fatty changes. In addition there are subtle bilateral low signal intensity lines running longitudinally of both sides of the sacrum in keeping with sacral insufficiency fractures

of the radiotherapy treatment can also provide a guide as to whether the stricture is benign or malignant as stricture formation from radiotherapy is a late complication of radiation treatment occurring after several months and persisting years after completion of radiotherapy treatment (Capps et al. 1997).

Musculoskeletal

As discussed in the earlier section of expected changes in the bones, the earliest changes detectable in the bones are seen on MR imaging and are the replacement of the marrow by fat. This change occurs in 90% of patients by 8 weeks following radiation treatment (Blomlie et al. 1995). Following this there is a spectrum of changes that occur to the cellular bone which gradually changes from fatty changes only, to radiation-induced osteitis and patchy areas of lysis and sclerosis and ultimately to insufficiency fractures from normal stresses subjected to this abnormal bone texture (Fig. 142.15).

The most common sites for insufficiency fractures to occur following pelvic radiotherapy are the sacrum and pubic rami. As the bone texture is abnormal in these areas, the normal healing process of a fracture is hampered and therefore nonunion and aseptic necrosis

are known complications of these fractures. If the patient is symptomatic, plain film is the first line of investigation, which may demonstrate both the fracture line and the abnormal bone texture. However, insufficiency fractures are often subclinical and should be specifically looked for on the follow-up MR or CT examination of patients who are known to have undergone pelvic radiotherapy treatment. On CT examination the abnormal bone texture is readily demonstrated as well as the breach of the cortex of the fracture. On MR examination the changes of the insufficiency fracture may be seen earlier before there is frank breach of the cortex as MR can detect edema of the bone marrow. This is seen as high signal intensity on T2-weighted images. For the fracture line, the T1-weighted images should be carefully evaluated for the fracture, which is of low signal intensity. Insufficiency fractures are commonly symmetrical and therefore if one is detected careful evaluation of the opposite side should be undertaken for any subtle signs of impending insufficiency fracture (Sugimura and Okizuka 2002). Bone scintigraphy is often used in addition for these cases as it is very sensitive for the detection of fractures. The characteristic H-shaped pattern of increased radionuclide uptake occurring across the sacrum is a typical finding in bilateral insufficiency fractures of the sacral ala (Figs. 142.16 and 142.17) (Tai et al. 2000).

In addition to changes of the cellular bone, radiotherapy can also cause changes of the muscles included in the pelvic radiotherapy field. This can be seen as high signal intensity on T2-weighted images and increased enhancement following intravenous contrast medium and reflects myositis of the affected striated muscle.

Fistulae

The expected findings of fibrosis and loss of definition of the soft tissue planes seen following radiation treatment can sometimes progress to include tissue necrosis and breakdown of adjacent anatomical soft tissue planes which can lead to the formation of complex fistulae in the pelvis. These are typically seen as late complications of radiotherapy because it takes time for the necrosis and breakdown of the tissues to occur. Fistulae are connection of one epithelial surface to another and can occur between any epithelial surfaces in the pelvis but due to the position of the radiotherapy

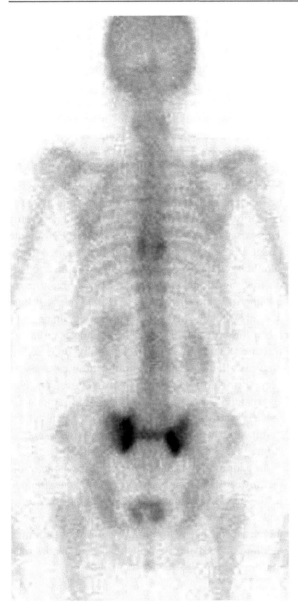

Fig. 142.16 Posterior acquisition of bone scintigraphy examination demonstrating increased uptake in the pelvis in an "H" shape consistent with the Honda sign of bilateral fractures of the sacral ala

field in treatment of gynecological malignancy are most commonly seen between the bladder and vagina, and the vagina and rectum. The small bowel may also be involved and there may also be a fistulous tract to the skin surface.

Malignant disease, can also invade adjacent soft tissue planes resulting in a fistulous tract and

therefore, it is also important to consider the possibility of recurrent disease and assess for any evidence of tumor invasion.

MR and CT examination both have differing strengths and weaknesses for identifying fistulae. On routine single-phase venous CT examinations, it can be difficult to directly visualize the fistulous tract but indirect signs of fistulae can be identified, such as the presence of air or oral contrast medium in the urinary bladder or renal collecting systems (Narayanan et al. 2009). CT can also demonstrate focal thickening of the bladder or bowel wall, which may be suspicious but definitely not diagnostic for the involved area of abnormality (Narayanan et al. 2009). Dedicated CT examinations for the assessment of fistulae can be very helpful by providing dynamic direct evidence of a functionally patent fistula. The administration of contrast medium via a foley catheter in the urinary bladder can readily demonstrate a vesicovaginal fistula as can the administration of rectal contrast medium for enteric fistulae (Fig. 142.18). For the assessment of more complex ureteral or vesical fistulae excretory phase imaging may also be of benefit. Three-dimensional reconstruction of the CT images should also be standard practice to optimize visualization.

MR imaging has the benefit of better delineating the soft tissue planes and adjacent walls of the viscera and therefore is the investigation of choice for demonstration of complex pelvic fistulae (Fig. 142.19) (Narayanan et al. 2009; Healy et al. 1996; Outwater and Schiebler 1993). High-resolution T2-weighted sequences performed in multiple planes allow for the identification of the optimal plane for fistula detection. This is usually the sagittal plane. Heavily T2-weighted sequences or fat-saturated T2-weighted sequences are helpful in the detection of the fistulous tract, which is seen as high signal intensity compared to the surrounding structures. The administration of intravenous gadolinium on T1-weighted images also increases the detection of the fistulous tract by demonstrating enhancement of the walls of the tract (Semelka et al. 1997). Conventional radiographic dynamic imaging studies, such as the use of water-soluble enemas, cystograms, and vaginograms, may also be helpful in demonstrating the fistula if there is a specific question. The increased use of CT imaging, however, has meant that these dynamic procedures can also be performed in CT with the added benefit of three-dimensional reconstruction.

Fig. 142.17 Axial CT image (**a**), reformatted sagittal CT image (**b**), and sagittal T1-weighted image following intravenous gadolinium (**c**) of a patient post radiotherapy complaining of intermittent fecal discharge per vaginum. The uterus is air filled (*white arrow*, **a** and *asterisk*, **b**) with a possible air-filled tract between the rectum and uterus demonstrated on sagittal reformatted images (*white arrow*, **b**). The sagittal post-gadolinium MR image (**c**) clearly demonstrates the fistulous tract between the uterus and bowel wall as well as the increased bowel wall thickening at this site in keeping with post-radiotherapy changes

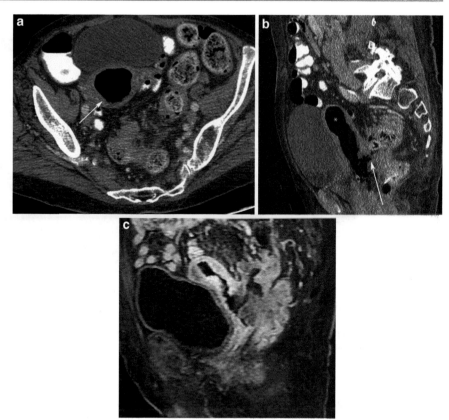

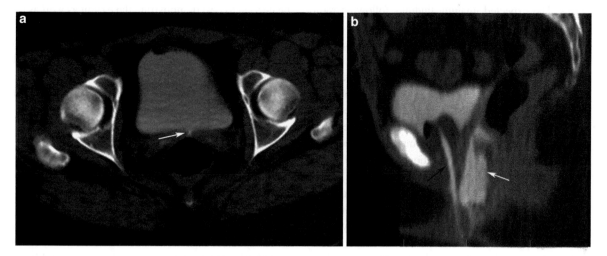

Fig. 142.18 Axial (**a**) and reformatted sagittal (**b**) CT images following CT cystogram with instillation of contrast medium via urinary catheter (*black arrow*, **b**) into the urinary bladder. Axial images demonstrate the narrow fistula between the urinary bladder and the vagina (*white arrow*, **a**) with contrast medium filling the vagina (*white arrow*, **b**) from the fistulous connection

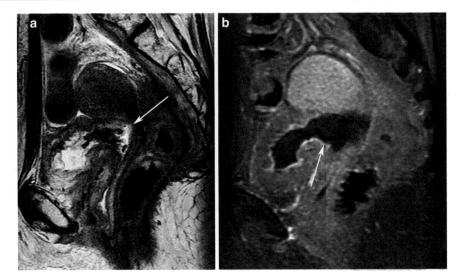

Fig. 142.19 Sagittal T2-weighted (**a**) and T1-weighted following gadolinium (**b**) MR images following radiotherapy for cervical carcinoma. The T2-weighted image (**a**) demonstrates the low signal atrophic appearances of the cervix in keeping with post-radiotherapy changes and a possible connection between the cervix and the bladder (*white arrow*, **a**). Following intravenous gadolinium (**b**) the fistulous tract is well demonstrated from cervix to urinary bladder with increased enhancement of the wall of the tract (*white arrow*, **b**)

Appropriateness of Different Imaging Modalities

Imaging follow-up after radiotherapy treatment for gynecological malignancy is typically with MR imaging to assess the local disease response in the pelvis and with CT examination to assess for evidence of distant metastases. The expected imaging findings following radiotherapy have been discussed with those that are seen on both CT and MR examinations such as enteritis, colitis, and cystitis as well as those that are best seen on MR such as fatty bone marrow changes. As the radiation field is localized to the pelvis and affects the soft tissue planes, most of the expected changes are more readily visualized on MR imaging. However, the appearances on both CT and MR imaging are important to recognize to allow for correct interpretation of the findings on follow-up imaging studies.

The imaging of complications following radiotherapy depends upon if the patient is symptomatic and then is guided by their symptoms. Many of the radiotherapy complications are detected incidentally on follow-up imaging and therefore we have discussed their appearances on routine MR and CT imaging. In the case of the unwell symptomatic patient with fever and abdominal pain following chemotherapy, CT examination is the investigation of choice as it readily demonstrates the bowel wall thickening and distribution of bowel involvement seen in typhlitis as well as the detection of those patients with transmural bowel wall necrosis and impending perforation. In the complication of radiation-induced pelvic fistulae, a combination of imaging modalities may be needed to best demonstrate the extent as well as the function of fistulae. Nuclear medicine imaging also has a role in the assessment of the post-radiotherapy patient with back pain or who is asymptomatic with suspicious MR appearances by having a high sensitivity for the detection of insufficiency fractures on bone scintigram.

Summary of Key Features/"Pearls to Remember"

- In addition to the tumor, the adjacent soft tissues are likely to undergo fibrotic changes. This may result in both appearing of low signal intensity and indistinguishable from each other particularly in the first 6 months following radiotherapy.

- In advanced cervical carcinoma where there was initial parametrial invasion, intravenous contrast medium can be helpful in distinguishing between radiotherapy-induced parametrial fibrosis and residual or recurrent disease. Fibrosis enhances later than tumor and tends to enhance homogeneously.
- The reconstitution of the normal low signal intensity cervical stroma is the most reliable indicator of a tumor-free post-radiation cervix.
- In premenopausal patients undergoing pelvic radiotherapy the function of the ovaries may be maintained by surgically placing them out of the radiation field; this is called ovarian transposition.
- Transposed ovaries can be mistaken for peritoneal disease because of their abnormal anatomical location, usually in the paracolic gutters. Careful interrogation for the presence of follicles is helpful to avoid this pitfall.
- MRI shows the earliest changes of radiotherapy damage to the urinary bladder: the bullous submucosal edema is seen as high signal intensity on T2-weighted images while the bladder wall is of normal thickness (<5 mm).
- Bone marrow fatty conversion, which occurs in the radiation field, results in very well-defined signal changes due to the boundary of the radiation field.
- The detection of a fistulous tract following radiotherapy may be better visualized following the administration of intravenous gadolinium on T1-weighted images.
- Recurrent disease, which invades the adjacent organs, can also cause a fistulous tract as well as soft tissue changes due to radiation alone. Careful evaluation for the presence of a soft tissue mass or other features of malignancy such as lymphadenopathy should therefore be routinely performed.
- Enteritis of the small bowel typically involves the more fixed terminal ileum and on CT examination appears as bowel wall thickening and submucosal edema. Chronic changes of fibrosis can lead to stenotic segments of small bowel which in turn may cause small bowel obstruction.
- Typhlitis (neutropenic colitis) following chemotherapy typically affects the cecum and ascending colon resulting in segmental circumferential bowel wall thickening with surrounding fat stranding and free fluid.

- In the long term after radiotherapy the urinary bladder is small volume and unable to fully distend because of its fibrotic wall. Perforation of the bladder is a recognized late complication following radiotherapy which is rare but a life-threatening event.
- The ureteric stricture from radiation treatment is smoothly tapered and can clearly be demonstrated on delayed CT examination following intraveneous contrast medium which opacifies the ureters.
- The most common sites of insufficiency fractures are the sacrum and pubic rami.
- Nonunion and aseptic necrosis of insufficiency fractures occurs because the abnormal bone texture cannot heal normally.

References

Addar MH, Stuart GC, Nation JG, Shumsky AG. Spontaneous rupture of the urinary bladder: a late complication of radiotherapy-case report and review of the literature. Gynecol Oncol. 1996;62(2):314–16.

Addley HC, Vargas HA, Moyle PL, Crawford R, Sala E. Pelvic imaging following chemotherapy and radiation therapy for gynecologic malignancies. Radiographics. 2010;30:1843–56.

Arrive L, Chang YC, Hricak H, Brescia RJ, Auffermann W, Quivey JM. Radiation – induced uterine changes: MR imaging. Radiology. 1989;170(1 Pt 1):55–8.

Barnes EA, Thomas G, Ackerman I, Barbera L, Letourneau D, Lam K, Makhani N, Sankreacha R. Prospective comparison of clinical and computed tomography assessment in detecting uterine perforation with intracavitary brachytherapy for carcinoma of the cervix. Int J Gynecol Cancer. 2007;17:821–6.

Blomlie V, Rofstad EK, Skjonsberg A, Tvera K, Lien HH. Female pelvic bone marrow: serial MR imaging before, during, and after radiation therapy. Radiology. 1995;194:537–43.

Capps G, Fulcher A, Szucs R, Turner M. Imaging features of radiation-induced changes in the abdomen. Radiographics. 1997;17:1455–73.

De Graef M, Karam R, Juhan V, Daclin PY, Maubon AJ, Rouanet JP. High signal in the uterine cervix on T2-weighted MR imaging sequences. Eur Radiol. 2003;13(1):118–26.

Delaney G, Jacob S, Barton M. Estimation of an optimal radiotherapy utilization rate for gynecologic carcinoma. Part I – Malignancies of the cervix, ovary, vagina and vulva. Cancer. 2004;101(4):671–81.

Donner CS. Pathophysiology and therapy of chronic radiation-induced injury to the colon. Dig Dis. 1998;16:253–61.

Feeney DD, Moore DH, Look KY, Stehman FB, Sutton GP. The fate of the ovaries after radical hysterectomy and ovarian transposition. Gynecol Oncol. 1995;56:3–7.

Flueckiger F, Ebner F, Poschauko H, Tamussino K, Einspieler R, Ranner G. Cervical cancer: serial MR imaging before and after primary radiation therapy – a 2 year follow-up study. Radiology. 1992;184:89–93.

Georg P, Georg D, Hillbrand M, Kirisits C, Potter R. Factors influencing bowel sparing in intensity modulated whole pelvic radiotherapy for gynaecological malignancies. Radiother Oncol. 2006;80:19–26.

Healy JC, Phillips RR, Rezneck RH, Crawford RA, Armstrong P, Shepherd JH. The MR appearances of vaginal fistulas. AJR Am J Roentgenol. 1996;167:1487–9.

Hoeffel C, Crema MD, Belkacem A, Azizi L, Lewin M, Arrive L, Tubiana JM. Multi-detector row CT: spectrum of diseases involving the ileocaecal area. Radiographics. 2006;26:1373–90.

Hricak H, Swift PS, Campos Z, Quivey JM, Gildengorin V, Goranson H. Irradiation of the cervix uteri: value of unenhanced and contrast-enhanced MR imaging. Radiology. 1993;189:381–8.

Hricak H, Akin O, Sala E, Ascher S, Levine D, Reinhold C. Chapter 3. In: Diagnostic imaging: gynecology. Salt Lake City: AMIRSYS; 2006. p. 51.

Iyer R, Jhingran A, Sawaf H, Libshitz H. Imaging findings after radiotherapy to the pelvis. AJR Am J Roentgenol. 2001;177:1083–9.

Kehoe S. Treatments for gynaecological cancers. Best Pract Res Clin Obstet Gynaecol. 2006;20(6):985–1000.

Mark RJ, Poen J, Tran LM, Fu YS, Heaps J, Parker RG. Postradiation sarcoma of the gynecologic tract: a report of 13 cases and a discussion of radiation-induced gynecologic malignancies. Am J Clin Oncol. 1996;19:59–64.

Narayanan P, Nobbenhuis M, Reynolds KM, Sahdev A, Reznek RH, Rockall AG. Fistulas in malignant gynecologic disease: etiology, imaging, and management. Radiographics. 2009;29:1073–83.

Outwater E, Schiebler ML. Pelvic fistulas: findings on MR images. AJR Am J Roentgenol. 1993;160:327–30.

Portelance L, Chao KS, Grigsby PW, Bennet H, Low D. Intensity – modulated radiation therapy (IMRT) reduces small bowel, rectum, and bladder doses in patients with cervical cancer receiving pelvic and para-aortic irradiation. Int J Rad Oncol Biol Phys. 2001;51:261–6.

Sella T, Mironov S, Hricak H. Imaging of transposed ovaries in patients with cervical carcinoma. AJR Am J Roentgenol. 2005;184:1602–10.

Semelka RC, Hricak H, Kim B, Forstner R, Bis KG, Ascher SM, Reinhold C. Pelvic fistulas: appearance on MR images. Abdom Imaging. 1997;22:91–5.

Sugimura K, Okizuka H. Postsurgical pelvis: treatment follow-up. Radiol Clin North Am. 2002;40(3):659–80.

Tai P, Hammond A, Van Dyk JV, Stitt L, Tonita J, Coad T, Radwan J. Pelvic fractures following irradiation of endometrial and vaginal cancers – a case series and review of literature. Radiother Oncol. 2000;56:23–8.

Vincens E, Balleyguier C, Rey A, Uzan C, Zareski E, Gouy S, Pautier P, Duvillart P, Haie-Meder C, Morice P. Accuracy of magnetic resonance imaging in predicting residual disease in patients treated for stage IB2/II cervical carcinoma with chemoradiation therapy: correlation of radiologic findings with surgicopathologic results. Cancer. 2008;113(8):2158–65.

Viswanathan AN. The frank Ellis memorial lecture: the use of three-dimensional imaging in gynaecological radiation therapy. Clin Oncol. 2008;20:1–5.

Weber T, Sostman H, Spritzer C, Ballard R, Meyer G, Clarke-Pearson D, Soper J. Cervical carcinoma: determination of recurrent tumour extent versus radiation changes with MR imaging. Radiology. 1995;194:135–9.

Yankelevitz DF, Henschke CI, Knapp PH, Nisce L, Yi Y, Cahill P. Effect of radiation therapy on thoracic and lumbar bone marrow: evaluation with MR imaging. AJR Am J Roentgenol. 1991;157(1):87–92.

Helen Clare Addley and Caroline Reinhold

Patient Management

Patient management for gynecological malignancy depends upon the origin of the primary tumor and the grade and stage of disease. The options are between surgery alone, surgery and the addition of oncological therapy such as chemotherapy or radiotherapy, or chemoradiotherapy alone. The management for patients undergoing chemoradiotherapy is discussed in detail in the preceding chapter.

Patients who undergo surgical management for gynecological malignancy are further stratified into different surgical groups depending upon the surgical procedure (Fig. 143.1). A multidisciplinary approach is used to discuss the radiological and histopathological findings of each patient with both surgical and oncological teams. In deciding upon the most appropriate surgical approach for a patient, not only the imaging findings and histopathology need to be discussed, but also clinical information about the patient such as wish to preserve fertility and parity.

Imaging plays a crucial role in the assessment of whether surgery is a suitable option for a patient, and if that is the case, whether routine surgery needs to be modified for example, to include lymphadenectomy. In the postoperative patient, follow-up imaging is crucial to assess if there is evidence of residual or recurrent disease as well as to identify any surgical complications, which would result in a change in patient management.

H.C. Addley (✉) • C. Reinhold
Department of Radiology, McGill University Health Center,
Montreal General Hospital, Montreal, Quebec, Canada

Patients undergoing simple hysterectomy or oophorectomy for benign gynecological disease are subject to the same postsurgical complications as patients with malignancy who undergo the same procedure, and therefore, will also be discussed in this chapter. Patients with cesarean sections performed for either emergency or routine delivery of a neonate do not undergo routine imaging follow-up but the appearances post Cesarean section and ensuing complications will be discussed in this chapter for the sake of completeness.

Surgical Options

Treatment stratification for surgery depends upon benign versus malignant disease and in malignancy on the grade, stage, and organ of origin of the malignancy. In endometrial cancer, early stage disease (Stage 1A) and grades 1–2 is treated with simple hysterectomy. Advanced stage endometrial cancer or grade 3 disease is treated with radical hysterectomy and lymph node sampling with adjuvant radiotherapy (Frei et al. 2000). In cervical cancer, surgery is considered if the size of the tumor is less than 4 cm in greatest diameter and either confined to the cervix (stage 1) or beyond the uterus but negative for parametrial extension (stage 2A) (FIGO Committee 2009). Pelvic sidewall invasion is therefore important to assess for in the pretreatment MR examination and would stratify the patient to undergo radiation treatment instead of surgical treatment. The radiologist should therefore be vigilant in the assessment for hydronephrosis, ureteral wall thickening, tumor less than 3 mm from the pelvic sidewall, and greater than

B. Hamm, P. R. Ros (eds.), *Abdominal Imaging*, DOI 10.1007/978-3-642-13327-5_185,
© Springer-Verlag Berlin Heidelberg 2013

Fig. 143.1 Schematic diagram demonstrating the normal anatomy of the female pelvis (**a**). Schematic diagrams (**b**–**e**) demonstrating the structures in blue removed during different surgical procedures. In trachelectomy (**b**) the cervix is removed with anastomosis of the body of the uterus to the vagina. In hysterectomy the uterus and cervix are removed without the ovaries (**c**) or in TAH + BSO with the ovaries (**d**). In pelvic exenteration (**e**) a combination of the pelvic organs are removed with urinary diversion in anterior exenteration and formation of colostomy in posterior exenteration

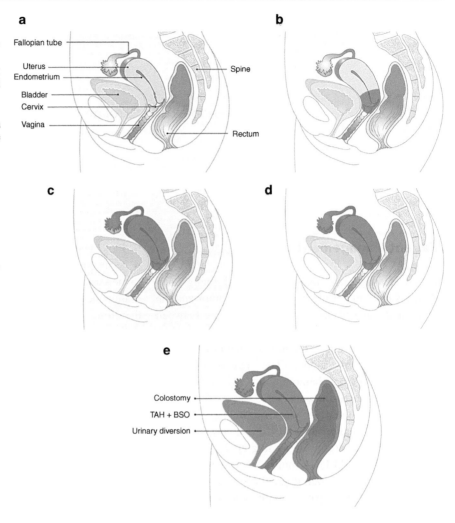

90° vessel encasement (Togashi et al. 1998). The surgical options for cervical cancer include trachelectomy, which is a fertility-sparing technique as well as hysterectomy. In ovarian cancer, total abdominal hysterectomy (TAH) and bilateral salpingo-oophorectomy (BSO) is the surgical treatment offered with or without omentectomy. Careful detection of peritoneal deposits and their location is important as these can often be resected in primary debulking surgery with certain exceptions at non-resectable sites such as the root of the mesentery. Lymphadenopathy above the level of the renal hilum, however, is important to recognize on preoperative ovarian cancer imaging, as neoadjuvant chemotherapy prior to surgery may be preferred over primary surgery (Kyriazi et al. 2010; Tsolakidis et al. 2010).

Hysterectomy

Hysterectomy is one of the most common abdominal procedures performed on female patients. There are different variations of the surgical technique depending mainly on the type and stage of the pathology being treated.

Total abdominal hysterectomy consists of resection of the body and cervix of the uterus as well as transection of the vagina near the cervical os. The vaginal apex is sutured creating a small cuff. The utero-sacral and cardinal ligaments are sutured to this cuff to provide added support. There is little disturbance of the ureters and trigone of the bladder as they are not removed from their beds (Thompson 1992). In modified radical (extended) hysterectomy the cervix, paracervical tissues, and upper vagina are removed. The ureters are dissected to the vesico-ureteric junction and retracted laterally to allow resection of the parametrial and paracervical tissues medial to them.

Radical abdominal hysterectomy involves removal of the uterus, upper third of the vagina, paracervical, parametria, and upper paravaginal tissues. All uterine ligaments are resected and all lymph nodes distal to and including the common iliac chains are removed. Para-aortic lymphadenectomy caudal to the renal hila is also sometimes performed. The standard procedure for ovarian carcinoma includes bilateral salpingo-oophorectomy and omentectomy.

The clinical evaluation of patients post hysterectomy is often limited therefore imaging plays a crucial role, which complements physical examination. The CT and MR appearance is similar after total and radical hysterectomy. The uterus is absent, and on axial images the opposed vaginal fornices are visualized as a thin line of soft-tissue density. Nodularity or fullness may be present on CT or T1 weighted MR images, and this should not be interpreted as a lesion (Fig. 143.2) (Sugimura and Okizuka 2002). The normal vaginal cuff is a symmetrical or minimally asymmetrical linear structure posterior to the bladder, usually surrounded by fat (Kasales et al. 1995). Its smooth, low signal intensity muscular wall is best

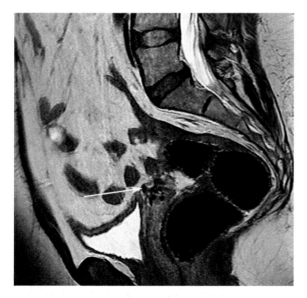

Fig. 143.2 Sagittal T2-weighted image of patient following hysterectomy. The normal vaginal vault can have a slightly nodular outline with presence of low signal intensity areas in keeping with signal voids due to surgical clips (*white arrow*)

visualized on T2-weighted MR images, although in some cases intermediate to low signal intensity on T2-weighted images will result from fibrous scar tissue (Jeong et al. 2003). Ultrasound may also be used for the evaluation of the vaginal cuff, which is usually seen as a homogeneously hypoechoic linear structure with a central thin echogenic line representing the vaginal mucosa. The size of the cuff varies with the patient's age and the exact surgical procedure and commonly shows some Doppler flow (Stein et al. 2006). Metallic clips along the pelvic sidewall can be detected at the site of lymph node dissection with CT. At MR imaging, these may appear as low-signal-intensity foci.

Trachelectomy

In 1994 a French surgeon, Daniel Dargent, developed the technique of a radical vaginal trachelectomy and pelvic lymphadenectomy to allow young women with early cervical cancer to have the potential to remain fertile and carry a child to birth (Dargent and Mathevet 1995). This technique has now been reproduced all over the world with reported lower mortality and morbidity with comparable curative rates to the traditional hysterectomy (Covens et al. 1999). Radical trachelectomy is a potentially curative surgical procedure for stage 1B1 or lower carcinoma of the cervix in women wishing to preserve their fertility. The technique involves a proximal vaginotomy, cervical resection, paracervical, and paravaginal dissections with laparoscopic bilateral lymph node dissections. The uterus is preserved, with an end-to-end anastomosis of the uterus to the remainder of the vaginal vault. A cerclage suture can be placed at the distal uterus to maintain uterine competency and hence fertility.

Successful pregnancy rates published are promising with up to 79% pregnancy rate reported in the women who wanted to conceive following radical trachelectomy (Sonoda et al. 2008). However, these pregnancies must be considered high risk with overall miscarriage rate of 13% –19% in the first and second trimesters respectively (Dursun et al. 2007; Rodriguez et al. 2001).

MR imaging is crucial in the preoperative assessment to determine the patient's eligibility for undergoing trachelectomy. As well as the stage of the cervical cancer, which needs to be stage 1A or 1B, the tumor size should be less than 2 cm unless it is exophytic in which case it can be up to 3 cm. In addition, the distance of the tumor from the internal os has to be at least 1 cm or greater to allow the surgeon enough distance to create an anastomosis (Bipat et al. 2011).

The best imaging modality for the post trachelectomy patient is MRI. Ultrasound and CT are not helpful in defining the anatomy or for assessment of early recurrence. T2-weighted MRI is the image sequence of choice, not only for the normal postoperative appearances, but also for normal postoperative variants, which are important to recognize and not to confuse with disease recurrence. There are a number of normal postoperative appearances, which must be appreciated on imaging. An end-to-end anastomosis between the corpus uteri and the vaginal vault is seen in approximately 45% of cases. The formation of a neo-fornix of the vagina is seen in approximately 50%. This is a posterior extension of the vaginal wall forming a posterior neo-fornix at the site of the utero-vaginal anastomosis (Fig. 143.3). This appearance does not change overtime and there is no abnormal

soft tissue to suggest recurrence (Hricak et al. 2006). The anastomotic sutures or the uterine cerclage suture can both give susceptibility artifacts in approximately 20% of cases. This is usually most pronounced in the fast spin echo T2-weighted sequences. Depending on the position of the artifacts, it may be difficult to exclude recurrence on imaging alone thus clinical examination is important (Sonoda et al. 2008).

Diffuse vaginal wall thickening with abnormal increased signal intensity on T2-weighted imaging can occur in approximately 5–10% of cases. This most likely represents postoperative change which gradually resolves by 1 year but it can be difficult to distinguish from infiltrating vaginal recurrence and therefore a biopsy may be required (Hricak et al. 2006). Isthmic stenosis may occur as early as 3 months after surgery in approx 2% of patients and manifests itself as secondary amenorrhea and hematometra (Sonoda et al. 2008). Exaggeration of the parametrial and pelvic venous plexus can be seen in approximately 10% of cases. No cause for this has been found and they are usually asymptomatic but irreversible (Hricak et al. 2006).

Pelvic Exenteration

Pelvic exenteration is performed in patients with persistent and recurrent disease or disease that does not respond to radiotherapy. It consists of radical en bloc resection of multiple endopelvic and exopelvic organs. In total exenteration, the uterus, vagina, bladder, urethra, and rectum are removed together with all the pelvic supporting and connective tissues. Partial exenteration may be anterior, with preservation of the rectum, or posterior with preservation of the bladder and urethra (Fig. 143.4). The introduction of new surgical techniques such as total mesovisceral excision and laterally extended endopelvic resection might increase the rate of surgical resections with clear margins even for tumors fixed to the pelvic sidewall (except the area of the sciatic foramen), which was previously regarded as a contraindication for pelvic exenteration (Höckel and Dornhöfer 2006).

Imaging appearances will reflect the surgical technique and the organs removed, with the potential spaces in the pelvis usually filled by bowel. In partial exenterations, the rectum may adopt a more anterior position or the bladder may extend more posteriorly than preoperatively.

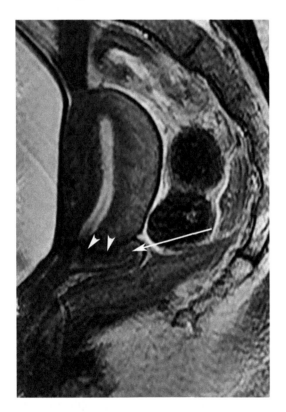

Fig. 143.3 Sagittal T2-weighted image of a patient post trachelectomy demonstrating normal appearances of the posterior neo-fornix (*white arrow*) and the site of the utero-vaginal anastomosis (*white arrowheads*)

Cesarean Section

Cesarean sections are percutaneous pelvic incisions through the anterior uterine wall into the endometrial cavity performed on an elective or emergency basis for delivery of the neonate. Preoperative imaging is usually by ultrasound only unless there is abnormal positioning of the placenta. Surgical techniques differ in the type of incision that is performed but postoperative imaging does not distinguish between the different surgical techniques. In the long term following a Cesarean section, a scar defect can be visualized usually in the lower uterine segment and the scar is also seen in the subcutaneous tissue on MR imaging. The subcutaneous scar is seen as a low signal intensity line on T2-weighted images and is most easily identified in the sagittal plane.

Postsurgical Complications

Following surgery, there are minor complications that can occur such as the formation of hematoma and lymphoceles, which need to be interpreted correctly

and not mistaken for recurrent disease. In addition, other complications seen following surgery may affect patient management such as pelvic abscess formation, fistulae, or adjacent visceral injury. These major complications are more likely to be seen in the symptomatic patient and therefore the imaging modality should be tailored to the most appropriate investigation.

Hematoma

Postoperative hematoma can occur from any gynecological surgical treatment and the incidence rate is difficult to define as many asymptomatic small collections are only seen on follow-up imaging. Severe hemorrhagic events are uncommon, only occurring in 2.1–3.1% of hysterectomies (Mäkinen et al. 2001). On CT acute hematoma has increased attenuation (hyperdense) due to aggregated fibrin, with Hounsfield units of 50–80 (Fig. 143.5). After 2–3 weeks the attenuation decreases and the lesion becomes hypodense. In the chronic phase, hematoma may appear like a simple cyst, with Hounsfield units equivalent to that of water.

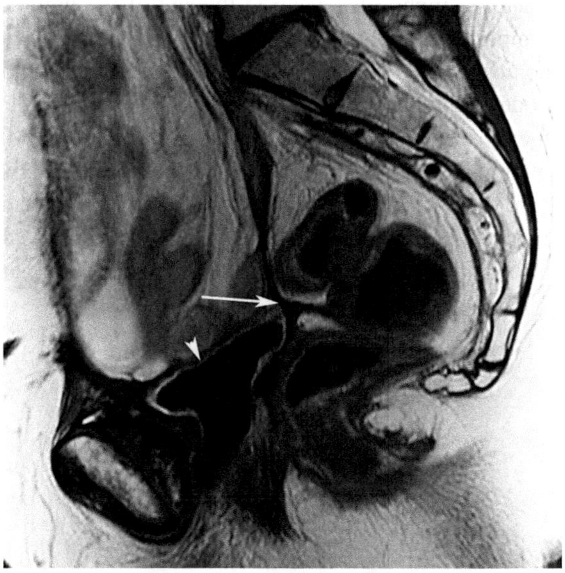

Fig. 143.4 Sagittal T2-weighted image post anterior exenteration. There are post hysterectomy appearances with absence of the uterus and cervix and low signal intensity line in their bed (*white arrow*). The urinary bladder has been replaced with an air-filled cavity following urinary diversion. The air-filled urinary bladder is seen as low signal intensity on the T2-weighted image (*white arrowhead*)

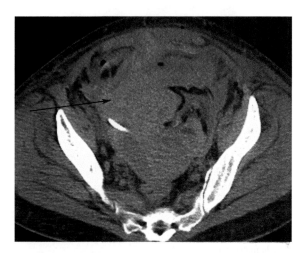

Fig. 143.5 Axial CT image of patient who had undergone TAH + BSO 24 h previously with a drop in hemoglobin level. Intermediate attenuation free fluid is seen in the pelvis consistent with hematoperitoneum as well as more dense material in the midline (*black arrow*) consistent with pelvic hematoma. The surgical drain can be seen to the right of the midline in the hematoma and was draining blood. Few bubbles of extraluminal gas are in keeping with recent postsurgical appearances

Hematoma on MRI can have a variable imaging appearance depending on the time elapsed from the onset of bleeding. In the acute phase, deoxyhemoglobin is of low or iso intensity on both T1 and T2-wighted imaging. Subacutely extracellular methemoglobin is of increased signal intensity on both T1 and T2-weighted imaging (Fig. 143.6). Chronic hematoma typically demonstrates the characteristic concentric ring sign, a dark peripheral rim on both T1 and T2-weighted images and a bright inner ring on T1-weighted images due to hemosiderin formation (Fig. 143.7) (Hahn et al. 1987).

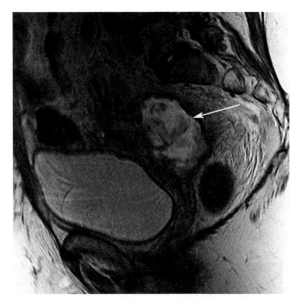

Fig. 143.6 Sagittal T2-weighted image following hysterectomy demonstrates a mixed signal intensity oval area (*white arrow*) in the pelvis with mainly high signal contents but wispy intermediate signal areas consistent with subacute hematoma

Lymphocele

Lymphadenectomy has an important role in the management of gynecological malignancies both for the assessment of lymph node status (Kim et al. 2004) and in the prevention of nodal recurrence (Milam et al. 2007; Lim et al. 2008). One of the most common postoperative complications of lymphadenectomy is a lymphocele, a fluid filled cyst without an epithelial lining which may occur in 12–24% of patients that undergo radical lymphadenectomy (Yang et al. 2004). It usually becomes detectable 3–8 weeks after surgery but may persist for up to a year. Symptoms depend on the size, location, and presence of super added infection (Pastore et al. 2007) Differentiation of lymphoceles from other postoperative complications such as hematoma, abscess, cystic tumor recurrence, or necrotic lymph nodes is important as the clinical management is different. Differentiating these on imaging alone can be difficult and aspiration or drainage of the collection with biochemical analysis can be helpful in making the final diagnosis (Kim et al. 1999).

Imaging demonstrates an elliptical fluid filled structure, which has thin walls that are typically unilocular unless complicated by infection or hemorrhage. Lymphoceles occur at the site of the previous lymph nodes dissection and imaging can very well demonstrate them following the anatomical lymph node chains within the pelvis, and are therefore commonly seen as bilateral structures (Fig. 143.8). On MR imaging, the cystic contents of the lymphocele give homogeneous high signal appearances on T2-weighted images (Fig. 143.9). The T1-weighted images should also be assessed for evidence of high signal intensity

Fig. 143.7 Axial T1-weighted image (**a**) and coronal T2-weighted image (**b**) of a chronic hematoma post trachelectomy. On both the T1-weighted image and T2-weighted image the rim of the hematoma is very dark (*white arrow*, **a**) in keeping with hemosiderin. The contents of the hematoma are darker on the T1-weighted image (*asterisk*, **a**) than the T2-weighted image in keeping with chronic blood product contents

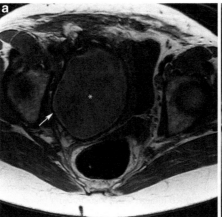
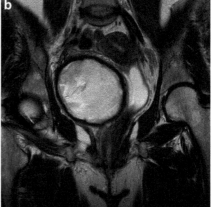

which is consistent with hemorrhage to avoid the pitfall of interpreting heterogeneity of signal as malignant disease. The presence of enhancing soft tissue would suggest tumor recurrence (Kim et al. 1999) and not a simple lymphocele.

Abscess and Endometritis

Infections following pelvic surgery occur in up to 13% of patients and are mostly related to the urinary tract and the surgical wound. Deep abscess formation is

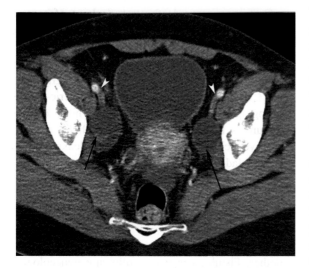

Fig. 143.8 Axial CT image following pelvic lymph node dissection demonstrates bilateral lymphoceles as bilateral well-defined fluid attenuation structures (*black arrows*) adjacent to the pelvic sidewalls in the position of the lymph node chains adjacent to the external iliac vessels (*white arrowheads*)

relatively rare (0.1–0.6%). In the early stages, there is bacterial proliferation and neutrophil accumulation in infected tissues, which is followed by liquefactive necrosis. On CT examination, there is initially a soft-tissue density mass that subsequently develops into a central area of water attenuation surrounded by a peripheral high attenuation rim that frequently enhances following intravenous contrast medium. Air is sometimes present within the abscess, and this may be a feature of colonization with gas-forming organisms or communication with the gastrointestinal (GI) tract (Fig. 143.10).

On MR imaging, an abscess initially appears as intermediate signal intensity on T1WI and high signal intensity on T2WI. With progression, air, necrosis, and liquefaction give a heterogeneous appearance that is associated with other non-specific signs of inflammation such as thickening or obliteration of adjacent fascial planes and displacement of surrounding structures (Sugimura and Okizuka 2002).

Although MR imaging clearly demonstrates the adjacent soft-tissue planes and pelvic structures, if percutaneous intervention is considered a possibility then CT or ultrasound examination should be performed. Deep pelvic abscesses are often not amenable to drain percutaneously via an anterior approach and therefore if a transgluteal approach is to be used the patient can be turned prone on the CT scanner and the drain inserted under CT guidance. Alternatively, a transvaginal approach can be used in selected patients.

Endometritis is inflammation of the endometrium and is seen as a complication following Cesarean

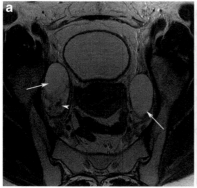
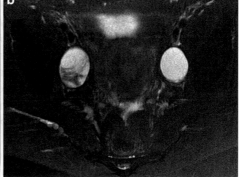

Fig. 143.9 Coronal T2-weighted image (**a**) and axial heavily T2-weighted image (**b**) of a patient post trachelectomy and pelvic lymph node clearance with bilateral lymphoceles. The lymphoceles are seen on the T2-weighted images as well-defined elliptical structures with high signal contents (*white arrows*). The lymphocele on the right is complicated with areas of wispy low signal intensity within it in keeping with hemorrhage (*white arrowhead*, **a**)

section. Patients typically complain of lower abdominal pain and fever a few days following the procedure. CT examination following the administration of intravenous contrast medium is the investigation of choice as it clearly demonstrates any additional abscess or fluid collection either between the uterus and the anterior abdominal wall or within the endometrial cavity (Fig. 143.11).

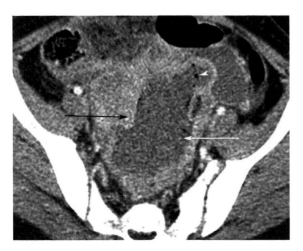

Fig. 143.10 Axial CT image demonstrating large fluid attenuation area (*white arrow*) within the pelvis with a thick enhancing rim (*black arrow*). Appearance is consistent with a deep pelvic abscess with small bubbles of gas seen within the abscess (*white arrowhead*), which do not rise anteriorly within the abscess to give a gas-fluid level because of the complex thick nature of the abscess fluid contents

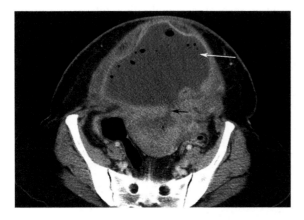

Fig. 143.11 Axial CT image of patient post Cesarean section with wound dehiscence of the uterine wall (*black arrow*) and a connection of fluid attenuation between the uterine cavity and a large subcutaneous abscess collection (*white arrow*) containing mostly fluid and a few bubbles of air with enhancing walls

Urinary Tract Injury

The incidence of urinary tract injury during gynecological surgery varies between 0.2 and 4% (Ibeanu et al. 2009). Risk factors include a large uterus, cystocele, ectopic vesico-ureteric junction as well as previous radiotherapy and surgery (Dandolu et al. 2003). The type of gynecological surgery is also important, with patients undergoing radical hysterectomy with lymph node dissection at higher risk of urinary tract injury, than patients with benign disease undergoing TAH (Paspulati and Dalal 2010).

Cystoscopy may demonstrate leakage of contrast material from an injured bladder, and some authors suggest that its routine intraoperative use increases the early pickup rate of this complication. Intravenous urogram (IVU) or contrast-enhanced CT urography are used to demonstrate iatrogenic ureteric leaks. Cystography or CT cystography where contrast medium is instilled via the foley catheter are both sensitive techniques for demonstrating leaks from the urinary bladder.

Fistulae

A fistula is a connection from one epithelial surface to another. Fistulae can occur following gynecological surgery due to the disruption of the normal anatomical planes, and if injury to the urinary tract or bowel occurs. They are also more likely to occur following radiotherapy and this is discussed in the preceding chapter. Although fistulae tend to be a late complication following radiotherapy, fistulae following surgery alone can also be seen as an early complication. Fistulae following gynecological surgery are most commonly vesicovaginal, involving the posterior bladder wall (Fig. 143.12). Fistulous tracts can also be more complex, however, and involve small bowel as well as pelvic cavities or abscesses, which may occur following more extensive surgery such as pelvic exenteration.

Youssef syndrome occurs following Cesarean section when there is fistula between the urinary bladder and uterus with patients presenting with vaginal urine leak, cyclic haematuria, and amenorrhea (Paspulati and Dalal 2010). As with patients who develop a fistula following radiotherapy, imaging can be tailored according to symptoms with CT cystography

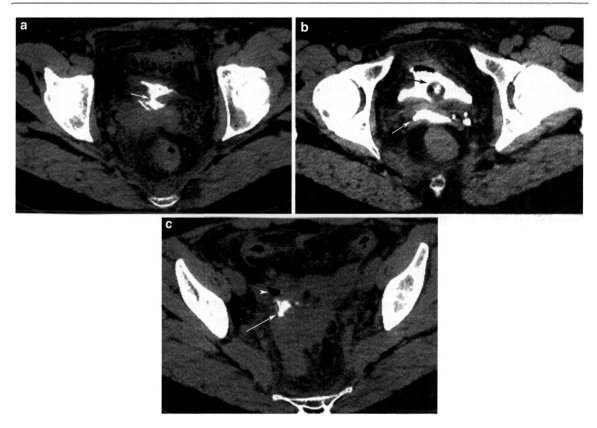

Fig. 143.12 Selected axial CT images from a CT cystogram following instillation of contrast medium into the urinary bladder. Patient is postoperative laparoscopic hysterectomy day two with continuous fluid leak from the vagina. CT cystogram demonstrates connection between the urinary bladder and vagina (*white arrow*, **a**) with contrast medium seen in both the urinary bladder with catheter in situ (*black arrow*, **b**) and the vagina (*white arrow*, **b**) as well as contrast medium (*white arrow*, **c**) and air (*white arrowhead*, **c**) seen in a pelvic collection just cranial to the bladder and vagina

or rectal contrast administration, as well as pelvic MR imaging, which may better delineate the fistulous tract.

Bowel Injury and Obstruction

Injury to the small or large bowel may occur during gynecological surgery and the risk is similar between laparoscopic and open procedures. The small bowel is more at risk during laparoscopic procedures and the rectum during vaginal hysterectomies (Paspulati and Dalal 2010). If bowel injury is suspected clinically, CT examination is the investigation of choice and will readily demonstrate intraperitoneal free air, the amount of which is important to assess in the early postoperative period as it may be in keeping with normal postoperative appearances. The administration of oral contrast or rectal contrast medium is helpful in such patients as contrast medium extravasation may be demonstrated and therefore localize the area of perforation.

Adhesions may occur as a late complication of any surgical procedure and adhesions may cause tethering of bowel loops and ultimately bowel obstruction. The surgical procedures, which are the most invasive such as the TAH and radical hysterectomies, are more likely to cause problems with adhesions than procedures, which are minimally invasive such as the laparoscopic hysterectomies. CT examination is the investigation of choice as it will demonstrate the caliber of the dilated, obstructed bowel, will identify the point of transition, and if the bowel obstruction is partial CT will demonstrate oral contrast medium distal to the transition site. The complications of bowel obstruction are also readily identified on CT examination such as perforation and bowel ischemia.

Scar Endometriosis

Endometrial implants at the site of the abdominal scar may occur as a late complication of surgery. This is most typically seen following Cesarean section, but may be seen following any type of gynecological surgery where there is a percutaneous scar. The patients present with a mass at the site of the scar and may complain of pain (Fig. 143.13).

On ultrasound imaging, the endometrial implant is demonstrated as a non-specific mass with mixed echogenicity and blood flow on color Doppler imaging (Fig. 143.14). CT examination is also non-specific. MR imaging is the investigation of choice as it may demonstrate high signal contents on T1-weighted imaging consistent with hemorrhage. The T2-weighted signal contents are typically variable and the deposit enhances following intravenous gadolinium (Fig. 143.15). As the imaging findings may also be seen in other diagnoses such as desmoid tumor or chronic hematoma at the scar site, biopsy, or excision is usually necessary (Blanco et al. 2003). As most of the implants are readily identified on ultrasound imaging and are superficial, ultrasound guided biopsy is a safe and convenient method.

Wound Dehiscence

Wound dehiscence following gynecological surgery contributes significantly to patient morbidity and increases patient stay in hospital and therefore risk of further complications. Patient factors contribute to poor wound healing such as obesity and diabetes mellitus. Imaging can be helpful in ensuring that there is no additional abscess formation or underlying subcutaneous collection. In the case of wound dehiscence occurring following Cesarean section, MR imaging may be more helpful than CT imaging as it demonstrates the layers of the uterus and therefore demonstrates if the entire uterine wall is dehiscent (Paspulati and Dalal 2010).

Appropriateness of Different Imaging Modalities

Postoperative imaging of the patient following gynecological surgery depends upon whether the imaging is for routine follow-up or for the symptomatic patient. In patients undergoing surgery for gynecological

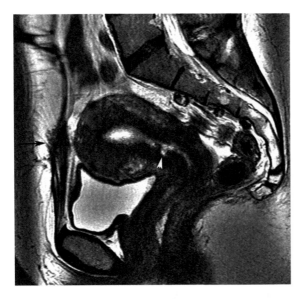

Fig. 143.13 Sagittal T2-weighted image years following Cesarean section with low signal intensity seen at the site of the subcutaneous scar (*black arrow*) and the high signal defect at the site of uterine section in the uterine wall (*white arrowhead*)

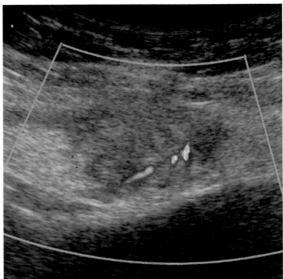

Fig. 143.14 Ultrasound color Doppler image in a patient post Cesarean section with palpable lump at the site of the scar. Ultrasound demonstrates a hypoechoic solid area in the subcutaneous tissues which contains blood flow. The appearances on ultrasound are non-specific but as ultrasound demonstrates the area well, following other investigations such as MRI, a biopsy can be obtained under ultrasound guidance if needed

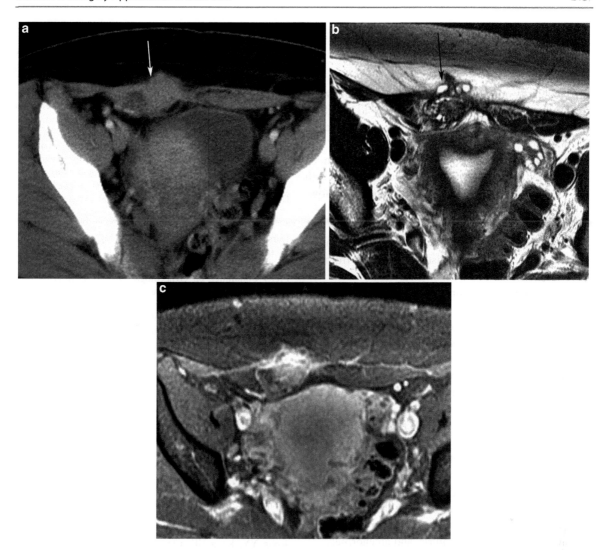

Fig. 143.15 Axial CT image (**a**) and MR T2-weighted image (**b**) and MR T1-weighted image following intravenous gaolinium (**c**) of the same patient as in Fig. 143.14 with palpable lump at site of Cesarean section scar. The CT examination demonstrates non-specific soft-tissue attenuation mass (*white arrow*, **a**) intimately related to the scar site. On MR imaging the signal characteristics are typical for endometriosis with high signal cystic areas and low signal surrounding areas (*black arrow*, **b**) with definite enhancement following intravenous contrast medium (**c**). Although the MRI appearances are suggestive of scar endometriosis, definitive diagnosis of endometriosis was made in this patient following ultrasound guided biopsy

malignancy, imaging follow-up is typically with MR imaging to assess the local site of where the primary disease had arisen and with CT imaging to assess for any distant disease. The expected findings, therefore, following the different surgical procedures should be known for both MR and CT examinations. For the patient undergoing surgery for benign gynecological disease, routine imaging follow-up is rarely performed.

Imaging of the symptomatic postoperative patient, whether for benign or malignant disease, is based upon the patient's symptoms and concern of a possible complication. CT imaging is the investigation of choice for the assessment of possible hematoma, abscess, urinary tract injury, and bowel injury. For the more detailed assessment of the pelvic organs and soft tissues, MR imaging may be very helpful in delineating a fistulous tract. MR imaging is also helpful in the assessment of possible scar endometriosis and for assessment of the uterine wall in the case of post Cesarean uterine wall dehiscence.

Summary of Key Features/"Pearls to Remember"

- Nodularity or fullness at the vaginal vault following hysterectomy may be present on CT or T1 weighted MR images, and should not be interpreted as a lesion.
- Metallic clips along the pelvic sidewall can be detected at the site of lymph node dissection with CT. At MR imaging, these may appear as low-signal-intensity foci.
- Trachelectomy criteria: stage 1A or 1B, tumor size less than 2 cm unless it is exophytic in which case it can be up to 3 cm and distance of tumor from the internal os must be 1 cm or greater.
- Differentiation of lymphocoeles from other postoperative complications such as hematoma, abscess, cystic tumor recurrence, or necrotic lymph nodes is important as the clinical management is different.
- Air is sometimes present within an abscess, and this may be a feature of colonization with gas-forming organisms or communication with the gastrointestinal (GI) tract.
- Patients undergoing radical hysterectomy with lymph node dissection are at higher risk of urinary tract injury than patients with benign disease undergoing TAH.
- Youssef syndrome occurs following Cesarean section when there is fistula between the urinary bladder and uterus with patients presenting with vaginal urine leak, cyclic haematuria, and amenorrhea.
- The small bowel is more at risk during laparoscopic procedures and the rectum during vaginal hysterectomies.
- Endometriosis implant may occur at the site of the scar following gynecological surgery and may require biopsy or excision for diagnosis.
- In the case of wound dehiscence occurring following Cesarean section, MR imaging may be more helpful than CT imaging as it demonstrates the layers of the uterus and therefore demonstrates if the entire uterine wall is dehiscent.

References

Bipat S, van den Berg RA, van der Velden J, Stoker J, Spijkerboer AM. The role of magnetic resonance imaging in determining the proximal extension of early stage cervical cancer to the internal os. Eur J Radiol. 2011;78(1):60–4.

Blanco RG, Parithivel VS, Shah AK, Gumbs MA, Schein M, Gerst PH. Abdominal wall endometriomas. Am J Surg. 2003;185(6):596–8.

Covens A, Shaw P, Murphy J, et al. Is radical trachelectomy a safe alternative to radical hysterectomy for patients with stage 1A-B carcinoma of the cervix? Cancer. 1999; 86:2273–9.

Dandolu V, Mathai E, Chatwani A, Harmanli O, Pontari M, Hernandez E. Accuracy of cystoscopy in the diagnosis of ureteral injury in benign gynecologic surgery. Int Urogynecol J Pelvic Floor Dysfunct. 2003;14(6):427–31.

Dargent D, Mathevet P. Schauta's vaginal hysterectomy combined with laproscopic lymphadenectomy. Baillieres Clin Obstet Gynaecol. 1995;9:691–705.

Dursun P, LeBlanc E, Nogueira MC. Radical vaginal trachelectomy (Dargent's operation): a critical review of the literature. Eur J Surg Oncol. 2007;33(8):933–41.

FIGO Committee on Gynecologic Oncology. Revised FIGO staging for carcinoma of the vulva, cervix and endometrium. Int J Gynecol Obstet. 2009;105:103–4.

Frei KA, Kinkel K, Bonel HM, Lu Y, Zaloudek C, Hricak H. Prediction of deep myometrial invasion in patients with endometrial cancer: clinical utility of contrast-enhanced MR imaging – a meta-analysis and Bayesian analysis. Radiology. 2000;216:444–9.

Hahn PF, Saini S, Stark DD, Papanicolaou N, Ferrucci Jr JT. Intraabdominal hematoma: the concentric-ring sign in MR imaging. AJR Am J Roentgenol. 1987;148:115–19.

Höckel M, Dornhöfer N. Pelvic exenteration for gynaecological tumours: achievements and unanswered questions. Lancet Oncol. 2006;7(10):837–47.

Hricak H, Akin O, Sala E, Ascher S, Levine D, Reinhold C. Chapter 3. In: Diagnostic imaging: gynecology. Salt Lake City: AMIRSYS; 2006. p. 51.

Ibeanu OA, Chesson RR, Echols KT, Nieves M, Busangu F, Nolan TE. Urinary tract injury during hysterectomy based on universal cystoscopy. Obstet Gynecol. 2009;113(1):6–10.

Jeong YY, Kang HK, Chung TW, Seo JJ, Park JG. Uterine cervical carcinoma after therapy: CT and MR imaging findings. Radiographics. 2003;23(4):969–81.

Kasales CJ, Langer JE, Arger PH. Pelvic pathology after hysterectomy. A pictorial essay. Clin Imaging. 1995;19(3):210–17.

Kim JK, Jeong YY, Kim YH, Kim YC, Kang HK, Choi HS. Postoperative pelvic lymphocele: treatment with simple percutaneous catheter drainage. Radiology. 1999;212:390–4.

Kim HY, Kim JW, Kim SH, Kim YT, Kim JH. An analysis of the risk factors and management of lymphocele after pelvic lymphadenectomy in patients with gynaecologic malignacies. Cancer Research and Treatment. 2004; 36:377–83.

Kyriazi S, Kaye SM, deSouza NM. Imaging ovarian cancer and peritoneal metastases – current and emerging techniques. Nat Rev Clin Oncol. 2010;7(7):381–93.

Lim CS, Alexander-Sefre F, Allam M, Singh N, Aleong JC, Al-Rawi H, Jacobs IJ. Clinical value of immunohistochemically detected lymphovascular space invasion in early stage cervical carcinoma. Ann Surg Oncol. 2008;15(9):2581–8.

Mäkinen J, Johansson J, Tomás C, Tomás E, Heinonen PK, Laatikainen T, Kauko M, Heikkinen AM, Sjöberg J.

Morbidity of 10 110 hysterectomies by type of approach. Hum Reprod. 2001;16(7):1473–8.

Milam MR, Frumovitz M, dos Reis R, Broaddus RR, Bassett Jr RL, Ramirez PT. Preoperative lymph-vascular space invasion is associated with nodal metastases in women with early-stage cervical cancer. Gynecol Oncol. 2007;106(1):12–15.

Paspulati RM, Dalal TA. Imaging of complications following gynecologic surgery. Radiographics. 2010;30:625–42.

Pastore M, Manci N, Marchetti C, et al. Late aortic lymphocele and residual ovary syndrome after gynecological surgery. World J Surg Oncol. 2007;5:146.

Rodriguez M, Guimares O, Rose PG. Radical abdominal trachelectomy and pelvic lymphadenectomy with uterine conservation and subsequent pregnancy in the treatment of early invasive cervical cancer. Am J Obstet Gynecol. 2001;185(2):370–4.

Sonoda Y, Chi DS, Carter J, Barakat RR, Abu-Rustum NR. Initial experience with Dargent's operation: the radical vaginal trachelectomy. Gynecol Oncol. 2008;108(1):214–19.

Stein MW, Grishina A, Shaw RJ, Roberts JH, Ricci ZJ, Adachi A, Freeman K, Koenigsberg M. Gray-scale and color Doppler sonographic features of the vaginal cuff and cervical remnant after hysterectomy. AJR Am J Roentgenol. 2006;187(5): 1372–6.

Sugimura K, Okizuka H. Postsurgical pelvis: treatment follow-up. Radiol Clin North Am. 2002;40(3):659–80, viii.

Thompson JD. Hysterectomy. In: Thompson JD, Rock JA, editors. Te Lind's operative gynecology. 7th ed. Philadelphia: JB Lippincott; 1992. p. 663–738.

Togashi K, Morikawa K, Kataoka ML, Konishi J. Cervical cancer. J Magn Reson Imaging. 1998;8:391–7.

Tsolakidis D, Amant F, Van Gorp T, Leunen K, Neven P, Vergote I. Diaphragmatic surgery during primary debulking in 89 patients with stage IIIB-IV epithelial ovarian cancer. Gynecol Oncol. 2010;116(3):489–96.

Yang DM, Jung DH, Kim H, et al. Retroperitoneal cystic masses: CT, clinical, and pathologic findings and literature review. Radiographics. 2004;24:1353–65.

144

Benign Conditions of the Vagina and Vulva

Nishat Bharwani and Rachel Connor

Introduction

Benign conditions of the vagina and vulva are relatively common clinical presentations. However, they are not common indications for imaging as many of these abnormalities can be confidently diagnosed on the basis of clinical history, examination, and biopsy where necessary. These conditions may be observed as incidental findings on imaging performed for other reasons or when the vagina or vulva is involved in a more extensive disease process. This chapter will discuss and illustrate the imaging appearances of acquired conditions encompassing inflammatory processes and benign tumors.

Acquired Anomalies of the Vagina and Vulva

Acquired Vulval Cysts

Bartholin Gland Cyst

The Bartholin glands are located in the posterolateral portion of the lower vagina behind the labia minora and are the female equivalent of the male Cowper glands.

N. Bharwani (✉)
Imaging, Bart's Cancer Centre, King George V Wing St Bartholomew's Hospital, West Smithfield, London, UK

Department of Radiology, St Mary's Hospital, Imperial College Healthcare NHS Trust, London, UK

R. Connor
South Glasgow University Hospitals, The Victoria Infirmary, Glasgow, UK

The ducts open onto the posterolateral vestibules on both sides, at the 4 o'clock and 8 o'clock positions. Bartholin gland cysts are the most common vulval cysts and develop as a result of ductal occlusion and retention of secretions (Fig. 144.1) (Lopez et al. 2005). The cause of obstruction is rarely apparent. Cysts can become secondarily infected resulting in Bartholinitis where patients present with a painful vulval mass. Causative organisms include genitourinary tract anaerobes, gram-negative bacilli, and *Neisseria gonorrhoeae*.

Bartholin's cysts are usually unilateral, nontender, tense, palpable masses in the labia majora measuring 1–4 cm in diameter (Kier 1992). Diagnosis is usually clinical; however, they can be visualized on perineal ultrasound but will not be seen on transabdominal or transvaginal ultrasound due to their location. They are often detected incidentally on MRI in women undergoing imaging for unrelated reasons. On T1-weighted sequences, they return low signal intensity when they contain simple fluid or intermediate to high signal intensity when they contain protein, mucin, or hemorrhage. Bartholin duct cysts are usually of uniformly high T2-weighted signal intensity (Kier 1992; Kozawa et al. 2008). Uncomplicated cysts have thin walls and do not enhance following intravenous contrast medium. Thickening of the wall with irregular contrast enhancement and high signal intensity in the surrounding tissues due to edema suggests superimposed Bartholinitis.

Skene Duct Cyst

The paired Skene's or periurethral glands are homologous to the prostate gland in males. They lie lateral to the urethral meatus and their ducts open onto the vulva on either side of the meatus. Skene duct cysts develop

B. Hamm, P. R. Ros (eds.), *Abdominal Imaging*, DOI 10.1007/978-3-642-13327-5_198,
© Springer-Verlag Berlin Heidelberg 2013

Fig. 144.1 Bartholin's cyst. Sagittal (**a**), coronal (**b**), axial (**c**) T2-weighted, and (**d**) axial T1-weighted MR images demonstrating a Bartholin's gland cyst (*white arrow*). T2-weighted images show a thin-walled high-signal-intensity structure lying below the pelvic diaphragm and symphysis pubis. The cyst is of high signal intensity on T1- and T2-weighted imaging indicating complex proteinaceous content

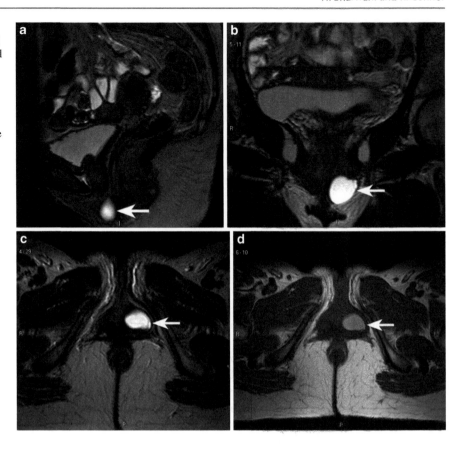

as a result of ductal occlusion and are usually asymptomatic and discovered incidentally. On imaging they typically appear as oval or round vulval masses that are hyperintense on T2-weighted imaging and of variable signal intensity on T1-weighted imaging depending on their contents (Hahn et al. 2004).

Acquired Vaginal Cysts

Vaginal Inclusion (Epidermal) Cyst

Vaginal epidermal or inclusion cysts result from the obstruction of a sebaceous gland due to mucosa trapped by surgical procedures such as episiotomy, colporrhaphy, or trauma including childbirth. They are the commonest acquired cystic lesions of the vagina and as they enlarge, symptoms may develop. They are generally found in the lower posterior or lateral vaginal wall. Imaging features are the same as simple cystic structures elsewhere with high T2-weighted and low T1-weighted signal intensity on MRI (Fig. 144.2).

Urethral Diverticulum

Urethral diverticula are a relatively common finding among women with chronic genitourinary conditions, such as recurrent infections, post-void dribbling, and dyspareunia. Due to their clinical presentation, location, and imaging findings, they are often an important differential for cystic lesions of the vulva and vagina. Urethral diverticula are outpouchings of tissue from the urethra into the urethrovaginal potential space (Fig. 144.3). Most are derived from dilated paraurethral ducts or glands and can extend inferiorly to present as a vulval "lump."

Urethral diverticula usually arise from the posterolateral wall in the mid-urethra at the level of the symphysis pubis. Larger diverticula can wrap around the urethra in a horseshoe configuration (Fig. 144.4). They are best visualized on MRI and return high signal intensity on T2-weighted sequences with variable signal intensity on T1-weighted

Fig. 144.2 Vaginal inclusion cyst. Sagittal (**a**) and axial (**b**) T2-weighted MR images demonstrating a large vaginal inclusion cyst (*white arrow*) extending over the full length of the vagina. Note is made of peri-urethral collagen (*white arrowheads*)

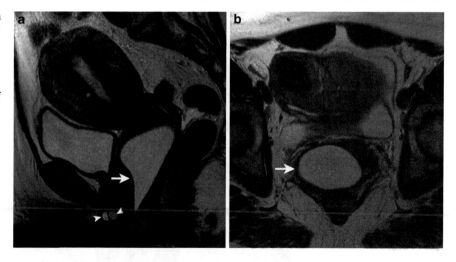

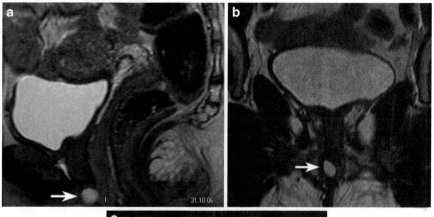

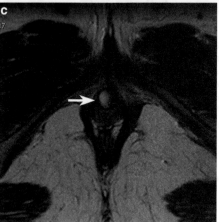

Fig. 144.3 Urethral diverticulum. Sagittal (**a**), coronal (**b**), and axial (**c**) T2-weighted images demonstrating a high T2-weighted signal intensity "cystic" perineal lesion in the periurethral region. This lesion was shown to be a urethral diverticulum; however, the imaging differential would include a Gartner's duct cyst or Skene's duct cyst

sequences depending on the contents (Hahn et al. 2004). The most important diagnostic feature is demonstration of a communication between the lesion and the urethra although this is often challenging. Differentiation from other perineal cystic lesions is important as surgical options differ and urethral diverticula require more complex surgery with urethral reconstruction.

Fig. 144.4 Horseshoe urethral diverticulum. Sagittal (**a**) and axial (**b**) T2-weighted images with corresponding sagittal (**c**) and axial (**d**) post-contrast T1-weighted fat-suppressed images demonstrating a large urethral diverticulum arising from the posterior urethral wall at the level of the symphysis pubis. The diverticulum (*white arrow*) extends into the urethrovaginal space and wraps around the urethra

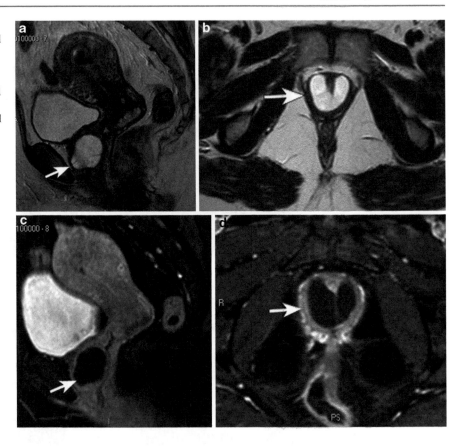

Fig. 144.5 Entero-vaginal fistula. Coronal (**a**) and sagittal (**b**) CT reconstructions demonstrating a fistulous tract (*white arrow*) between a loop of inflamed bowel (*white arrowheads*, **a**) and the upper vagina. Contrast material is seen to extend along the length of the vagina (Images courtesy of Dr E Sala, Addenbrooke's Hospital, Cambridge, UK)

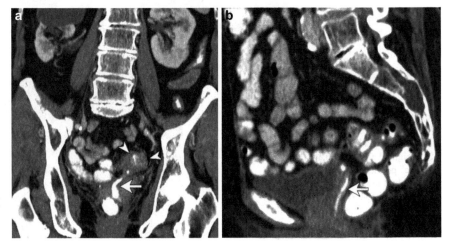

Vaginal/Vulval Fistula

Fistulas can form between the vagina and/or vulva and neighboring urethra, bladder, and bowel. The most common primary causes are surgical or obstetric trauma, radiation damage, and inflammatory bowel disease

(Fig. 144.5). The presence of a fistula is a clinical diagnosis, although imaging can demonstrate the tract and aid in surgical planning. Information regarding the presence of a fistulous tract has traditionally been obtained from vaginography, barium studies, or excretory urography. However, additional information regarding extraluminal

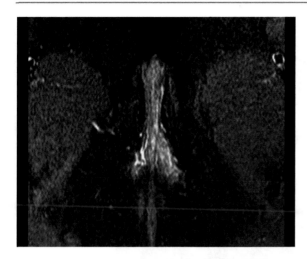

Video 144.1 Ano-vulval fistula in Crohn's disease. Stacked MR images demonstrating an ano-vulval fistula in a patient with Crohn's disease. Axial STIR sequences eloquently map the course of a left sided fistula with an internal opening in the 3 o'clock position and an external opening onto the left labia majora

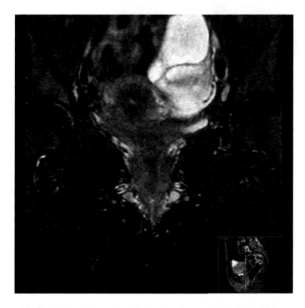

Video 144.2 Ano-vulval fistula in Crohn's disease. Stacked MR images demonstrating an ano-vulval fistula in a patient with Crohn's disease. Coronal STIR sequences eloquently map the course of a left sided fistula with an internal opening in the 3 o'clock position and an external opening onto the left labia majora

disease and the underlying pathology is best demonstrated with CT and MRI. MRI is often the first-line imaging modality due to the multi-planar imaging capabilities, ability to demonstrate the course and relationships of multiple fistulae and any associated complications (Narayanan et al. 2009). High resolution, heavily T2-weighted sequences are exquisitely sensitive to any fluid within a fistulous tract (see Videos 144.1 and 144.2). Delayed contrast medium enhanced T1-weighted fat-suppressed sequences help in the detection of those fistulae which do not contain fluid at the time of imaging and where active inflammatory change and granulation tissue lining the tract enhance aiding detection and characterization.

Crohn's disease is a chronic granulomatous inflammatory bowel disease that can affect any part of the gastrointestinal tract from mouth to anus. Gynecological involvement is common and can be difficult to diagnose, particularly when it precedes active bowel disease (Feller et al. 2001). Crohn's disease is seen to primarily or secondarily involve the vulva in 2% of patients (Fig. 144.6) (Vettraino and Merritt 1995) and entero-vaginal fistulas account for 9% of Crohn's fistulae. Cutaneous changes may occur before the onset of bowel symptoms and the area of involvement may extend to the perineal and perianal area. Localized or generalized labial edema, with erosions and multiple painful ulcers of variable severity, may be observed. Ulcers may be solitary, deep, and necrotic, possibly leading to formation of fistulae (Burgdorf 1981). Perianal and rectovaginal fistulae are common complications (Maconi et al. 2007).

Fistulae can also occur following trauma which most commonly occurs during prolonged childbirth. Diagnosis is usually clinical and imaging is rarely required in this situation. In some cases, MRI can be useful in delineation of suspected fistulae prior to further management.

Radiation Change

The vagina and vulva are often in the radiation field used for the treatment of pelvic malignancies. Acute changes (in the first 6 months) are usually transient and reversible and include mucosal and intramuscular edema manifest as high signal intensity on T2-weighted imaging (Grigsby et al. 1995). Mild chronic changes include mucosal atrophy where the vaginal wall returns low signal intensity on T2-weighted imaging and can be associated with narrowing and shortening of the vaginal canal. More severe late radiation changes include vaginal stenosis, ulceration, and necrosis which can

Fig. 144.6 Vulval fistula. Axial (**a**) and coronal (**b**) T1-weighted and axial STIR (**c**) MR images in a patient with Crohn's disease. MRI demonstrates a fistulous tract opening out onto the left side of the vulva (*arrows*). Note high signal intensity fluid within the tract on the STIR image

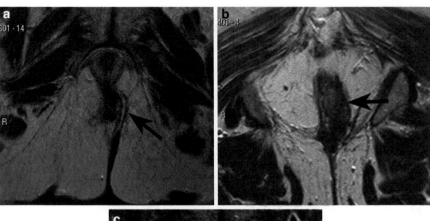

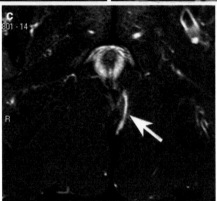

result in secondary fistula formation (Figs. 144.7 and 144.8). These late changes often occur at a very delayed stage after radiotherapy and are therefore unexpected. Imaging with PET/CT or MRI with diffusion-weighted and dynamic contrast-enhanced sequences can help to differentiate between recurrent tumor and radiation necrosis as the underlying cause for secondary fistula formation.

Endometriosis

Endometriosis is a condition in which endometrial tissue is found outside the uterus and most commonly involves the ovaries but can involve any pelvic organ (Chamie et al. 2011). In the vagina, endometriosis may develop at the site of a previous operation or as primary implants. Nodularity of the posterior vaginal fornix may represent endometriotic implants of the posterior cul-de-sac and may eventually erode or grow into the vaginal mucosa. Deposits can extend further inferiorly to involve the rectovaginal space which lies between the posterior wall of the vagina and anterior wall of the rectum

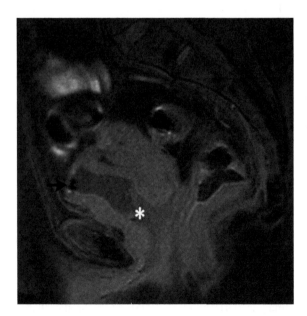

Fig. 144.7 Vesico-vaginal fistula. Sagittal post-contrast T1-weighted fat-suppressed MR image in a patient with recurrent cervical carcinoma previously treated with radiotherapy. A wide fistula tract (*) is seen between the upper vagina and posterior bladder wall. Note is made of gas in the thick-walled urinary bladder (*black arrow*)

Fig. 144.8 Rectovaginal fistula. Sagittal (**a**) and axial (**b**) T2-weighted MR images in a patient previously treated with radiotherapy for rectal carcinoma. A large fistula is seen between the posterior vaginal wall and anterior rectal wall (*black arrow*). Post-radiotherapy changes are also noted in the urinary bladder (*black arrowheads*, **a**) (Images courtesy of Dr E Sala, Addenbrooke's Hospital, Cambridge, UK)

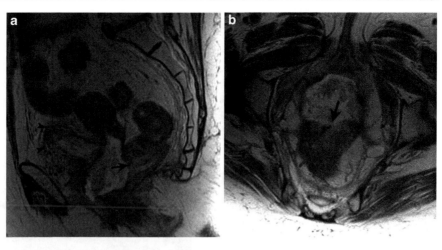

Fig. 144.9 Vaginal endometriotic deposit. Coronal T1-weighted (**a**) and coronal T1-weighted fat-suppressed (**b**) MR images demonstrating a high-signal-intensity mass involving the right superior vagina (*arrowheads*). Note the increase in conspicuity of these blood products on the fat-suppressed image (**b**) (Images courtesy of Dr S Babar, Imperial College Healthcare NHS Trust, London, UK)

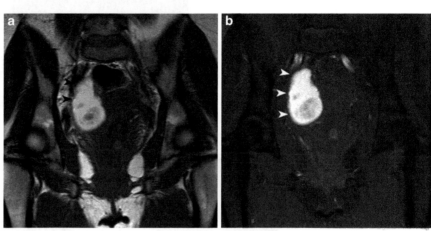

below the level of the peritoneal reflection. The inferior two thirds of this space, the rectovaginal septum, can be involved in deep pelvic endometriosis. When visualized colposcopically, implants generally appear dark blue or brown but can be white when associated with fibrosis. The diagnosis is usually made clinically and following biopsy. However, on imaging with MRI, vaginal deposits can be suspected in the presence of pelvic endometriosis elsewhere or diagnosed as a result of T1- and T2-weighted characteristics. Small, symptomatic lesions are treated by excision or laser vaporization. However, large lesions arising in the posterior cul-de-sac and extending into the posterior vaginal fornix may require laparotomy to accomplish excision.

On transvaginal ultrasound, vaginal endometriotic plaques are hypoechoic when compared to myometrium. MRI is increasingly being employed in complex cases to guide surgical management preoperatively and to delineate the presence and

anatomy of disease involving the vagina. With MRI, deposits characteristically return low signal intensity on T2-weighted imaging, intermediate signal intensity on T1-weighted imaging, and exhibit enhancement following contrast medium administration (Chamie et al. 2011). Acute hemorrhage can be easily identified on MRI as high T1-weighted signal intensity which can be made more conspicuous following fat suppression (Figs. 144.9 and 144.10). Associated fistulous tracks can be demonstrated by MRI where high signal intensity fluid is seen on STIR and T2-fat-saturated sequences.

Foreign Body

On occasion, foreign bodies can be seen in the vagina, (Fig. 144.11). These may be iatrogenic, e.g., vaginal pessary/retained surgical swabs, or non-iatrogenic,

Fig. 144.10 Vaginal endometriosis. Axial T2-weighted (**a**), T1-weighted (**b**), and fat-suppressed T1-weighted (**c**) images demonstrating an endometriotic deposit in the vagina (*white arrow*) which returns low T2-weighted signal intensity and high T1-weighted signal intensity in keeping with acute hemorrhage. A further deposit is noted in the urethra (*white arrowhead*)

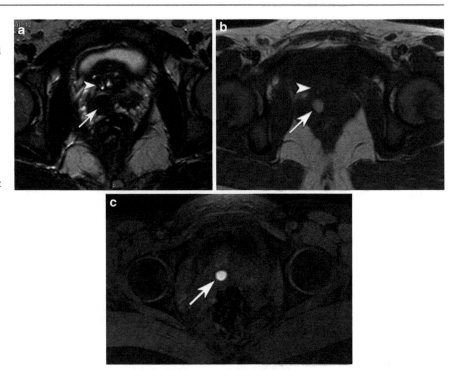

Fig. 144.11 Ring pessary. Sagittal T2-weighted (**a**) and sagittal T1-weighted fat-suppressed (**b**) MR images showing a vaginal ring pessary (*white arrowheads*)

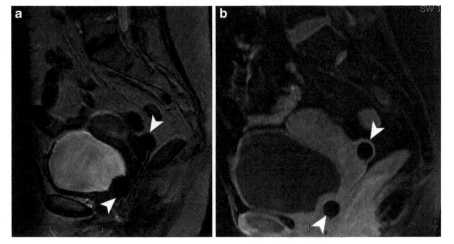

e.g., penetrating injury/intentional placement/abuse. Depending on the material inserted, the body may mount an inflammatory response resulting in an inflammatory mass or granuloma which may increase in size over time. The first-line imaging modality is a plain abdominal radiograph. CT and MRI can be employed for foreign bodies deep in the vagina or to evaluate complications such as perforation and abscess formation.

Benign Vulval and Vaginal Tumors

Neoplasms of the vulva and vagina are uncommon and the frequency of benign lesions ranges from rare to very rare. Most vaginal tumors produce no symptoms until a significant size is reached. Symptoms and signs may include a sensation of pressure, dyspareunia,

Fig. 144.12 Vulvo-vaginal leiomyoma. Sagittal T1-weighted (**a**), sagittal T1-weighted fat-suppressed (**b**), and axial T2-weighted (**c, d**) MR images in a 30-week pregnant female demonstrating a vaginal leiomyoma which is enlarging during pregnancy and demonstrates increasing internal T2-weighted signal intensity. The leiomyoma extends into the right labia majora from the lower right anterolateral vagina and displaces the urethra anteriorly and to the left (**c**, *white arrowhead*). Incidental note is made of an ovarian dermoid (**a, b** *black arrow*) which shows signal dropout on fat-suppressed image (**b**)

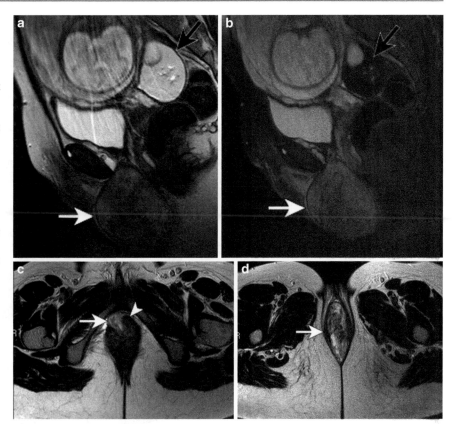

vaginal or urethral obstruction, or vaginal bleeding. However, most lesions will be detected during a routine exam in the asymptomatic patient. As is true for any neoplasm, biopsy provides a definitive diagnosis; however, etiology can be suggested on the basis of imaging findings.

Lipoma

As elsewhere involving cutaneous tissue, vulval lipomas can present as well-defined pedunculated masses, non-pedunculated vulvar swellings, or mimic ambiguous genitalia (Oh et al. 2009). They can occur at any age and have been reported in the newborn. Imaging reveals a mass with internal fat characteristics.

Leiomyoma

Leiomyomas are rarely seen in the vagina and vulva. When seen in the vagina they are usually located in the midline anterior wall although they can occur anywhere (Shimada et al. 2002). In the vulva, they are the most common benign solid tumor identified (Figs. 144.12 and 144.13). These lesions are benign smooth muscle neoplasms, usually solitary and in many cases asymptomatic.

Radiologically they resemble leiomyomata of other origins; on ultrasound they are seen as a well-defined hypoechoic masses. On MRI, they are typically of homogeneous low signal intensity on T1- and T2-weighted imaging similar to myometrium with homogeneous enhancement following contrast medium administration. As with leiomyomata elsewhere they can undergo degeneration resulting in varied signal characteristics (see Table 144.1): hyaline degeneration demonstrates low signal intensity on T2-weighted images; myxoid and cystic degeneration demonstrate high signal intensity on T2-weighted imaging and red degeneration demonstrate peripheral or diffuse high signal intensity on T1-weighted sequences and variable signal intensity on T2-weighted imaging with or without a low signal intensity rim (Murase et al. 1999; Allison 2007).

Fig. 144.13 Vaginal
leiomyoma. Sagittal
T2-weighted (**a**), axial
T2-weighted (**b**), and sagittal
post-contrast T1-weighted
fat-suppressed (**c**) images
demonstrating a large
enhancing leiomyoma arising
from the anterior vaginal wall
(*white arrows*) and displacing
the urethra anteriorly (*white
arrowhead*)

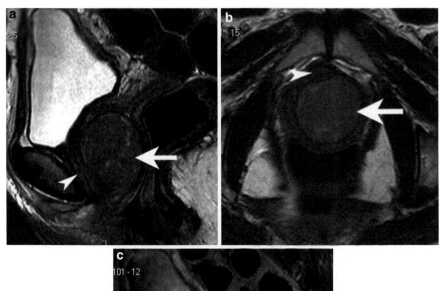

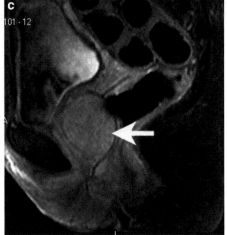

Table 144.1 Degenerating leiomyomata – typical signal intensity (SI) characteristics on MRI (Allison 2007; Murase et al. 1999)

Type of degeneration	T1-weighted sequences	T2-weighted sequences
Hemorrhagic	Diffusely increased SI	Diffuse low SI
Red/carneous	Early: increased SI; Late: high SI rim	Low SI rim with variable SI centrally
Cystic	Low SI in cystic spaces	High SI in cystic spaces
Hyaline	Variable, maybe high SI	Low SI
Calcific	Punctate signal voids	Punctate signal voids
Myxoid	Variable SI	High SI
Edema	Diffuse low SI	High SI

Fibroepithelial Polyp

Fibroepithelial polyps of the vagina are uncommon
and usually asymptomatic. They are usually small
and may be multiple. During pregnancy, these lesions
may become enlarged, very edematous, and bizarre in
appearance.

Lymphangioma

Lymphangiomas are benign tumors of the lymphatic
vessels. Vulvar lymphangiomas (lymphangioma
circumspectum) are rare (Fig. 144.14) and may be
congenital or acquired (Vlastos et al. 2003), and in such
cases they may represent a rare complication of radiation

Fig. 144.14 Vulval lymphangioma. Sagittal T2-weighted (**a**) and coronal T1-weighted (**b**) MR images in a 14-year-old female demonstrating a large vulval lymphangioma (*white arrow*)

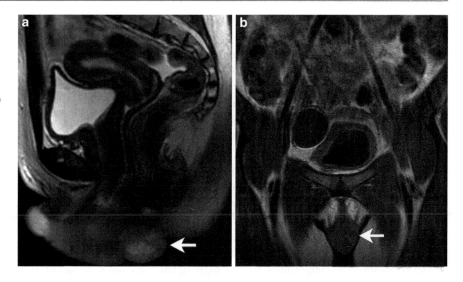

Fig. 144.15 Vulval hemangioma. Sagittal (**a**) and coronal (**b**) STIR images demonstrating a right vulval hemangioma. STIR images demonstrate serpiginous high-signal-intensity vessels extending into the right labia majora. T1-weighted images (not shown) showed intermediate signal intensity channels which enhanced avidly following intravenous contrast medium administration

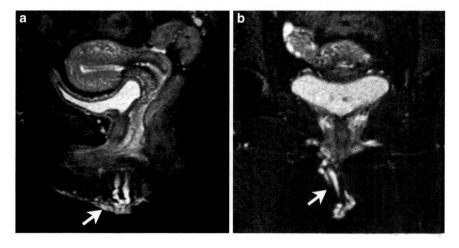

therapy (Tulasi et al. 2004). Congenital lymphangiomas are unusual tumors that readily cross and/or invade fascial planes and anatomical "compartments" (cf. cystic hygromas in the neck).

Ultrasound generally demonstrates a thin-walled, fluid-filled, multi-septated structure. The septae and walls are of variable thickness and contents range from being anechoic when simple fluid is present to demonstrating fluid-fluid levels in the presence of hemorrhage. On MR imaging, the cystic components of larger tumors are hyperintense on T2-weighted sequences with variable T1-weighted signal intensity according to the protein content of the fluid. Fluid-fluid levels may be seen if hemorrhage is present.

Cavernous Hemangioma

Cavernous hemangiomas are benign tumors of vascular endothelium that enlarge by active proliferation of endothelial cells due to unknown factors. They usually arise in infancy and can involve either the vagina or vulva. Vulvar hemangiomas often involve the labia majora, posterior commissure, and clitoris. Hemangiomas tend to grow until the age of 2 years before they either start to involute or simply stop growing (Siegelman et al. 1997). They can be seen as part of the Klippel-Trénaunay syndrome where patients can present with vaginal bleeding (Kanterman et al. 1996).

Hemangiomas are seen as complex masses on ultrasound with low resistance arterial flow on color Doppler evaluation. Phleboliths may cause posterior acoustic shadowing when present. On CT, hemangiomas demonstrate phlebolithic calcification and enhance avidly following contrast medium administration. MRI is the optimal imaging tool as it allows characterization and also delineation of the extent of the abnormality. Lesions return intermediate signal intensity on T1-weighted imaging with peripheral areas of high signal intensity due to intralesional fat. On T2-weghted imaging, they have a lobulated appearance due to vascular spaces containing stagnant blood and return high signal intensity. STIR often demonstrates the slow flow in the large vascular channels as serpiginous foci of high signal intensity (Fig. 144.15). Fluid-fluid levels may be present (Kanterman et al. 1996; Griffin et al. 2008). Following contrast medium enhancement, hemangiomas enhance avidly.

Conclusion

The diagnosis of benign conditions of the vagina and vulva is predominantly clinical as these areas are easily accessible for examination. However, imaging, particularly MRI, is playing a greater role in the evaluation of these lesions. It is particularly important in depicting anatomy and to aid surgical planning to minimize surgical resection and reduce iatrogenic effects on sexual function and pelvic floor dysfunction.

References

Allison SJ. Leiomyoma, degeneration. In: Hricak H, Akin O, Sala E, Ascher SM, Levine D, Reinhold C, editors. Diagnostic imaging: gynecology. Salt Lake City: Amirsys; 2007. pp. 110–114.

Burgdorf W. Cutaneous manifestations of Crohn's disease. J Am Acad Dermatol. 1981;5:689–95.

Chamie LP, Blasbalg R, Pereira RM, Warmbrand G, Serafini PC. Findings of pelvic endometriosis at transvaginal US, MR imaging, and laparoscopy. Radiographics. 2011;31: E77–100.

Feller ER, Ribaudo S, Jackson ND. Gynecologic aspects of Crohn's disease. Am Fam Physician. 2001;64:1725–8.

Griffin N, Grant LA, Sala E. Magnetic resonance imaging of vaginal and vulval pathology. Eur Radiol. 2008;18: 1269–80.

Grigsby PW, Russell A, Bruner D, Eifel P, Koh WJ, Spanos W, Stetz J, Stitt JA, Sullivan J. Late injury of cancer therapy on the female reproductive tract. Int J Radiat Oncol Biol Phys. 1995;31:1281–99.

Hahn WY, Israel GM, Lee VS. MRI of female urethral and periurethral disorders. AJR Am J Roentgenol. 2004;182:677–82.

Kanterman RY, Witt PD, Hsieh PS, Picus D. Klippel-Trenaunay syndrome: imaging findings and percutaneous intervention. AJR Am J Roentgenol. 1996;167:989–95.

Kier R. Nonovarian gynecologic cysts: MR imaging findings. AJR Am J Roentgenol. 1992;158:1265–9.

Kozawa E, Irisawa M, Heshiki A, Kimura F, Shimizu Y. MR findings of a giant Bartholin's duct cyst. Magn Reson Med Sci. 2008;7:101–3.

Lopez C, Balogun M, Ganesan R, Olliff JF. MRI of vaginal conditions. Clin Radiol. 2005;60:648–62.

Maconi G, Ardizzone S, Greco S, Radice E, Bezzio C, Bianchi PG. Transperineal ultrasound in the detection of perianal and rectovaginal fistulae in Crohn's disease. Am J Gastroenterol. 2007;102:2214–9.

Murase E, Siegelman ES, Outwater EK, Perez-Jaffe LA, Tureck RW. Uterine leiomyomas: histopathologic features, MR imaging findings, differential diagnosis, and treatment. Radiographics. 1999;19:1179–97.

Narayanan P, Nobbenhuis M, Reynolds KM, Sahdev A, Reznek RH, Rockall AG. Fistulas in malignant gynecologic disease: etiology, imaging, and management. Radiographics. 2009;29(4):1073–83.

Oh JT, Choi SH, Ahn SG, Kim MJ, Yang WI, Han SJ. Vulvar lipomas in children: an analysis of 7 cases. J Pediatr Surg. 2009;44:1920–3.

Shimada K, Ohashi I, Shibuya H, Tanabe F, Akashi T. MR imaging of an atypical vaginal leiomyoma. AJR Am J Roentgenol. 2002;178:752–4.

Siegelman ES, Outwater EK, Banner MP, Ramchandani P, Anderson TL, Schnall MD. High-resolution MR imaging of the vagina. Radiographics. 1997;17:1183–203.

Tulasi NR, John A, Chauhan I, Nagarajan V, Geetha G. Lymphangioma circumscriptum. Int J Gynecol Cancer. 2004;14:564–6.

Vettraino IM, Merritt DF. Crohn's disease of the vulva. Am J Dermatopathol. 1995;17:410–3.

Vlastos AT, Malpica A, Follen M. Lymphangioma circumscriptum of the vulva: a review of the literature. Obstet Gynecol. 2003;101:946–54.

Malignant Conditions of the Vulva

145

Hebert A. Vargas, T. Barrett, and Evis Sala

Introduction

The vulva is a triangular soft tissue structure within the perineum, bounded by the symphysis pubis anteriorly, the anal sphincter posteriorly, and the ischial tuberosities laterally. It is comprised of the mons pubis, labia majora, labia minora, clitoris, vestibular bulb, vestibular glands, and vestibule of the vagina. Cancer affecting the vulva accounts for approximately 3–5% of all female genital malignancies (Sankaranarayanan and Ferlay 2006; Siegel et al. 2011). In this chapter, we discuss the clinical features and different imaging modalities used to define the extent of primary or recurrent disease in patients with vulvar cancer. Imaging techniques include sentinel node imaging for lymph node assessment, MRI mainly for local staging, CT or PET-CT for the assessment of distant disease, and ultrasound, which is often utilized for image-guided biopsy procedures.

Etiology and Pathology

One of the main risk factors for vulval carcinoma is older age, with the peak incidence occurring in the 65–75 year age group, although the number of younger women with invasive disease is increasing, possibly due to an increase in the prevalence of human papillomavirus (HPV) infection (Saraiya et al. 2008). Squamous cell carcinoma (SCC) accounts for >85% of cases. Verrucous carcinoma is a variant of SCC with a better prognosis; it is well differentiated, slow growing, and does not metastasize. The remaining histological subtypes include melanoma (approximately 5%) and rarer entities such as Bartholin gland carcinoma, basal cell carcinoma, sarcoma, and endodermal sinus tumor (Flanagan et al. 1997; Parker et al. 2000; Ulutin et al. 2003).

Clinical Features, Diagnosis, and Staging

Clinical presentation is typically with vulvar pain, pruritus, or bleeding. Imaging plays no role in initial diagnosis, as the lesions are usually readily visible and accessible to biopsy. Despite this, there is often a delay in diagnosis due to failure to seek medical attention or initial medical treatment for symptom control (e.g., topical estrogens or corticosteroids) (Jones and Joura 1999). Vulvar carcinoma primarily spreads via the lymphatic system. The primary lymph drainage is to the superficial then deep femoral and inguinal nodes and subsequently the pelvic nodes. Lateralized lesions generally drain to the ipsilateral groin. Isolated pelvic node involvement without ipsilateral inguinal node involvement is rare (Stehman and Look 2006). Lesions that are close to the midline can drain to either side. Lymphatic drainage pathways from the clitoris directly to the pelvis have been described; however, it is unusual for clitoral lesions to involve the pelvic nodes unless the inguinal nodes are involved

H.A. Vargas (✉)
Radiology Department, Memorial Sloan-Kettering Cancer Center, New York, NY, USA

T. Barrett
Department of Radiology, School of Clinical Medicine, Addenbrooke's Hospital and University of Cambridge, Cambridge, UK

E. Sala
Memorial Sloan-Kettering Cancer Center, New York, NY, USA

B. Hamm, P. R. Ros (eds.), *Abdominal Imaging*, DOI 10.1007/978-3-642-13327-5_201,
© Springer-Verlag Berlin Heidelberg 2013

Table 145.1 FIGO and TNM and group staging of primary vulvar cancer (Pecorelli 2009)

TNM	Stage	Vulva
Tis	0	The cancer is not growing into the underlying tissues. This stage, also known as *carcinoma in situ*, is not included in the FIGO system
T1	I	Tumor confined to the vulva or perineum
T1a	IA	$\leq$2 cm in size with stromal invasion $\leq$1 mm
T1b	IB	$\leq$2 cm in size with stromal invasion >1 mm
T2	II	Tumor >2 cm in size confined to the vulva or perineum
T3	III	Tumor of any size, with adjacent spread (lower one-third urethra, lower one-third vagina, anus)
T4	IVA	Tumor invades other regional structures (upper two-third urethra, upper two-third vagina), bladder mucosa, rectal mucosa, or fixed to pelvic bone
N1a	IIIA	Tumor has spread to one or two lymph nodes, each <5 mm in size. *T stage T1 or T2*
N1b	IIIA	Tumor has spread to one lymph node $\geq$5 mm. *T stage T1 or T2*
N2a	IIIB	Tumor has spread to three or more lymph nodes, each <5 mm. *T stage T1 or T2*
N2b	IIIB	The tumor has spread to two or more lymph nodes with each area of spread 5 mm or greater. *T stage T1 or T2*
N2c	IIIC	Positive node of any size with extracapsular spread
N3	IVA	Fixed or ulcerated inguinofemoral lymph nodes
M1	IVB	Spread to any distant site, including pelvic lymph nodes

(Eriksson et al. 1984). Lymph node involvement is the single most important prognostic factor (Hacker et al. 1983; Homesley 1994) and is directly related to size of the primary lesion and the depth of stromal invasion. The lymphatic supply to the vulva is rich, thus nodal metastases occur at an early stage. The FIGO staging system takes these factors into account (Table 145.1) (Pecorelli 2009), although it should be noted vulvar melanoma follows the melanoma staging system. Hematogenous spread and spread by direct extension of the primary tumor to adjacent structures may also be seen, although this occurs infrequently, especially in early stage disease.

Management of Primary Vulvar Carcinoma

Patients with biopsy-proven vulvar carcinoma are initially staged clinically on the basis of history and physical examination. However, physical examination is only accurate in approximately 25% of patients for

the detection of metastatic inguinofemoral nodes (Homesley et al. 1993).

The mainstay of treatment for vulvar carcinoma is radical surgery. The introduction in the first half of the twentieth century of radical vulvectomy with en bloc bilateral inguinofemoral and pelvic lymphadenectomy (Basset-Way operation) resulted in an increase in overall survival from 20% to over 60%. Despite the improvement in outcomes, the operation was associated with significant comorbidities such as wound infection and disruptions, lymphocoele formation, and lymphedema. More recently, radical vulvectomy has been replaced with wide local excision of the vulvar lesion to achieve a 1-cm gross margin, which is considered sufficient to address the primary lesion. Standard practice across many centers is to perform an ipsilateral groin node dissection through a separate incision. Bilateral dissection is performed if there is a midline lesion or if the ipsilateral nodes are positive. Adequate operation on the vulva results in 85–90% local control of disease, even among patients with positive lymph nodes.

Vulvar Carcinoma Recurrence

Recurrent vulvar cancer affects approximately one-third of patients, and 80% of recurrence occur in the first 2 years following primary treatment (Crosbie et al. 2009). The predominant site of recurrence is on the vulva, even when radical operations are performed (Podratz et al. 1982). The risk of local recurrence increases as a function of depth of invasion and primary lesion size. Recurrences at the local site are three times as common as recurrences in the groin, pelvis, or distant sites, and many are amenable for re-excision (Stehman and Look 2006). Excision of groin nodal recurrences may be of some benefit if the femoral vessels are not involved. Distant recurrences are rare, representing approximately 5% of all recurrences, and are associated with a dismal prognosis.

Role of Imaging and Impact on Patient Management

The main role of imaging in primary and recurrent vulvar carcinoma is to define the extent of disease, mainly to detect the presence of metastatic lymph nodes thus guiding the need for and extent

Fig. 145.1 MRI of stage 3b vulvar cancer. Axial T2-weighted (**a**), axial diffusion-weighted using b values of 0 and 1,000 s/mm^2 (**b**), and sagittal T2-weighted images (**c**) show a vulval tumor (*black arrow*) which appears as intermediate signal intensity on T2 images and of high signal intensity on DW images (restricted diffusion). The tumor involves the anterior perineum, extends into the perianal fat (*white arrows* in **a** and **b**), and invades the urethra and lower third of the vagina (*white arrows* in **c**)

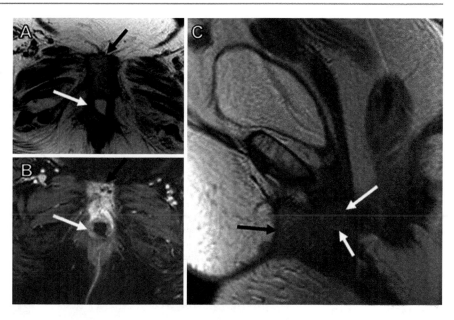

of lymphadenectomy. The imaging appearances of primary and recurrent disease are similar. Imaging also plays a role in evaluating the features of the primary lesion (e.g., depth of tumor involvement) and assessing for locally advanced disease (defined as cases where radical surgical excision of the vulva would be insufficient to remove the cancer with adequate surgical margins) and involvement of adjacent anatomical structures such as the urethra, bladder, rectum, or anal sphincter, which if present, requires more aggressive intervention such as pelvic exenteration combined with chemo- and radiation therapy.

MRI

Vulval tumors are typically isointense to muscle on T1-weighted images and show intermediate-to-high signal intensity on T2-weighted imaging (Sohaib et al. 2002); Fig. 145.1. As the perineal region is rich in fat, tumors are generally easier to recognize using fat-suppressed T2-weighted images; however, small primary tumors may not be readily detected on MRI. Occasionally, it may also be challenging to discriminate whether tumors originate from the right or left labia on MRI. Contrast-enhanced MR sequences serve to aid detection of primary lesions and have been shown to increase staging accuracy from 75% to 85% (Kataoka et al. 2010). Tumors may also demonstrate restricted diffusion on diffusion-weighted

MRI; Fig. 145.1. Vulvar melanoma may demonstrate increased signal intensity on T1-weighted images. The most commonly used MRI criterion for lymph node metastases is the short-axis diameter of a node. However, the reported sensitivity of this approach is low (around 40–50%) (Sohaib et al. 2002). Other parameters may prove more helpful. For example, a short/long axis ratio >75% resulted in the highest accuracy for prediction of lymph node metastases (Kataoka et al. 2010). MRI, like CT, is unable to detect micrometastatic lymph node involvement. However, the aim of imaging in patients eligible for the sentinel node procedure is to exclude gross nodal involvement and not to detect very small metastases. MR lymphography using iron-particle contrast agents may be a promising tool in this scenario, as it has been shown to increase sensitivity for detecting nodal metastases in other gynecological malignancies (Rockall et al. 2005); however, such trials are lacking for vulvar cancer.

Sentinel Node Imaging

The sentinel lymph node (SLN) is defined as the first node or group of nodes that drain the primary tumor. If the sentinel node contains metastases, then a complete dissection is undertaken. SNL imaging is indicated for diagnostic purposes in clinically low stage vulvar cancer, i.e., patients with clinically negative inguinal nodes and tumor size <4 cm (Levenback et al. 2009).

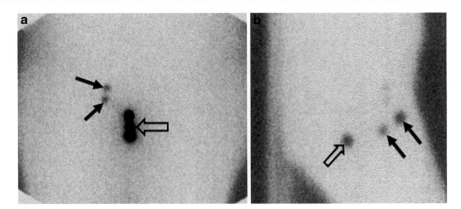

Fig. 145.2 Sentinel node lymphoscintigraphy in a patient with ulcerated vulval melanoma. Gamma camera images acquired anteriorly (**a**) and in the right lateral position (**b**) after four intradermal injections of 0.055 mCi-filtered 99mTechnetium-

sulfur colloid around the primary vulval lesion demonstrate uptake at the injection sites in the right vulva (*open arrows*) and within two draining lymph nodes in the right inguinal region (*arrows*)

Fig. 145.3 SPECT-CT lymphoscintigraphy in a patient with squamous cell carcinoma of the vulva. (**a**) Axial CT following intravenous contrast demonstrates an enhancing lesion of the vulva (*arrow*). Fused SPECT-CT in the axial (**b**) and coronal planes (**c**) performed immediately after intradermal injection of 99mTechnetium-sulfur colloid around the lesion. Tracer uptake is seen at the injection site (*open arrow* in **c**) and within a right inguinal sentinel node (*arrow* in **b** and **c**). Subsequent sentinel node histology was negative

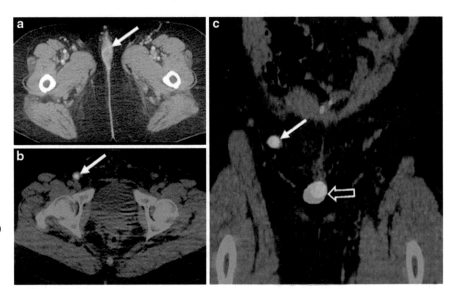

SNL detection can by either dye based or scintigraphy based (^{99m}Tc-colloidal sulfur). Although 2-D planar scintigraphy with multiple views has been traditionally employed (Fig. 145.2), 3-D single-photon emission computed tomography (SPECT) with or without CT or MRI is being increasingly utilized. The fusion of SPECT with CT or MRI offers advantages over planar SPECT imaging alone, providing more accurate information regarding the number and anatomical localization of nodes (Fig. 145.3). A recent study showed that in 27% of patients where planar imaging showed a single focus of uptake, fused imaging showed further grouped individual nodes or additional separate localizations (Beneder et al. 2008).

Ultrasound

Ultrasound is useful to evaluate for nodal involvement, especially in cases where large inguinofemoral metastases obstruct lymphatic flow, which thereby bypasses the sentinel node (de Hullu et al. 2004). Typical ultrasound features are similar to metastatic nodes in other anatomical regions, namely, increase in size (e.g., larger than 5 mm in short-axis diameter), rounded shape, irregular contour, and loss of normal internal configuration (i.e., loss of the fatty hilum). Some authors suggest that patients with enlarged and/or suspicious inguinofemoral lymph nodes should

Fig. 145.4 CT of Stage 1b squamous cell carcinoma of the vulva. (**a**) Axial CT shows an enhancing soft tissue mass of the vulva (*arrow*). (**b**) Fused axial FDG PET-CT at the same level demonstrates avid tracer uptake within the primary lesion (*arrow*); SUVmax = 14.2. (**c**) Coronal PET image confirms uptake within the primary lesion (*arrow*), but with no evidence of spread to the local lymph nodes or distal metastases; physiological uptake is noted within the bowel, liver, and bladder

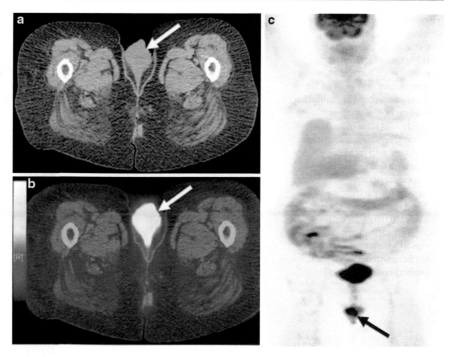

Fig. 145.5 CT showing recurrent squamous cell carcinoma of the vulva. Axial (**a**) and coronal (**b**) CT images show an irregular enlarged left inguinofemoral lymph node (*arrows*); ultrasound-guided biopsy confirmed disease recurrence. The patient had previously been treated with a left radical hemi-vulvectomy; clips are seen bilaterally within the inguinal regions, from prior lymph node dissection

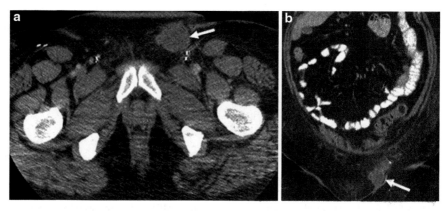

undergo fine needle aspiration cytology (FNAC) and be excluded from sentinel node biopsy when FNAC shows metastatic disease (Oonk et al. 2010). A major advantage of ultrasound is that it is a cheap, widely available, and simple technique that is well tolerated; however, it is very operator dependant.

Computed Tomography

The main advantage of CT over ultrasound is that it can provide additional information on deep pelvic nodes and distant metastases. CT also benefits from faster acquisition times which limit artifact from respiratory motion and bowel peristalsis compared to other modalities. The primary tumor may be visualized as an area of soft tissue density in the vulva (Fig. 145.4). Detection of nodal involvement relies heavily on size (Fig. 145.5). It has been reported that the sensitivity and specificity of CT for the detection of nodal metastases (58% and 75%, respectively) is lower than for ultrasound-guided FNAC performed on the largest or most abnormal looking lymph node in each groin (80% and 100%, respectively) (Land et al. 2006).

Fig. 145.6 FDG PET-CT of recurrent squamous cell carcinoma of the vulva. (a) Maximum intensity projection PET image shows tracer uptake at the site of the primary tumor and at multiple vertebral bodies, the right scapula, and right gluteal muscle group. The findings are consistent with local recurrence and distal metastases; hydronephrosis accounts for the increased activity seen in the right kidney. (b) Coronal PET-CT image concurrently acquired helps to localize tracer uptake, seen here within two of the vertebral bodies (*arrows*)

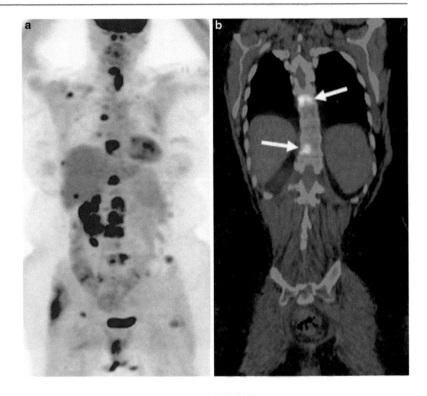

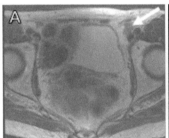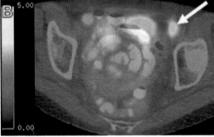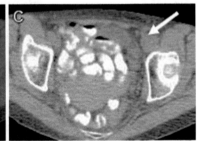

Fig. 145.7 MRI and PET-CT of recurrent squamous cell carcinoma of the vulva. Axial T2-weighted MRI (**a**), axial fused PET-CT (**b**), and axial unenhanced CT (**c**) images. MRI and CT show an irregular lymph node (*arrows* in **a** and **c**), which demonstrates high tracer uptake on PET-CT (**b**). Metastatic disease was subsequently confirmed at biopsy

Positron Emission Tomography

Positron emission tomography (PET) is performed using several radiotracers such as ^{18}F-Fluorodeoxyglucose (FDG), and when combined with CT can be used to provide both functional and anatomical information (Fig. 145.4). Its main advantages are a large (whole-body) field of view, which is particular useful for identifying distant metastases (Fig. 145.6). Both the primary tumor and metastatic sites demonstrate increased radiotracer uptake. A recent review on PET in gynecological cancer found a sensitivity of 67–75% and a specificity of 62–95% for detection of inguinofemoral lymph node metastases but only two studies have involved PET in patients with vulvar cancer (Grigsby 2009); Fig. 145.7. Some of the limitations of PET/CT include radiotracer uptake within reactive non-metastatic lymph nodes, and uptake within the urinary tract or leakage of urine in the perineum masking or mimicking metastases.

Conclusion

Vulvar cancer is diagnosed clinically, and treatment is usually surgical. Imaging plays a critical role as the extent of surgery and need for adjuvant or neoadjuvant therapy is adjusted according to the extent of disease on imaging (e.g., wide local excision of tumor versus pelvic exenteration).

Pearls to Remember

- Vulvar cancer accounts for approximately 3–5% of all female genital malignancies. Risk factors include older age and human papillomavirus infection, and the majority of cases (>85%) are squamous cell carcinomas.
- Lymph node involvement is the single most important prognostic factor and is directly related to size of the primary lesion and the depth of stromal invasion.
- Primary lymph drainage is to the superficial then deep femoral and inguinal nodes and subsequently the pelvic nodes.
- Imaging modalities are used to define the extent of primary or recurrent disease in patients with vulvar cancer.
- Treatment is surgical. Identification of locally advanced disease is critical as it affects the extent of surgery (e.g., need for pelvic exenteration) and adjuvant or neoadjuvant therapy.
- Sentinel node imaging can be dye based or scintigraphy based and is indicated for diagnostic purposes in clinically low stage vulvar cancer (clinically negative inguinal nodes and tumor size <4 cm).
- Ultrasound-guided fine needle aspiration or core biopsy can help prove nodal metastatic disease or recurrence.
- Fat-saturated T2-weighted MR imaging and contrast-enhanced sequences are used for assessment of local invasion.
- CT has traditionally been used to assess more distal disease, while PET-CT shows promise for improving sensitivity for detecting nodal disease.

References

Beneder C, Fuechsel FG, Krause T, Kuhn A, Mueller MD. The role of 3D fusion imaging in sentinel lymphadenectomy for vulvar cancer. Gynecol Oncol. 2008;109(1):76–80.

Crosbie EJ, Slade RJ, Ahmed AS. The management of vulval cancer. Cancer Treat Rev. 2009;35(7):533–9.

de Hullu JA, Oonk MH, Ansink AC, Hollema H, Jager PL, van der Zee AG. Pitfalls in the sentinel lymph node procedure in vulvar cancer. Gynecol Oncol. 2004;94(1):10–5.

Eriksson E, Eldh J, Peterson LE. Surgical treatment of carcinoma of the clitoris. Gynecol Oncol. 1984;17(3):291–5.

Flanagan CW, Parker JR, Mannel RS, Min KW, Kida M. Primary endodermal sinus tumor of the vulva: a case report and review of the literature. Gynecol Oncol. 1997;66(3):515–8.

Grigsby PW. Role of PET in gynecologic malignancy. Curr Opin Oncol. 2009;21(5):420–4.

Hacker NF, Berek JS, Lagasse LD, Leuchter RS, Moore JG. Management of regional lymph nodes and their prognostic influence in vulvar cancer. Obstet Gynecol. 1983;61(4):408–12.

Homesley HD. Lymph node findings and outcome in squamous cell carcinoma of the vulva. Cancer. 1994;74(9):2399–402.

Homesley HD, Bundy BN, Sedlis A, et al. Prognostic factors for groin node metastasis in squamous cell carcinoma of the vulva (a Gynecologic Oncology Group study). Gynecol Oncol. 1993;49(3):279–83.

Jones RW, Joura EA. Analyzing prior clinical events at presentation in 102 women with vulvar carcinoma. Evidence of diagnostic delays. J Reprod Med. 1999;44(9):766–8.

Kataoka MY, Sala E, Baldwin P, et al. The accuracy of magnetic resonance imaging in staging of vulvar cancer: a retrospective multi-centre study. Gynecol Oncol. 2010;117(1):82–7.

Land R, Herod J, Moskovic E, et al. Routine computerized tomography scanning, groin ultrasound with or without fine needle aspiration cytology in the surgical management of primary squamous cell carcinoma of the vulva. Int J Gynecol Cancer. 2006;16(1):312–7.

Levenback CF, van der Zee AG, Rob L, et al. Sentinel lymph node biopsy in patients with gynecologic cancers expert panel statement from the International Sentinel Node Society Meeting, February 21, 2008. Gynecol Oncol. 2009;114(2):151–6.

Oonk MH, de Hullu JA, van der Zee AG. Current controversies in the management of patients with early-stage vulvar cancer. Curr Opin Oncol. 2010;22(5):481–6.

Parker LP, Parker JR, Bodurka-Bevers D, et al. Paget's disease of the vulva: pathology, pattern of involvement, and prognosis. Gynecol Oncol. 2000;77(1):183–9.

Pecorelli S. Revised FIGO staging for carcinoma of the vulva, cervix, and endometrium. Int J Gynaecol Obstet. 2009;105(2):103–4.

Podratz KC, Symmonds RE, Taylor WF. Carcinoma of the vulva: analysis of treatment failures. Am J Obstet Gynecol. 1982;143(3):340–51.

Rockall AG, Sohaib SA, Harisinghani MG, et al. Diagnostic performance of nanoparticle-enhanced magnetic resonance imaging in the diagnosis of lymph node metastases in patients with endometrial and cervical cancer. J Clin Oncol. 2005;23(12):2813–21.

Sankaranarayanan R, Ferlay J. Worldwide burden of gynaecological cancer: the size of the problem. Baillieres Best Pract Res Clin Obstet Gynaecol. 2006;20(2):207–25.

Saraiya M, Watson M, Wu X, et al. Incidence of in situ and invasive vulvar cancer in the US, 1998–2003. Cancer. 2008;113(10 Suppl):2865–72.

Siegel R, Ward E, Brawley O, Jemal A. Cancer statistics, 2011. CA: A Cancer J. Clin.. 2011;61(4):212–36.

Sohaib SA, Richards PS, Ind T, et al. MR imaging of carcinoma of the vulva. AJR Am J Roentgenol. 2002;178(2):373–7.

Stehman FB, Look KY. Carcinoma of the vulva. Obstet Gynecol. 2006;107(3):719–33.

Ulutin HC, Zellars RC, Frassica D. Soft tissue sarcoma of the vulva: a clinical study. Int J Gynecol Cancer. 2003;13(4):528–31.

Non-squamous Malignant Disease of the Vagina

146

E. J. O'Donovan, P. Narayanan, and S. A. Sohaib

Introduction

This chapter reviews the clinical and imaging features of other malignant diseases involving the vagina but excluding primary vaginal squamous cell carcinoma (see ▶ Chap. 147). These other malignancies are a very heterogeneous group and very rare apart from secondary malignancy affecting the vagina. The data and descriptions of these other primary malignancies are limited to case reports or small case series. The diagnosis and staging of these other primary tumors are similar to primary squamous cell vaginal cancer. The diagnosis is made at examination under anesthesia (EUA) and biopsy of the macroscopic lesion. These tumors are staged using the clinical FIGO staging system. However, the treatment, prognosis, and imaging are dependent on the underlying histology of the primary.

Adenocarcinoma

Primary vaginal adenocarcinomas are the second most common primary cancer of the vagina after squamous cell cancer. They represent between 5% and 15% of primary vaginal cancers (Sulak et al. 1988; Nasu et al. 2010). The infrequency of these lesions may be secondary to the relatively small number of glandular structures in the normal vagina. The cause for primary vaginal adenocarcinoma is unknown but it is thought to arise from areas of vaginal adenosis but may also arise in foci of endometriosis, Wolffian rest remnants, and periurethral glands.

Various histologic subtypes of vaginal adenocarcinoma are recognized including clear cell, endometrioid, mucinous, and serous type. *Clear cell adenocarcinoma* is characterized by cells with clear cytoplasm. This tumor occurs in young women whose mothers took diethylstilbestrol (DES) during pregnancy. Diethylstilbestrol (DES) is a synthetic estrogen that was used during the 1950s–1970s in the treatment of threatened miscarriage. In utero exposure to DES increases the risk of clear cell carcinoma by 40-fold (Hatch et al. 1998). Since the use of DES was discontinued nearly 40 years ago the occurrence of DES-related vaginal adenocarcinoma has become even rarer. Women with DES-related clear cell adenocarcinoma typically present in their teens and 20s (Sulak et al. 1988).

DES unrelated clear cell carcinomas occur in middle-aged and elderly women like the other rare subtypes of adenocarcinoma (Sulak et al. 1988). *Endometrioid adenocarcinomas* arise on a background of vaginal endometriosis and most cases are located at the vaginal apex (Staats et al. 2007; Nomoto et al. 2010). *Mucinous adenocarcinomas* are characterized by mucin-producing cells (Saitoh et al. 2005; Nasu et al. 2010).

Adenocarcinoma of the vagina tends to occur on the anterior wall of the proximal/upper third of the vagina which corresponds to the most frequent site of adenosis. The tumor can appear macroscopically as a plaque-like, polypoid, papillary, or ulcerated lesion. Sometimes the areas of visible tumor appear discrete but microscopic examination usually reveals its continuity in the submucosa. Like squamous cell vaginal cancer, most patients present with vaginal bleeding or discharge and less commonly with urinary symptoms.

E.J. O'Donovan • P. Narayanan • S.A. Sohaib (✉)
Department of Diagnostic Imaging, Royal Marsden Hospital, London, UK

B. Hamm, P. R. Ros (eds.), *Abdominal Imaging*, DOI 10.1007/978-3-642-13327-5_200,
© Springer-Verlag Berlin Heidelberg 2013

Therapy for adenocarcinoma is similar to that of primary squamous vaginal cancer. The treatment choices tend to be influenced by the extent of the disease and institutional preferences. Early stage disease may be treated by radical hysterectomy, vaginectomy, and lymphadenectomy. Radiotherapy is effective for early disease but is usually reserved for more advanced disease. The results of these therapies do not appear to be as successful when compared with the management of squamous cell carcinoma of the vagina (Nasu et al. 2010).

Imaging of Primary Vaginal Adenocarcinoma

The role of imaging in adenocarcinoma is similar to that of squamous cell vaginal cancer (see ▶ Chap. 147). It is important to exclude other potential primary sites of disease before accepting the diagnosis of primary vaginal adenocarcinoma. There is very little data on the imaging appearance of primary vaginal adenocarcinoma. MR imaging with its excellent soft tissue contrast is the most useful imaging technique at visualizing the primary lesion (Parikh et al. 2008). The tumor is not readily seen on CT unless it is bulky.

The appearance of primary vaginal adenocarcinoma at MR imaging can be as a localized lobulated high signal intensity mass or as diffuse circumferential mural thickening of the vaginal wall (Fig. 146.1) (Parikh et al. 2008). It may appear as homogenously hyperintense on T2-weighted imaging and isointense to muscle on T1-weighted imaging. The high T2 signal intensity is secondary to mucin and this enables better demonstration of the low signal intensity vaginal wall which can therefore show invasion into the paravaginal tissues. The high signal intensity on T2-weighted images also helps distinguish adenocarcinoma from squamous cell carcinoma which is more intermediate signal on T2-weighted imaging. The enhancement is found to be variable following administration of intravenous Gadolinium contrast medium.

Mesenchymal Tumor/Sarcoma

Primary vaginal sarcoma comprises approximately 2–3% of all malignant primary vaginal neoplasia (Ciaravino et al. 2000). The commonest type

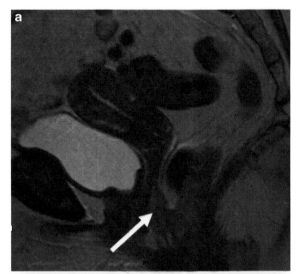
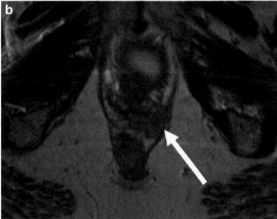

Fig. 146.1 Vaginal adenocarcinoma in a 67-year-old woman. (a) Sagittal and (b) high-resolution axial T2-weighted images show an intermediate signal intensity vaginal mass (*arrow*) which extends through the vagina and abuts the left levator muscle

of vaginal sarcoma is leiomyosarcoma followed by rhabdomyosarcoma with other types being extremely rare.

Vaginal Leiomyosarcoma

The most common vaginal soft tissue sarcoma is leiomyosarcoma which accounts for less than 2% of all vaginal cancers (Umeadi et al. 2008). Leiomyosarcoma of the vagina arises from smooth muscle cells. The etiology of vaginal leiomyosarcoma is unknown although it may occur after genital tract radiotherapy (Yang et al. 2009). It is postulated that it

Fig. 146.2 Vaginal leiomyosarcoma in a 68-year-old lady who presented with the feeling of a vaginal mass. (**a**) Sagittal, (**b**) axial, and (**c**) coronal T2-weighted images show a large heterogeneous signal intensity mass which has replaced the vagina. The mass contains focal areas of high and low signal intensity and abuts but does not invade the left pelvic side wall (*arrow*). On the (**d**) axial T1-weighted image the tumor is of relatively homogenous signal intensity

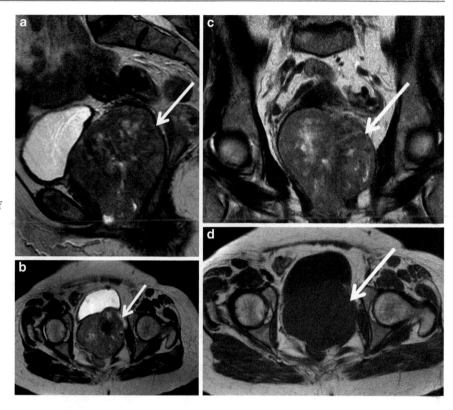

may also represent the malignant transformation of a vaginal leiomyoma (Miyakawa et al. 1985). Macroscopically they appear as a bulky submucosal locally infiltrating mass ranging from 3 to 10 cm. They are most commonly thought to arise from the rectovaginal septum or the posterior vaginal wall, mainly involving the upper vagina, but may occur anywhere (Yang et al. 2009). Microscopically vaginal leiomyosarcomas are identical to those found elsewhere in the body.

The age of presentation is wider than that of adenocarcinoma or melanoma of the vagina occurring between the ages of 25 and 86 years with an average age of presentation of 47 years (Ciaravino et al. 2000). Most patients present incidentally at vaginal examination, either for nonspecific symptoms or during routine gynecological examination. However, they can present with pain, vaginal discharge, bleeding, or difficulty in micturition. Primary vaginal leiomyosarcoma is aggressive with early hematogenous spread (Ciaravino et al. 2000). Local extension into the cervix, parametria and lymph nodes are common.

There is no consensus guideline on its management although radical surgical removal is generally recommended as the treatment of choice. If diagnosed early surgical excision may produce cure. Otherwise extensive surgery including vaginectomy may be performed with or without adjuvant chemo/radiotherapy (Umeadi et al. 2008). These sarcomas are not particularly radiosensitive although postoperative radiotherapy has been used in the management of soft tissue sarcomas to reduce local regional recurrence (Ciaravino et al. 2000). The prognosis is poor as the tumor has often disseminated by the time of presentation and recurrent disease is common (Yang et al. 2009). The 5-year survival rate is reported as being approximately 36% (Ciaravino et al. 2000).

On imaging, these tumors tend to appear as a bulky mixed solid and cystic mass arising out of the pelvis centered on the vagina (Fig. 146.2). They may show homogenous low signal intensity on T1- and heterogeneous high signal intensity on T2-weighted imaging due to pockets of necrosis (Parikh et al. 2008). The presence of acute hemorrhage results in pockets of high signal intensity on T1-weighting. On STIR sequences they are reported as having very high signal intensity, similar to the appearance of skeletal metastases from uterine leiomyosarcoma (Parikh et al. 2008). Enhancement characteristics are reported as

Fig. 146.3 A 10-year-old girl with recurrent vaginal rhabdomyosarcoma. (**a**) Sagittal and (**b**) axial T2-weighted images show a vaginal mass (*arrow*) at the introitus which is of intermediate to high signal intensity. (**c**) High-resolution axial T2-weighted image shows anterior extension (*arrow*) of the lesion to invade the urethra. The lesion (*arrow*) is of high signal on the (**d**) coronal STIR sequence image

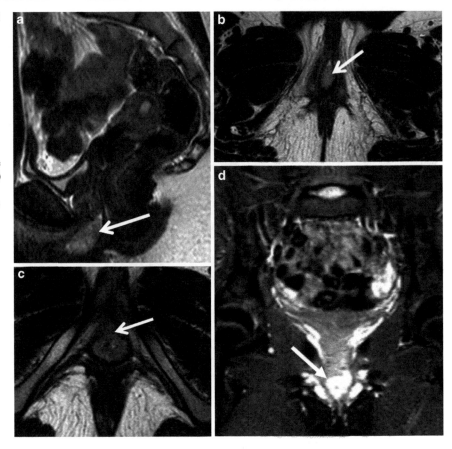

heterogeneous following the administration of intravenous gadolinium (Shadbolt et al. 2001; Yang et al. 2009). In comparison, vaginal leiomyomas appear as a well-circumscribed homogenous hypointense mass on T1- and T2-weighted images with homogenous enhancement following gadolinium (Shadbolt et al. 2001; Yang et al. 2009).

Vaginal Rhabdomyosarcoma

Rhabdomyosarcoma of the lower genital tract tends to occur in childhood and has a peak incidence in the second decade with patients aging from 13 to 30 (Ghaemmaghami et al. 2008). Lower genital tract rhabdomyosarcoma generally presents with a vulval, vaginal, or perineal mass, with or without vaginal bleeding. As skeletal muscle is not normally found in the genital tract, rhabdomyosarcomas are thought to arise in primitive mesenchymal tissue capable of forming rhabdomyoblasts. The intergroup

rhabdomyosarcoma study group (IRSG) recognizes embryonal, alveolar, and undifferentiated types of rhabdomyosarcoma. The imaging characteristics of rhabdomyosarcoma are nonspecific with low signal intensity on T1- and high signal on T2-weighted imaging (Fig. 146.3) (Allen et al. 2007). Sometimes a pseudocapsule is seen which can be low signal on both sequences. If there is heterogeneity in the lesion this may be secondary to necrosis and hemorrhage. Administration of intravenous gadolinium may result in heterogeneous enhancement.

Sarcoma botryoid is a subtype of embryonal rhabdomyosarcoma which develops in girls up to the age of 6 years. This sarcoma often presents with soft nodules that protrude from the vagina like a bunch of grapes or polypoid mass, and some may present with vaginal bleeding (Ghaemmaghami et al. 2008). This subtype has a more favorable outcome when compared with the alveolar and the rarest undifferentiated types. These tumors show areas of bright T2 signal within the lesions, intermixed with areas of lower T2 signal tissue, and show considerable enhancement. These imaging findings are reflective of the histologic architecture of these lesions, which are composed of separate myxoid and subepithelial cellular zones (Kobi et al. 2009).

Other Sarcomas

Other rare malignant primary sarcomatous tumors which have been described in the vagina include angiosarcoma which is sometimes found arising as a complication of radiation therapy (Takeuchi et al. 2005), alveolar soft part sarcoma, endometrioid stromal sarcoma, carcinosarcoma, and Ewing's sarcoma/PNET. Malignant mixed mesodermal tumor is a very rare tumor with an appearance similar to that of the mixed mesodermal tumor of the uterine corpus. Spindle cell synovial sarcoma is a rare aggressive soft tissue tumor arising from mesenchymal or epithelial cells. These lesions are usually well-defined masses resulting in the displacement of adjacent structures. On MR imaging they are very high signal intensity masses with focal areas of low signal on the T2-weighted images. On T1-weighted images they are of heterogeneous intermediate signal intensity. The MR imaging features correspond with the of synovial sarcomas of the extremities (Parikh et al. 2008).

Vaginal Melanoma

Primary vaginal melanomas are a rare, non-cutaneous form of melanoma. They account for less than 0.5–2% of melanomas in women and less than 3% of all vaginal malignancies, vulval melanomas being more common (Fan et al. 2001; Baloglu et al. 2009). Most appear in white postmenopausal women older than 60 years of age (Baloglu et al. 2009). The most common symptom is vaginal bleeding due to superficial ulceration of the mass, vaginal discharge or less frequently with symptoms of pelvic pain and a vaginal mass.

Malignant melanoma is mostly located in the inferior one third of the vagina (Fan et al. 2001; Baloglu et al. 2009) and has a predilection for the anterior and lateral walls. Macroscopically they are a brown/black, mucosal or submucosal nodular, pedunculated papillary or lobulated mass. Although they are usually pigmented, the amelanotic type, devoid of pigment,

accounts for 5% of vaginal melanomas. Primary vaginal melanomas may also contain both pigmented and nonpigmented areas (Fan et al. 2001). Necrosis and ulceration are often seen which may mimic squamous cell carcinoma. Microscopically the tumors usually comprise of sheets of cells which vary in morphological appearance. Occasionally tumor cells may infiltrate the submucosa.

Treatment for vaginal malignant melanomas includes surgery, radiotherapy, chemotherapy, and immunotherapy. Radiotherapy can be applied adjuvantly after surgery or for those tumors that cannot be removed surgically. The prognosis is worse than that of cutaneous melanomas with the 5-year survival rate ranging from 5% to 25% (Baloglu et al. 2009). Tumor size has been defined as the most important prognostic factor determining survival (Baloglu et al. 2009).

The role of imaging in vaginal melanoma is to supplement the clinical evaluation of the primary and to define the distant disease spread. In terms of the primary lesion, melanomas have a distinct appearance on MR imaging. Melanin results in shortening T1 and T2 relaxation times due to its paramagnetic effects. This combined with the paramagnetic effects of methemoglobin from intratumoral necrosis or hemorrhage results in melanoma characteristically having high signal intensity on T1- and low signal intensity on T2-weighted images. The MR imaging features of vaginal melanomas vary according to the melanin concentration and presence of hemorrhage. For this reason some primary vaginal melanomas appear as typical high signal intensity lesions on T1- and low signal intensity on T2-weighted images or as intermediate to high signal intensity on T1- and intermediate to high signal intensity on T2-weighted images (Fig. 146.4) (Moon et al. 1993; Fan et al. 2001; Kim et al. 2003). The signal intensity of most tumors on T2-weighted imaging is higher than that of the adjacent muscles. Amelanotic melanomas appear as low signal intensity on T1- and intermediate to high signal intensity on T2-weighted images. The absence of high signal intensity on T1-weighted imaging should, therefore, not preclude the diagnosis of malignant melanoma (Chang et al. 1988; Kim et al. 2003). Melanomas are much more clearly demonstrated on fat-suppressed images with brighter signal as the dynamic range becomes narrower allowing the detection of subtle differences (Fan et al. 2001).

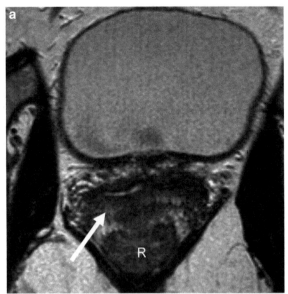

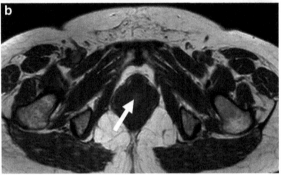

Fig. 146.4 Vaginal melanoma in a 78-year-old woman who presented with postmenopausal bleeding. (**a**) High-resolution axial T2-weighted images show the tumor involving the posterior vaginal wall with infiltration into the rectovaginal septum (*arrows*, *R* = rectum). On the (**b**) T1-weighted images there is a high signal intensity area (*arrow*) within the mass which suggests the presence of melanin

Nodal staging for cutaneous melanoma when there is no clinical evidence of regional nodal metastasis is usually assessed by sentinel lymph node biopsy, which is typically performed following intraoperative lymphatic mapping. Vaginal melanoma can be managed in a similar fashion and lymphoscintigraphy may be of value in such cases (Kim et al. 2006; Dhar et al. 2007). If there is clinical suspicion of regional adenopathy, ultrasound of the groin with fine-needle aspiration (FNA) or biopsy can be performed (Sohaib and Moskovic 2003).

In evaluating distant disease, one needs to appreciate that the spread in melanoma disease is highly unpredictable (Patnana et al. 2011). Cutaneous melanomas can metastasize to almost any organ and as vaginal melanoma originates from melanocytes of the vaginal mucosa, which are not different from those which give rise to cutaneous melanoma, metastatic spread is likely to be similar. CT is currently the most widely used technique for tumor staging, surveillance, and assessment of therapeutic response (Patnana et al. 2011). In cutaneous melanoma, metastases are predominantly FDG-avid, and therefore, combined FDG-PET CT is likely to provide most accurate evaluation of the extent of disease (Swetter et al. 2002; Oudoux et al. 2004; Strobel et al. 2007).

Vaginal Lymphoma

Lymphoma involving the vagina may be seen in up to 40% of autopsies on women with disseminated lymphoma (McNicholas et al. 1994). However, primary pelvic lymphoma accounts for approximately 1.5% of primary extranodal lymphoma (Trenhaile and Killackey 2001). In a review of 9,500 cases of female lymphoma, only four cases of primary vaginal lymphoma were identified (Chorlton et al. 1974). Primary vaginal lymphomas are diffuse large B-cell type and tend to occur in younger women. High-stage non-Hodgkin's lymphoma involving the vagina are also usually diffuse large B-cell type and tend to affect postmenopausal women (Vang et al. 2000).

The most common presenting features of pelvic/vaginal lymphoma are abnormal vaginal bleeding, pelvic pain, and pelvic masses. These tumors can mimic squamous cell carcinoma of the cervix both clinically and histologically; so it is vital to consider lymphoma in the diagnosis. This is especially important as the treatment for the two conditions is very different, surgery being unnecessary in lymphoma (Perren et al. 1992). Other misdiagnoses may include sarcoma, poorly differentiated carcinoma, and chronic inflammation (Trenhaile and Killackey 2001). The treatment for lymphoma usually involves chemotherapy with or without radiation. As with all lymphomas, the stage of disease is the single most important factor in determining outcome and management. The Ann Arbor system for staging extranodal lymphomas is generally felt to be more useful than the FIGO system as FIGO does not take into account the status of regional lymph nodes, but use of FIGO in parallel can give useful information on tumor bulk.

Once a diagnosis of vaginal/pelvic lymphoma has been made, the role of imaging is related to the management of the lymphoma. The imaging features on ultrasound of vaginal lymphoma are described as a well-defined, bulky mass of medium to low echogenicity (McNicholas et al. 1994). On CT the lesions have been described as having a lobulated often bulky contour with a CT density similar to that of muscle (McNicholas et al. 1994). On MR imaging the mass is usually of low signal intensity on T1- and is usually intermediate to high signal intensity on T2-weighted imaging. Heterogeneous signal on T2-weighted images is usually the result of necrosis. Vaginal lymphoma usually demonstrates homogenous contrast enhancement. With successful treatment the disease becomes less cellular and more fibrotic which results in decreasing T2 signal intensity (McNicholas et al. 1994). To our knowledge there are no specific reports on the appearance of vaginal lymphoma on FDG-PET. FDG-PET is now routinely used in the staging of lymphoma with active disease being FDG-avid.

Other Primary Vaginal Malignancies

There are other histological types of primary vaginal carcinomas such as small cell cancers (Kaminski et al. 2003), and germ cell tumor (e.g., yolk sac tumor). These are extremely rare with little in terms of imaging description.

Vaginal Metastases

Secondary malignancies of the vagina are far more common than primary tumors and account for greater than 80% of all vaginal tumors (Merino 1991). After the ovary, the vagina is the commonest site in the female genital tract for metastatic deposits (Mazur et al. 1984; Chagpar and Kanthan 2001). The vast majority of vaginal metastases occur secondary to direct extension from adjacent tumor into the vagina. The tumors most commonly resulting in this contiguous spread are cervical, endometrial, vulval, bladder, ovarian, and rectal carcinomas. Much more rarely metastases in the vagina may be from extragenital

tumors such as colonic adenocarcinoma, renal carcinoma, breast and melanoma, with rarer case reports of pancreas, thyroid, and small bowel (Mazur et al. 1984). These vaginal metastases may occur as a consequences of hematogenous spread.

Secondary involvement from squamous cell cancer is from cervical cancer in the majority followed by vulval cancer (Parikh et al. 2008). Adenocarcinoma vaginal metastases in the anterior wall and upper third arise from the upper genital tract, while lesions in the posterior wall and the lower third arise from the gastrointestinal tract (Parikh et al. 2008). Approximately 80% of vaginal metastases occur within the first 3 years after the primary tumor and two thirds occur after surgical removal of the primary lesion.

The management of secondary malignancy to the vagina is dependent on the underlying primary tumor and amount of metastatic disease. Imaging is performed to define the extent of local and distant disease. In general, both the primary and metastatic tumors demonstrate similar imaging characteristics on CT, MRI, and PET imaging. On MR imaging, secondary malignant involvement is usually low to intermediate signal intensity on T1- and high to intermediate signal intensity on T2-weighted imaging. On PET imaging, if the primary tumor is FDG-avid, then the metastatic lesions are also likely to be FDG-avid and well seen on FDG-PET CT.

Metastases from Gynecological Malignancy

Cervical cancer commonly involves the vagina, due to the position of the cervix. The proximal two thirds of the vagina is most commonly involved and occasionally the distal third may be involved in very advanced cases. Spread to the vagina is by direct contiguous spread. Skip lesions into the distal vagina may be seen in recurrent cervical cancer (Parikh et al. 2008). The signal intensity of cervical metastatic vaginal disease is typically intermediate to high on T2- and low on T1-weighted MR images. As most cervical cancers are FDG-avid, metastases in the vagina are FDG-avid on FDG-PET/CT.

In *uterine cancer*, vaginal involvement is uncommon and tends to occur in locally advanced disease. Spread of the disease is either by contiguous direct extension or from tumor seeding from the uterus into the vagina. Hence the whole vagina should be

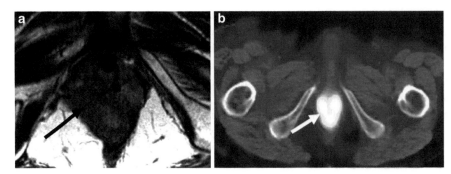

Fig. 146.5 Endometrial cancer recurrence in the vagina in a 65-year-old woman. (**a**) Axial T2-weighted images show a large intermediate signal intensity vaginal mass (*arrow*) which is invading the rectum posteriorly. On (**b**) FDG-PET-CT the mass (*arrow*) is markedly FDG-avid but there are no other sites of metastatic disease

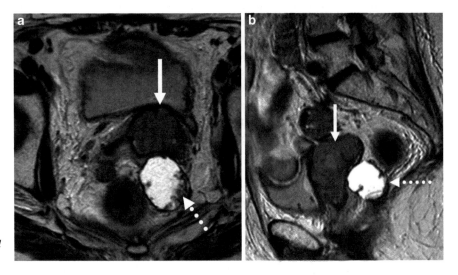

Fig. 146.6 Vaginal metastases from ovarian cancer in a 70-year-old woman. (**a**) High-resolution axial T2-weighted and (**b**) sagittal T2-weighted images show the vaginal metastasis (*arrow*) as a large mass of intermediate signal intensity expanding the vaginal vault. Note also a predominantly cystic peritoneal deposit posterior to the vagina (*dotted arrow*)

examined when staging uterine cancer on imaging. Rarely, spread into the peritoneal cavity may occur in endometrial cancer and involve the peritoneal reflection on the vaginal fornix, but this is more commonly seen in ovarian cancer. Most metastases are endometrial adenocarcinomas and appear as ill-defined heterogeneous signal intensity masses on T2-weighted MR images invading through the low T2 signal of the vaginal wall, and are low signal intensity on T1-weighted MR images (Fig. 146.5) (Parikh et al. 2008). In recurrent endometrial cancer, the vagina, in particular the vault, is one of the most common sites of disease (Sohaib et al. 2007). Vaginal metastases from uterine leiomyosarcomas and carcinosarcomas have similar appearances to that of primary tumor from which they have spread (Cantisani et al. 2003).

Ovarian cancer undergoes peritoneal spread and involves the vagina when disease invades it from the peritoneal cavity (Fig. 146.6). The pouch of Douglas is the most dependent part of the peritoneum, and tumor deposits at this site may extend into the vaginal vault. This occurs in primary and recurrent ovarian cancer. Involvement is seen on sagittal images either on reformatted CT or better still on T2-weighted MR images.

In patients who have undergone hysterectomy as part of their treatment for their gynecological malignancy, it is not possible on imaging to distinguish between a new vaginal primary carcinoma or a vaginal metastasis from the original cancer for which the patient had the hysterectomy, for example, cervical cancer. In such cases careful review of clinical history and pathology is required.

Metastases from Non-gynecological Malignancies

Rectum and bladder cancer may involve the vagina in locally advanced disease or if there is local relapse following treatment. The imaging appearance reflects that of the local tumor. True metastases, that is, hematogenous from extragenital cancers are very rare and most commonly occur from adenocarcinoma of the colon and breast (Chagpar and Kanthan 2001). In *colonic cancer*, vaginal metastases when present are usually found in the face of grossly disseminated metastatic disease, which carries with it a very poor prognosis. The presentation may be of an abnormal vaginal discharge and a friable mass in the anterior vagina (Chagpar and Kanthan 2001). *Breast cancer* may metastasize to any organ and to the female reproductive system. The ovaries are the most common site but cases of vaginal metastases have also been reported (Pineda and Sall 1978). *Renal cell carcinoma* may metastasize to the vagina and rarely is the presenting feature with vaginal bleeding (Tarraza et al. 1998; Queiroz et al. 1999). Vaginal metastases occur more frequently from left-sided renal cancer (Tarraza et al. 1998).

Summary

Apart from secondary malignancy to the vagina, non-squamous cell malignancy of the vagina is very rare. Hence, there is limited information on the natural history, optimal treatment, and imaging characteristics. However, the principles of imaging are similar to primary squamous cell cancer of the vagina. The local extent and definition of the disease is best assessed by MR imaging due to its exceptional soft tissue contrast resolution. This aids in diagnosis, staging, and treatment of the lesion related to the vaginal disease. CT or PET-CT is of value in the assessment of distant or recurrent disease.

References

Allen SD, Moskovic EC, et al. Adult rhabdomyosarcoma: cross-sectional imaging findings including histopathologic correlation. AJR Am J Roentgenol. 2007;189(2):371–7.

Baloglu A, Bezircioglu I, et al. Primary malignant melanoma of the vagina. Arch Gynecol Obstet. 2009;280(5):819–22.

Cantisani V, Mortele KJ, et al. Vaginal metastasis from uterine leiomyosarcoma. Magnetic resonance imaging features with pathological correlation. J Comput Assist Tomogr. 2003;27(5):805–9.

Chagpar A, Kanthan SC. Vaginal metastasis of colon cancer. Am Surg. 2001;67(2):171–2.

Chang YC, Hricak H, et al. Vagina: evaluation with MR imaging. Part II. Neoplasms. Radiology. 1988;169(1):175–9.

Chorlton I, Karnei Jr RF, et al. Primary malignant reticuloendothelial disease involving the vagina, cervix, and corpus uteri. Obstet Gynecol. 1974;44(5):735–48.

Ciaravino G, Kapp DS, et al. Primary leiomyosarcoma of the vagina. A case report and literature review. Int J Gynecol Cancer. 2000;10(4):340–7.

Dhar KK, Das N, et al. Utility of sentinel node biopsy in vulvar and vaginal melanoma: report of two cases and review of the literature. Int J Gynecol Cancer. 2007;17(3):720–3.

Fan SF, Gu WZ, et al. Case report: MR findings of malignant melanoma of the vagina. Br J Radiol. 2001;74(881):445–7.

Ghaemmaghami F, Karimi Zarchi M, et al. Lower genital tract rhabdomyosarcoma: case series and literature review. Arch Gynecol Obstet. 2008;278(1):65–9.

Hatch EE, Palmer JR, et al. Cancer risk in women exposed to diethylstilbestrol in utero. JAMA. 1998;280(7):630–4.

Kaminski JM, Anderson PR, et al. Primary small cell carcinoma of the vagina. Gynecol Oncol. 2003;88(3):451–5.

Kim H, Jung SE, et al. Case report: magnetic resonance imaging of vaginal malignant melanoma. J Comput Assist Tomogr. 2003;27(3):357–60.

Kim W, Menda Y, et al. Use of lymphoscintigraphy with SPECT/CT for sentinel node localization in a case of vaginal melanoma. Clin Nucl Med. 2006;31(4):201–2.

Kobi M, Khatri G, et al. Sarcoma botryoides: MRI findings in two patients. J Magn Reson Imaging. 2009;29(3):708–12.

Mazur MT, Hsueh S, et al. Metastases to the female genital tract. Analysis of 325 cases. Cancer. 1984;53(9):1978–84.

McNicholas MM, Fennelly JJ, et al. Imaging of primary vaginal lymphoma. Clin Radiol. 1994;49(2):130–2.

Merino MJ. Vaginal cancer: the role of infectious and environmental factors. Am J Obstet Gynecol. 1991;165(4 Pt 2):1255–62.

Miyakawa I, Yasuda H, et al. Leiomyosarcoma of the vagina. Int J Gynaecol Obstet. 1985;23(3):213–6.

Moon WK, Kim SH, et al. MR findings of malignant melanoma of the vagina. Clin Radiol. 1993;48(5):326–8.

Nasu K, Kai K, et al. Primary mucinous adenocarcinoma of the vagina. Eur J Gynaecol Oncol. 2010;31(6):679–81.

Nomoto K, Hori T, et al. Endometrioid adenocarcinoma of the vagina with a microglandular pattern arising from endometriosis after hysterectomy. Pathol Int. 2010;60(9):636–41.

Oudoux A, Rousseau T, et al. Interest of F-18 fluorodeoxyglucose positron emission tomography in the evaluation of vaginal malignant melanoma. Gynecol Oncol. 2004;95(3):765–8.

Parikh JH, Barton DP, et al. MR imaging features of vaginal malignancies. Radiographics. 2008;28(1):49–63. quiz 322.

Patnana M, Bronstein Y, et al. Multimethod imaging, staging, and spectrum of manifestations of metastatic melanoma. Clin Radiol. 2011;66(3):224–36.

Perren T, Farrant M, et al. Lymphomas of the cervix and upper vagina: a report of five cases and a review of the literature. Gynecol Oncol. 1992;44(1):87–95.

Pineda A, Sall S. Metastasis to the vagina from carcinoma of the breast. J Reprod Med. 1978;20(5):243–5.

Queiroz C, Bacchi CE, et al. Cytologic diagnosis of vaginal metastasis from renal cell carcinoma. A case report. Acta Cytol. 1999;43(6):1098–100.

Saitoh M, Hayasaka T, et al. Primary mucinous adenocarcinoma of the vagina: possibility of differentiating from metastatic adenocarcinomas. Pathol Int. 2005;55(6):372–5.

Shadbolt CL, Coakley FV, et al. MRI of vaginal leiomyomas. J Comput Assist Tomogr. 2001;25(3):355–7.

Sohaib SA, Moskovic EC. Imaging in vulval cancer. Best Pract Res Clin Obstet Gynaecol. 2003;17(4):543–56.

Sohaib SA, Houghton SL, et al. Recurrent endometrial cancer: patterns of recurrent disease and assessment of prognosis. Clin Radiol. 2007;62(1):28–34. discussion 35–6.

Staats PN, Clement PB, et al. Primary endometrioid adenocarcinoma of the vagina: a clinicopathologic study of 18 cases. Am J Surg Pathol. 2007;31(10):1490–501.

Strobel K, Dummer R, et al. High-risk melanoma: accuracy of FDG PET/CT with added CT morphologic information for detection of metastases. Radiology. 2007;244(2):566–74.

Sulak P, Barnhill D, et al. Nonsquamous cancer of the vagina. Gynecol Oncol. 1988;29(3):309–20.

Swetter SM, Carroll LA, et al. Positron emission tomography is superior to computed tomography for metastatic detection in melanoma patients. Ann Surg Oncol. 2002;9(7):646–53.

Takeuchi K, Deguchi M, et al. A case of postirradiation vaginal angiosarcoma treated with recombinant interleukin-2 therapy. Int J Gynecol Cancer. 2005;15(6):1163–5.

Tarraza Jr HM, Meltzer SE, et al. Vaginal metastases from renal cell carcinoma: report of four cases and review of the literature. Eur J Gynaecol Oncol. 1998;19(1):14–8.

Trenhaile TR, Killackey MA. Primary pelvic non-Hodgkin's lymphoma. Obstet Gynecol. 2001;97(5 Pt 1):717–20.

Umeadi UP, Ahmed AS, et al. Vaginal leiomyosarcoma. J Obstet Gynaecol. 2008;28(5):553–4.

Vang R, Medeiros LJ, et al. Non-Hodgkin's lymphoma involving the vagina: a clinicopathologic analysis of 14 patients. Am J Surg Pathol. 2000;24(5):719–25.

Yang DM, Kim HC, et al. Leiomyosarcoma of the vagina: MR findings. Clin Imaging. 2009;33(6):482–4.

Squamous Cell Carcinoma of the Vagina

147

P. Narayanan and S. A. Sohaib

Introduction

Malignant involvement of the vagina occurs most commonly from metastatic spread and the most common sites of metastatic disease are from direct local invasion from the female urogenital tract. Primary vaginal carcinoma should only be diagnosed if other gynecological malignancies have been excluded. Primary vaginal carcinomas are defined as arising solely from the vagina with no involvement of the external cervical os superiorly or the vulva inferiorly (Beller et al. 2006). The importance of this definition lies in the different clinical approaches in the treatment of cervical and vulval carcinoma.

Primary carcinomas of the vagina are very uncommon tumors comprising approximately 1–3% of all gynecologic malignancies (Creasman 2005). They rank fifth in frequency among the gynecologic cancers behind carcinoma of the ovary, uterus, cervix, and vulva. The commonest primary malignant tumor arising in the vagina is squamous cell carcinoma comprising approximately 85% of all malignant primary vaginal neoplasms. The histological distinction between squamous cell carcinoma and non-squamous malignancy of the vagina (see ► Chap. 146) is very important because the two groups represent very distinct diseases, each with differing pathogenesis, natural history, management, and imaging. This chapter reviews the clinical and imaging features of primary squamous cell cancer of the vagina.

P. Narayanan • S.A. Sohaib (✉)
Department of Diagnostic Imaging, Royal Marsden Hospital, London, UK

Aetiology and Pathology

The underlying aetiology of vaginal cancer is most commonly related to infection with the human papillomavirus (HPV) as well as some other sexually transmitted infections. HPV is present in the majority of vaginal tumors, and in a recent survey, about 60% of invasive and 80–90% of in situ vaginal squamous cell carcinomas contain HPV DNA (Daling et al. 2002). Presence of HPV16 antibodies increases risk for invasive tumors by up to 6 times and by 13 times for in situ tumors (Carter et al. 2001; Daling et al. 2002). Genital warts (associated with HPV infection) are also associated with an increased risk for in situ vaginal cancer by almost sixfold, but the association with invasive tumors is less clear (Daling et al. 2002; Madsen et al. 2008). Presence of antibodies to the herpes simplex virus type 2 is associated with an increased risk of vulval and vaginal cancer and precancer (Hildesheim et al. 1997; Daling et al. 2002). There is also an increased risk for vaginal cancer and precancer in HIV-positive women (Chaturvedi et al. 2009).

Other aetiological factors for primary squamous cell cancer include chronic irritation from procidentia, pessary, or frequent vaginal douching (Schraub et al. 1992). Unlike some other gynecological malignancy, vaginal squamous cell cancer is not related to reproductive factors or exogenous hormones.

Vaginal intraepithelial neoplasia (VAIN) is classified in a similar manner to cervical intraepithelial neoplasia (CIN), relating to grade and loss of stratification and nuclear atypia. VAIN 1 or mild dysplasia is categorized as a low grade squamous intraepithelial lesion while VAIN 2 and 3 are termed as high grade squamous intraepithelial neoplasia (Duong and Flowers 2007).

B. Hamm, P. R. Ros (eds.), *Abdominal Imaging*, DOI 10.1007/978-3-642-13327-5_199,
© Springer-Verlag Berlin Heidelberg 2013

Fig. 147.1 FIGO stage II
squamous cell carcinoma in
a 71-year-old woman with
postmenopausal bleeding.
(**a**) Sagittal and (**b**) axial
T2-weighted images show
a vaginal mass which has
breached the posterior vaginal
wall and extends to the sub-
vaginal tissues (*white arrows*).
On the left, the anterior and
posterior vaginal walls are
closely opposed and intact and
retain their low T2W signal
intensity appearance
(*dashed arrow*)

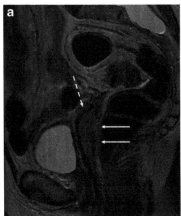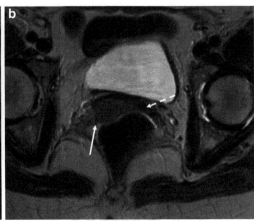

VAIN may precede the development of vaginal carcinoma and is predominantly found in patients over
the age of 60. Risk factors for the development of
VAIN include HPV infection, previous pelvic irradiation, immunosuppression, and a previous hysterectomy for cervical cancer (Duong and Flowers 2007).
VAIN is seen in the upper vagina near the vaginal cuff
and often with concomitant vulval or cervical lesions.
Progression rates of treated VAIN of 2–5% have
been reported, although these rates vary according
to the treatment used (Sillman et al. 1997; Dodge
et al. 2001). While a PAP smear can detect VAIN,
the rarity of the disease would make screening for
vaginal cancer an inefficient use of resources, even
in patients with previous cervical neoplasia (Cooper
et al. 2006).

Primary vaginal squamous cell carcinoma has
a predilection for involvement of the posterior wall
of the upper third of the vagina (Fig. 147.1). Squamous cell vaginal cancer initially tends to spread
superficially within the vaginal wall and later invades
the paravaginal tissues. It tends to spread early, by
direct invasion of the bladder/urethra anteriorly and
rectum posteriorly. The disease metastasizes primarily by lymphatic and hematogenous routes. Lymphatic drainage and, hence, nodal involvement is
dependent on the anatomic location of the primary
cancer. Generally, the upper two thirds of the vagina
drain into deep pelvic nodes. The lower third drains
into femoral and inguinal nodes. Hematogenous
spread is unusual and occurs late and the most common sites of distant spread include the lungs, liver,
and bony skeleton.

Clinical Features

Primary vaginal squamous cell carcinoma occurs predominantly in postmenopausal women in the 6th and
7th decades of life. Presentation is usually with vaginal
bleeding (65–80%), discharge (30%), urinary symptoms (20%), pelvic pain (15–30%), or a feeling of
a mass in the vagina (10%) (Dixit et al. 1993). Up to
30% of patients may be asymptomatic and may be
diagnosed during routine examination or smear.
Advanced disease may produce urinary symptoms
such as urinary retention or hematuria when the
tumor is anteriorly located, while posterior tumors
can present with rectal symptoms such as tenesmus
and constipation.

Diagnosis and Staging

The diagnosis of invasive disease is made at examination under anesthesia (EUA) and biopsy of the macroscopic lesion. The EUA should include careful
inspection of the whole vagina, cervix, a combined
vaginal and rectal examination to detect extra vaginal
spread, and cystoscopy. The biopsy should be full-
thickness biopsy for accurate histological diagnosis.
This clinical assessment also forms the staging of
vaginal cancer. Vaginal carcinoma, as with all gynecological malignancies, is staged according to the
International Federation of Gynecology and Obstetrics
(FIGO) staging system (see Table 147.1 and 147.2)
(Oncology 2009). The correlation of FIGO and TNM

Table 147.1 FIGO classification of vaginal cancer (Oncology 2009)

FIGO stage	Description	TNM category
0	Carcinoma in situ	Tis
I	Tumor confined to the vagina	T1
II	Tumor invades paravaginal tissues but not the pelvic side wall	T2
III	Tumor extension to the pelvic side wall	T3
IVa	Tumor extends beyond the true pelvis and invades the bladder, urethra, or rectum	T4
IVb	Distant metastases	M1

Table 147.2 TNM staging of vaginal cancer (Sobin et al. 2009)

Primary tumor	
TX	Primary tumor cannot be assessed
T0	No evidence of primary tumor
Tis 0	Carcinoma in situ
T1/I	Tumor confined to vagina
T2/II	Tumor invades paravaginal tissues but not to pelvic wall
T3/III	Tumor extends to pelvic wall
T4/IVA	Tumor invades mucosa of the bladder or rectum and/or extends beyond the true pelvis
Regional lymph nodes (N)	
NX	Regional lymph nodes cannot be assessed
N0	No regional lymph node metastasis
N1/IVB	Pelvic or inguinal lymph node metastasis
Distant metastasis (M)	
M0	No distant metastasis
M1/IVB	Distant metastasis

Table 147.3 Correlation of FIGO and TNM staging

FIGO			
	T	N	M
0	Tis	N0	M0
1	T1	N0	M0
2	T2	N0	M0
3	T1	N1	M0
	T2	N1	M0
	T3	N0	M0
	T3	N1	M0
4a	T4	Any N	M0
4b	Any T	Any N	M1

staging is shown in Table 147.3 (Sobin et al. 2009). The FIGO staging has been recently updated in 2009 for carcinoma of the cervix, endometrium, and vulva but there have been no changes to the staging of vaginal carcinoma (Oncology 2009). As with cervical cancer, the FIGO staging of the vaginal cancer is clinical. Approximately 33% of women will be stage I at presentation, 20% stage II, 26% stage III, and 20% stage IV (Hellman et al. 2006).

Treatment and Prognosis

Several treatment options exist for patients with squamous cell vaginal carcinomas, including radiation therapy, surgery, combination therapy with radiation and surgery, and chemotherapy (Creasman 2005).

Radiotherapy is delivered using a combination of external beam radiotherapy and either interstitial or intracavity brachytherapy. Treatment is tailored to the extent of disease, with small localized tumors receiving high doses of radiation with brachytherapy for local control. In advanced disease, the radiotherapy treatment includes the pelvic nodes in upper vaginal tumors and the inguino-femoral nodes for lower vaginal tumors. Systemic chemotherapy with cisplatin may be given with radiotherapy if patients are fit enough. Surgery may be preferred in small tumors. Lesion in the upper third of the vagina involving the posterior wall can undergo a hysterectomy and partial vaginectomy. Localized tumors of the lower third of the vagina can be excised with a partial vulvectomy and inguinal lymphadenectomy. Adjuvant radiotherapy may be used after surgery for vaginal cancer to reduce the likelihood of recurrence. Where radical radiotherapy has failed exenterative surgery may result in cure for some patients (Tjalma et al. 2001).

Stage is the most important prognostic factor as it relates to the spread of the disease through the vagina and involvement of the other local structures. High grade tumor which tends to be associated with both large tumors and increased depth of penetration also has a poor prognosis. Presence of lymph node involvement is also an adverse prognostic feature. Other factors that predict poor survival include tumor size of >4 cm and advanced patient age at diagnosis (Hellman et al. 2006). Exophytic tumors have been shown to have a better prognosis compared with tumors which have an ulcerative or circumferential growth pattern (Hellman et al. 2006). The more recent of the reports have suggested better overall outcomes with 70% 5-year survival for stage 1 disease and better than 50% 5-year survival for advanced stage cancer (Creasman 2005).

Imaging of Vaginal Cancer

Due to the rarity of the vaginal cancer there is relatively little data on imaging in primary vaginal cancer (Parikh et al. 2008). Despite this, imaging does have many important roles in managing such patients. The diagnosis of vaginal cancer can be easily done by biopsying the gross lesion. However, before a diagnosis of primary vaginal cancer is made it is important to rule out disease from adjacent organs (e.g., the cervix) involving the vagina. In this regard imaging is very important and MRI provides the best delineation of the pathology within the pelvis.

Once a diagnosis of primary vaginal cancer has been made, staging according to the FIGO system is clinical (see above) and similar to staging for cervical cancer. However, advanced imaging techniques can be used to supplement the clinical evaluation in order to determine the management of these patients. Here again MR imaging of the pelvis is the imaging technique of choice. MRI can provide details not readily assessed at examination under anesthesia (EUA). MRI is better than CT for the preoperative staging as it gives better delineation of the local extent of the vaginal tumor due to its superior soft tissue contrast resolution. MRI has a higher sensitivity for identifying clinically occult pelvic extension into other pelvic organs, e.g., bladder or rectum (Siegelman et al. 1997). MRI is crucial in demonstrating the location of the tumor, determining parametrial extension, and detecting pelvic side wall involvement and spread to the bladder/urethra, rectum, and lymph nodes. Furthermore, MRI can be of value in depicting pelvic anatomy for surgical and radiotherapy planning. Similarly, in the follow-up of patients to determine treatment response or to identify recurrent disease, MRI of the pelvis provides the most local information to manage the patient. For assessing metastatic disease CT or FDG PET-CT should be used but where the likelihood of distant disease is low chest radiographs may suffice.

MRI

The normal vaginal wall is of low T2W signal intensity and the paravaginal fat is of high signal on both T1 and T2W sequences (see ▶ Chap. 148). Squamous cell carcinomas are best visualized on T2 weighted images on which they appear of homogenous intermediate signal intensity. Occasionally they are heterogenous with areas of high T2W signal intensity; this implies tumoral necrosis and a more poorly differentiated carcinoma. Most vaginal tumors are macroscopically visualized as ulcerating lesions and less commonly appear as a fungating mass or as an annular constricting mass. On MRI, ulcerating lesions are seen as ill-defined irregular masses. The fungating type of carcinoma appears as a well-defined lobulated mass while the annular type as a circumferential thickening.

MR imaging can be used to stage vaginal cancer. In a retrospective study of 25 patients with primary vaginal carcinoma, MRI identified over 95% of primary vaginal tumors, enabled radiological staging which correlated with outcome (Taylor et al. 2007). Stage I disease (i.e., tumor is confined to the vagina) appears as an intermediate signal intensity mass on T2 weighted images within the vagina with preservation of the low signal vaginal wall. Disruption of the low signal vaginal wall or the presence of intermediate signal intensity within the high signal paravaginal fat would lead to a diagnosis of extravaginal spread, that is, stage II disease (Fig. 147.1). High-resolution axial T2W images perpendicular to the long axis of the vaginal canal provide optimal views to allow the evaluation of integrity of the vaginal wall. Stage III disease can be diagnosed on MRI when the vaginal mass is seen to extend to the low T2W signal intensity pelvic side wall muscles (Fig. 147.2).

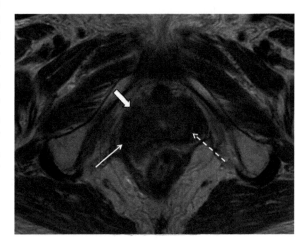

Fig. 147.2 FIGO stage III squamous cell cancer in a 68-year-old woman with a vaginal discharge and bleeding. Axial T2-weighted image shows a vaginal mass which is of intermediate signal intensity relative to muscle. This breaches the right posterolateral vaginal wall (*thin arrow*) with extension to the right levator muscle (*thick arrow*), i.e., pelvic side wall. The left posterior vaginal wall is intact and retains its low signal intensity (*dashed arrow*)

Fig. 147.3 FIGO stage IV squamous cell cancer in a 55-year-old with postmenopausal bleeding. (**a**) Sagittal and (**b**) axial T2-weighted images show a vaginal mass of intermediate signal intensity (*white arrow*). There is bullous edema of the bladder (*dashed arrow*). The presence of this feature in itself does not indicate bladder invasion. There is, however, disruption of the normal low signal intensity of the posterior bladder wall signifying bladder serosal and muscle invasion. (**c**) The axial T2-weighted image shows that this is stage IV disease by the fact that the vaginal tumor engulfs the urethra (*dashed arrow*)

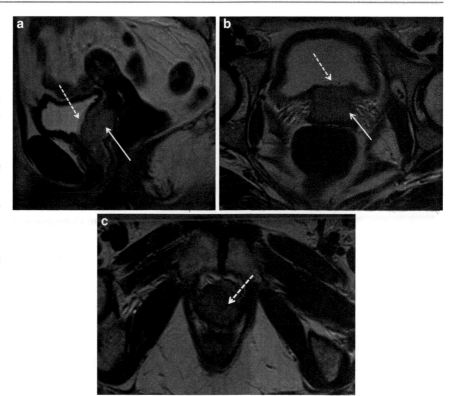

This is often best identified on axial and coronal T2W sequence. In stage IV disease, the tumor extends to the rectum or bladder with loss of the low T2W signal intensity wall of these structures. In order to diagnose stage IV disease, there has to be extension into the mucosa. The presence of bullous edema within the bladder or disease within the mesorectal fat does not constitute stage IV disease (Fig. 147.3).

MRI is also of value in the evaluation of complications of vaginal carcinomas such as vesicovaginal and rectovaginal fistulae. These are best demonstrated on sagittal and axial (high-resolution) planes both on T2-weighted and STIR sequences where they appear as tracts of high signal intensity (Fig. 147.4) (Narayanan et al. 2009). Fistulae may arise as a result of direct extension of tumor or from previous radiotherapy and often require urinary or bowel diversion procedures for palliation. MRI can elegantly demonstrate the site and course of the fistulous tract to aid with surgical management.

In the treated pelvis, MRI also has the ability to differentiate tumor recurrence from scarring and treatment-related changes. Scarring and fibrosis generally appear of low T2-weighted signal intensity whereas recurrent tumor is usually of intermediate or high T2-weighted signal and tumor has a mass-like appearance (Fig. 147.4). Enhancement following intravenous gadolinium may also help but inflammatory change in scar tissue may also enhance and require a biopsy.

CT and FDG PET-CT

CT is primarily used in vaginal cancer to image distant metastatic disease. In a patient who cannot undergo MRI (e.g., due to pacemaker), CT can be used to evaluate the extent of local disease. FDG PET-CT has been shown to be more sensitive and specific than CT and MRI in the detection of para-aortic and pelvic lymph nodes in cervical carcinoma. However, there is limited data on vaginal cancer. A prospective study of 23 patients with vaginal carcinoma compared CT and FDG-PET in vaginal carcinoma (Lamoreaux et al. 2005). The primary tumor was visualized with CT in 9% of patients whereas FDG-PET identified 100% of primary lesions, though PET does not provide the anatomical detail of MRI for T-staging of the disease. All lymph nodes identified on CT were also identified with FDG-PET. In addition, FDG-PET was able to identify four additional foci of

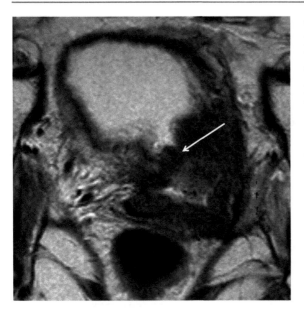

Fig. 147.4 Vesicovaginal fistula in a 56-year-old woman with recurrent squamous vaginal cancer. Oblique axial T2-weighted image shows a fistula (*arrow*) between the necrotic recurrent vaginal tumor and the bladder

potential nodal metastasis. As patients were referred for radiotherapy, pathological confirmation of nodal status could not be obtained, and therefore, the authors were unable to provide a sensitivity/specificity of FDG-PET based on their findings. The combined images from FDG PET-CT may provide better definition of metastatic disease than CT alone.

Other Imaging Techniques

Ultrasound has a limited role in imaging vaginal cancer. As in vulva cancer, it may be of use in the detection of pathological inguinal lymph nodes and has the benefit of offering the potential for fine needle aspiration at the time of ultrasound examination (Sohaib and Moskovic 2003).

Identification of sentinel lymph nodes has been investigated in patients with cervical and vulval carcinoma but reports in vaginal carcinoma are limited. A prospective study of 14 patients with vaginal carcinoma (50% had squamous carcinoma) who underwent preoperative lymphoscintigraphy found that there was no relationship between sentinel node location and the location of the tumor or histologic subtype (Frumovitz et al. 2008). They concluded that the primary tumor

did not always behave in an anatomically predicted pattern and advocated sentinel node lymphoscintigraphy as part of the initial workup in patients with vaginal carcinoma. In this study, due to the unexpected pattern of drainage, 33% of women had their radiation treatment field altered subsequent to lymphoscintigraphy. However, this needs further study.

Summary

Primary squamous cell vaginal carcinoma is a relatively rare gynecologic malignancy which is clinically staged using the FIGO staging system. Imaging, particularly MR imaging, plays an invaluable role in assessment of disease location and extent, in treatment planning, response assessment, and in the evaluation of complications of the disease.

References

Beller U, Benedet JL, et al. Carcinoma of the vagina. FIGO 26th annual report on the results of treatment in gynecological cancer. Int J Gynaecol Obstet. 2006;95(Suppl 1):S29–42.

Carter JJ, Madeleine MM, et al. Human papillomavirus 16 and 18 L1 serology compared across anogenital cancer sites. Cancer Res. 2001;61(5):1934–40.

Chaturvedi AK, Madeleine MM, et al. Risk of human papillomavirus-associated cancers among persons with AIDS. J Natl Cancer Inst. 2009;101(16):1120–30.

Cooper AL, Dornfeld-Finke JM, et al. Is cytologic screening an effective surveillance method for detection of vaginal recurrence of uterine cancer? Obstet Gynecol. 2006;107(1):71–6.

Creasman WT. Vaginal cancers. Curr Opin Obstet Gynecol. 2005;17(1):71–6.

Daling JR, Madeleine MM, et al. A population-based study of squamous cell vaginal cancer: HPV and cofactors. Gynecol Oncol. 2002;84(2):263–70.

Dixit S, Singhal S, et al. Squamous cell carcinoma of the vagina: a review of 70 cases. Gynecol Oncol. 1993;48(1):80–7.

Dodge JA, Eltabbakh GH, et al. Clinical features and risk of recurrence among patients with vaginal intraepithelial neoplasia. Gynecol Oncol. 2001;83(2):363–9.

Duong TH, Flowers LC. Vulvo-vaginal cancers: risks, evaluation, prevention and early detection. Obstet Gynecol Clin North Am. 2007;34(4):783–802, x.

Frumovitz M, Gayed IW, et al. Lymphatic mapping and sentinel lymph node detection in women with vaginal cancer. Gynecol Oncol. 2008;108(3):478–81.

Hellman K, Lundell M, et al. Clinical and histopathologic factors related to prognosis in primary squamous cell carcinoma of the vagina. Int J Gynecol Cancer. 2006;16(3):1201–11.

Hildesheim A, Han CL, et al. Human papillomavirus type 16 and risk of preinvasive and invasive vulvar cancer: results from a seroepidemiological case–control study. Obstet Gynecol. 1997;90(5):748–54.

Lamoreaux WT, Grigsby PW, et al. FDG-PET evaluation of vaginal carcinoma. Int J Radiat Oncol Biol Phys. 2005; 62(3):733–7.

Madsen BS, Jensen HL, et al. Risk factors for invasive squamous cell carcinoma of the vulva and vagina–population-based case–control study in Denmark. Int J Cancer. 2008; 122(12):2827–34.

Narayanan P, Nobbenhuis M, et al. Fistulas in malignant gynecologic disease: etiology, imaging, and management. Radiographics. 2009;29(4):1073–83.

Oncology FCOG. Current FIGO staging for cancer of the vagina, fallopian tube, ovary, and gestational trophoblastic neoplasia. Int J Gynaecol Obstet. 2009;105(1):3–4.

Parikh JH, Barton DP, et al. MR imaging features of vaginal malignancies. Radiographics. 2008;28(1):49–63. quiz 322.

Schraub S, Sun XS, et al. Cervical and vaginal cancer associated with pessary use. Cancer. 1992;69(10):2505–9.

Siegelman ES, Outwater EK, et al. High-resolution MR imaging of the vagina. Radiographics. 1997;17(5):1183–203.

Sillman FH, Fruchter RG, et al. Vaginal intraepithelial neoplasia: risk factors for persistence, recurrence, and invasion and its management. Am J Obstet Gynecol. 1997;176(1 Pt 1): 93–9.

Sobin LH, MK G, et al., editors. TNM classification of malignant tumours. New York: Wiley-Liss; 2009.

Sohaib SA, Moskovic EC. Imaging in vulval cancer. Best Pract Res Clin Obstet Gynaecol. 2003;17(4):543–56.

Taylor MB, Dugar N, et al. Magnetic resonance imaging of primary vaginal carcinoma. Clin Radiol. 2007;62(6):549–55.

Tjalma WA, Monaghan JM, et al. The role of surgery in invasive squamous carcinoma of the vagina. Gynecol Oncol. 2001;81(3):360–5.

M. J. Soo, N. Bharwani, and Andrea G. Rockall

Introduction

Detecting and evaluating abnormalities of the female vagina and vulva are difficult on imaging due to the limitations inherent in each modality, radiation safety issues, and perhaps cultural restrictions. Computed tomography (CT) does not play a significant role in imaging the vagina and vulva due to poor soft tissue resolution of perineal anatomy. Although ultrasound and magnetic resonance imaging (MRI) often play complimentary roles, MRI is now the predominant imaging modality. It is often superior to both ultrasound and CT because of its ability to produce nondegraded multi-planar images and superior contrast resolution without the use of ionizing radiation. MRI is also noninvasive and allows visualization of the female reproductive organs in their orthotopic positions.

Anatomy Overview

The vagina is a fibromuscular tube measuring approximately 8 cm in length and is lined by estrogen-sensitive stratified squamous epithelium. The vaginal

M.J. Soo
Imaging, Bart's Cancer Centre, King George V Wing, St Bartholomew's Hospital, London, UK

N. Bharwani
Imaging, Bart's Cancer Centre, King George V Wing St Bartholomew's Hospital, West Smithfield, London, UK

Department of Radiology, St Mary's Hospital, Imperial College Healthcare NHS Trust, London, UK

A.G. Rockall (✉)
Imperial College Healthcare NHS Trust, London, UK

canal length can vary from 6.5 to 12.5 cm (Lloyd et al. 2005). The vagina has three functions: as an excretory duct for the uterus, female organ of copulation, and part of the birth canal. It extends superiorly and posteriorly from the vestibule of the vulva to surround the cervix of the uterus. The anterior and posterior walls of the vagina are in apposition with folded mucosal surfaces which form rugae that are more prominent in premenopausal women (Suh et al. 2003).

For anatomical purposes, the vagina is divided into the upper, middle, and lower parts. The upper part is derived from the Müllerian ducts, which descend cephalocaudally, also forming the uterus, cervix, and fallopian tubes. The middle and lower parts of the vagina originate from the urogenital ducts, from two sinovaginal tubercles which fuse to form the vaginal plate under the influence of the Müllerian ducts (Hopkins et al. 2000). The upper part of the vagina corresponds to the anterior and posterior fornices that lie above and behind the base of the bladder. The middle part corresponds to the level of the bladder base while the lower part lies just posterior to the urethra (Fig. 148.1). The upper part of the vagina is supported by levator ani muscles together with transverse cervical, pubocervical, and sacrocervical ligaments. The middle part is supported by the urogenital diaphragm while the lower part of the vagina lies within the perineum (Grant et al. 2010).

The arterial blood supply to the vagina is via a network of vessels formed by anatomoses between the vaginal and uterine branches of the internal iliac arteries (Griffin et al. 2008). Venous drainage is via pelvic venous plexuses that drain into the internal iliac veins. Posteriorly, the vaginal and uterine plexuses form part of the rectovaginal septum (Grant et al. 2010).

B. Hamm, P. R. Ros (eds.), *Abdominal Imaging*, DOI 10.1007/978-3-642-13327-5_197,
© Springer-Verlag Berlin Heidelberg 2013

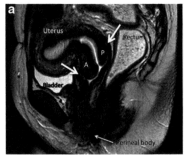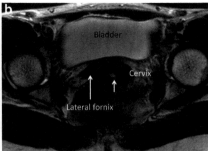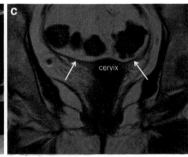

Fig. 148.1 Normal appearance of the vaginal fornices on T2WI: (**a**) Sagittal image demonstrates the anteverted uterus and the anterior (*A*) and posterior (*P*) lips of the cervix. The anterior and posterior vaginal fornices (arrows) are of low T2 signal intensity and insert into the cervix. Note the high signal intensity of the vaginal mucosa and endoluminal fluid on T2WI.

Note the low T2 signal intensity of the perineal body. (**b**) Axial image demonstrates the normal appearance of the right lateral vaginal fornix (*long arrow*) at the level of the cervix (*short arrow*). Note the high signal intensity within the endocervical canal (*short arrow*) on T2WI. (**c**) Coronal T2WI demonstrates the transverse cervical ligaments (*arrows*)

Fig. 148.2 Normal appearance of the vulva on axial T1WI (**a**) and T2WI (**b**). The paired labia minora (*short white arrow*) lie medial to the paired labia majora (*long white arrow*)

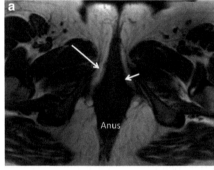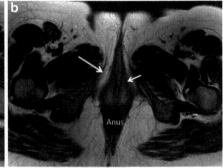

The lymphatic drainage of the vagina is dependent on its anatomical parts: upper part drains into the internal and external iliac nodes, middle part to the internal iliac nodes, and the lower part to the medial group of the superficial inguinal lymph nodes (Griffin et al. 2008).

The vulva forms the external female genitalia and is comprised of the mons pubis, labia majora and minora, clitoris, vestibular bulb, vestibular glands, and the vestibule of the vagina. It is bounded by the symphisis pubis anteriorly, the anal sphincter posteriorly, and ischial tuberosities laterally (Grant et al. 2010). Arterial blood supply of the vulva is derived from the internal and external pudendal arteries while its lymphatics drain into the superficial inguinal lymph nodes (Griffin et al. 2008). The labia majora are two mounds of soft tissue on each side with the labia minora arising medially (Fig. 148.2). The latter form the dorsal hood of the clitoris anteriorly. The vestibular bulbs are paramedian in location, run parallel to the clitoral crura, and surround the urethra and vaginal canal anterolaterally

(Suh et al. 2003). The paired bulbs serve as paravaginal erectile tissue during sexual arousal (Fig. 148.3).

Imaging Techniques and Appearances

MRI

Patients are imaged supine with a phased-array pelvic coil to ensure good signal-to-noise ratio. A partially distended bladder may be helpful in displacing distal bowel loops from the pelvis (Griffin et al. 2008). The practice of administering an anti-peristaltic agent via an intramuscular or intravenous injection may be used in selected patients, particularly in cases where the upper vagina is the site of interest. Sagittal, axial, and coronal or axial oblique T2 signal intensity sequences are essential in imaging the vagina with thin sectional slices to reduce partial volume effect. An endoluminal coil may be used to produce high-resolution images of

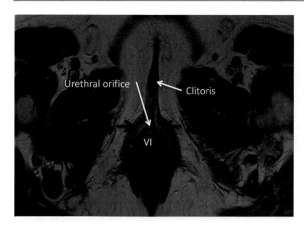

Fig. 148.3 T2WI of vulva: Intermediate signal intensity of the paired vestibular bulbs (*black arrows*) in axial view. They run parallel to surround the urethral orifice (*long white arrow*) and vaginal introitus anterolaterally. *VI* vaginal introitus

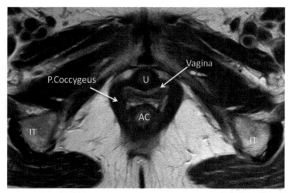

Fig. 148.4 Normal anatomical appearances of the adult female pelvis on T1WI in the axial plane at the level of the ischial tuberosities. The urethra and anal canal both have a target appearance. The vagina has intermediate signal intensity. The pubo-coccygeus muscle is of low signal intensity and forms part of the levator ani muscle complex (*U* urethra, *AC* anal canal, *IT* ischial tuberosity)

the vagina and its immediate surroundings, with the disadvantage of having a small field of view, but this is not widely used (Griffin et al. 2008). Intravenous gadolinium is frequently administered to enhance the labia, vestibular bulbs, clitoris, urethra, cervix, rectum, and vaginal mucosa to provide high level of anatomical delineation. Optimal contrast enhancement is seen in the delayed phase of 6–9 min post administration (Suh et al. 2003). The entire examination requires approximately 30 min of patient cooperation and a regular breathing pattern (Church et al. 2009). It is important to consider this factor when selecting children for this examination.

Normal Anatomical Appearances

T1-weighted images are usually performed in the axial plane with a large field of view. T1-weighted images show high signal intensity in adipose tissues, proteinaceous or mucinous fluid, and blood products, while the remaining soft tissues have a fairly homogenous signal (Church et al. 2009) (Fig. 148.4). This sequence is best for identifying lymphadenopathy, bone marrow changes, and separation of the pelvic structures from surrounding structures. The axial T1 sequence with fat suppression aids in identifying proteinaceous or hemorrhagic material, especially in cases of obstructed congenital utero-vaginal anomalies. This sequence also acts as a pre-contrast baseline prior to gadolinium administration. T2-weighted images provide clear delineation of pelvic structures and often characterize pathology (Griffin et al. 2008) (Fig. 148.5).

Vagina

The vagina usually appears as an H or W-shaped structure in axial slices on both T1- and T2-weighted sequences (Fig. 148.5). On T1-weighted imaging, the mucosal layer and the vaginal lumen are of low signal intensity, followed by a low-intensity muscularis layer and a higher-intensity adventitial layer on T1 and T2 which contains blood vessels and fat (Suh et al. 2003) (Fig. 148.6). The vaginal mucosal layer is best seen on T2- weighted images in which it returns high signal intensity (Fig. 148.5), corresponding with the low signal intensity on T1-weighted images, with enhancement post intravenous contrast administration (Grant et al. 2010). The mucosal layer is thicker and of higher signal intensity on T2-weighted images in the neonate and mid-secretory phase of the menstrual cycle in adults which parallels estrogen levels (Griffin et al. 2008). Endoluminal secretions within the vaginal vault will return a high signal on T2-weighted images and corresponding low signal on T1-weighted images (Church et al. 2009). The submucosal and muscularis layer return low signal intensities in both T1 and T2 sequences. The vaginal venous plexuses that contain slow flowing blood within the adventitial layer of the vagina (Fig. 148.6) will return higher signal intensities on T2-weighted images than T1 (Griffin et al. 2008).

Cervix and Vaginal Fornices

The superior aspect of the vagina inserts into the cervix (Fig. 148.1b). The anterior and posterior

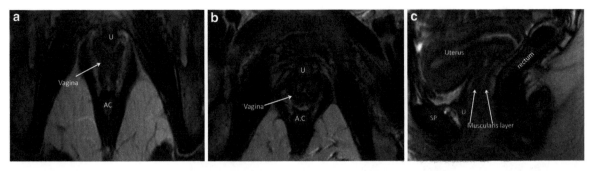

Fig. 148.5 T2WI: Normal appearances of the vagina and surrounding structures in the oblique axial (**a**), axial (**b**), and sagittal (**c**) views. Normal H-shaped (**a**) and W-shaped (**b**) vagina. The vaginal mucosa and endoluminal fluid return high signal intensity compared with low signal intensity from the muscularis layer. The outer adventitial layer has intermediate to high signal intensity on T2WI. *AC* anal canal, *U* urethra, *SP* symphysis pubis

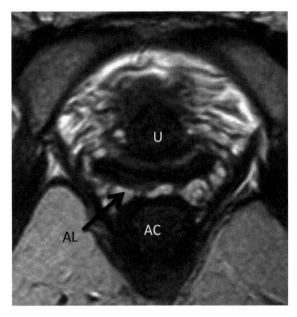

Fig. 148.6 Axial T2WI with small field of view demonstrating the high signal intensity of the adventitial layer which contains the venous plexus. *AL* adventitial layer, *U* urethra, *AC* anal canal

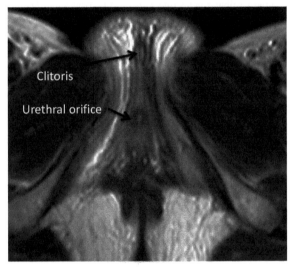

Fig. 148.7 Axial T2WI demonstrating the normal position of the clitoris in relation to the urethra

fornices may be seen as folds of vagina adjacent to the cervix on the sagittal images. The cervix may be more difficult to identify in postmenopausal women due to its small size and indistinct margins (Suh et al. 2003).

Vulva

The labia minora and majora can be identified on T1 and T2 W images, with the labia minora lying medially (Fig. 148.2).

Bartholin's Glands and Clitoris

The Bartholin's glands are located at the posterior lateral aspect of the vaginal introitus (at the 4 and 8 o'clock positions). The clitoris (Fig. 148.7), lying just anterior to the urethral meatus, is well delineated on T1-weighted post-contrast images, appearing as a wishbone-shaped structure anterior to the paired bulbs, which surround the target-like urethra and the vagina. The clitoris and vestibular bulbs enhance brightly following contrast administration (Suh et al. 2003).

Ultrasound

The patient is scanned transabdominally with a full bladder using a curvilinear probe (with caudal angulation in both transverse and longitudinal scans)

Fig. 148.8 Normal appearance of the vagina on a transabdominal sonogram. The vagina is seen as a triple line echo structure with an echogenic mucosal layer and hypoechoic muscularis layer. (**a**) Normal longitudinal appearance of the vagina. (**b**) Normal transverse appearance of the vagina

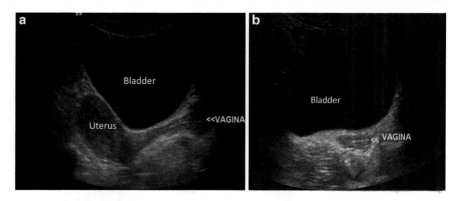

(Lloyd et al. 2005). The length and thickness of the vagina vary according to the fullness of the bladder and rectum. The combined thickness of the anterior and posterior wall should not exceed 1 cm (Lloyd et al. 2005). The transvaginal approach can be used to accurately assess vaginal wall thickness but is otherwise limited as a diagnostic tool (Panayi et al. 2010). The normal vagina is seen as triple line echoes with a mucosal layer that is highly echogenic and a muscularis layer that is moderately hypoechoic (Fig. 148.8). In difficult cases, a transperineal approach with an empty bladder may be tried to gain better visualization of the vagina (Lloyd et al. 2005).

Ultrasound is not widely used in evaluating the vulva, apart from the assessment of groin nodes in the case of vulval carcinoma.

Computed Tomography (CT)

There is poor soft tissue resolution of the anatomical structures of the perineum on CT and thus this is not the optimal imaging method. Patients are imaged supine and axial images are obtained and viewed using a 5 mm slice reconstruction or multi-planar reformatted images for the evaluation of a vaginal abnormality. Un-opacified bowel loops may mimic a mass lesion in the pelvis, thus 500–1,000 ml of oral contrast may be given an hour before scanning to minimize this effect. In selected patients, a vaginal tampon is useful in outlining the vaginal canal. The demarcations of the uterine body, cervix, and vagina are not shown well on CT when compared to MRI.

Congenital Anomalies of the Vagina

The vagina is derived from fusion of two embryological structures, the Müllerian duct and the urogential sinus. The upper two thirds of the vagina derive from the Müllerian ducts which descend cephalocaudally, also forming the uterus, cervix, and fallopian tubes. The lower third of the vagina derives from the urogenital ducts, from two sinovaginal tubercles which fuse to form the vaginal plate under the influence of the Müllerian ducts. Congenital anomalies may result from nondevelopment or fusion defects of the Müllerian ducts and may be associated with other Müllerian duct anomalies. Müllerian duct anomalies have been reported to occur in 1–5% of women (Carrington et al. 1990). There is also a frequent association with renal anomalies due to the close proximity of the Müllerian and Wolffian ducts during embryological development. MRI is the modality of choice for complete anatomical mapping and is also accurate in determining the presence of associated abnormalities.

Vaginal Agenesis

Vaginal agenesis may be partial or complete (Fig. 148.9). It is categorized under Müllerian duct anomalies. It occurs in approximately 1 in 5,000 women (Semelka et al. 1997). The commonest cause for vaginal agenesis is Mayer-Rokistansky-Kuster-Hauser (MRKH) syndrome (1 in 4,500 females). It is divided into two clinical subtypes: Type 1 is characterized by an isolated agenesis or hypoplasia of the proximal two thirds of the vagina with normal ovaries,

Fig. 148.9 A 22-year-old female presented with primary amenorrhea, pelvic pain, and vaginal agenesis on examination. She was subsequently diagnosed to have MRKH syndrome: Axial (**a**) and sagittal (**b**) T2W images demonstrate complete absence of the vagina and uterus. The space that is normally occupied by the vagina is partly replaced by adipose tissue (*white arrows*). *SP* symphisis pubis, *U* urethra, *AC* anal canal

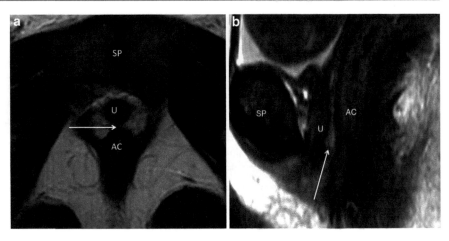

fallopian tubes, and external genitalia. Type 2 is associated with other abnormalities of the urinary tract in 40% of cases. In addition, there may be abnormalities involving the cardiovascular, skeletal, or auditory systems (Morcel et al. 2007).

Other causes of vaginal agenesis or hypoplasia include gonadal dysgenesis (Turner syndrome 45 XO), androgen insensitivity syndrome (CAIS), and male pseudohermaphroditism, which are commonly associated with ambiguous external genitalia.

This anomaly is best seen on MRI on high-resolution T2-weighted sequences. If vaginal and uterine remnants are present, the documentation of their presence is important in future surgical management of these patients.

Vaginal Atresia

Vaginal atresia arises due to failure of the primitive urogenital sinus to develop and results in the absence of the lower third of the vagina. There is low vaginal obstruction with fibrotic tissue replacing the lower third and associated secondary hematometrocolpos. The upper two thirds of the vagina, the uterus, and ovaries are present.

On imaging, there is distension of the vagina and endometrial cavity due to trapped secretions and the lower third of the vagina is replaced by fibrous tissue which extends to the introitus. The vagina is generally more distensible than the endometrial cavity. On ultrasound, the contents of the distended vagina/endometrial cavity have a variable appearance ranging from

anechoic to low-level echoes to echogenic depending on their composition (hemorrhagic material or inspissated secretions). On MRI, T1-weighted imaging with fat suppression allows appreciation of the presence of blood products which remain of high signal intensity and T2-weighted sequences show fluid of low to intermediate to high signal intensity depending on the age of blood products and may demonstrate fluid/debris levels.

Imperforate Hymen

An imperforate hymen is the most frequently encountered obstructive anomaly of the vagina (Scanlan et al. 1990). There is distal vaginal obstruction by a thin endodermal membrane at the level of the introitus which is thought to be due to failure of the sinovaginal bulbs to completely canalize. As a result, there is very low vaginal obstruction with preservation of vaginal length and a "bulging" membrane is seen at the introitus. Patients with a complete imperforate hymen tend to present at menarche with symptoms of hematocolpos. Imaging is rarely required as the diagnosis is usually clinically apparent. However, occasionally imaging is performed for assessment of an enlarging pelvic mass in a pre-menarchal patient.

When imaging is performed, often with perineal ultrasound, imaging appearances are similar to those seen with vaginal atresia; however, the vagina is distended along its entire length to the level of the introitus. The persistent membrane is often difficult to visualize.

Vaginal Septa

Congenital vaginal septa can be either transverse or longitudinal. They may occur in isolation or in the presence of other Müllerian duct developmental malformations. The septum is best seen on T2-weighted images as a low-signal-intensity structure. Longitudinal vaginal septae are best visualized in either coronal or axial planes (Grant et al. 2010).

A transverse septum is formed by the failure of vertical fusion of the down-growing Müllerian duct systems with the up-growing urogenital sinus and is not associated with other Müllerian duct anomalies (Burgis 2001) (Siegelman et al. 1997) (Grant et al. 2010). A transverse septum is seen in 1 in 2,100 to 1 in 72,000 females, can occur at any level within the vagina, and can be complete or incomplete (Burgis 2001). It is seen most commonly at the upper to middle third junction but can be seen at the junction of the middle and lower thirds of the vagina in 15% of patients. Patients with complete transverse septum usually present during adolescence with primary amenorrhea, cyclical pelvic pain, and occasionally a palpable pelvic mass. The latter two symptoms indicate the presence of functioning endometrium which gives rise to retained menstrual secretions (hematometrocolpos). Symptoms of incomplete transverse septum usually present later on in life with symptoms of dyspareunia or dysmenorrhea.

Imaging features are similar to those seen with vaginal atresia and an imperforate hymen except that a transverse septum can be appreciated within the vagina. MRI demonstrates the level and thickness of the septum which are important features in planning further surgical management.

Longitudinal vaginal septae are thought to develop as a consequence of either failure of lateral fusion of the Müllerian duct systems, resulting in duplication of the uterus, cervix (uterus didelphys), and vagina, or from incomplete resorption of the vaginal septum, which can involve varying lengths of the vagina and may also be obstructive (Siegelman et al. 1997). Longitudinal vaginal septae are seen in up to 75% of uterine didelphys in which there is complete duplication of the uterine horn and cervix (Griffin et al. 2008).

MRI is the optimal modality to depict vaginal septae, duplicated cervix, and uterus. T2-weighted sequences may be planned in the oblique coronal and axial planes, in relation to the vagina, cervix, and uterus. The anatomy of the anomaly and any site of obstruction can be demonstrated. The septum is seen as a thin, longitudinal low-signal-intensity structure that extends through the vagina over varying lengths (Fig. 148.11).

Congenital Vaginal Cysts

Vaginal cysts may be congenital or acquired and may be seen incidentally on MRI.

Gartner's duct cysts develop as a result of incomplete regression of the mesonephric or Wolffian duct during fetal development (Griffin et al. 2008). When present, these cysts may be multiple and are located submucosally along the anterolateral aspects of the upper vagina (typically above the level of the symphysis pubis) (Fig. 148.10). These cysts are usually small and asymptomatic, requiring no further treatment. Larger cysts in the vaginal fornix may extend to the lateral aspects of the cervix causing dyspareunia and require treatment. It is important to be aware of the association between Gartner's duct cysts and metanephric abnormalities such as unilateral renal agenesis, renal hypoplasia, and ectopic urethral insertion (Currarino 1982).

In contrast to Gartner's duct cysts, paramesonephric or Müllerian duct cysts have a Müllerian duct origin. These cysts may be found anywhere in the vagina but are often seen anterolaterally and frequently contain mucus. Imaging characteristics are similar to those of Gartner duct cysts and the distinction between these entities is irrelevant clinically (Fig. 148.12).

On ultrasound, these cysts are well-defined anechoic or hypoechoic masses in the anterior vaginal wall. Occasionally they can contain internal echoes due to hemorrhage or proteinaceous content. They do not demonstrate color Doppler flow.

On MRI, a vaginal cyst will typically return low-signal-intensity on T1-weighted images and high-signal-intensity on T2 when they contain simple fluid. Occasionally, there are intermediate to high signal intensities seen on T1-weighted images that suggest the presence of proteinaceous or hemorrhagic content within (Griffin et al. 2008). Uncomplicated cysts have thin walls and do not enhance following intravenous contrast medium. Thickening of the wall and contrast enhancement suggests superimposed infection (Kier 1992).

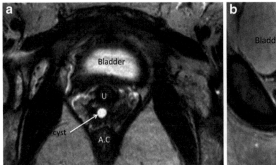 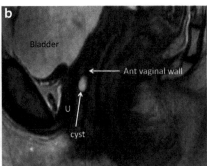

Fig. 148.10 T2WI demonstrating an incidental finding of a vaginal cyst (Gartner duct type): (**a**) Axial T2WI showing a rounded structure of high signal intensity (similar to the bladder) at the anterolateral wall of the vagina. (**b**) Sagittal T2WI of the same patient further demonstrating the position of the Gartner cyst in relation to the anterior vaginal wall. *U* urethra, *AC* anal canal

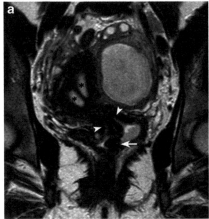 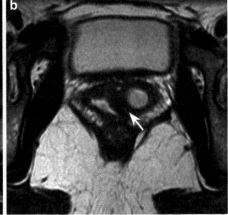

Fig. 148.11 Longitudinal vaginal septum in a patient with uterus didelphys. Coronal (**a**) and axial (**b**) T2-weighted MR images demonstrating a longitudinal vaginal septum (*white arrow*) in a patient with failure of fusion of the lateral Müllerian ducts, resulting in duplication of the uterus (*), cervix (*white arrowheads*), and vagina

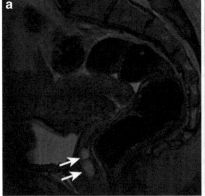 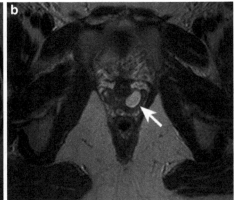

Fig. 148.12 Müllerian duct or paramesonephric cyst. Sagittal (**a**) and axial (**b**) T2-weighted MR images demonstrating two Müllerian duct cysts (*white arrows*). Two thin-walled cystic structures are seen in the right anterolateral vaginal wall at the level of the lower third of the vagina

Congenital Vulval Cysts

Cyst of the Canal of Nuck

The canal of Nuck is an abnormal patent processus vaginalis in the female which extends anterior to the round ligament into the labia majora. This space can fill with peritoneal fluid resulting in a "cyst" or hydrocele. This corresponds to the site of an indirect inguinal hernia. On ultrasound, these structures are typically seen as cystic collections lying superficial and medial to the pubic bone at the level of the superficial inguinal ring. On MRI, they are described as thin-walled fluid-filled structures that run along the course of the round ligament (Park et al. 2004).

Vaginal/Vulval Involvement in Congenital Anomalies of Other Organ Systems

Ectopic Ureter

Faulty embryogenesis can result in an ectopic ureter which can drain into any structure derived from the Wolffian duct or at sites of ectopic Wolffian duct tissue. Approximately 80% of all ectopic ureters are associated with duplicated collecting systems and the more cephalad system is usually the one that drains ectopically.

The ectopic ureter may insert into the vagina which results in urinary incontinence and patients present with characteristic clinical symptoms. Imaging is used to confirm the presence of an ectopic ureter, to assess the remainder of the renal tract, to delineate the course of the ureter, and to plan further management. Intravenous urography is often employed as the initial imaging modality. Cross-sectional techniques such as CT urography and MR urography provide further information regarding the kidney and allow further surgical planning.

Imaging in Relation to Patient Management

Congenital vaginal anomalies are fairly uncommon. They can be isolated or part of a complex anomaly affecting other parts of the reproductive tract, urinary

system, and even cardiovascular system. The spectrum of imaging investigations that are used should encompass these possibilities.

Fertility is commonly affected with congenital vaginal anomalies, therefore it is important to consider and manage the psychological implications for the patient and her family. Many patients first present with symptoms at puberty or later as teenagers. Their age and mental maturity needs to the taken into account when planning treatment as well as timing of various stages of treatment. Psychological preparation of the patient is essential and usually requires multidisciplinary involvement.

Vaginal Agenesis

Vaginal and uterine agenesis is seen in Mayer-Rokitansky-Kuster-Hauser syndrome (MRKH) and much less commonly in incomplete androgen insensitivity syndrome (CAIS) (Quint et al. 2010). In all women with suspected MRKH, associated congenital anomalies of the urinary tract, abdominal wall, skeleton, etc., need to be ruled out prior to definitive treatment. Counseling is the first step, especially with regards to fertility issues and future fertility options. The imaging requirements can be discussed with the patient. Image findings may indicate whether a conservative approach (such as vaginal dilatation) is feasible (Quint et al. 2010). Surgical vaginal creation should only be considered in late adolescence and early adulthood, and good preoperative imaging may help surgical planning.

Vaginal Septum/Imperforate Hymen

Clinically, vaginal septa are classified into obstructive or non-obstructive. The former is usually diagnosed shortly after menarche. The symptoms include primary amenorrhea with cyclical pelvic/abdominal pain and occasionally a pelvic mass can be felt. An MRI scan prior to management should be done to evaluate the exact location and thickness of the septum in relation to an existing cervix. Imperforate hymen may present as a hymenal bulge at birth. Intervention is not indicated at this stage and the bulge will tend to resolve within 1–2 months (Quint et al. 2010).

Non-obstructive vaginal septa are rare and are commonly longitudinal. Patients typically present later in life with dyspareunia, infertility, and obstetrical complications (Quint et al. 2010). MRI may provide an anatomical guide for surgical planning. Resection of vaginal septa and imperforate hymen is usually performed in adolescent years as estrogenization will improve healing (Quint et al. 2010).

Pearls to Remember

- Magnetic resonance imaging (MRI) is the current predominant method of imaging of the vagina and vulva. It is superior in contrast resolution and provides direct multi-planar images.
- T1-weighted images are used for identifying lymphadenopathy, bone marrow changes, and differentiation of the pelvic structures from the surrounding fat. Retained blood products may also be identified.
- T2-weighted images usually delineate anatomy and characterize pathology.
- Assessment of the vagina using ultrasound is usually performed transabdominally and occasionally via transperineal approach. Trans-vaginal approach is limited to the assessment of vaginal wall thickness and evaluation of cysts.
- The commonest cause for vaginal agenesis is Mayer-Rokistansky-Kuster-Hauser (MRKH) syndrome and is often associated with renal anomalies.
- Vaginal septa are seen on T2-weighted images.
- Congenital vaginal cysts are usually asymptomatic and an incidental finding on MRI. They usually do not require treatment unless symptomatic.
- In the presence of a congenital vaginal anomaly, full delineation of the pelvic anatomy using MRI is important for planning of a patient's management.

References

Burgis J. Obstructive Müllerian anomalies: case report, diagnosis, and management. Am J Obstet Gynecol. 2001;185:338–44.

Carrington BM, Hricak H, Nuruddin RN, Secaf E, Laros Jr RK, Hill EC. Müllerian duct anomalies: MR imaging evaluation. Radiology. 1990;176:715–20.

Church DG, Vancil JM, Vasanawala SS. Magnetic resonance imaging for uterine and vaginal anomalies. Curr Opin Obstet Gynecol. 2009;21(5):379–89.

Currarino G. Single vaginal ectopic ureter and Gartner's duct cyst with ipsilateral renal hypoplasia and dysplasia (or agenesis). J Urol. 1982;128:988–93.

Grant LA, Sala E, Griffin N. Congenital and acquired conditions of the vulva and vagina on magnetic resonance imaging: a pictorial review. Semin Ultrasound CT MR. 2010;31(5):347–62.

Griffin N, Grant LA, Sala E. Magnetic resonance imaging of vaginal and vulval pathology. Eur Radiol. 2008;18(6):1269–80.

Hopkins KL, Nino-Murcia M, Friedland GW, et al. Miscellaneous congenital anomalies of the genitourinary tract. In: Pollack HM, McClennan GL, editors. Clinical urography. 2nd ed. Philadelphia: W. B Saunders; 2000. p. 892–911.

Kier R. Nonovarian gynecologic cysts: MR imaging findings. Am J Roentgenol. 1992;158:1265–9.

Lloyd J, Crouch NS, Minto CLK, Liao LM, Creighton SM. Female genital appearance: "normality" unfolds. BJOG. 2005;112(5):643–6.

Morcel K, Camborieux L, Guerrier D. Mayer-Rokitansky-Kuster-Hauser (MRKH) syndrome. Orphanet J Rare Dis. 2007;2:13.

Panayi DC, Digesu GA, Tekkis P, Fernando R, Khullar V. Ultrasound measurement of vaginal wall thickness: a novel and reliable technique. Int Urogynecol J. 2010;21(10):1265–70.

Park SJ, Lee HK, Hong HS, Kim HC, Kim DH, Park JS, Shin EJ. Hydrocele of the canal of Nuck in a girl: ultrasound and MR appearance. Br J Radiol. 2004;77:243–4.

Quint EH, McCarthy JD, Smith YR. Vaginal surgery for congenital anomalies. Clin Obstet Gynecol. 2010;53(1):115–24.

Scanlan KA, Pozniak MA, Fagerholm M, Shapiro S. Value of transperineal sonography in the assessment of vaginal atresia. Am J Roentgenol. 1990;154:545–8.

Semelka RC, Ascher SM, Reinhold C. Female urethra and vagina. In: Semelka RC, editor. MRI of the abdomen and pelvis: a text atlas. North Carolina: Wiley-Liss; 1997. p. 571–8.

Siegelman ES, Outwater EK, Banner MP, Ramchandani P, Anderson TL, Schnall MD. High-resolution MR imaging of the vagina. Radiographics. 1997;17:1183–203.

Suh DD, Yang CC, Cao Y, Garland PA, Maravilla KR. Magnetic resonance imaging anatomy of the female genitalia in premenopausal and postmenopausal women. J Urol. 2003;170(1):138–44.

Marie Cassart

Introduction

Imaging modalities are essential in fetal medicine. The routine follow-up of fetuses is achieved by ultrasound (US) which is and remains the first level screening technique.

Complementary imaging is mandatory in various clinical situations either to clarify an US diagnosis or to precise a prognosis. *Fetal magnetic resonance imaging* (MRI) and *fetal computed tomography* (CT) are therefore performed in selected indications following US (Coakley et al. 2004; Ruano et al. 2004). Undoubtedly, the main field of investigations for fetal MRI is the central nervous system (CNS) (Huisman et al. 2002; Blaicher et al. 2003; Brown et al. 2004), but recently, its use has been significantly extended to thoraco-abdominal indications to precisely depict pulmonary or urogenital malformations, characterizing masses and analyzing the digestive tract (Farhataziz et al. 2005; Shinmoto and Kuribayashi 2003; Hill et al. 2005).

Fetal CT is used in the evaluation of the fetal skeleton in carefully selected indications. Although sonography has proved reliable for the prenatal detection of skeletal abnormalities (Doray et al. 2000), the precise diagnosis of a dysplasia is often difficult to make before birth (especially in the absence of a familial history).

In the following pages, we will describe the respective MRI and CT procedures in the fetus, precise their indications and interest in antenatal diagnosis.

M. Cassart
Department of Medical Imaging (FEA, AM and MC) and Fetal Medicine (RL), University Clinics of Brussels, Erasme Hospital, Brussels, Belgium

Fetal MRI

Fetal MRI is widely accepted as a good complementary imaging modality to US in antenatal diagnosis (Laifer-Narin et al. 2007). Several factors have contributed to its progressive widespread use. First, US is sometimes insufficient in establishing a correct diagnosis (and/or prognosis) related to poor sonographic conditions (maternal obesity, fetal position, twin pregnancies). MRI provides a larger field of view, a better contrast resolution and is not affected by bone shadowing or other conditions of poor US resolution (anamnios). Second, the images provided are more "readable" than US images for non radiologists; this facilitates communication inside the medical staff and clarifies the information delivered to the parents. Third, the important contribution of fetal MR in the diagnosis and prognosis helps for maternal counseling and pre- and postnatal management. Consequently, fetal MRI has become a commonly used modality for antenatal imaging. Nevertheless, its cost and limited accessibility remain a barrier to a more widespread use (Levine 2004).

Technique

Fetal MRI is generally performed on a 1.5-T magnet. All acquisitions are obtained with a phased array body coil. The patients comfortably installed supine are generally not sedated. If sedation is administered, it consists in 1 mg of flunitrazepam 20 min before the examination starts. Feet entry into the scanner is useful in cases of claustrophobia. The mainstay of fetal MRI is T2-weighted sequences which allow rapid acquisitions

B. Hamm, P. R. Ros (eds.), *Abdominal Imaging*, DOI 10.1007/978-3-642-13327-5_129,
© Springer-Verlag Berlin Heidelberg 2013

minimizing fetal motion artifacts. Such sequences yield good image contrast for the fetal anatomy of the brain and body. For the fetal brain, the most commonly used sequences are turbo spin-echo sequences (TR/TE, 5,324/140 msec) without mother respiratory triggering. Each sequence includes 20 sections that are acquired within 19 s. Those sequences are performed in three orthogonal planes according to the fetal head. In order to assess intracranial hemorrhage, a T1 sequence is used (TR/TE, 18/6.9 ms; angle, 22°, inversion time, 1,354 ms, shot duration 2,574 ms; 13 sections with 5 mm thickness; number of excitations, six; duration, 4 min). This sequence is acquired in one orientation only. Diffusion tensor imaging is frequently performed in neurological indications. This imaging modality can assess microstructural changes of fetal cerebral white matter related to maturation and myelination. In the future, parenchymal lesions due to abnormal metabolism or insufficient blood supply could be detected by proton MR spectroscopy which is not presently performed on a routine basis (Kim et al. 2008; Guimiot et al. 2008). For the fetal abdomen, we perform single shot T2 weighted sequences (TR/TE: 661/80 ms) respiratory triggered in three orthogonal planes. We also always perform T1 weighted sequences (TE: 2.3 ms, TR: 4.5 ms, angle: 10°, FOV: 400 × 300, acquisition duration:16 s) in at least two planes (including a sagittal plane) to visualize the digestive tract. These T1 sequences necessitate maternal apnea. Because of fetal movement, each sequence acts as a scout for the next sequence. The field of view is 340 mm in order to avoid wrap-around artifacts and slice thickness is 3–4 mm. The acquisitions are completed in no more than 30 min.

So far, no deleterious effects have been demonstrated even with high magnetic fields. Nevertheless, MRI should be avoided in the first trimester. Gadolinium chelates cross the placenta and are ingested by the fetus through the amniotic fluid. The potential risk on the fetus is not known, therefore, we do not use contrast agent in fetal imaging.

Indications

The fetal MRI indications are numerous and increasing with time. In the present text, we will separately describe the indications for fetal brain from fetal abdomen and focus on the most commonly encountered indications in daily practice. As said above and as a general statement

MRI is indicated when: the sonographic data are equivocal or inconclusive (poor US conditions) or when the detection of associated anomalies (to a known malformation) may change the fetal prognosis and/or the pregnancy management (mode and site for delivery and level and type of neonatal care unit).

Fetal Brain MRI

Most often, the main fetal cerebral anomalies are detected on US (callosal agenesis, brain tumor, or hemorrhage). Several series have shown that MRI is superior to US in assessing cortical maturation and dysplasia, migrational anomalies, midline, and posterior fossa anomalies. It also accounts for a better evaluation of subependymal (heterotopias, tubers) and parenchymal lesions. Therefore, the role of MRI in the evaluation of the fetal brain is mainly focused on the detection of anomalies possibly overlooked by US (brain maturation, gyration, etc.) that could modify the prognosis of the pregnancy.

The most common indications of fetal CNS MRI include:

Fetuses with known anomalies whose prognosis depends on associated lesions undetectable by US:
- Ventriculomegaly (to find an etiology).
- Midline anomalies (to better visualize the midline structures – corpus callosum, midline cyst, etc.).
- Posterior fossa malformations (to precisely analyze the anatomy of the vermis).
- Micro (simplified gyral pattern) and macrocephaly (true megalencephaly) (to analyze the gyration).
- Tumors (to try to characterize them and better define their extension).

Fetuses at risk of CNS anomalies with a normal US scan:
- Familial history of brain malformation (known as being possibly overlooked by US such as subtle gyration or posterior fossa anomalies).
- Viral infections (gyration or white matter anomalies).
- Fetal cardiac rhabdomyomas (to exclude tuberous sclerosis).
- Pregnancies with an increased risk of cerebral ischemia (monochorionic twin pregnancy with twin-twin transfusion, etc.).

Fig. 149.1 (a) Coronal T2-weighted slice of a 30-week-old fetus with a midline arachnoïd cyst. (b) The cyst interfered with the normal development of the corpus callosum which is incompletely developed

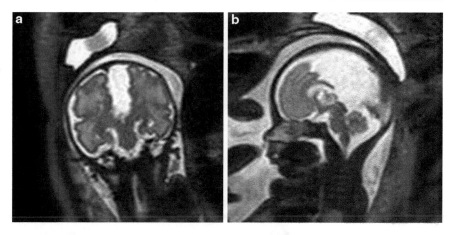

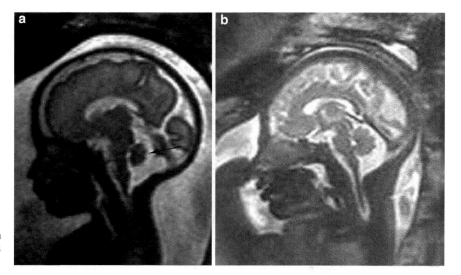

Fig. 149.2 (a) A vermian hypoplasia in a 28-week-old fetus (*arrow*). (b) Midsagittal T2 weighted slice on the brain of a normal 31-week-old fetus for comparison

Ventriculomegaly is defined as a transverse diameter of the ventricular atrium at the level of the glomus of the choroid plexus superior to 10 mm. It constitutes the most frequent indication for fetal brain MRI. Its incidence ranges between 0.3 and 1.5 in 1,000 births. MRI is of utmost importance to orient toward a malformative, destructive, or isolated dilatation (Benacerraf et al. 2007). Most of the cases are isolated (71%) and carry a better prognosis. The cases with associated anomalies (29%) are secondary to infections, destructive lesions (hemorrhagic or ischemic), developmental, or chromosomal anomalies (13 or 18 trisomy) for which the prognosis is poorer.

Midline anomalies mainly concern the corpus callosum and include malformations like total or partial callosal agenesis or hypoplasia. This diagnosis relies on US, the role of MRI is to detect possibly

overlooked associated anomalies that worsen the prognosis (Dill et al. 2009) (i.e., neuronal migration anomalies, posterior fossa anomalies, cortical atrophy, etc.). Midline anomalies also include arachnoïd cysts that can be very huge and interfere with the commissural structures development (Fig. 149.1).

Posterior fossa malformations carry a poor prognosis. Fetal US can diagnose malformations as early as the second trimester but a precise diagnosis is often difficult to ascertain. MRI is a good complementary investigation for the posterior fossa as it allows imaging in three orthogonal planes with a precise cerebellar biometry leading to the difficult diagnosis of cerebellar and/or vermian agenesis or hypoplasia (Guibaud 2004) (Fig. 149.2). The superior contrast resolution of MRI also accounts for a better delineation of the brainstem very difficult to visualize on US.

Fig. 149.3 (a) Axial
T2-weighted slice of
a 31-week-old fetus with
congenital cytomegalovirus
infection. The MRI
demonstrates extended
gyration anomalies, with
bilateral sylvian opercular
dysplasia. (b) Normal fetus at
the same gestational age for
comparison

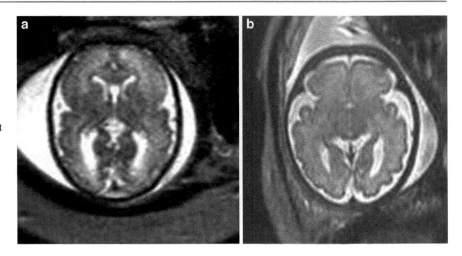

Micro- and macrocephaly are rare developmental anomalies associated with poor prognosis. In both situations a precise visualization of the fetal brain is mandatory to detect neuronal migration and gyration anomalies that may result in microcephaly with simplified gyration carrying a very poor prognosis (Desir et al. 2008) or hemimegalencephaly very difficult to depict on US.

Fetal cerebral tumors are usually reported during the third trimester and carry a poor prognosis with a global postnatal survival of only 28%. The definite diagnosis of these lesions generally relies on histology. Yet making a tentative diagnosis during fetal life using MRI may be clinically important to provide the parents with information regarding the prognosis and to discuss the management of pregnancy (Cassart et al. 2008).

Cytomegalovirus is the most common agent responsible for congenital infection. It affects 0.2–2% of live birth. The prenatal diagnosis relies on viral culture on amniotic fluid and IgM on fetal blood sampling. In cases attesting the fetal infection, a negative US examination is still associated to 20% of neurological sequelae including sensorineural hearing loss.

The typical neuroradiological findings are calcifications, migrational anomalies (Fig. 149.3), disturbed myelination, and cerebellar hypoplasia. In this context, MRI could play an interesting role in detecting gyration and neuronal migration anomalies or posterior fossa malformations (Benoist et al. 2008).

Tuberous sclerosis is an autosomal dominant multisystemic disorder which affects the skin, brain, heart, and other organs. The estimated prevalence is approximately one case per 6,000–10,000 individuals. The cardiac rhabdomyoma(s) detected on fetal US lead

to suspicion of the diagnosis even when there is no family history. MRI better than US can depict CNS hamartomas or subependymal tumors that confirm the suspected diagnosis. This improves the genetic counseling and prenatal diagnosis of patients.

Parenchymal abnormalities secondary to hemorrhagic or ischemic lesions are often visualized with US, but the precise extension of the parenchymal involvement may be overlooked or underestimated, notably in the centrum semiovale and the temporal lobes. Calcified leucomalacia may appear as faint hyperechogenicity which may be missed, whereas MR sequences are more conspicuous. Diffusion weighted imaging might play an important role in the detection of diffuse white matter abnormalities.

Fetal Body MRI

Chest

Fetal thoracic anomalies that are most often investigated by MRI include diaphragmatic hernias, bronchopulmonary malformations, and thoracic masses.

– *Congenital diaphragmatic hernia* affects one upon 2,400–3,000 live births. US allows to establish the diagnosis and is able to approximate the content of the hernia. The prognosis of such a malformation when isolated relies on its side, time of discovery, content (position of the liver), and residual lung volume. In this context, MRI is a good complementary tool that helps in establishing the prognosis (Jani et al. 2008). Thanks to its better contrast resolution, MRI is interesting first to define the content

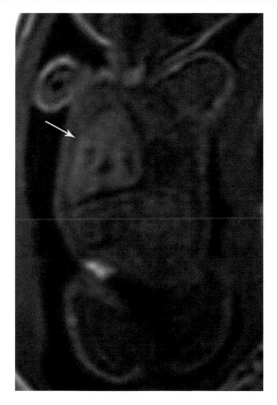

Fig. 149.4 Coronal T1-weighted slice of a 28-week-old fetus with left congenital diaphragmatic hernia. The slightly hyperintense liver is herniated in the thorax (*arrow*)

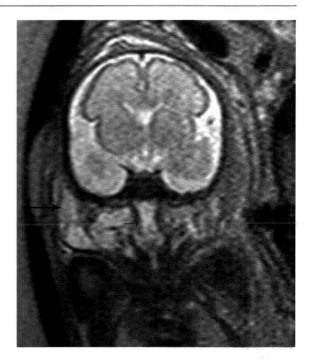

Fig. 149.5 Coronal T2-weighted slice on a 28-week-old fetus presenting a cervical lymphangioma (*long arrow*). The interest of MR is to demonstrate that the laryngeal structures are not involved (*short arrow*)

of the hernia, which is an important information for the surgeon and second to precise the volume of liver herniated in the thorax (T1 images) (Fig. 149.4) which is considered by some authors as an interesting prognostic parameter. The residual lung volume can be evaluated by planimetry on T2 weighted sequences and again is useful in predicting the respiratory function at birth. Both parameters are of interest in predicting survival (Jani et al. 2008).

– *Bronchopulmonary malformations* include congenital cystic adenomatoid malformation and sequestration. These lesions are diagnosed by US because of their typical hyperechoïc pattern; the differentiation between the two conditions relies on the detection of a systemic arterial vessel characterizing the sequestration. This vessel is often better demonstrated with US than with MRI.

The contrast between the malformation and the adjacent normal lung is higher with MRI which allows a better evaluation of its extension and potential mass effect on adjacent mediastinal structures. MRI is also used to measure the volume of the unaffected lung and to appreciate the regression of the lesion with time.

– *Cervicothoracic masses* may infiltrate and/or compress the pharyngeal and mediastinal structures inducing occlusion of the respiratory tract that can be fatal at birth. The most commonly encountered masses are cystic lymphangiomas (Fig. 149.5) and teratomas.

The airways are better visualized with MRI that may help in attesting about their integrity. In case of involvement of the airways by the mass, it is not possible with either method to differentiate extrinsic compression from infiltration. Possible spinal extension of a cervical and/or thoracic mass may be missed by US and is well depicted by MRI.

Abdomen

Nine percent of fetal malformations are of gastrointestinal origin. MRI may help in characterizing the lesion and therefore establish a prognosis.

– *The digestive tract* can be visualized by MR from the esophagus to the distal colon. In the third trimester, the small bowel filled with ingested amniotic fluid appears hyperintense on T2 weighted sequences and the colon filled with meconium, appears hyperintense on T1 weighted sequences (Saguintaah et al. 2002). Therefore, MRI may help in locating digestive tract occlusions. When *esophageal atresia* is suspected on US (polyhydramnios, and/or absent or small size stomach), we perform MRI dynamic acquisitions focused on the fetal esophagus to follow spontaneous swallowing of the fetus. If an esophageal pouch is seen, the diagnosis is confirmed, if the continuity of the esophagus is demonstrated during fetal swallowing, the diagnosis can be definitely excluded (Langer et al. 2001).

Small bowel occlusion occurs in one upon 3,000 births and is secondary to atresia or volvulus. The diagnosis is again most frequently established during the third trimester. The most common sites affected are the proximal jejunum and distal ileum. The US signs are dilated loops (>10 mm) and polyhydramnios. MRI can therefore be used to better define the level of the occlusion according to the signal of the dilated loop and the presence of normally filled proximal or distal loops (Fig. 149.6). The presence of unused microcolon attests of a small bowel atresia (Garel et al. 2006; Veyrac et al. 2004).

- *Abdominal masses*

Abdominal cystic masses are frequently encountered; they may originate from the digestive or genitourinary tract or correspond to cystic tumors. The role of antenatal imaging is to establish an early diagnosis in order to reassure the parents in cases of benign and reversible lesions (ovarian cysts) or to prepare them to a difficult postnatal management in cases of complex anatomical malformations (cloacal malformations) or tumors. The differential diagnosis of abdominal cystic masses includes lymphangioma, cystic teratoma, mesenteric cyst, ovarian cyst, duplication cyst, choledochal cyst, and meconial pseudo cyst. In some situations, the US is conclusive and no complementary imaging modality is necessary. If the diagnosis is not fixed on US data, MRI is then generally performed. MRI may be useful in the differential diagnosis as it can provide information on the content of the mass (hemorrhagic, liquid, etc.) and help to precise its nature and detailed anatomic relationships with adjacent organs. *Lymphangioma* appears like a mass that can be cystic or solid, sometimes with

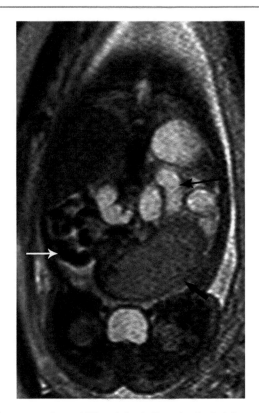

Fig. 149.6 Coronal T2 weighted slice of a fetal abdomen at 32 weeks. The proximal small bowel loops are dilated and filled with amniotic fluid (*thin black arrow*). The distended small bowel has intermediate signal content (*thick black arrow*). The distal loops are collapsed or filled with dehydrated meconium (*thin white arrow*). This entails us to diagnose a midgut atresia

vascular components. The mass is infiltrative, it compresses and encases the vascular structures which may present serous, chylous, or bloody contents. The abdominal location is rare (5%). The diagnosis is generally established on US. MR is useful to precise the extension of the lesion. *Teratomas* affect 1/35–40,000 live births, it mostly concerns female fetuses. Most are benign but 10% become malignant. Teratomas can be cystic, solid, or mixed tumors; the solid component is often highly vascularized sometime inducing fetal high-output heart failure or intracranial ischemia. Arguments for benignity are: the early diagnosis, important cystic components, and extra pelvic extension. The role of MRI is to characterize the mass and to depict its effect on the urinary tract and other abdominal organs (Avni et al. 2002) (Fig. 149.7). Thanks to their specific signal,

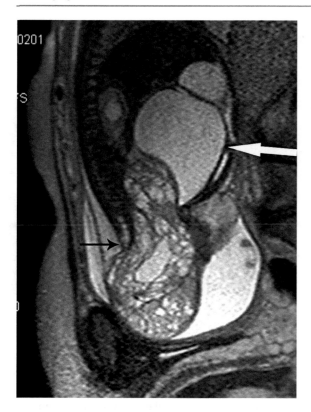

Fig. 149.7 Sagittal T2 weighted image of a huge sacro-coccygeal teratoma with intra medullar canal involvement (*black arrow*) and secondary hydrometrocolpos (*white arrow*)

MRI may properly localize the mass in relation to the bladder, the uterus, the rectum, and the spine. *Ovarian cyst* is a classical finding, it can be uni- or bilateral and is related to maternal hormonal status. The cyst can be hemorrhagic and even rupture in the abdomen. *The duplication cyst* is encountered in 1 upon 4,500 autopsies. It is mainly located in the terminal ileum but can be found anywhere along the digestive tract from the esophagus to the rectosigmoid. The postnatal complications which are numerous including intussusceptions, torsion, hemorrhage, or malignant degeneration can be obviated by antenatal diagnosis (Foley et al. 2003). The *choledochal cyst* is a sub hepatic cyst located on the main bile duct. It is associated to a decreased bile excretion in utero. It can be associated to biliary atresia which significantly worsen the prognosis and is impossible to diagnose in utero. The diagnosis is important to establish promptly because of the possible complications (cholangitis, hepatic fibrosis, etc.). MRI better than US can demonstrate

the anatomical relationships of the cyst with the biliary tree and therefore confirm the diagnosis and the type of choledochal cyst. The precise diagnosis of these abdominal lesions will facilitate planning for delivery and neonatal management.

– *Genitourinary tract*

Most urinary tract abnormalities may be detected by US. MRI may be helpful for detecting small cysts, particularly those located in the medulla (Cassart et al. 2004). It can better characterize bilateral anomalies and can provide an overview of the whole urinary tract. In cases with *huge urinary tract dilatation* filling the entire fetal abdomen, US may be insufficient in characterizing the anomaly. Thanks to its larger field of view, MRI better differentiates dilated pyelo-caliceal cavities from ureters and bladder, helping in precisely depicting the malformation.

In cases of enlarged bladder, T1 MRI sequences showing a normal colon can easily exclude a megacystis-microcolon syndrome which is one of the differential diagnosis of a fetal megacystis that carries a very poor prognosis (Cassart et al. 2004) (Fig. 149.8). In cases of *suspected renal agenesis*, the presence of a hypoplastic solitary kidney may be difficult to assess in poor US condition due to oligohydramnios or anamnios. MRI can affirm or exclude the presence of renal parenchyma and therefore help in the decision of interrupting or continuing the pregnancy. Thanks to its good contrast resolution, MRI can help in differentiating the urinary from the digestive tract in *complex genitourinary tract malformations* leading to a precise anatomical description of the anomaly. This entails a more conspicuous prognostic evaluation.

Fetal CT

Skeletal dysplasias are a heterogeneous group of conditions which affect bone development and result in various anomalies in shape and size of the skeleton. Around 250 different entities are described, of which many are exceedingly rare. The prevalence of these dysplasias in the newborn has been estimated about 3–4 per 10,000 and the overall frequency of skeletal dysplasias among perinatal death is about 9 per 1,000. Despite recent advances in fetal imaging, these

Fig. 149.8 (a) Sagittal T2 weighted slice of a fetus with megabladder. (b) Sagittal T1 weighted slice, the hyperintense colon is of normal size allowing to exclude a megabladder-microcolon association

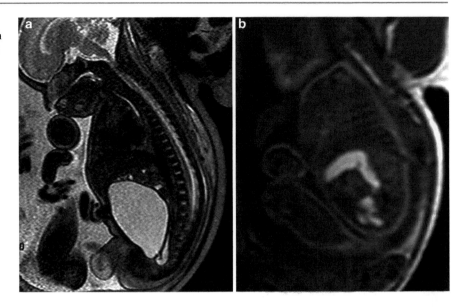

dysplasias remain a diagnostic challenge. The characterization of a dysplasia is often difficult due to their various phenotypic presentations, the variable gestational age at discovery and often, the lack of precise molecular diagnosis. This is a clinically relevant issue as skeletal dysplasias may be associated with severe disability and may even be lethal.

In this context, CT plays a key role. We will first describe the technique of acquisition and analysis, then precise the indications and the diagnostic contribution of CT in the antenatal assessment of skeletal malformations (Cassart 2010).

Technique

– *Acquisition*

The CT should always be performed after a detailed ultrasound examination. The US findings should be known by the radiologist performing the CT in order to focus on specific skeletal parts or bone segments during the post processing work-up. We perform the acquisitions on a computed tomography multislice 16 scanner (Siemens, Erlangen, Germany) set with the following parameters: 40 mAs, 120 KV, 16 slices per rotation, pitch 0.75, and slice thickness 0.75 mm. This corresponds to a mean irradiation dose given to the fetus of 3.12 mGy (CTDIw) which is similar to the irradiation exposure of conventional fetal standard radiological examinations

(3 mGy) (Hurwitz et al. 2006). The acquisition lasts about 20 s and is performed during maternal apnea to prevent kinetic artifacts that can mimic fractures or bone deformations. A total of 350–500 images per fetus are stored for further analysis. After segmentation and removal of the maternal pelvic bones, post processing consists in 2D and 3D reconstructions of the entire fetal skeleton using maximum intensity projection. This procedure is performed with the inspace software in the Leonardo Workstation (Siemens). The whole process takes about 20 min (Cassart et al. 2007).

– *Analysis of the images*

The 2D-CT reconstructions include axial slices on the skull base obtained in order to appreciate the inner ear bony structures. Axial slices on the spine are also realized to evaluate the ossification of the vertebral bodies and posterior arches. On each segment of the skeleton, slices are specifically angulated in order to give the best view of the bone shape and structure (cortical/medullar bone ratio). In the long bones, the metaphyseal shape is analyzed (Fig. 149.9). The 3D reconstructions allow moving the fetus in the three-dimensional space to appreciate the global proportions and morphological deformities (curved bones, short ribs, spinal shortening, disruptions, etc. . . .) (Fig. 149.10).

In our experience, CT demonstrates additional, but also specific skeletal findings that can be overlooked by US. It mainly concerns the vertebral

Fig. 149.9 (a) 2D reconstruction of femoral bones in a 24 weeks old fetus affected by a spondylo-metaphyseal dysplasia showing abnormal metaphyseal cupping. (b) Normal aspect of the metaphysis on a 2D slice of a normal femoral bone of a 28 weeks old fetus

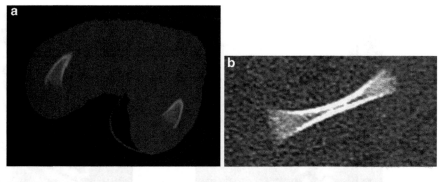

Fig. 149.10 (a) 3D reconstructions of a fetal skeleton at 30 weeks of GA showing the normal proportions between the spine and the long bones. (b) A 30 weeks old fetus with a Desbuquois dyplasia showing the abnormal proportion between the spine and the legs and arms. All the joints are disrupted (ankles, knees, elbows, etc.)

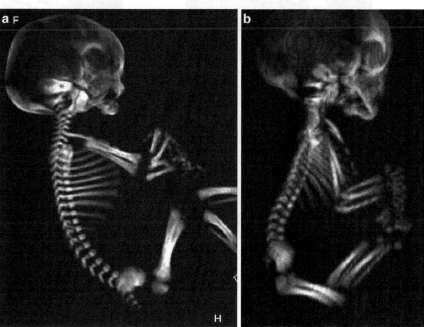

column (vertebral body shape) (Fig. 149.11), the pelvic bones shape, the ossification points, and possible synostosis. These abnormalities are often inconspicuous on US, but may be of great importance in establishing a precise diagnosis.

Indications

CT is an irradiating technique; therefore, its use on fetal imaging should be obviously restricted to cases for which US and genetic data are inconclusive in diagnosing or excluding a specific skeletal dysplasia (Table 149.1). Often genetic testing is too long to be performed before birth that is why CT may orient the diagnosis and sometimes help in targeting the genetical analyses. The cases referred should be restricted to

situations in which the diagnosis is likely to impact on the follow-up of the pregnancy (termination) or the neonatal work-up. The indications encountered most frequently in clinical practice are: long bone shortening (there should at least be 5 weeks delay in the GA). It must be kept in mind that the vast majority of fetuses with mild shortened long bones do not present skeletal dysplasia, abnormal bone measurements being related to intra uterine growth restriction (associated with oligohydramnios, pathological Doppler studies), or normal variant (small parents). In those fetuses, as mentioned above, no complementary investigation is necessary.

Other indications concern small thorax (leading to pulmonary hypoplasia and lethality); long bone deformities (curvature, fractures) with or without metaphyseal shape anomalies; and joint deformities (disruption).

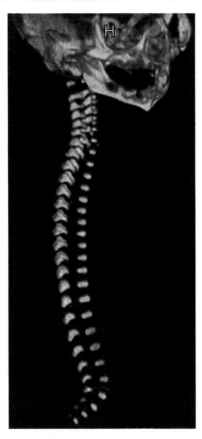

Fig. 149.11 3D reconstruction of a 24 weeks old fetus presenting platyspondylia

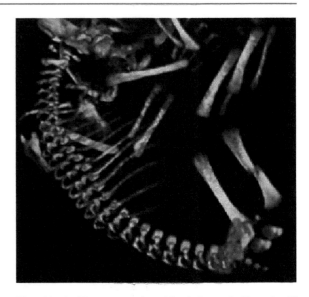

Fig. 149.12 3D reconstruction of the skeleton of a 30 weeks old fetus. The "fractured" femur is a movement artifact

Table 149.1 Indications for fetal CT

1. Long bones shortening (more than 5 weeks of growth retardation)
2. Long bones deformities (bowing, angulation, etc.)
3. Joint deformities (disruption)
4. Metaphyseal deformities (flared, irregular shape, cupping, etc.)
5. Epiphyseal anomalies (absent, punctuate epiphysis)
6. Thoracic hypoplasia (short ribs, short thorax, barrel shape thorax, etc.)
7. Spinal deformities (angulation, suspected platyspondyly)
8. Abnormal skull shape (clover leave skull, scaphocephaly, frontal bossing)
9. Abnormal facial bones (micro-retrognathy)

CT is helpful in better depicting the suspected malformation. Cranial deformities (clover leaf skull, frontal bossing, etc.) are also good indications for which CT can help in visualizing the cranial vault sutures. Spinal angulations incompletely fixed by US should be referred to CT in order to better depict the segmentation anomalies (hemivertebras, fused vertebras, butterfly shape vertebra, platyspondyly).

Limitations

The examination should ideally be performed during the third trimester once organogenesis is completed and bone mineralization is sufficient. This time restriction depreciates the impact of the technique in antenatal diagnosis. In poor prognosis cases with possible termination of pregnancy as an outcome and since some are already detected during the second trimester, we sometimes perform it earlier (from 26 weeks of GA). Additionally, the image quality is dependent on fetal immobility which is also more easily obtained late in pregnancy. Noteworthy, false images of skeletal deformities or fractures can be secondary to such fetal movements (Fig. 149.12).

CT is still often insufficient for the precise and complete visualization of the fetal extremities (hands and feet) and for the quantification of bone mineralization due to lack of normal data. At present time, there are no data about fetal bone density on CT correlated with gestational age. Such measurements would be helpful in the diagnosis of bone diseases affecting mineralization like osteopetrosis or conversely like osteogenesis imperfecta for which the actual diagnosis on imaging mostly relies on inconstant bone fractures.

Conclusion

In selected cases, MRI and CT are good complementary imaging modalities to US. MRI brings additional structural, anatomical, and topographic information that improves the diagnosis and therefore clarifies the prognosis of the pregnancy. CT helps in depicting a skeletal malformations or characterizing a suspected skeletal dysplasia. Consequently, those examinations help in counseling the parents and entail a better management of the newborn.

References

Avni FE, Guibaud L, Robert Y, et al. MR imaging of fetal sacrococcygeal teratoma: diagnosis and assessment. AJR. 2002;178:179–83.

Benacerraf BR, Shipp TD, Bromley B, et al. What does magnetic resonance imaging add to the prenatal sonographic diagnosis of ventriculomegaly? J Ultrasound Med. 2007;26:1513–22.

Benoist G, Salomon LJ, Molho M, et al. Cytomegalovirus-related fetal brain lesions: comparison between targeted ultrasound examination and magnetic resonance imaging. Ultrasound Obstet Gynecol. 2008;32:900–5.

Blaicher W, Prayer D, Bernaschek G. Magnetic resonance imaging and ultrasound in the assessment of the fetal central nervous system. J Perinat Med. 2003;31:459–68.

Brown SD, Estroff JA, Barnewolt CD. Fetal MRI. Appl Radiol. 2004;33(2):9–25.

Cassart M. Suspected fetal skeletal malformations or bone diseases: how to explore? Pediatr Radiol. 2010;40(6):1046–51.

Cassart M, Massez A, Metens T, et al. Complementary role of MRI after sonography in assessing bilateral urinary tract anomalies in the fetus. AJR. 2004;182(3):689–95.

Cassart M, Massez A, Cos T, et al. Contribution of three dimensional computed tomography in the assessment of skeletal dysplasia. Ultrasound Obstet Gynecol. 2007;29(5):537–43.

Cassart M, Bosson N, Garel C, et al. Fetal intracranial tumors: a review of 27 cases. Eur Radiol. 2008;18(10):2060–6.

Coakley FV, Glenn OA, Qayyum A, et al. Fetal MRI: a developing technique for the developing patient. AJR. 2004;182:243–52.

Desir J, Cassart M, David P, et al. Primary microcephaly with ASPM mutation shows simplified cortical gyration with antero-posterior gradiant pre- and post natally. Am J Med Genet. 2008;146:1439–43.

Dill P, Poretti A, Boltshauser E, et al. Fetal magnetic resonance imaging in midline malformations of the central nervous system and review of the literature. J Neuroradiol. 2009;36(3):138–46.

Doray B, Favre R, Viville B, et al. Prenatal sonographic diagnosis of skeletal dysplasias. A report of 47 cases. Ann Genet. 2000;43:163–9.

Farhataziz N, Engels JE, Ramus RM, et al. Fetal MRI of urine and meconium by gestational age for the diagnosis of genitourinary and gastrointestinal abnormalities. AJR. 2005;184:1891–7.

Foley PT, Sithasanan N, Mc Ewing R, et al. Enteric duplications presenting as antenatally detected abdominal cysts: is delayed resection appropriate? J Pediatr Surg. 2003;38:1810–3.

Garel C, Dreux S, Philippe-Chomette P, et al. Contribution of fetal magnetic resonance imaging and amniotic fluid digestive enzyme assays to the evaluation of gastrointestinal tract abnormalities. Ultrasound Obstet Gynecol. 2006;28(3):282–91.

Guibaud L. Practical approach to prenatal posterior fossa abnormalities using MRI. Pediatr Radiol. 2004;34:700–11.

Guimiot F, Garel C, Fallet-Bianco C, et al. Contribution of diffusion-weighted imaging in the evaluation of diffuse white matter ischemic lesions in fetuses: correlations with fetopathologic findings. AJNR. 2008;29:110–5.

Hill BJ, Bonnie NJ, Qayyum A, et al. Supplemental value of MRI in fetal abdominal disease detected on prenatal sonography: preliminary experience. AJR. 2005;184:993–8.

Huisman TA, Wisser J, Martin E, et al. Fetal magnetic resonance imaging of the central nervous system. Eur Radiol. 2002;12:1952–61.

Hurwitz LM, Yoshizumi T, Reiman RE, et al. Radiation dose to the fetus from MDCT during early gestation. AJR. 2006;186:871–6.

Jani J, Cannie M, Sonigo P, et al. Value of prenatal magnetic resonance imaging in the prediction of post natal outcome in fetuses with diaphragmatic hernia. Ultrasound Obstet Gynecol. 2008;32:793–9.

Kim DH, Chung SW, Vigneron DB, et al. Diffusion-weighted imaging of the fetal brain in vivo. Magn Reson Med. 2008;59:216–20.

Laifer-Narin S, Budorick NE, Simpson LL. Platt LD fetal magnetic resonance imaging: a review. Curr Opin Obstet Gynecol. 2007;19(2):151–6.

Langer JC, Hussain H, Khan A, et al. Prenatal diagnosis of oesophageal atresia using sonography and magnetic resonance imaging. J Pediatr Surg. 2001;36:804–7.

Levine D. Fetal magnetic resonance imaging. J Matern Fetal Neonatal Med. 2004;15(2):85–94.

Ruano R, Molho M, Roume J, Ville Y. Prenatal diagnosis of fetal skeletal dysplasias by combining two-dimensional and three-dimensional ultrasound and intrauterine three-dimensional helical computer tomography. Ultrasound Obstet Gynecol. 2004;24:134–40.

Saguintaah M, Couture A, Veyrac C, et al. MRI of the fetal gastro intestinal tract. Pediatr Radiol. 2002;32:395–404.

Shinmoto H, Kuribayashi S. MRI of fetal abdominal abnormalities. Abdom Imaging. 2003;28:877–86.

Veyrac C, Couture A, Saguintaah M, Baud C. MRI of fetal GI tract abnormalities. Abdom Imaging. 2004;29(4):411–20.

Ultrasound During the Second and Third Trimester

150

Fred E. Avni, Rosine Lejeune, Anne Massez, and Marie Cassart

Introduction

As for any Ultrasound (US) examination, obstetrical US is very dependant on the skill and knowledge of the examinator as well as on the patient "insonation" qualities.

For the latter choosing and optimizing the equipment is essential.

For transabdominal US examination, a curvilinear 3.5–7 MHz transducer is currently used. A vaginal 5–12 MHz probe is used for vaginal examinations.

The equipment must be customized for obstetrical examination including all necessary curves and measurements. Pulsed and Color Doppler are clearly useful tools.

More recently, 3D-4D modes have been applied and provide selective additional information (Benoit and Chaoni 2005).

Properly used, obstetrical US has been proved safe and without any harmful complications for the developing fetus (Torhoni et al. 2009).

The examinations should be performed following a well structured and standardized method. The mother-to-be should be installed comfortably; the examinator should check the reason for examination, features helping establishing the age of the pregnancy, and any other influencing the course of the pregnancy.

The examination should end by a report with clear conclusions and recommendations as useful for the US and clinical follow-up.

Ultrasound Examination of the Second Trimester

Introduction

Even though the first trimester US examination is also intended to detect morphological anomalies, the second trimester examination remains for most professionals "the" morphological examination. It should be as standardized as possible and every sonographer/sonologist knows that he/she has to follow a "check list" in order to fulfill recommendations.

The examination includes three parts: evaluation of (1) the fetal growth (biometry), (2) fetal morphology, and (3) fetal environment. In the vast majority of cases, the examination will be normal and the conclusions reassuring for the parents.

Yet, in about 1% of cases an anomaly will be detected with a wide spectrum of severity (from mild to incompatible with postnatal life).

Once an anomaly is detected, the role of the examinator will be to establish its diagnosis and prognosis by detecting the presence of associated malformations. The antenatal work-up will also define the need for complementary examination and subsequent follow-up of the pregnancy.

Each examination should end by a report that includes clear conclusions and adapted recommendations; so that, the parents can be adequately advised.

F.E. Avni (✉)
Department of Medical Imaging, Erasme Hospital, Brussels, Belgium

R. Lejeune • A. Massez • M. Cassart
Department of Medical Imaging (FEA, AM and MC) and Fetal Medicine (RL), University Clinics of Brussels, Erasme Hospital, Brussels, Belgium

B. Hamm, P. R. Ros (eds.), *Abdominal Imaging*, DOI 10.1007/978-3-642-13327-5_128,
© Springer-Verlag Berlin Heidelberg 2013

Fig. 150.1 Routine measurements. (**a**) Biparietal: transverse scan of the fetal head. The scan displays the septum pellucidum (*) midline and lateral ventricle (*arrow*). The crosses are placed on the external limit and internal limit of the proximal and distal parietal bones. The *dotted line* is intended to measure the cerebral circumference. (**b**) Abdominal circumference: transverse scan of the fetal abdomen through the liver, stomach, and vertebral body (*arrow*). The circumference (*dotted line*) is measured automatically. (**c**) Femur: the femoral diaphysis shaft is measured between crosses; both proximal and distal hypoechoic cartilaginous epiphyses are visualized

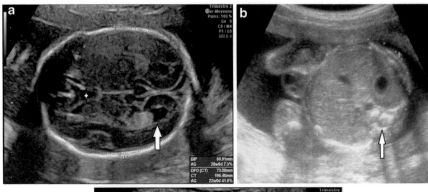

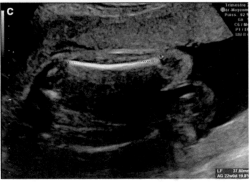

The Sonographic Evaluation of a Normal Second Trimester Pregnancy

Establishing the Fetal Gestational Age

The second trimester examination is performed around 20–22 weeks last menstrual period (LMP). The determination of the gestational age (GA) (in weeks LMP) is easy under the condition that a first trimester examination had been performed and that a GA was established through the measurement of the CRL (Crown–Rump Length), whose error is less than 4 days. Another way of establishing the GA, is to be base its calculation upon the first day of the LMP (only if a precise date is known).

If none of these data is available, the GA can be approximated through the age corresponding to the 50th centile of the abdominal circumference (Verburg et al. 2008; Degani 2001).

Fetal Size and Growth

The evaluation of the fetal size and growth is based on the measurements of:

1. The fetal biparietal diameter: obtained on a transverse scan of the fetal head displaying the midline, the 3rd ventricle and the septum pellucidum complex. The measurement is performed from the external limit of the proximal parietal bone till the internal limit of the distal one (Fig. 150.1a).

2. The abdominal circumference: measured on a transverse scan of the fetal abdomen that displays the stomach, liver, umbilical vein, and a vertebral body (Fig. 150.1b).

3. The femoral diaphyseal length: measured on a sagittal scan of the thigh that displays the entire femoral diaphysis including the cartilaginous epiphysis at each extremity (Fig. 150.1c).

These three measurements are compared to tables that display the expected values for the gestational age and express them in centiles. Normal values are those included between the 10 and 90th centiles. Many supplementary measurements can be performed as needed whenever there is any echographic doubt or a specific requirement (for instance head circumference in case of dolichocephaly) (Fig. 150.1a).

If a first trimester examination had been performed, the growth can be assessed by comparison with this previous examination. Conversely, the second trimester evaluation will be the basis for the examination performed in the third trimester.

Table 150.1 Recommendations (Based on Salomon et al. 2011)

1. Head:
   - Calvarium contours
   - Aspect and size of lateral ventricles
   - Aspect of midline falx
   - Cavum septum pellucidum
   - Aspect of posterior fossa and cerebellum
   - Thalami
2. Face:
   - Both orbits
   - Median profile – nasal bones
   - Upper lip
   - Mouth
3. Chest/Heart:
   - Activity – beats/min
   - Position
   - Four chambers
   - Symmetry of chambers
   - Aortic and pulmonary outflow tract
   - Diaphragm
   - Lungs – echogenicity
4. Abdomen:
   - Position of stomach
   - Aspect of intestines
   - Aspect of abdominal wall/cord insertion site
5. Urinary tract:
   - Aspect and volume of the bladder
   - Localisation, size and appearance of the kidneys
6. Extremities:
   - Presence of four members
   - Three parts to each members
   - Digits
7. Spine: aspects of vertebra on transverse and sagittal views
8. Evaluation of amniotic fluid volume
9. Placenta
   - Appearance
   - Position
10. Umbilical cord: three vessels
11. External Genitalia:
    - Penis – scrotum
    - Labia major and minor

Fetal Morphology

Recommendations have been published by various scientific societies (Salomon et al. 2011). They define the minimal requirements that must be checked during the examination (Table 150.1). For many organs, tables showing the evolution of their size and growth throughout the pregnancy are available and can be used as useful.

For each item there must be a conclusion drawn: "item seen" and "normal."

Head

Many anatomical landmarks (midline, 3rd ventricle, basal ganglia, cavum septum pellucidum) will already be seen on the biparietal axial scan. Slight variations and inclinations around this scan will enable to visualize properly the lateral ventricles (with measurement of the atrium) and the posterior fossa (with the cerebellum and cisterna magna) (Monteguado and Timor-Trisch 2009) (Fig. 150.2a).

A mid sagittal scan is mandatory for the visualization of the corpus callosum (Fig. 150.2b) and a coronal view is helpful for the visualization of the Sylvian fissures.

Face

A superficial frontal view will visualize the continuity of the upperlip and nose/nostrils (Fig. 150.3). Whenever useful a mid sagittal scan will display the fetal nasal bone and fetal profile. 3-D and 4D rendering may easy this visualization (Benoit and Chaoni 2005).

Chest

The lungs are best demonstrated on sagittal scans where they display their typical triangular uniformly echogenic shape. Their echogenicity is (slightly) above the one of the liver and should be the same for both lungs (as seen on a transverse scan).

A lateral sagittal scan allows to verify the diaphragmatic continuity (Blaas and Eik-Nes 2008) (Fig. 150.4).

For the heart, two views are essential: the four chambers view showing the symmetry of the ventricles and aorta and the aorta/pulmonary artery view (Fig. 150.5a, b). Both are obtained on an axial scans. The latter view is slightly above the first one.

The continuity between the left ventricle and aorta must be verified. The position of the pulmonary veins entering the right atrium is another important anatomical item. The heart rate ranges from 120 to 160 beats per minute (Lee et al. 2008).

Abdomen

The stomach is always present to the left of the midline in its normal situation and is easily demonstrated (Fig. 150.1b). Variations in its volume are usual. The small bowel is visualized as slightly echogenic tubular structures occupying a large part of the upper abdomen (Fig. 150.4). Continuity of anterior wall of the abdomen as well as the entrance of the umbilical vessels within the abdomen will confirm the absence of any abdominal wall defect (Blaas and Eik-Nes 2008).

Fig. 150.2 Fetal head.
(**a**) Transverse scan, oblique
compared to Fig. 150.1a,
showing the cerebelluml (*C*)
and posteria fossa. (**b**) Sagittal
scan displaying the corpus
callosum (*arrows*)

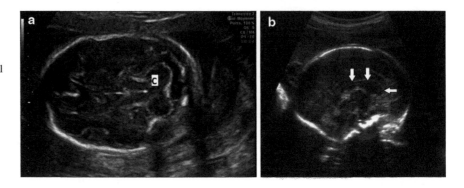

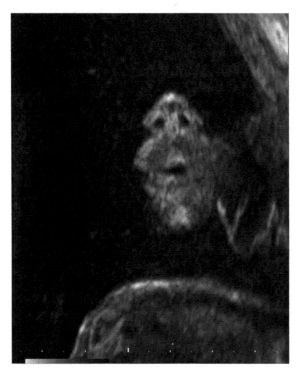

Fig. 150.3 Fetal face. Frontal view through the lips and nostrils

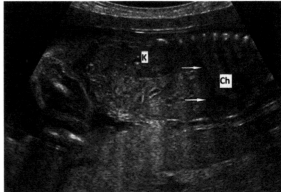

Fig. 150.4 Fetal trunk. Sagittal scan displaying the chest (*Ch*),
hypoechoic curvilinear diaphragm (*arrows*), one kidney (*K*) and
hypoechoic small bowel loops (cystic appearance with
hyperechoic rim)

Urinary Tract

The urinary bladder and the kidneys are important
landmarks. The bladder has a characteristic round
and cystic appearance and is located within the fetal
pelvis (Fig. 150.6), the two umbilical arteries run at
both lateral sides. The kidneys are slightly hyperechoic
and a corticomedullary differentiation (CMD) is
commonly seen (Fig. 150.6). The kidneys are best
demonstrated on parasagittal and axial scans (Blaas
and Eik-Nes 2008).

Extremities

For each extremity, the presence and size of the three
segments must be checked. At this stage, it is easy to
display all digits in hands and feet (Fig. 150.7).

Spine

The evaluation of the spine must be obtained in all
three axis: sagittal, frontal, and transverse in order to
visualize each vertebra, the physiological curvatures
and the continuity of the dorsal skin (Monteguado and
Timor-Trisch 2009) (Fig. 150.8).

Genitalia

The fetal sex can be determined through the visualization of the penis and scrotum in boys (Fig. 150.9), the
labia major and minor in girls (Pinette et al. 2003).

Fig. 150.5 Fetal heart.
(**a**) Four-chambers view.
Typical symmetrical
appearance of the two
ventricles and two atria.
(**b**) Aorta/pulmonary crossing
view. The pulmonary artery
divides and surrounds the
aorta (*arrow*). The lungs
appear laterally as
symmetrical echogenic
masses

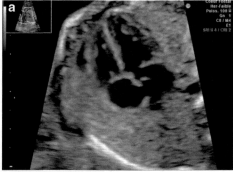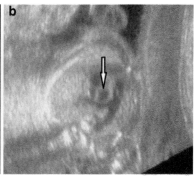

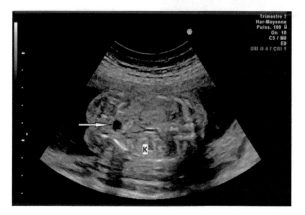

Fig. 150.6 Fetal bladder: sagittal scan of the fetal abdomen.
The bladder appears as a cystic structure (*arrow*). One kidney is
also visualized (*K*)

Fetal Environment and Well-Being

It is important to verify the amount of the amniotic
fluid volume and the placenta localisation
(Fig. 150.10) (normally positioned or low lying). The
amniotic fluid volume is usually evaluated subjectively. The relation of the lower end of the placenta
and the internal cervical should be verified. It should
remain at least 2.5 cms. The closure of the uterine
internal cervix os should be verified.

Fetal well-being is assessed by the demonstration of
its mobility, heart rate swallowing movements, and
micturition (Marino 2004).

Any maternal anatomical abnormality (i.e., ovarian
cyst, fibroid) should be reported as well.

Report and Recommendations

The report must include conclusions about biometry
and morphology, as well as about fetal environment.

Any organ not well seen or any doubt about its
normal appearance should be checked at the subsequent examination.

Abnormal Second Trimester Pregnancy

The second trimester examination can demonstrate
abnormalities in relation with fetal size/growth, or
lead to the discovery of morphological anomalies.

In most cases, complementary procedures will be
necessary in order to demonstrate associated genetic or
infectious anomalies.

Abnormal Size – Growth

Intrauterine Growth Retardation (IUGR) and small
fetal size are defined by a biometry showing measurements below the 10th centile.

IUGR is unusual during the second trimester; therefore, the first step should be to control the GA and the
measurements. If a IUGR is confirmed, this finding
should raise a suspicion of malformative syndrome,
a genetic syndrome or a materno-fetal infection. In
most cases, other anomalies will be present as well
(Ott 2006).

Conversely, macrosomia (above 90th centile), at
this stage is very unusual as well. Maternal diabetes
or genetic syndromes that include overgrow would be
suspected (i.e., Beckwith–Wiedemann).

Abnormal Morphology
Head and Neck

During the second trimester, the most common abnormality of the Central Nervous System (CNS) is
ventriculomegaly defined by a width of the atrial diameter above 10 mm (Fig. 150.11).

A ventriculomegaly can be isolated or associated to
other malformations of the CNS, mainly of the midline
(agenesis of the corpus callosum, Dandy–Walker

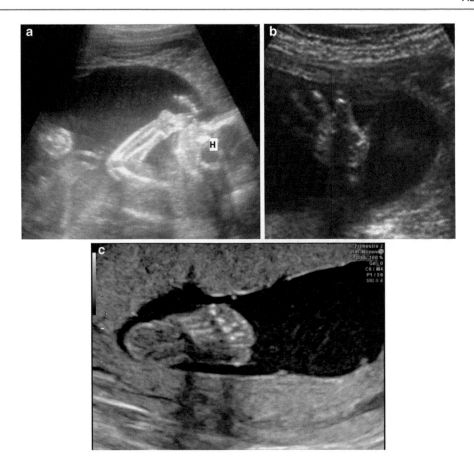

Fig. 150.7 Fetal extremities. (**a**) Foreamen. Scan displays the elbow, radius and cubitus, and wrist (*H* fetal head). (**b**) Hand. (**c**) Foot

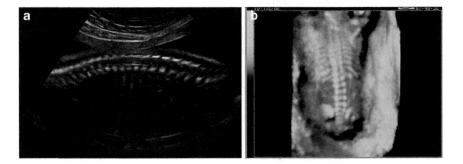

Fig. 150.8 Fetal spine.
(**a**) Sagittal view of the entire spine. (**b**) 3-D rendering

sequence, etc.). A ventriculomegaly can also be related to a feto-maternal infection or to a spinal developmental anomaly (see below).

Agenesis of the corpus callosum can be partial or complete. In such malformation, the ventricles are mainly dilated in the occipital horns. The Dandy-Walker sequence includes a cystic dilatation of the 4th ventricle with an abnormal insertion of the teratonious cerebellum and a (partial) agenesis of the cerebellar vermis. Other anomalies of the CNS include anencephaly,

encephalocele, subarachnoid cyst and very rare second trimester tumors (Garel et al. 2003).

Tumors may be discovered at the level of the neck as well (i.e., cystic lymphangioma or teratoma). Lymphangioma appear as cystic and septated masses. Teratoma contains more echogenic components. They have a high potential of rapid growth and their evolution should be controlled closely. MR Imaging will be necessary to determine the extent of all these anomalies (see below) (Kamil et al. 2008).

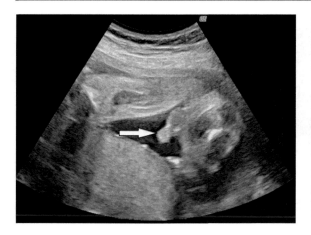

Fig. 150.9 Fetal genitalia. Male sex: the penis and scrotum are visible (*arrow*)

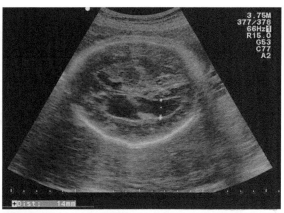

Fig. 150.11 Ventriculomegaly. Transverse scan of fetal head. The lateral ventricle atrium (between *crosses*) measures 14 mm. No other anomaly is visualized

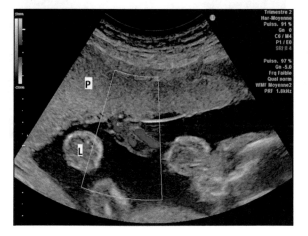

Fig. 150.10 Placenta (*P*), umbilical cord (Color Doppler), and amniotic fluid are displayed. *L* fetal limbs

Facial anomalies should be detected during the second trimester examination. These include cleft palate and facial cleft (uni- or bilateral). They are best seen in axial scans; 3D US help for their assessment (Rotten and Levaillant 2004).

Chest

Anomalies of the chest include bronchopulmonary malformations (BPM), cardiac malformations, diaphragmatic hernia, and pleural effusion.

- BPM include a spectrum of anomalies, the most common being Cystic Adenomatoïd Malformation (CAM), Sequestration (S), and bronchogenic cyst. The latter appears as a unilocular cystic lesion that can be observed everywhere in the chest.

CAM and S appear as an echogenic mass displacing the mediastinal structures (Fig. 150.12a).

Both (mainly CAM) may contain cystic parts. A S will typically display a feeding artery arising from the aorta. In most cases, a spontaneous involution of CAM and S (at least partial) will occur during the development of the pregnancy (Cavoretto et al. 2008) (Fig. 150.12b).

- Cardiac malformations include a wide spectrum of entities.

Not all of them will be diagnosed in utero. The aim of the second trimester examination is to detect the most severe ones that will necessitate emergency management at birth or cases that may be terminated due to their severity. Many will be detected on the four chambers view (Tegmander et al. 2006).

Univentricular heart, small left ventricle, and atrioventricular canal can be easily characterized (Fig. 150.13). Tetratology or Fallot and transposition of great vessels may be more difficult to diagnose.

Rarely cardiac tumors can be diagnosed in utero. They appear as echogenic masses and correspond to rhabdomyoma. These echogenic masses should raise the diagnosis of tuberous sclerosis and induce complementary fetal MR Imaging of the CNS.

Abnormal heart beating may occur without underlying malformation and is usually benign.

- A diaphragmatic hernia is a classical discovery of the second trimester examination through the demonstration of the intrathoracic position of the fetal

Fig. 150.12 Congenital cystic adenomatoid malformation. (**a**) At 22 weeks: transverse scan of fetal chest. The fetal heart (*H*) is displaced by an echogenic mass (*M*) corresponding to the malformation. (**b**) At 32 weeks: the volume of the malformation has dramatically reduced and the heart is back to its midline position

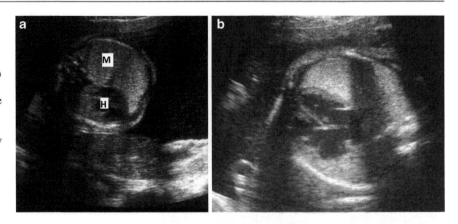

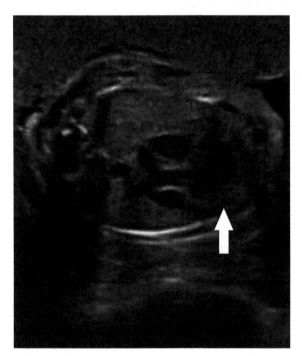

Fig. 150.13 Small left ventricle. Transverse scan of the fetal heart. Four-chamber view. The left ventricle (*arrow*) is clearly smaller

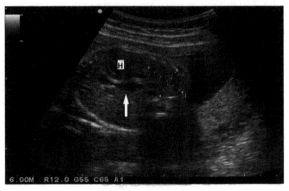

Fig. 150.14 Left diaphragmatic hernia. Transverse scan of the fetal chest. The stomach (*arrow*) and other digestive structures have herniated into the fetal chest. The heart (*H*) is displaced. The measurements drawn correspond to the residual right compressed lung

Fetal Abdomen and Abdominal Wall Malformations

Anomalies of the fetal abdomen detected during the second trimester include the non visualization or a small fetal stomach potentially related to an esophageal atresia, abdominal wall defects and ascitis.

In case of esophageal atresia, the dilated upper pouch may be difficult to visualize (Brantberg et al. 2007). MR Imaging may help. Polyhydramnios will be an associated finding. An intestinal obstruction can be easily overlooked as, there is little amniotic fluid distending the bowel during the second trimester (one exception is the meconium ileus in which the small bowel loops appear clearly hyperechoic) (Shawis and Antao 2006).

Abdominal wall defects include omphalocele (Fig. 150.15) and gastroschisis (laparoschisis). An omphalocele corresponds to the herniation of digestive

stomach (Fig. 150.14) (and/or other abdominal viscera). Once detected, the evaluation of the anomaly must be global (look for other malformations, chromosomal analysis, assessment of pulmonary hypoplasia, . . .) in order to define the potential prognosis. A close follow-up is needed (Gorincour et al. 2006).

– Pleural effusions are also classical findings and usually associated with materno-fetal infection or fetal anemia.

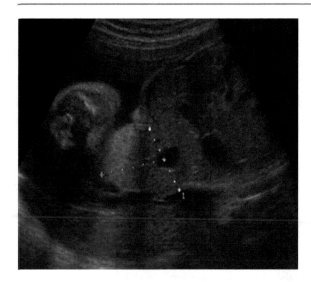

Fig. 150.15 Omphalocele. Transverse scan of the fetal abdomen. A liver herniation is visible (delimited by the *crosses*)

structures or the liver through the umbilical cord. The hernia may be small or large. It is potentially associated with chromosomal anomalies (Martin 1998). A gastroschisis corresponds to a para-umbilical hernia of the small bowel or colon: the bowel loops float freely within the amniotic cavity. It is less commonly associated with genetic anomalies.

Ascitis may be related to materno-fetal infection. It can be associated with pleural effusion and cystic hygroma of the neck.

Bladder and Kidneys Anomalies

Renal malformations are very common; the range of diseases is wide. The kidney may be absent (agenesis), ectopic, dilated, cystic, or dysplastic. The diagnosis of urinary tract dilatation is based on the measurement of the renal pelvis on a transverse scan of the fetal abdomen. Dilatation is considered above 5 mm. Visualizing the ureter is always abnormal (Fig. 150.16a, b).

Renal cysts are unusual at this stage (except multicystic dysplastic kidney) (Fig. 150.17) but cystic kidneys may be observed under the pattern of enlarged echogenic kidneys (see below).

Bladder anomalies include non visualization related to absent urine production (< renal disease) or abnormal bladder morphology (bladder exstrophy) due to non- closure of its anterior wall. The latter is a very important diagnosis since postnatal morbidity is very important. Conversely, the bladder can be too large due to bladder outlet obstruction (i.e., due to posterior urethral valves) (Fig. 150.16c) (Yiee and Wilcox 2008).

Spine and Spinal Canal

The second trimester is an important period for the detection of non-closure of the spinal canal (spina bifida) and other dysraphisms. Spina bifida may express itself under various aspects depending on the type of anomaly and its level. The posterior arch of one or several vertebral body will be absent, the spinal canal wide, and there may or may not be a meningocele associated. Cases without meningocele are more difficult to diagnose. The skin defect must be checked on transverse and sagittal scans (Fig. 150.18).

Depending on the type of anomaly, there will be associated CNS anomalies (Chiari II malformation and/or ventriculomegaly) (Appasamy et al. 2006; Ghi et al. 2006).

Another classical diagnosis is the saccrococcygeal teratoma that appears as a mass of variable size, at the level of the fetal buttocks. The tumor can invade the fetal pelvis and has a great growth potential. It has to be monitored closely (Swamy et al. 2008).

Skeletal Anomalies

The basis for the diagnosis of a skeletal anomaly, especially osteochondrodysplasia, is the length of the femur which is one of the systematic measurements performed during the second trimester examination. This length is expressed in standard deviations from the mean.

A femur at -4SD is highly suspicious for fetal dwarfism. The shorter the femur, the higher the suspicion. In order to precise the diagnosis, further steps include measurements of the other segments of the extremities, shape of long bones (Fig. 150.19), aspect of the spine and skull. The role of the examination would be to differentiate between lethal and non lethal osteochondrodysplasias.

Noteworthy, a small femur can be indicative of IUGR and also of a genetic anomaly.

Other skeletal malformations include amputations anomalies (amniotic band syndrome), segmentation anomalies (polydactyly), or malformations of the extremities (i.e., Clubfoot: the foot and tibia will be seen in the same scan) (Ruano et al. 2004; Digher et al. 2008).

Fig. 150.16 Fetal uropathies.
(**a**) Hydronephrosis –
transverse scan of fetal
abdomen showing marked
unilateral renal dilatation (*).
Arrow indicates vertebra.
(**b**) Dilated ureter (*U*) oblique
view of the fetal abdomen.
(**c**) Oblique view of the fetal
abdomen showing the
distended obstructed bladder
(*B*) (*H* fetal head)

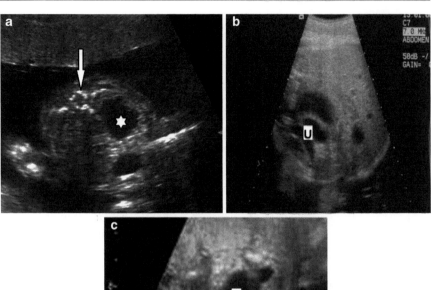

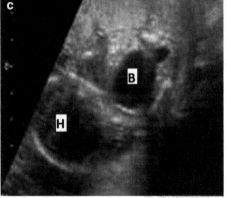

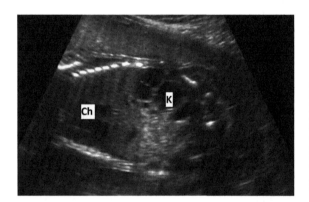

Fig. 150.17 Multicystic dysplastic kidney (MDK). Sagittal
scan of the fetal trunk. A typical MDK (*K*) is visualized. *Ch*
fetal chest

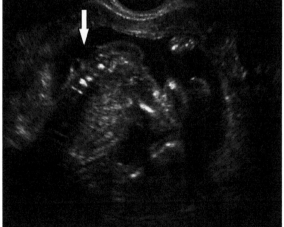

Fig. 150.18 Open spina bifida. Sagittal scan of the fetal buttocks. A small meningocele is visible (*arrow*) (vaginal approach)

Genetic Scan

Many major fetal malformations are in relation
with genetic abnormalities and should prompt a
chromosomalanalysis. There are also many more
subtle abnormalities that are soft markers for
chromosomal anomalies as well. The combination of
several of the soft markers increases the risk
(Table 150.2) (Smith-Bind Man et al. 2007).

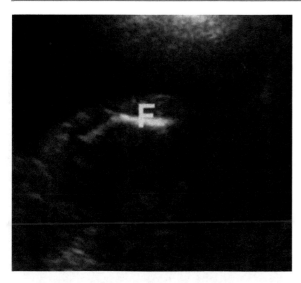

Fig. 150.19 Campometric dysplasia. Typical bowing of the femoral shaft (*F*)

Table 150.2 Genetic scan second trimester

(a) Major signs: → chromosomal analysis mandatory
  – CNS malformation
  – Cardiac malformations
  – Duodenal atresia
  – Omphalocele
  – Thickened nuccal folds
  – Any association of malformations

(b) Minor signs: → combination of two or more minor signs → chromosomal analysis
  – Absence or shortening of the nasal bones
  – Frontal bossing
  – Cardiac echogenic spot
  – Hyperechoic small bowel
  – Sandal gap
  – Short femur or humerus
  – Thick cystic placenta
  – Bilateral pyelectasis

Fetal Environmental Anomalies

Hydramnios is an unusual finding during the second trimester. It may be related to esophageal atresia, diaphragmatic hernia and cardiac malformations. Oligohydramnios can be associated with an IUGR, a major renal malformation or materno-fetal infection.

Management and Recommendations

Once a fetal anomaly has been diagnosed the pregnancy becomes a high risk one.

The work-up and management must then be adapted to the type of anomaly and its severity in order to precise the diagnosis and define the prognosis.

Complementary examinations usually include chromosomal analysis and fetal blood sampling looking for materno-fetal infection. MR Imaging or fetal CT should be performed as necessary (see Chapter M. Cassart).

US follow-up will become an important part of the surveillance of the pregnancy.

Normal and Abnormal Third Trimester Obstetrical Ultrasound Examination

Introduction

The sonographic examination that is performed during the third trimester (around 32 weeks) is very important: on one hand, it is (should be) the continuation of the one performed during the second trimester and therefore intended to verify the good evolution of the pregnancy; on the other, it is an examination by itself and as such, it has to be conducted as systematic and detailed as the second trimester one.

At this stage, the sonographic evaluation of the pregnancy must again include a part of measurements, an evaluation of the fetal morphology, and well-being as well as an assessment of the fetal environment (placenta, amniotic fluid volume, and cervix length).

The aims of the third trimester examination are therefore to assess normal development, to detect abnormal intrauterine growth, fetal malformations, and abnormal placentation.

In case of the detection of an abnormality (growth, morphology, or environment), the examination will evolve from a screening test to the work-up and management of a pregnancy at risk with potentially increased perinatal morbidity or mortality. The sonographic follow-up will be an essential tool for the surveillance of such pregnancies.

The Sonographic Evaluation of a Normal Third Trimester Pregnancy

Fetal Gestational Age

The determination of the fetal gestational age (GA) is calculated on the basis of the second trimester examination conclusions.

If the exact GA is not available, it must be estimated on the basis of the combination of the different measurements obtained. The US examination is most usually performed using a transabdominal approach. It should first verify fetal mobility and heart beating rate.

Fetal Lye

The examination evaluates fetal lye in the maternal uterus (cephalic, breech, or transverse presentation).

Fetal Growth

The evaluation of the normal fetal growth and size is assessed through measurements (similar to the second trimester) of the fetal biparietal diameter, abdominal circumference, and femoral length. All these measurements should be performed on appropriate and meticulous fetal scans, very similar to those performed in the second trimester.

The measurements must be compared to expected values for the gestational age and expressed in percentiles. They are considered within normal values if they are included between the 10th and 90th percentiles. Several complementary measurements can be performed whenever necessary.

If possible, the normality of fetal growth/size must be confirmed by comparison with the second trimester conclusions.

The fetal weight is determined by integrating several of these measurements and is visually measured automatically by the US equipment (Verburg et al. 2008; Deganis 2001).

Fetal Morphology

The sonographer or sonologist must comply with recommendations in order to fulfill the aims of the examination. As mentioned, several scientific societies have published lists of organs that must be imperatively visualized during the examination (Table 150.1).

For each item, the structure must not only be visualized, but also defined as normal by the examinator (Salomon et al. 2011).

Head and Face

Similarly to the second trimester, axial, sagittal, and frontal views are necessary.

An axial scan is mainly useful to visualize the midline complex, lateral ventricles, the posterior fossa, and Sylvian fissures; sagittal scans are useful to visualize the corpus callosum and lateral ventricles. Frontal views may be useful for assessing the correct operculation of the

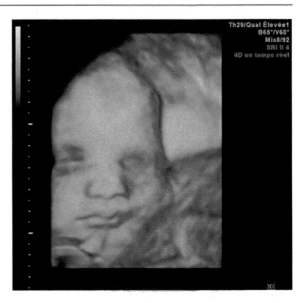

Fig. 150.20 3-D surface rendering of the fetal face

Sylvian fissures (Monteguado and Timor-Trisch 2009). Transvaginal examination may be useful in selected cases (vertex or very low cephalic presentation).

The fetal face should be examined as completely as possible: including the upper lip and nostrils (on axial scan) as well as the fetal profile (on a sagittal scan) (Benoit and Chaoni 2005). 3-D-4D rendering is helpful as well (Fig. 150.20).

Chest

Sagittal and transverse scans aim to assess the form and echogenecity of the lungs; the diaphragm must be visualized entirely (see Fig. 150.13b). The heart and mediastinal vessels must be controlled (four chambers view, crossing vessels/aorta/pulmonary artery) as defined during the second trimester (Blaas and Eik-Nes 2008; Lee et al. 2008).

Abdomen

The visualization of the stomach is an essential landmark, the intestine (filled with liquid), the colon (filled with hypoechoic meconium), and liver are easily demonstrated (Fig. 150.21).

The kidneys display a characteristic C.M. differentiation, they can be measured; the renal cortex should not be more echogenic than the liver after 32 weeks. The bladder is another normal landmark of pelvis, it is relatively large especially in girls when the filling/emptying cycle is slowing (Blaas and Eik-Nes 2008) (Fig. 150.22).

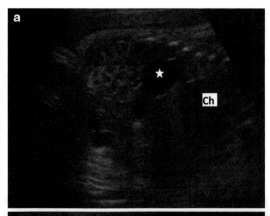

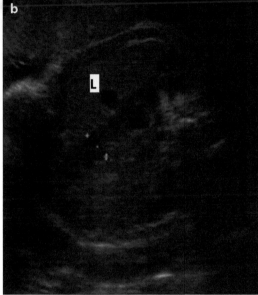

Fig. 150.21 Fetal digestive tract. (**a**) Small bowel and stomach. Oblique view of the fetal abdomen. The stomach (*) is visualized above the small bowel filled with fluid. *Ch* fetal chest. (**b**) Transverse colon (between *crosses*) filled with hypoechoic meconium (*L* liver)

Spine and Skeletal Systems

The spine should be displayed in its entire length, verifying the normal curvatures, the position, and integrity of each vertebra. The various long bones of the upper and lower limbs should be visualized, the hands and feet are more difficult to assess at this stage (Monteguado and Timor-Trisch 2009).

Fetal Gender

The fetal sex can be confirmed easily through the visualization of the penis and scrotum or the labia major and minor and uterus (Pinette et al. 2003) (Fig. 150.23).

Fetal Environment and Well-Being

The biometrical and morphological evaluations must be completed by the assessment of fetal well-being and environment.

Well-being is globally evaluated through demonstration of the fetal mobility, heart beating rate, swallowing, eye movements, and micturition (Marino 2004).

Fetal environment assessment includes evaluation of the amniotic fluid volume (the amniotic fluid volume can be assessed through measuring the fluid compartments within the amniotic pouches punch), placental insertion (the placenta lower end should be at more than 25 mm from internal os), and cervical length measurement (it should be above 32 mm length) (Fig. 150.24).

Abnormal Third Trimester Pregnancy

Abnormal Growth

The fetal growth is a dynamic process customized to each fetus that progress during the entire duration of the pregnancy, alternating periods of rapid and slower growth.

There are many factors that intervene to ensure normal growth some are related to fetal environment, other to the placentar–fetal complex or to maternal features. Furthermore, some genetic factors influence growth as well (i.e., familial shortness).

All must be considered when evaluating the fetal growth.

Detecting abnormal growth patterns is one among the most important aims of obstetrical ultrasound examination as both growth retardation and macrosomia are associated with increased perinatal morbidity and mortality (Ott 2006).

Intrauterine Growth Retardation (IUGR)

IUGR is defined by fetal measurements below the 10th centile for gestational age especially for the abdominal circumference. Most usually, IUGR is detected during the third trimester. Growth retardation is easier to detect when the growth profile of the fetus had been assessed by US during the 2d trimester and when the third trimester measurements show that growth follows abnormal centiles curves.

IUGR can be asymmetrical (sparing the cerebral – biparietal diameter – growth) or symmetrical

Fig. 150.22 Urinary tract. (a) Fetal bladder (*B*). Sagittal scan of the fetal abdomen. (b) Kidney. Sagittal scan showing the kidney (*K*) with a typical corticomedullary differentiation. The scan displays the echogenic lung (*L*) and the hypoechoic diaphragm (*arrows*)

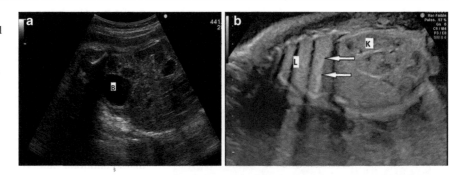

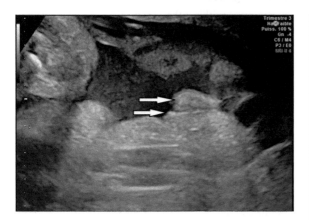

Fig. 150.23 Fetal genitalia. Female labia major (*arrows*)

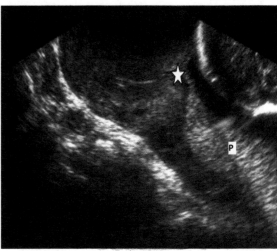

Fig. 150.24 Low insertion of a posterior placenta endovaginal approach. The hyperechoic placenta (*P*) abuts the internal os (*)

(involving the whole fetus). Cases with symmetrical IUGR (and those detected during the second trimester) carry a poorer prognosis and have an increased perinatal morbidity–mortality rates (Ott 2006).

Doppler analysis has been shown to be of great interest for the detection of an IUGR in a population at risk (i.e., those with previous IUGR); its yield has not been demonstrated in a low risk population. Using pulsed Doppler at the level of the various vessels of the feto-maternal circulation, the resistive index (RI) can be measured.

The Doppler analysis is classically performed at the level of the uterine arteries. The presence of a prediastolic notch after 26 weeks favors the diagnosis of IUGR.

Doppler evaluation will be essential not only for the initial evaluation but also for the prognosis of the IUGR during follow-up examinations.

Once detected a global evaluation of the fetus as well as complementary examinations (chromosomalanalysis, fetal blood sampling...) are necessary in order to determine the etiology of the IUGR.

For the follow-up, US examinations must be perfomed every 2 weeks to verify fetal growth and the evolution of the Doppler indices particularly at the level of the umbilical, and anterior cerebral arteries. A progressive increase of the RI (above 0.8) or even a reverse diastolic flow at the level of the umbilical artery are factors suggesting increased perinatal risk and could induce earlier extraction.

Measuring the biometry every 15 days and assessment of fetal well-being will be essential as well (Urban et al. 2007).

Macrosomia

Macrosomia is defined by an abdominal circumference above the 90th centile some consider the 95th centile (or even the 97th centile) or above an estimated weight of 4,000 g. The fetal weight can be estimated through a formula combining biparietal, AC and fetal length. Nowadays, an estimated weight is automatically calculated by most equipments.

Fig. 150.25 Fetal CNS tumor. Transverse scan of the fetal head. There is a large heterogeneous mass (*M*) in the midline (= teratoma)

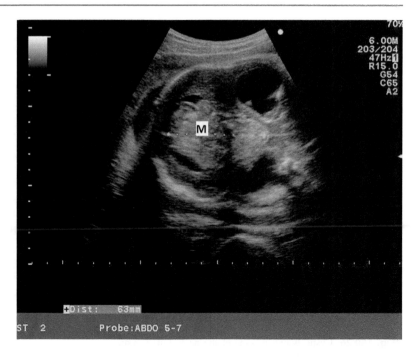

Macrosomia is clearly associated with maternal diabetes; the origin may be genetic and there may be associated overgrowth syndromes (like Beckwith–Wiedemann Syndrome).

Fetuses with macrosomia will be followed by US to determine the best timing of delivery.

Abnormal Morphology

Most major malformation would have been detected during the second trimester and the third trimester examination is intended to monitor their evolution. Some malformations could have been overlooked and detected only during the third trimester examination (yet, on the basis of the same characteristics as during the second trimester).

Still for some, the detection and characterization of an anomaly will be easier during the third trimester examination.

Head and Neck

During the third trimester, a ventricular dilatation is also defined by an atrial measurement above 10 mm. The dilatation can be isolated or combined with other CNS malformations especially midline or posterior fossa malformations (Garel et al. 2003). Microcephaly is an important diagnosis of the third trimester and should be considered if the cerebral circumference measures <P3 for the gestational age.

Most cerebral tumors and vascular malformations will be detected only during the third trimester. Tumors will act as a space occupying lesion and will have devastating compressive consequences on the developing brain. Teratomas and glioblastomas are the most common (yet rare) tumors. Their prognosis is poor (Fig. 150.25).

Vascular malformations (Galen vein aneurysm) will also have devastating consequences on the developing brain. Color Doppler analysis is mandatory for their evaluation.

Cerebral hemorrhage can occur at any GA and may determine parenchymal destruction and subsequent ventricular dilatation. Hemorrhage appears as en echogenic mass that should not be misinterpreted as tumor. Fetal MR Imaging will be helpful for the differential diagnosis.

Cerebral lesions secondary to materno-fetal infection are variable in appearance. On US examination, they may appear as calcifications, parenchymal lesions, gyration anomalies, and ventricular dilatation (Kamil et al. 2008).

Orofacial tumors (lymphangioma or teratoma) are important to diagnose and follow-up as these tumors may grow considerably during the third trimester and prevent normal birth (EXIT procedure). They display a mixed pattern with echogenic and cystic parts (Digher et al. 2011) (Fig. 150.26).

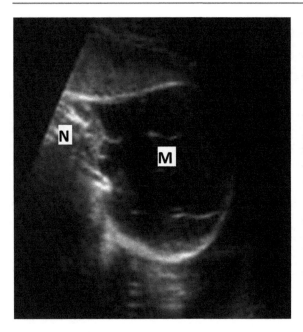

Fig. 150.26 Cystic lymphangioma of the neck. Large cystic septated mass (*M*) at the lateral part of the neck (*N*)

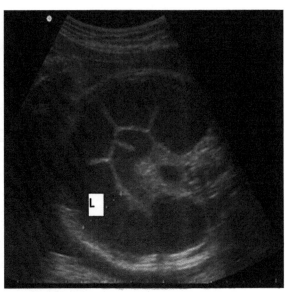

Fig. 150.28 Intestinal obstruction. Transverse scan of the fetal abdomen showing distended bowel loops (*L*)

Chest

During the third trimester, the bronchopulmonary malformations usually reduce in size and may even not be detectable anymore; this does not necessarily mean that they have completely disappear and a postnatal assessment is still mandatory (Fig. 150.13b). On the contrary, some thoracic tumors may grow and determine mediastinal shift and/or ana-sarca (i.e., teratoma or lymphangioma). They also will need a close follow- up (Cavoretto et al. 2008).

Cardiac malformations may be more difficult to assess due to fetal lye. The features of a malformation are the same as in the second trimester. The presence of cardiomegaly would be a sign of heart failure (Tegmander et al. 2006).

Pleural effusion may be part of fetal hydrops, infection, and chylothorax.

Abdomen

Intestinal obstruction is diagnosed mainly during the third trimester rather than in the second trimester as the obstructed intestine progressively dilates; yet, the level of obstruction is not necessarily obvious and fetal MR Imaging may be necessary to locate this level. Most cases correspond to duodenal atresia, to small bowel atresia and obstruction associated or not to meconium peritonitis (Shawis and Antao 2006) (Fig. 150.28).

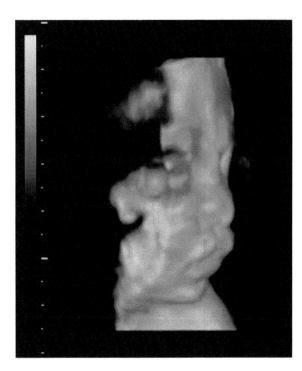

Fig. 150.27 Upper lip cleft assessed by 3-D surface rendering US

Upper lip and soft palate malformations can be discovered during the third trimester helped by 3D-US (Fig. 150.27).

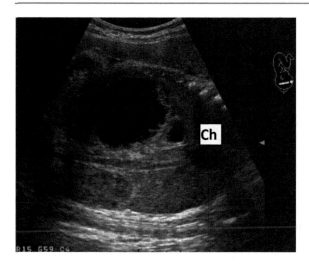

Fig. 150.29 Fetal ovarian cyst. Transverse/oblique scan of the fetal abdomen showing a large cystic mass. *Ch* fetal chest

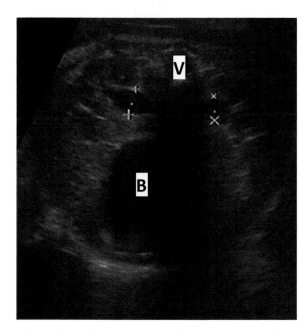

Fig. 150.30 Fetal reflux. Transverse scan of the fetal abdomen shows bilateral renal dilatation (the renal pelves are measured between the *crosses*) and enlarged bladder (*B*). *V* vertebra

Table 150.3 Urinary tract malformations

1. Ureteropelvic junction obstruction
2. Ureterovesical junction obstruction
3. Vesicoureteric reflux
4. Posterior uretral valves
5. Renal duplication
6. MDKD

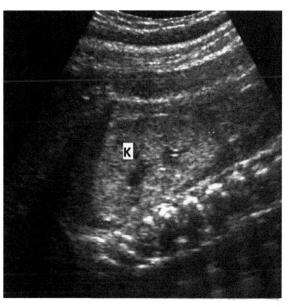

Fig. 150.31 Polycystic recessive kidney disease. Sagittal scan of a kidney (both were affected). The kidney (*K*) appears hyperechoic without corticomedullary differentiation

dilatation is defined by a renal pelvis AP diameter above 7 mm, a visible ureter or an enlarged bladder (Fig. 150.30). The differential diagnosis will be based on the demonstration of the level of obstruction and the status of the renal parenchyma (Dahmen-Elias et al. 2005; Feldman et al. 2001) (Table 150.3). The kidneys can also be affected by various congenital cystic diseases determining renal enlargement and parenchymal hyperechogenicity (Fig. 150.31).

The differential diagnosis will be based upon the US patterns and familial history (Table 150.4) (Avni and Hall 2010).

Spine and Spinal Canal

Spinal malformations are more difficult to demonstrate during the third trimester. Occasionally, spina bifida or vertebral segmentation anomalies would be depicted on US but they will be better characterized on MRI and fetal CT.

Cystic tumor or tumor-like conditions may develop in the fetal abdomen; in girls, an ovarian cyst is the main diagnosis to consider during the third trimester (Fig. 150.29). In boys, duplication or mesenteric cysts are the main diagnosis to consider (Hyett 2008; Heiling et al. 2002).

Urinary tract anomalies are among the most common malformations detected in utero. Urinary tract

Table 150.4 Differential diagnosis of hyperechoic kidneys

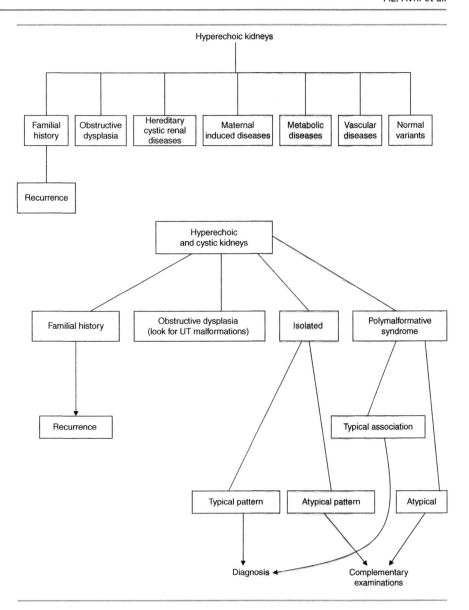

As mentioned above, the diagnosis and the growth of a sacrococcygeal teratoma would be important to follow during the third trimester as it may enlarge dramatically and induce perinatal complication (Fig. 150.32).

The mass is usually large with a wide spectrum of the US appearances from completely cystic and septated to diffusely echogenic. The intrapelvic component may be difficult to objectivate by US and MR imaging is helpful (Swamy et al. 2008).

Skeletal System

The femoral length measurement is again the basis for the detection of a skeletal malformation. Other features leading to such detection are bones deformities, spinal anomalies, chest/abdomen discrepancies, and "depressible cranium."

The main feature is the so-called short femur. Most authors consider a short femur as a measurement below P5. The diagnosis during the third trimester is more difficult to differentiate. First, a short femur can correspond to a constitutional short femur (familial). Second, a short femur can be associated with an IUGR.

Lastly, a short or a very short femur can result from various osteochondrodysplasia, most of which would have been detected during the second trimester examination.

Fig. 150.32 Sacrococcygeal teratoma. (**a**) Sagittal scan. A large cystic mass (*M*) has developped at the extremity of the sacrococcygeal spine (*arrow*). (**b**) Transverse/oblique scan. The cystic tumor extends towards the posterior fetal pelvis

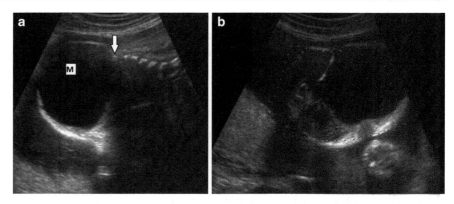

One diagnosis that may typically become obvious only during the third trimester is. Achondroplasia where the shortening of the femur becomes obvious after 28 weeks.

In complex cases of other osteo-chondrodysplasia, a precise diagnosis will not be established in utero by US and CT may help.

External Genitalia Anomalies

In the male fetus, a hydrocele or undescended testis should not be considered as abnormal. Hypospadias can be detected due to shortening of the penis and widening of its end. As an isolated finding, it does not carry a poor diagnosis.

In the female fetus, the labia major or/and minor may appear physiologically large and should not be misinterpreted as a sign of ambiguous genitalia.

In case of well demonstrated ambiguous genitalia, the adrenals should be verified in order to demonstrate hypertrophy associated to adenogenital syndrome.

Abnormal Environment

The Placenta and Cord

The placenta insertion is an important part of the third trimester examination. A placenta praevia is defined by a lower limit below 2.5 cms distance of the internal os.

A marginal placenta abuts the inner opening of cervix, and a central praevia covers the entire internal os with no free way to a normal delivery. The mother bladder should be filled in order to optimize the visualization of the lower limit of the placenta. In selected cases, a vaginal approach should be necessary.

The cord insertion on the placenta should also be checked; peripheral (velamentous) insertion carriers an increased risk of bleeding during delivery.

Abnormal placentations are other conditions necessitating skill and complementary examinations such as fetal MR Imging.

A placental hematoma is an acute condition necessitating prompt extraction. It will not be always demonstrated in US (Bauer and Bonanno 2009).

Abnormal Fluid Volume

Polyhydramnios can be associated with numerous malformations especially intestinal obstruction but is primary in over 90% of cases.

Oligohydramnios is related to be IUGR or abnormal fetal urine production.

Report and Recommendations

At the end of the examination, the sonologist or sonographer should provide a complete and comprehensive report of what was assessed.

The conclusions can be:
- All items were seen, the growth is normal.
- All items were not seen: should be checked.
- Growth is abnormal: to be controlled.
- An abnormality has been found: to be controlled after birth or to be controlled in utero.
- Complementary work-up needed.

The Case of Twin Pregnancies

Twin pregnancies necessitate special surveillance as they have an increased risk for malformations and complications. The complications are related to vascular anastomosis between umbilical vessels within the placenta. Determining chorionicity is important and is usually achieved during the first trimester examination.

Once a twin pregnancy has been diagnosed; US has an important role for its surveillance.

Twin fetuses should grow at the same rate up to 30 weeks.

Afterwards, a discrepancy may develop.

Complications are higher in monochorionic and mortality has been reported as high as 30–70% pregnancies.

Major complications include the twin–twin transfusion syndrome where there is an asymmetry in the twin growth (over 20% difference) and oligohydramnios in one fetus.

Another complication is related to fetal death in utero and eventually ischemic lesions in the survivor.

The increased risk necessitates a closer surveillance and potentially an early extraction (Monteguado and Roman 2005).

References

Appasamy M, Roberts D, Pilling D, Buxton N. Antenatal US and MR imaging in localizing the level of lesion in spina bifida with postnatal outcome. Ultrasound Obstet Gynecol. 2006;27:530–6.

Avni FE, Hall M. Renal cystic diseases: new concepts. Pediatr Radiol. 2010;40:939–46.

Bauer ST, Bonanno C. Abnormal placentation. Semin Perinatol. 2009;33:88–96.

Benoit B, Chaoni R. Development in 3-D US in obstetrics. Ultrasound Obstet Gynecol. 2005;26:309–15.

Blaas HG, Eik-Nes SH. US development of the normal foetal thorax and abdomen across gestation. Prenat Diagn. 2008;28:568–80.

Brantberg A, Blaas HGK, Hansen SE, Eik-Nes SH. Oesophageal obstruction: detection rate and outcome. Ultrasound Obstet Gynecol. 2007;30:180–7.

Cavoretto P, Molina F, Poggi S, Davenport M, Nicolaides KH. Prenatal diagnosis and outcome of echogenic fetal lung lesions. Ultrasound Obstet Gynecol. 2008;32:769–83.

Dahmen-Elias HA, Dejong TL, Stigler RH, Visser GH, Stontenbeek PH. Congenital renal tract anomalies: outcome and follow-up 40% cases detected between 1986 and 2002. Ultrasound Obstet Gynecol. 2005;25:134–43.

Degani S. Fetal biometry; clinical, pathological and technical considerations. Obstet Gynecol Surv. 2001;56:159–67.

Digher M, Fligner C, Chang E, Waner E, Dubinsky T. Fetal skeletal dysplasia: an approach to diagnosis with illustrate cases. Radiographics. 2008;28:1061–77.

Digher MK, Peterson SE, Dunbrinsky TJ, Perkins J, Cheng E. EXIT procedure: technique and indications with prenatal imaging parameters for assessment of airway patency. Radiographics. 2011;31:511–26.

Feldman DM, De Cambre M, Kong E, Bongida A, Jamil M, Mc Kerma P, Egan JF. Evaluation and follow-up of fetal hydronephrosis. J Ultrasound Med. 2001;20:1065–9.

Garel C, Luton D, Oury JF, Gressens P. Ventricular dilatations. Childs Nerv Syst. 2003;19:517–23.

Ghi T, Pilu G, Falco P. Prenatal diagnosis of open and closed spina bifida. Ultrasound Obstet Gynecol. 2006;28:899–903.

Gorincour G, Bouvenot J, Maurot MG, Chaumoire K, Garel C, Guibaud L, Rypens F, Avni F, Cassart M, Mangez-Laulone B, Brunelle F, Durand C, Eurin D. Prenatal diagnosis of congenital diaphragmatic hernia using MR imaging measurement of fetal lung volume. Ultrasound Obstet Gynecol. 2006;26:738–44.

Heiling KS, Chaoni R, Kirchmair F, Stadie S, Bollmann R. Fetal ovarian cysts: prenatal diagnosis, management and post-natal outcome. Ultrasound Obstet Gynecol. 2002;20:47–50.

Hyett J. Intra-abdominal masses: prenatal differential diagnosis and management. Prenat Diagn. 2008;28:645–55.

Kamil D, Tepelman J, Berg C, Herp A, Axt Fliedner R, Gembuch V, Geipel AI. Spectrum and outcome of prenatally diagnosed fetal tumors. Ultrasound Obstet Gynecol. 2008;31:296–302.

Lee W, Allan JS, Carvalho R, Chaani R, Copel J, Devore G, Hechner K, Munoz H, Nelson T, Paladinis D, Yagel S. ISVOG consensus statement: What constitute a fetal echocardiogram. Ultrasound Obstet Gynecol. 2008;32:239–42.

Marino T. US abnormalities of the amniotic fluid, membranes umbilical cord and placenta. Obstet Gynecol Clin North Am. 2004;31:177–200.

Martin RW. Screening for fetal abdominal wall defects. Obstet Gynecol Clin North Am. 1998;25:517–26.

Monteguado A, Roman AS. US in multiple gestations: twin and other multifetal pregnancies. Clin Perinatol. 2005;32:329–54.

Monteguado A, Timor-Trisch TE. Normal US development of the CNS from the 2nd trimester awards using 2D, 3D and transvaginal US. Prenat Diagn. 2009;29:316–99.

Ott WJ. US diagnosis of fetal growth restriction. Clin Obstet Gynecol. 2006;49:295–307.

Pinette MG, Wax JR, Blackstone J, Cartin P. Normal growth and development of fetal external genitalia demonstrated by US. J Clin Ultrasound. 2003;31:465–72.

Rotten D. Levaillant JM 2D and 3D US assessment of fetal face. Ultrasound Obstet Gynecol. 2004;24;402–11.

Ruano R, Molto M, Roume J, Ville Y. Prenatal diagnosis of fetal skeletal dysplasias by combining 2D and 3D US and intrauterine 3D helical CT. Ultrasound Obstet Gynecol. 2004;24:134–40.

Salomon LJ, Alfirevic Z, Berghella V, Bilando C, Hernandez-Andrade E, Johnsen SR, Kelache K, Leing KY, Malinger G, Mung H, Prefuno F, Toi A, Leer W. Practice guidelines for performance of the routine mid trimester fetal US scan. Ultrasound Obstet Gynecol. 2011;37:116–26.

Shawis R, Antao B. Prenatal bowel dilatation and the subsequent post-natal management. Early Hum Dev. 2006;82:297–303.

Smith-Bind Man R, Chu P, Goldberg JD. 2D trimester prenatal US for the detection of pregnancies at increased risk of Down syndrome. Prenat Diagn. 2007;27:235–544.

Swamy R, Embelton N, Hale J. Saccrococcygeal teratoma over two decades in birth prevalence, prenatal diagnosis and clinical outcomes. Prenat Diagn. 2008;28:1048–51.

Tegmander E, Williams W, Johansen OJ, Blaas HG, Eik-Nes SH. Prenatal detection of heart defects in a non-selected population of 30,149 fetuses: detection rates and outcomes. Ultrasound Obstet Gynecol. 2006;27:252–65.

Torhoni MR, Vedmedovska N, Merialdi M, Betran AR, Allen T, Gonzales R, Platt LD. Safety of US in pregnancy: who systematic review of the literature and meta-analysis. Ultrasound Obstet Gynecol. 2009;33:599–608.

Urban G, Vergain P, Ghidini A, Tortoli P, Ricci S, Patrizio P, Poidas MJ. State of the art: non invasive US assessment of the uteroplacental circulation. Semin Perinatol. 2007; 31:232–9.

Verburg BO, Steegers EAP, De Ridder M, Snijders RJM, Smith E, Hofman A, Moll HA, Jaddoe VWV, Wittemans JCM. New charts for US dating of pregnancy and assessment of fetal growth: longitudinal data from a population-based cohort study. Ultrasound Obstet Gynecol. 2008;31:388–96.

Yiee J, Wilcox D. Abnormalities of the fetal bladder. Semin Fetal Neonatal Med. 2008;13:164–70.

Ultrasound of the Fetus During the First Trimester

151

Mona Massoud, Jérôme Massardier, and Laurent Guibaud

Introduction

Ultrasound (US) examination at 11–14 weeks of gestation aims to confirm the gestational age, determinate chorionicity for multiple pregnancies, measure the nuchal translucency (NT) thickness to assess the risk of aneuploidy, and to visualize the basic anatomical structures of the fetus (Guidelines of the Fetal Medicine Foundation, London; http://www.fetalmedicine.com). Despite the lack of clear checklist for the ultrasound examination of the fetal anatomy, during the first trimester, several studies have described in great details the evolving anatomy of the fetus during this period. For transabdominal examination, a curvilinear 3.5–7 MHz is used; nevertheless, the vaginal 5–12 MHz transducer is currently used during the first trimester. Pulsed and Color Doppler are useful tools. Three-dimensional (3D) modes have been applied; its use is subject to a considerable heterogeneity (Ioannou et al. 2012).

First Trimester Ultrasound Examination

Determining Gestational Age (GA)

In a patient with a 28-day cycle, the GA is established on the first day of the last normal menstrual period. Embryologic dating begins with conception, 2 weeks later than the first day of the normal menstrual period. However, calculating GA on the basis of menstrual history is often risky since individual variations exist in the time of ovulation during the cycle. Thus, Robinson and Fleming in 1975 proposed the determination of the GA from the measurement of the Crown Rump Length (CRL) of the fetus with +/− 4.7 days of error, for the period covering 6–14 weeks' gestation. The maximal straight-line length is currently measured and one should use the average CRL measurements from three satisfactory images (Fig. 151.1). Then, the measurement is referred to published tables for estimation of GA. In women with unknown dates or when there is a difference greater than 7 days between the menstrual and ultrasound age, it is profitable to date the pregnancy by CRL. Once the gestational age is established, it should never be changed based on the measurements made later in pregnancy.

The measurement of the fetal Biparietal Diameter (BPD) and the abdominal circumference (AC) can be used for the determination of the GA, but these measurements are not more accurate than the CRL.

M. Massoud • J. Massardier
Center of Fetal Medicine, Hospital Femme Mère Enfant, Univeristé Claude Bernard, Lyon 1, France

L. Guibaud (✉)
Center of Fetal Medicine, Hospital Femme Mère Enfant, Univeristé Claude Bernard, Lyon 1, France

Department of Pediatric and Fetal Imaging, Hospital Femme Mère Enfant, Univeristé Claude Bernard, Lyon 1, France

B. Hamm, P. R. Ros (eds.), *Abdominal Imaging*, DOI 10.1007/978-3-642-13327-5_127,
© Springer-Verlag Berlin Heidelberg 2013

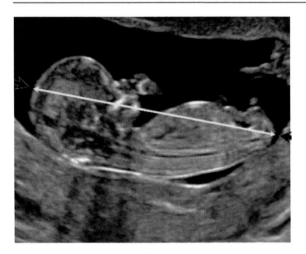

Fig. 151.1 Measurement of the crown rump length

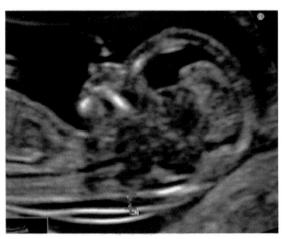

Fig. 151.2 Measurement of the nuchal translucency

Nuchal Translucency Screening for Trisomy 21 (Down Syndrome)

Nuchal translucency (NT) measurement has been established as the best imaging assessment for chromosomal abnormalities, thus making the 11–14 weeks gestation the first detailed US examination of the fetus (Snijders et al. 1998). NT refers to the normal subcutaneous fluid-filled space between the back of the fetal neck and the overlying skin. This space is normally small, and can be significantly increased in fetuses with Down syndrome. It is possible to obtain an accurate measurement of NT in the vast majority of fetuses between 10 and 14 weeks' gestation (CRL of 36–84 mm). The measurement requires optimal technique focusing on the following criteria (Abuhamad 2005) (Fig. 151.2):

- The fetus should be imaged in the midsagittal plane, ideally with the fetal spine down.
- The image should be adequately magnified so that only the fetal head, neck, and upper thorax fill the viewable area.
- The fetal neck should be neutral, with care being taken to avoid measurements in the hyperflexion or hyperextension positions.
- The skin of the fetal back should be clearly differentiated from the underlying amniotic membranes, either by visualizing separate echogenic lines or by noting that the skin lines move with the fetus.

- Measurement calipers should be placed on the inner borders of the echolucent space and should be perpendicular to the long axis of the fetus.
- Ultrasound and transducer settings should be optimized to ensure clarity of the image and in particular, the borders of the nuchal space.

There is a direct correlation between increasing NT and risk for Down syndrome, other aneuploidies, major structural malformations (mainly cardiac malformations), and adverse pregnancy outcomes.

Septated cystic hygroma corresponds to an enlarged NT extended along the entire length of the fetus and in which septations are clearly visible. It is highly associated to fetal aneuploidy or major structural fetal malformations.

Researches in first trimester have shown that pregnancies with fetal Down syndrome are associated with altered levels of certain maternal serum markers including elevated levels of total hCG and of the free β subunit of hCG (with a median multiple of the median (MoM) of 1.83 in affected cases) and lower levels of pregnancy-associated plasma protein A (with a median MoM of 0.38 in affected cases). A combined serum and sonographic screening protocol is proposed actually, with detection rates of 87%, 85%, and 82% at 11, 12, and 13 weeks' gestation respectively for a false-positive rate of 5% (FaSTER study, Malone et al. 2005).

Indeed, when the estimated risk of trisomy 21 is estimated as high, the parents are counseled, and an

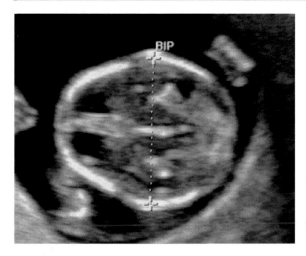

Fig. 151.3 Biparietal diameter measured on a transverse axial plane of the head

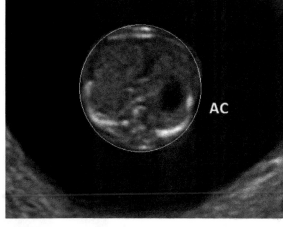

Fig. 151.4 Abdominal circumference

invasive diagnostic test, chorionic villus sampling or amniocentesis is proposed to assess the fetal karyotype.

Fetal Anatomy

Fetal Biometry

Although the measurement of the CRL is the most accurate parameter to determine the GA, the evaluation of the fetal growth can be assessed by the measurement of the following parameters:

- Biparietal diameter (BPD) is measured on a transversal axial plane of the fetus head, showing the falx cerebri, the third ventricle and the septum pellucidum complex. The cursors are positioned in the middle of near calvarial wall to middle of far calvarial wall (Fig. 151.3).
- Head circumference (HC) is measured in the same axial plane of the BPD, the cursors are positioned on the outer edge of the near calvarial wall and the outer edge of the far calvarial wall.
- Abdominal circumference (AC) is measured on a transverse plane of the fetal abdomen that displays the bifurcation of the left and right portal vein and the appearance of the lower ribs is symmetric. The ellipse is fit to the skin edge (Fig. 151.4).
- Femur length (FL) is measured in its long axis in a sagittal plane of the thigh (Fig. 151.5).

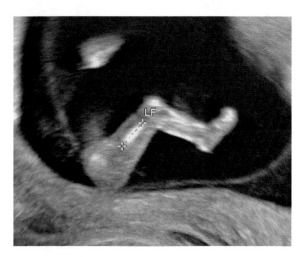

Fig. 151.5 Femur length

These measurements are compared to tables that express them in percentiles. Normal values are included between the 10th and 90th centiles. These measurements can allow the diagnosis of early onset of intrauterine growth restriction.

Fetal Morphology

Despite the lack of a clear checklist for fetal anatomy examination during the first trimester of pregnancy, several studies have evaluated the feasibility of measurement of the basic anatomical structure of the fetus during this period (von Kaisenberg et al. 2005; Souka et al. 2004).

- Skull and brain
  Axial view of the intactness of the cranium, the presence of the falx cerebri, the anterior and posterior horns of the lateral ventricles, and the butterfly shape of the choroid plexus (Fig. 151.6).
- Face
  Examination of the orbits and the presence of lenses and eyeballs. A view of the profile showing the maxillae and mandibules, the frontal bone, the nasal bone, and a frontal view for nostrils and upper and lower lips.

- Spine
  Examination of the alignment of the vertebrae and the complete vertebral column in sagittal, frontal, and axial planes with the skin covering the spine from the cervical to the sacral region (Fig. 151.7).
- Heart
  Examination of the four chamber view (two atria, two ventricles and the crux and atrioventricular valves).
- Abdomen
  Examination of the abdominal wall and the umbilical cord insertion on a sagittal view. The small bowel herniates physiologically through the left umbilical cord at around 8–9 weeks. During the 10th week, the intestine returns into the abdominal cavity. This reduction of the midgut herniation should have resolved before 12 weeks (Timor-Tritsch et al. 1989). The stomach is visualized on an axial view as a hypoechoic structure in the left abdomen (Fig. 151.4).
- Kidneys
  Visualization of the kidneys as hyperechoic structures with a hypoechoic center lateral to the spine. The bladder is the other cystic structure that should

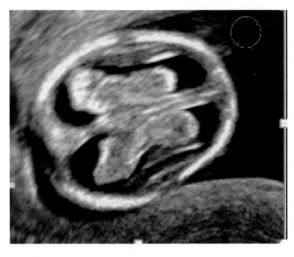

Fig. 151.6 Axial view of the cranium, with the falx cerebri, the butterfly shape of the anterior and posterior horns of the lateral ventricles

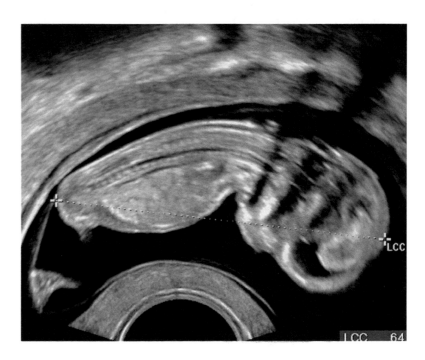

Fig. 151.7 Sagittal view of the fetus showing the integrity of the vertebral column and the skin covering the spine

Fig. 151.8 Bladder (*circle*) and kydneys (*arrows*)

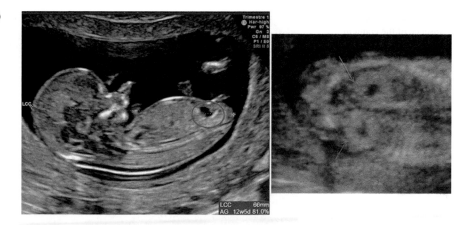

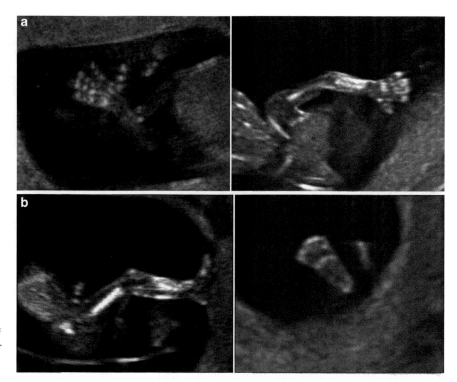

Fig. 151.9 (**a**) Fingers of the hand, humeri, radii, and ulnae. (**b**) The leg with the femur, tibiae, fibulae, and the foot

be visible during the first trimester. It is located medially in the fetal pelvis and is visible around 8–9 weeks. The bladder (Fig. 151.8) is surrounded by the two umbilical arteries, easily visualized on the color flow Doppler.

- Extremities (Fig. 151.9a, b)
  Examination of the long bones, femur, tibiae, fibulae, normal posture and shape of the feet and toes, humeri, ulnae, radii, and the normal posture and shape of hands and fingers.

Diagnosis of Fetal Anomalies (Excluding Nuchal Translucency) During the First Trimester

Although more than 80% of the most common structural defects are already present by 12 weeks' gestation, fetal ultrasound examination during the 11–14 weeks is used to screen mainly chromosomal abnormalities focusing especially on nuchal translucency measurement. Several studies (Carvalho et al. 2002;

Fig. 151.10 Anencephaly, absence of the cranium, irregular borders of the head

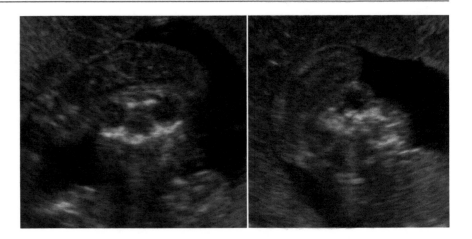

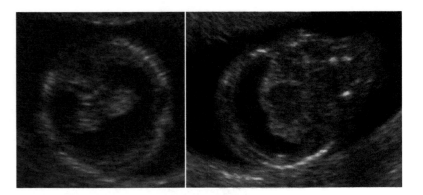

Fig. 151.11 Holoprosencephaly, absence of the falx cerebri, with a single ventricle and fused thalami

Taipale et al. 2004; Souka et al. 2006) have assessed the role of ultrasound in the detection of fetal anomalies in routine obstetric population during this period and showed that 38–50% of major structural defects (Syngelaki et al. 2012; Souka et al. 2006) could be detected. Some authors attribute this evolution to the use of the transvaginal probe during the ultrasound examination from 11 to 14 weeks' gestation (Timor-Tritsch et al. 1989), or the use of harmonic and compound imaging during the transabdominal scan (Von Kaisenberg et al. 2005).

- Cranium and brain
  - Anencephaly is characterized by the absence of development of the cranium with dystrophic brain tissue. The fetal head has irregular borders and not contained by bone (Fig. 151.10).
  - Encephalocele is a defect in the cranium through which intracranial contents herniate outside the skull.
  - Holoprosencephaly is a brain anomaly resulting from failure of cleavage of the prosencephalon into the cerebral hemispheres. Only the severe

forms of alobar holoprosencephaly are diagnosed during the first trimester, the falx cerebri is absent, there is a single primitive ventricle (holoventricle), and the thalami are fused in the midline with absence of the third ventricle. This anomaly is often encountered in trisomy 13 (Fig. 151.11).

- Neural tube
  - Open spina bifida refers to incomplete closure of the bony elements of the spine posteriorly. The defect of the neural tube is associated with separation of the posterior arch of the vertebrae, absence of posterior soft tissue, and is frequently associated to the cyst formed by the myelomeningocele. The skin defect is visualized on sagittal and transverse scans. The defect may vary in size. Only major forms of open spina bifida with large myelomeningoceles are diagnosed during the first trimester. These forms are often associated with the Arnold-Chiari II malformation (consequence of leakage of cerebrospinal fluid into the amniotic cavity and

hypotension in the subarachnoid spaces, leading to caudal displacement of the brain stem and obliteration of the cisterna magna). Chaoui et al. have shown that it is possible to diagnose the chiari malformation during the 11–13-week scan. In the midsagittal view of the fetal face, as used for the measurement of the NT, the fourth ventricle is easily visible; it presents as an intracranial translucency parallel to the NT that is delineated by two echogenic borders: the dorsal part of the brain stem anteriorly and the choroids plexus of the fourth ventricle posteriorly. (Chaoui et al. 2009) suggest that in fetuses with open spina bifida, the fourth ventricle is compressed and thus the intracranial translucency could not be visualized.

- Cardiac malformations

High nuchal translucency thickness is associated to a higher risk of cardiac defects. Recent studies have described early diagnosis of cardiac abnormalities such as double outlet right ventricle, hypoplastic left heart, transposition of the great arteries, atrioventricular septal defects, Tetralogy of Fallot, and pulmonary atresia. Fetal echocardiography using both transabdominal and transvaginal approaches at or before 16 weeks' gestation allowed distinction between normal or abnormal cardiac appearance. However, the earlier scan seems less accurate whereas some forms of cardiac malformations are not evident at the early onset of pregnancy and thus some of the late developing lesions may be undetectable during early evaluation. Therefore, cardiac exploration is usually performed at 18–22 weeks' gestation.

- Ventral wall defects

Omphalocele is defined as a midline abdominal wall defect with herniation of abdominal organs at the umbilical cord insertion (Sadler 1990) (Fig. 151.12). The herniated organs are covered by the peritoneum and the amnion. It consists, more probably, in a failure of the intestinal loops to integrate the abdominal cavity after 12 weeks' gestation, or a failure of the embryonic lateral folds to fuse in the midline (Sadler 1990). The ultrasound diagnosis is based on the visualization of the abdominal wall defect with the presence of intestine loops and/or liver and/or the stomach into the umbilical cord. Omphalocele is associated to aneuploidy in 35–40% of cases (trisomy 13, 18, 21 and Turner's syndrome) (Snijders et al. 1998);

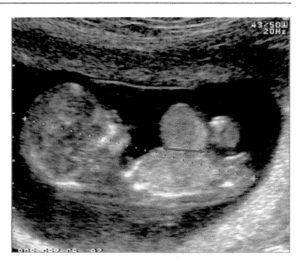

Fig. 151.12 Omphalocele

thus, it is frequently associated to a nuchal translucency or cystic hygroma during the first trimester sonography. Omphalocele is also known to be a part of different anomaly syndromes such as Beckwith-Wiedemann syndrome, Pentalogy of Cantrell, etc.

Early diagnosis of omphalocele is possible. Nevertheless, the prognosis is mainly related to associated structural anomalies which are detected at the second trimester screening in half of the cases (Blazer et al. 2004) and to chromosomal abnormalities. Transient omphaloceles have also been described which disappear during gestation. Usually these omphaloceles are of small size, containing only few intestinal loops (Blazer et al. 2004). In our experience, omphaloceles appear larger at the examination in the first trimester than at examination performed later in pregnancy. Fetuses with isolated omphalocele and normal karyotype carry most often a good prognosis. In contrast, omphaloceles of poor prognosis have also been reported in the first trimester in association to larger malformative complex either in case of Pentalogy of Cantrell (midline supra-umbilical abdominal wall defect and ectopia cordis) or omphalocele-extrophy-imperforate anus-spinal defects complex (OEIS).

Gastroschisis (Fig. 151.13) is a congenital ventral body wall defect characterized in evisceration of abdominal contents, mainly loops of the small bowel, occasionally spleen, liver, or genitourinary tract, typically located on the right side of a normally inserted umbilical cord. The incidence of gastroschisis has been increasing, during the last two decades. There are known factors associated to the increasing incidence

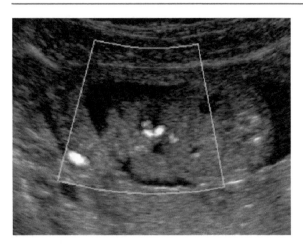

Fig. 151.13 Gastroschisis

of gastroschisis as young mother's age, low socioeconomic status, maternal smoking, and the use of vasoactive medications at the first trimester of pregnancy (Werler et al. 1992). Gastroschisis is commonly diagnosed during the first trimester ultrasound scan (Cullen et al. 1990), the typical sonographic features are multiple loops of bowel floating freely in the amniotic fluid to the right of the normal umbilical cord insertion. Gastroschisis can be diagnosed at 11 week's gestation since the physiological herniation should have returned to the peritoneal cavity (David et al. 2008). The main differential diagnosis is exomphalos. Other differential diagnoses include a cystic umbilical cord lesion, urachal cysts, bladder and cloacal extrophy, limb body wall complex, and Pentalogy of Cantrell. In the majority of cases, gastroschisis constitutes an isolated finding and the risk of aneuploidy is not increased. Several prognosis factors were proposed, such as bowel and gastric dilatations, polyhydramnios, and intrauterine restriction in growth. These criteria are difficult to evaluate during the first trimester. Thus, regular ultrasonographic controls are recommended to monitor fetal growth and the bowel status.

• Fetal abdominal cyst

Abdominal cysts diagnosed in the early pregnancy are rare. Indeed, abdominal cysts are frequently detected during the second and third trimester (McEwing et al. 2003) and there are only few articles, mainly case reports, describing abdominal cyst diagnosed in the first trimester. Moreover, their significance during early pregnancy remains often unclear since some of them disappear spontaneously in the second part of pregnancy. The majority of the prenatal

abdominal cysts are of renal origin (hydronephrosis, pelvicalyceal dilatation, multicystic dysplastic kidney, ureteric dilatation, and distended bladder). The most common extra-renal cysts are ovarian cysts, intestinal duplication cysts, mesenteric or omental cysts, choledochal cysts, adrenal cystic masses (hemorrhage, cystic neuroblastoma, subdiaphragmatic sequestration), and meconium pseudocysts. Less common causes include splenic and hepatic cysts, urachal cysts and hydrometrocolpos, cloacal dysgenesis sequence, etc. One should note that in large cystic mass detected in the first trimester, the origin of the lesion is often difficult to assess and requires regular sonograpic follow-up both to evaluate its evolution in size and to precise its anatomical location.

Umbilical cord cysts or pseudocysts, arising from the remnants of the allantois or omphalomesenteric duct, are most frequently located at the fetal end of the cord and can be detected in the early pregnancy. If they are uncommon (incidence 0.4–3%), they have often been reported in association to trisomies 13 and 18. The risk of aneuploidy is believed to be higher when the cyst is located near the placental or fetal end of the cord. However, the rate of chromosomal anomalies is significantly higher in the second and third trimesters than in the first trimester. Moreover, umbilical cord cysts detected in early pregnancy are more likely to resolve completely.

Finally, one should note that ovarian cyst, the most frequent prenatal cyst in female fetus, is not encountered in the first trimester, since its development is related to excessive stimulation by the maternal and the placental hormones in the second part of the pregnancy.

• Renal and bladder

   • Abnormal renal number: unilateral agenesis is suspected when the kidney is not visualized in the lumbar area. Bilateral renal agenesis is incompatible with extrauterine life and is associated to anhydramnios that is rarely visualized during the first trimester scan, since the renal production of urine as the main source of amniotic fluid starts after 18 weeks' getstation. This condition results in pulmonary hypoplasia and musculoskeletal abnormalities, the Potter's syndrome.

   • Abdominal cysts of renal origin detected in the first trimester are mainly megacystis (Fig. 151.14). Indeed, most cases of severe upper renal tract dilatation are not visible until the second trimester due to low fetal urine production (Rabinowitz et al. 1989). Megacystis at 11–13 weeks is defined by bladder length of 7 mm or more. It is found in about 1 in 1,500 pregnancies and in about 30% of cases, there is an associated aneuploidy, mainly trisomy 13 or 18 (Kagan et al. 2010). In the euploid group, the prognosis depends on bladder length; in 90% of cases with bladder length below 16 mm there is a spontaneous resolution of the megacystis, while there is usually a progression to severe obstructive uropathy in those with bladder length of 16 mm or more.

- Skeleton (Fig. 151.15)
  Evaluation of the long bones should include the measurements of all long bones, the degree of curvature. Osteochondrodysplasia is rarely diagnosed during the first trimester. Nevertheless, amputations anomalies (amniotic band syndrome), segmentation anomalies (polydactyly, ectrodactyly), or extremities malpositions are detectable abnormalities.
- Amniotic band syndrome
  This syndrome is characterized by deformities of the fetus including ventral wall defects, encephaloceles, and limb amputations.
- Body stalk anomaly
  This is characterized by the presence of a major abdominal wall defect, severe kyphoscoliosis, short umbilical cord, and rupture of the amniotic membranes so that half of the body lies in the amniotic cavity and the other half in the celomic cavity.

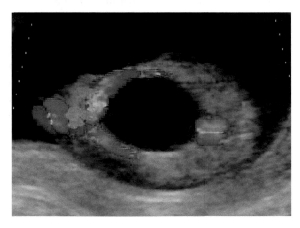

Fig. 151.14 Megacystis

The Particular Case of Twin Pregnancies

The determination of chorionicity and amniocity for twin pregnancy is crucial for the follow-up and in predicting complications of these pregnancies. First trimester is the best time to determine the chorionicity and amniocity in multiple gestations. The diagnosis is based on the number of gestational sacs, amnions, and yolk sacs (in the early US examination).

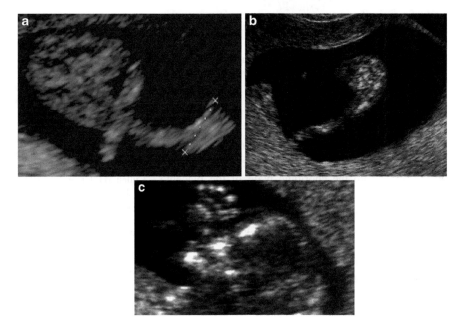

Fig. 151.15 (**a**) Talipes, (**b**) amputation of a member, (**c**) polydactyly

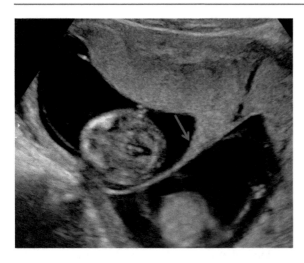

Fig. 151.16 Dichorionic-diamniotic placentation with the lambda sign (*arrow*)

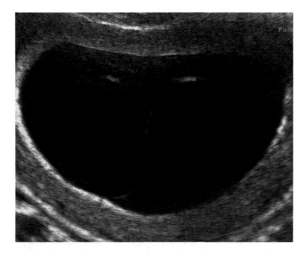

Fig. 151.17 Monochorionic-diamniotic placentation with the visualization of two amniotic sacs in early pregnancy

- Monochorionic-monoamniotic twins correspond to a single amniotic cavity.
- Dichorionic-diamniotic (Fig. 151.16) twins is likely when the groove between the membranes at the insertion into the chorionic plate of the placenta appears thick; it is called the "lambda sign."
- Monochorionic-diamniotic placentation is likely when the insertion of the membranes clearly joins the chorionic plate which is thin wispy; it is called "T" sign or the visualization of two amniotic sacs in the early pregnancy (Fig. 151.17).

It is possible to evaluate the thickness of the membrane to assess the chorionicity, a thick membrane is used to be seen in dichorionic-diamniotic placenta and a thin membrane in the monochorionic-diamniotic placenta.

The counting of the number of layers in the dividing membrane is also another marker. If two layers were seen, a monochorionic pregnancy is diagnosed while a dichorionic pregnancy is diagnosed when more than two layers are found.

Conclusion

The role of 11–14 weeks scan as an effective method of screening for aneuploidies is now well established. Recent studies have shown that this scan can identify many nonchromosomal major abnormalities which allow an early termination of pregnancy and thus giving the parents earlier reassurance when the fetal anatomy is explored. Nevertheless, knowing that a significant number of major anomalies have late onset and, thus, may not be detectable by the first trimester ultrasound, the second trimester anomaly scan remains necessary.

Acknowledgments Acknowledgments to Dr. Pierre Godard, Dr. Daniele Combourieu, and Dr. Marc Althuser for their contribution to the images.

References

Abuhamad A. Technical aspects of nuchal translucency measurement. Semin Perinatol. 2005;29:376.

Blazer S, Zimmer EZ, Gover A, Bronshtein M. Fetal omphalocele detected early in pregnancy: associated anomalies and outcomes. Radiology. 2004;232(1):191–5.

Carvalho MH, Brizot ML, Lopes LM, Chiba CH, Miyadahira S, Zugaib M. Detection of fetal structural abnormalities at the 11–14 week ultrasound scan. Prenat Diagn. 2002;22:1–4.

Chaoui R, Benoit B, Mitkowska-Wozniak H, Heling KS, Nicolaides KH. Assessment of intracranial translucency (IT) in the detection of spina bifida at the 11–13-week scan. Ultrasound Obstet Gynecol. 2009;34(3):249–52.

Cullen MT, Green J, Whetham J, Salafia C, Gabrielli S, Hobbins JC. Transvaginal ultrasonographic detection of congenital anomalies in the first trimester. Am J Obstet Gynecol. 1990;163:66–476.

David AL, Tan A, Curry J. Gastroschisis: sonographic diagnosis, associations, management and outcome. Prenat Diagn. 2008;28(7):633–44.

Ioannou C, Sarris I, Salomon LJ, Papageorghiou AT. A review of fetal volumetry: the need for standardization and definitions in measurement methodology. Ultrasound Obstet Gynecol. 2012. doi:10.1002/uog.9074.

Kagan KO, Stamboulidou I, Syngelaki A, Cruz J, Nicolaides KH. The 11–13-week scan: diagnosis and outcome of holoprosencephaly, exomphalos and megacystis. Ultrasound Obstet Gynecol. 2010;36:10–4.

Malone FD, Canick JA, Ball RH, Nyberg DA, Comstock CH, Bukowski R, Berkowitz RL, Gross SJ, Dugoff L, Craigo SD, Timor-Tritsch IE, Carr SR, Wolfe HM, Dukes K, Bianchi DW, Rudnicka AR, Hackshaw AK, Lambert-Messerlian G, Wald NJ, D'Alton ME. First- and Second-Trimester Evaluation of Risk (FASTER) research consortium. First-trimester or second-trimester screening, or both, for Down's syndrome. N Engl J Med. 2005; 353(19):2001–11.

McEwing R, Hayward C, Furness M. Fetal cystic abdominal masses. Australas Radiol. 2003;47(2):101–10.

Rabinowitz R, Peters MT, Vyas S, Campbell S, Nicolaides KH. Measurement of fetal urine production in normal pregnancy by real-time ultrasonography. Am J Obstet Gynecol. 1989;161:1264–6.

Sadler TW. Digestive system. In: Sadler TW, editor. Langman's medical embryology. 6th ed. Baltimore: Williams & Wilkins; 1990. p. 237–60.

Snijders RJM, Noble P, Sebire NJ, Souka AP, Nicolaides KH. UK multicentre project on assessment of risk of trisomy 21 bymaternal age and nuchal-translucency thickness at 10–14 weeks of gestation. Lancet. 1998;351:343–6.

Souka AP, Pilalis A, Kavalakis Y, Kosmas Y, Antsaklis P, Antsaklis A. Assessment of fetal anatomy at the 11–14-week ultrasound examination. Ultrasound Obstet Gynecol. 2004;24(7):730–4.

Souka PA, Kavalakis I, Antsaklis P, Papantoniou N, Mesogitis S, Antsaklis A. Screening for major structural abnormalities at the 11- to 14-week ultrasound scan. Am J Obstet Gynecol. 2006;194:393–6.

Syngelaki A, Chelemen T, Dagklis T, Allan L, Nicolaides KH. Challenges in the diagnosis of fetal non-chromosomal abnormalities at 11–13 weeks. Prenat Diagn. 2012;31(1):90–102. doi:10.1002/pd.2642.

Taipale P, Ammälä M, Salonen R, Hiilesmaa V. Two-stage ultrasonography in screening for fetal anomalies at 13–14 and 18–22 weeks of gestation. Acta Obstet Gynecol Scand. 2004;83:1141–6.

Timor-Tritsch IE, Warren WB, Peisner DB, et al. First trimester midgut herniation. A high frequency transvaginal sonographic study. Am J Obstet Gynecol. 1989;161:831.

von Kaisenberg CS, Kuhling-von Kaisenberg H, Fritzer E, Schemm S, Meinhold-Heerlein I, Jonat W. Fetal transabdominal anatomy scanning using standard views at 11 to 14 weeks' gestation. Am J Obstet Gynecol. 2005;192(2):535–42.

Werler MM, Mitchell AA, Shapiro S. First trimester maternal medication use in relation to gastroschisis. Teratology. 1992;45:361–7.

Index